NURSING CARE
of the
OLDER ADULT

NURSING CARE

of the

OLDER ADULT

THIRD EDITION

Edited by

Mildred O. Hogstel, Ph.D., R.N., C.

Abell-Hanger Professor of Gerontological Nursing

Harris College of Nursing

Texas Christian University

Fort Worth, Texas

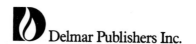 Delmar Publishers Inc.

NOTICE TO THE READER

Cover by: Mary E. Siener
Text design by: Karen Kunz Kemp

Delmar Staff:

Executive Editor: David Gordon
Associate Editor: Elisabeth F. Williams
Project Editor: Carol Micheli
Production Coordinator: Barbara A. Bullock
Art Manager: Russell Schneck
Art Coordinator: Brian Yacur
Design Coordinator: Karen Kemp

For information, address Delmar Publishers Inc.
3 Columbia Circle, Box 15-015
Albany, New York 12212

Copyright © 1994
by Delmar Publishers Inc.
The trademark ITP is used under license.

Printed in the United States of America
Published simultaneously in Canada by Nelson Canada, a division of the Thomson Corporation

3 4 5 6 7 8 9 10 XXX 00 99 98 97 96 95 94

Library of Congress Cataloging-in-Publication Data

Nursing care of the older adult / edited by Mildred O. Hogstel. — 3rd ed.

p. cm.
Includes bibiliographical references and index.
ISBN 0-8273-5121-6
1. Geriatric nursing. I. Hogstel, Mildred O.
[DNLM: 1. Geriatric Nursing. WY 152 N9745]
RC954.N884 1994
610.73165—dc20
DNLM/DLC
for Library of Congress   92-49248
                                                          CIP

Contents

Part 6 Special Concerns

List of Tables

List of Figures

To my father,
and in loving memory of
my mother,
my grandparents,
and so many other older
people who have touched
my life and taught
me so much

Contributors

Sister Rose Therese Bahr, A.S.C., Ph.D., R.N., F.A.A.N., formerly Professor of Nursing and Chair, Division of Community Health Nursing, School of Nursing, The Catholic University of America, Washington, DC

Patricia Bohannon, Ph.D., R.N., Dean, School of Nursing, Valdosta State College, Valdosta, Georgia

Marta Askew Browning, M.S., R.N., formerly Assistant Professor of Nursing, College of Allied Health, Temple University, Philadelphia, Pennsylvania

Mary Flo Bruce, Ph.D., R.N., Acting Coordinator of Baccalaureate Nursing Unit, Weber State University, Salt Lake City, Utah

Patricia F. Cheong, Director, Tarrant County Area Agency on Aging, Fort Worth, Texas

Linda Cox Curry, Ph.D., R.N., Associate Professor of Nursing, Harris College of Nursing, Texas Christian University, Fort Worth, Texas

Kathleen Ryan Fletcher, M.S.N., G.N.P., Assistant Professor of Nursing, University of Virginia School of Nursing, Charlottesville, Virginia

Howard Graitzer, D.O., F.A.C.O.I., Associate Professor of Medicine, Texas College of Osteopathic Medicine, Fort Worth, Texas

Elaine L. Gross, M.S.N., R.N., Assistant Professor of Nursing, College of Allied Health, Temple University, Philadelphia, Pennsylvania

Mildred O. Hogstel, Ph.D., R.N., C., Abell-Hanger Professor of Gerontological Nursing, Harris College of Nursing, Texas Christian University, Fort Worth, Texas

Allene Jones, M.N., R.N., Assistant Professor of Nursing, Harris College of Nursing, Texas Christian University, Fort Worth, Texas

Rhonda Keen-Payne, Ph.D., R.N., Associate Professor of Nursing, Harris College of Nursing, Texas Christian University, Fort Worth, Texas

Janice A. Knebl, D.O., F.A.C.P., Chief, Division of Geriatrics, Assistant Professor of Medicine, Department of Medicine, Texas College of Osteopathic Medicine, Fort Worth, Texas

Jeanette Lancaster, Ph.D., R.N., F.A.A.N., Dean, University of Virginia School of Nursing, Charlottesville, Virginia

Peggy Mayfield, M.S., R.N., A.N.P., Emeritus Associate Professor of Nursing, Harris College of Nursing, Texas Christian University, Fort Worth,Texas

Mira Kirk Nelson, Ed.D., R.N., C.G.N.P., Nurse Specialist, Division of Licensure and Certification, Texas Department of Health, Arlington, Texas

M. Kathryn Nichols, M.S., R.N., Emeritus Associate Professor of Nursing, Harris College of Nursing, Texas Christian University, Fort Worth, Texas

Carol A. Reynolds, Ph.D., R.N., C.E.N., Clinical Nurse Specialist, Department of Emergency Medicine, Harris Methodist Fort Worth, Fort Worth, Texas

Brenda Botts Riley, D.S.N., R.N., Associate Professor of Nursing, Troy State University, Troy, Alabama

Nell B. Robinson, Ph.D., R.D., L.D., Emeritus Professor, Department of Nutrition and Dietetics, Texas Christian University, Fort Worth, Texas

Kathy Ryals Simpson, M.S., R.N., Assistant Professor of Nursing, Mobile College School of Nursing, Mobile, Alabama

Carol A. Stephenson, Ed.D., R.N., Associate Professor of Nursing, Harris College of Nursing, Texas Christian University, Fort Worth, Texas

Joy Graham Stone, M.S.N., R.N., C.S.C., Psychiatric Clinical Nurse Specialist, private practice, Fort Worth, Texas

Laura Talbot, Ph.D., R.N., C., Assistant Professor of Nursing, Harris College of Nursing, Texas Christian University, Fort Worth, Texas

Mary Taylor-Martof, Ed.D., R.N., Assistant Professor of Nursing, University of Southwestern Louisiana College of Nursing, Lafayette, Louisiana

Preface

Mildred O. Hogstel

The purpose of this third edition is to update and expand the content of the first and second editions and to add new chapters that reflect the recent changes and growth in the dynamic field of gerontological nursing.

The core of knowledge about the nursing care of older adults is growing rapidly. This expansion is occurring, at least in part, because of the emphasis on the predicted growth of this population group in the last part of this century and because many nurses are concerned about increasing the quantity and improving the quality of nursing care for a group of people who need specialized care. The amount of material being written about gerontology and gerontological nursing is increasing every year in an attempt to meet this great need.

This book is intended to provide answers to many theoretical questions and practical problems in caring for and working with older adults in a variety of settings. Emphasis has been placed on the problems and needs of well older adults in the community as well as on sick older people in institutional settings, who have acute and chronic health problems.

There is a new chapter in this edition on wellness in old age—a major component of gerontological nursing. The chapter on psychological changes of the aging process has been broadened to include the overall psychosocial changes of aging. The chapter on psychosocial assessment has been revised with a strong emphasis on sociocultural aspects to consider in assessing older adults. The chapters on emergency care, hospital care, perioperative care, and critical care have been revised and strengthened to reflect current trends in these areas. There is also a new chapter on discharge planning and teaching older adults in a variety of settings.

Content on adapting the home environment for elder care in the home and new information on health insurance coverage for older adults have been added to the chapter on home care. A new chapter concentrates on family support with content on the rewards and burdens of caregiving by family members. The chapter on elder abuse has been completely rewritten with a broader perspective of the larger problem of maltreatment of older adults.

Gerontological nursing has become an important and expanding specialty field in nursing. Nursing students and practicing nurses are becoming more aware of and interested in the specialized study of the care of older adults. The trend is expected to continue. As nurses and students become more knowledgeable about and involved in gerontological nursing, they discover that it is a challenging and rewarding field and that there is much more to be learned.

This book is intended to be used by undergraduate nursing students in courses in medical–surgical nursing, community health nursing, and gerontological nursing. Graduate students, beginning study in gerontological nursing, will find here an overview of the field as well as topics not often found in most other sources, e.g., the care of older adults in emergency settings and surgery and the ethical and legal issues related to older adults. The nurse's role in recognizing, assessing, and presenting elder maltreatment is stressed. Practical and useful new information about legal problems older adults experience has also been provided. Copies of sample legal documents related to advance directives are included in the appendix. Several complete assessment guides also are in the appendix. The specific role of the nurse in legal issues related to caring for older people has been added. Suggestions for topics of study and nursing research as well as ideas for publications are offered, especially in areas that have little material in print.

Nurses who care for older adults in general hospitals, geropsychiatric units, extended care facilities, community health agencies, nursing homes, and other long-term care facilities, outpatient clinics, physicians' offices, day-care centers, home health agencies, private homes, and hospice environments will find this book a useful reference in their everyday practice. Supervisors responsible for the orientation, education, and evaluation of nursing staff and auxiliary personnel in these settings should also find helpful information and many ideas for inservice education programs.

In addition, administrators, managers, and professional social service workers in hospitals, community health agencies, long-term care facilities, nursing homes, senior centers, and retirement centers will find this book helpful in gaining a deeper understanding of their older clients. Gerontologists who are not nurses also will find many topics of interest in this text, along with concerns and questions that need to be explored further.

The words *patient* and *client* have been used throughout the book because nurses and other health-care personnel in various settings may prefer one term or the other. Also, the terms *older adults* and *older people* are generally used instead of terms such as the *aging* and the *aged* because the former imply more individualism and humanism than *the aging* or *the aged*, which can apply to many things besides people. In addition, *aged* implies a static state rather than a continually changing one and does not seem appropriate when referring to human beings who are in a constant state of change.

Sincere appreciation is expressed to all the contributing authors; to typists Susan Moore and Jessie McCoy; and to colleagues and peers who offered support and encouragement throughout the writing and editing of the manuscript. Most of all, however, appreciation is expressed to the many older patients, clients, friends, and family members who have provided numerous personal experiences, opportunities for new insights, and incentives for me to learn more and share more about the aging process. Their experiences continually motivate me to work toward improving the quality of health care and life for older people. It is hoped that this book will help nursing students, professional nurses, and others improve the health care they provide for a very large and increasing segment of our population.

Part 1

Introduction

1 An Overview of Gerontological Nursing

Sister Rose Therese Bahr

CHAPTER OUTLINE

FOCUS

This chapter introduces the reader to the specialized field of gerontological nursing, including its historical evolution and effect on the health care delivery system. Factors affecting this area of study are trends in demographics, federal legislation, and attitudes toward older people. The education, standards of practice, and specialized roles of gerontological nurses are explored.

OBJECTIVES

1. Trace the development of gerontological nursing as a specialty.

2. Explore the concept and effects of ageism.

3. Evaluate how nursing can improve the health care delivery system for older persons.

4. Identify recent federal legislation affecting the care of nursing home residents.

5. Discuss the educational preparation of gerontological nurses.

6. Differentiate the gerontological nurse practitioner and gerontological clinical nurse specialist according to education, function, and national certification.

7. Identify types of gerontological nursing content recommended for nursing curricula.

8. List clinical problems recommended for further research in the nursing care of older adults.

9. Evaluate the purpose and implementation of the American Nurses' Association Standards and Scope of Gerontological Nursing Practice.

10. Discuss prediction and future trends in gerontological nursing.

Gerontological nursing is recognized as a specialty within the ranks of American professional nurses (Bahr 1992). The acceptance of gerontological nursing as a specialty has not been won without a struggle. The battle continues against the attitudes of society generally and of the nursing profession specifically in terms of the negative stereotyping of older adults. Although the profession of nursing has involved the care of older people for decades, it was believed that no special education or knowledge was needed by people who practiced in this field. It is from this unpromising background that gerontological nursing has emerged as a respected branch of professional nursing.

In 1961 (Eliopoulos 1979), the specialty attained national recognition with the creation of its own division of nursing within the American Nurses' Association (ANA). Nurses in the United States who were aware of the population trends realized the importance of such a step. The charter members of the Division of Gerontological Nursing who were instrumental in its establishment deserve a great deal of credit for this visionary action.

The major topics addressed in an overview of gerontological nursing and the expanding scope of this practice in the United States include

1. the historical evolution of gerontological nursing practice, based on population statistics and how ageism in our society has affected the profession of nursing

2. the health care delivery system and the care of older adults

3. nursing education and the care of older adults with a perspective derived from

   a) studies of the attitudes and interests of nursing personnel and nursing students

   b) the increasing knowledge about gerontology and the use of this knowledge in the practice of nursing, aided by undergraduate and graduate programs in nursing

4. the delineation of various aspects of nursing care of older adults, including clinical practice based on

   a) the ANA *Standards of Nursing Practice*

   b) selected theories of nursing applied to the care of older adults

   c) the expanding scope of gerontological nursing in general and the roles of the clinical nurse specialist and the gerontological nurse practitioner in particular

5. trends in gerontological nursing and long-term care

EVOLUTION OF GERONTOLOGICAL NURSING AS A SPECIALTY

Florence Nightingale defined the profession of nursing on the battlefields of the Crimean War in 1853 (Kelly 1981; Lee 1987). Assuming leadership of a group of her female friends she requested to join her, she accepted the challenge of caring for battle weary and injured soldiers whose unique health needs resulted from their combat activities. This situation called for the most demanding and sympathetic nursing care. As the practice of nursing as a profession emerged, emphasis continued to be placed on the acute care (medical) model. In this model the nurse tended to those physical needs arising from illnesses and injuries that required emergency hospital care. With this foundation, for many decades professional nursing reaffirmed its position through educational programs that concentrated on acute care facilities as the clinical setting in which future nurses were educated. Because of this approach, which extended well into the twentieth century, nurses had difficulty accepting roles that extended beyond those within institutional walls. Administering care to people other than those with acute physical conditions was not recognized as a nursing function. This historical framework made it difficult to perceive gerontological nursing as a separate field of nursing practice.

Nursing as a human service profession enjoys its status in American society because such services are needed for the betterment of society's members. It may be said that "as society goes, so does a profession," when that profession is nursing. The United States is described as a youth-oriented nation. As a result the emphasis in nursing curricula is on caring for young mothers, infants, children, adolescents, and young adults in acute care situations. A substantial portion of the classroom and clinical requirements in the nursing curriculum is based on the needs of the younger segment of the patient population. All other persons are classified as adults, regardless of their unique needs and age categories.

This blurring of the adult years in the content and clinical nursing experience of education programs has contributed to establishing stereotypes that nursing students seeking socialization into the nursing profession find difficult to overcome. For many of these students, exposure to and encounters with older people have been extremely limited as our society has become more mobile.

Contact with older relatives—grandparents, uncles, and aunts—has been considerably reduced as the nuclear family constellation has taken precedence nationally. Thus many young people have not enjoyed the richness of a relationship with an older person and continue to think in terms of "young is beautiful; old is ugly and repulsive." The ideals of society, which embrace citizens from all cultures, philosophical ideologies, and persuasions, have contributed to the pervasive attitude that only the young are important to society and its growth. Consequently older persons have not enjoyed the favorable position to which they are entitled. It is often forgotten that in their earlier years they were the youth who contributed to the growth of America through their labors and efforts.

The turning point for the older American citizen was the institutionalization of the Social Security system in 1935 (Tedrow 1979). This legislation, based on a model adopted in Germany, mandated retirement from employment at the arbitrarily-set age of 65, regardless of the state of well-being of the older person. Retirees were made to feel they were no longer capable of performing at peak level and were forced to leave jobs they enjoyed and in which they could have continued for a number of years. Suddenly faced with an empty existence, the older person often quickly deteriorated to a point of needing care considered beyond the scope of the family. This situation gave rise to the concept of "nursing homes"—institutions where custodial care would be provided with little attention to the totality of the human personality and its potential for continued growth and a satisfying quality of life. Within the nursing home setting, little effort was made to support the positive aspects of the aging process. It was sufficient, in the minds of administrators and staff who had never been educated to understand the components of the aging process, to provide a facil-

ity where meeting the basic needs of oxygen, food, water, sleep, and security constituted the highest quality of care. This approach reflected the prevalent attitude of "ageism" in America.

AGEISM IN THE UNITED STATES

Butler (1974) described ageism as a "process of systematic stereotyping of and discrimination against people because they are old." This phenomenon, which emerged in the 1960s, can be seen in many areas of American life. Americans still tend to see the United States as a nation of young people, although recent statistics indicate the United States places sixth among the top fifteen nations that are considered "old" because of the increasing numbers of their aging citizens (United Nations Population Division, 1982). Figure 1-1 demonstrates the steady growth of the aging population in America.

Siegel and Taeuber (1986) noted that the projection for the aging population has been updated. Statistics now depict that, in contrast to the 28.5 million older persons in the United States in 1985, 34.9 to 64.6 million can be expected to be living at the turn of the century and through the year 2030.

The turning point for the United States came in the 1960s when the concept of zero population growth was introduced as a means of balancing the population. Gradually the birth rate decreased, but older people, because of better living conditions, health, and ability to finance retirement opportunities, lived longer, thus increasing the number and proportion of older citizens. Suddenly, awareness of older people and their lifestyles, their concerns, and their needs became a reality for a society unprepared to cope with this aging segment of society.

An awareness of the increasing numbers of older people has made members of various segments of the community realize the immensity and complexity of the problems facing them. Legislators, medical care personnel, health professional groups, housing authorities, building contractors, and transportation planners soon saw that businesses and delivery systems were not coping very well with the needs of older people who came under their domain. Older people themselves, gaining strength in numbers and unifying their efforts to bring about change, organized into such activist groups as the American Association of Retired Persons (AARP), National Retired

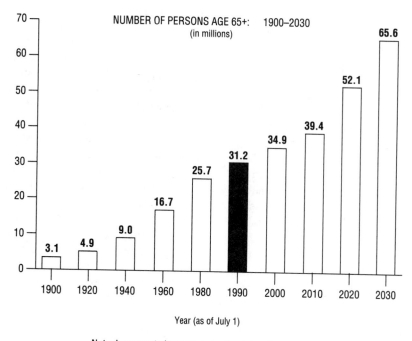

Figure 1–1   Number of persons 65+: 1900–2030 (in millions). Note that increments in year on horizontal scale are uneven. Source: *A Profile of Older Americans: 1991:* Prepared by the Program Resources Department, American Association of Retired Persons (AARP) and the Administration on Aging (AoA), US Department of Health and Human Services, 1991.

Teachers' Association (NRTA), Catholic Golden Age (CGA), and the Gray Panthers, an intergenerational organization that was spearheaded by Margaret Kuhn, a retired union organizer. Issues were raised in various forums by these groups. They spoke on behalf of older persons, requesting that attention be given to the needs of this growing segment of the population as well as to those of the younger members of society. For some time these demands were either ignored by the groups at which they were directed or written off as the passing whims of "little old ladies and men who didn't have their wits about them." However, government agencies were at last persuaded to investigate the conditions experienced by older people in the United States. Lobbying by activist groups and action stimulated by the older members of the Missouri legislature, known as the

"silver-haired legislators," and groups in other states resulted in laws, rules, and regulations that began to have an impact on various service agencies and institutions. It was discovered that abuse and lack of special concern were the order of the day in some settings where older adults were housed or served by various agencies.

From this investigation of alleged abuse, new insights were gleaned into the quality of life of many dependent older persons. Programs were created in many but not all communities. Limited funding brought headache and heartache to administrators who soon realized that once again older people were being denied benefits. Many more older clients sought assistance in order to live a marginally comfortable existence, but they found they had difficulty meeting the eligibility requirements of many agencies. Many programs projected by legislators were inappropriate for what older people wanted or needed, but in many instances those programs received the largest amounts of funding. As Kalish (1979) noted, a new ageism was prevalent. This more current attitude supplemented the former, not in reinforcing the stereotyping of older people but rather in the overemphasis on their behaviors (e.g., dependency and incapacity to meet their own needs so that societal programs overreacted in assuming all responsibility for older people rather than being in a supportive role). In addition, the new ageism pinpoints the issue of programs planned without sufficient emphasis on the benefits to be derived from the service provided older adults. This newer focus projects the attitude that others know better than older people themselves what is good for them. They were rarely consulted except through committee meetings or surveys. These sampling techniques did not necessarily give an accurate portrayal of what they needed, who could best provide the services, and how cost-effective these services were in terms of the results.

Kalish (1979) believes that older persons must be allowed to develop the same qualities and capabilities as other people, without being set apart from the rest of society. When given the freedom and assistance to do so, older people can realize the full potential of their personalities. This type of attitude allows older people to be themselves, not the faceless class prototype covered by a mask of senility, whether they are functioning fully and responsible for their own lives or whether, because of the ravages of time, they are suffering from deteriorating conditions that make them dependent on others for their care. Kalish (1979) pleaded that America move from the attitude of the new ageism to one in which human beings are treasured because they are human beings and precious to society regardless of age.

NURSING AND OLDER ADULTS

Nursing, a profession established to provide care for individuals and groups with a focus on health and its promotion has had its own biased attitudes and values about older adults. Nursing had little impact on the care of older people in the first part of the twentieth century because its main focus had been the young in a youth-oriented culture. Not until there

was a shift in societal emphasis, giving visibility to older people, did the nursing community begin to focus on this segment of the population with serious intent to upgrade the care in health care settings and resident housing units. Nursing shortages continue to exist in long-term care settings, where the residents, who have a greater acuity of illness because of Prospective Payment System legislation, require increasingly more skilled nursing care. However, the health care industry, with the help of the federal government and the prodding of the ANA, is slowly bringing greater professionalism to this area. The upgrading of nursing homes through federal regulations, such as the Omnibus Budget Reconciliation Act (OBRA) of 1987, has made employment of better prepared professional nurses and aides who are certified for certain tasks a possibility. Administrators of nursing homes, realizing that qualified nurses affect the quality of care for their residents, have begun to upgrade salaries and working conditions, making the nursing home a more attractive employment setting. Because of these changes a gradual increase in the number of professional nurses providing nursing care in nursing homes is evident. The 1992 membership in the ANA numbered approximately 180,000. Of that number, only 435 were reported as members of the Council of Gerontological Nursing (telephone conversation, ANA, Membership Department, January 21, 1992).

Ageism is an attitude that through education will gradually be eradicated. Older persons will then be valued members of society, appreciated by the nursing profession just as clients in other areas of nursing practice.

A HEALTH CARE DELIVERY SYSTEM FOR OLDER ADULTS

Awareness of a societal condition such as health care tends to focus attention on that issue by many constituencies (e.g., politicians). Studies undertaken by such groups as Health Systems Agencies (HSA) and the American Nurses' Association Health Care Reform Task Force (1991) indicate the need for change in the health care delivery system, particularly as it relates to the older citizen. An evaluation of this system is therefore useful.

The word *system* suggests that there is an orderly, efficient, well-staffed, well-financed approach to achieving some goal. When the word *system* is applied to the complex phenomenon of health care delivery for older adults, its impact is great. In the United States a true health care delivery system for older adults that is comprehensive in its offerings of health care services has not yet been implemented.

As reported earlier, the United States has, since the 1970s, attempted to come to grips with the situation of a larger population of older adults who are increasingly dependent on an organized plan of care for their survival and well-being. The cost of the care is so prohibitive that many people who could benefit from the care are excluded because of a fixed income or because inflation has played havoc with the value of their savings.

In addition to the lack of facilities, the medical care "system" lacks a philosophical base that would allow interested professionals to promote the health status of older adults, that is, use of a wellness model of health with explanation of what possible changes to anticipate as one ages. The medical profession has focused on the illness or the sick role of the person who seeks assistance, rather than on health and preventive aspects. Even the Medicare program is illness-oriented. It does not provide for payment of preventive care such as routine physical examinations. The medical profession has few practitioners who are trained in the specialties of geriatrics or gerontology. Because of the scarcity of personnel, subtle signs and professional systems often go undetected in the assessment of the older client. Such early detection could lead to treatment that would prevent further physical and mental deterioration of the client. This situation leads to a greater demand for hospital and nursing home beds, which are not readily available to many older adults who live on fixed incomes.

As a result of increased awareness of the plight of older adults, particularly those who live in the community and in their own homes, a number of health care services are now available to allow the older person to maintain a healthful life-style. Some of these services are

- *Home health care.* For the older client who needs monitoring of such conditions as hypertension, diabetes, and medication regimen, this service, provided by an increasing number of private and public agencies, brings a professional nurse into the home. Daily, weekly, or monthly visits are provided with fees determined by the economic status of the client and federal regulation agency policies.

- *Home-delivered meals.* Older people who are unable to shop for groceries or prepare a major meal may have one meal a day brought to their homes by a catering service provided through the local Area Agency on Aging. These meals are well balanced, hot, and nutritious. The service brings another person into the home, an important part of the older person's socialization process; it also affords the opportunity for another person to monitor the condition of the client. However, the service is mainly provided on weekdays; the problem of providing meals on the weekends remains. Also, bad weather may prevent the delivery of meals, creating a hardship for the client, particularly if he or she is diabetic and needs a special daily diet. Dry pack meals are available in some locations for storage in the homes of those who have no means to obtain food during bad weather.

- *Day-care programs.* The older person, whether ambulatory or in a wheelchair, may benefit from the opportunity to socialize with peers in a day-care program, which is usually operated in a facility such as a health care institution or senior center. In the program, older adults are encouraged to care for themselves, so that they learn to draw on their own potential for independence, health, and well-being. Such an emphasis helps them use their own abilities to maintain meaning in their lives, helping others by sharing their experiences, talents, knowledge, skills, and themselves as a resource in caring for another human being.

- *Adult foster care programs.* This service is available for those older persons who may need some live supervision in their daily living habits. Some older adults suffer from memory loss in terms of self-care practices (bathing, eating, taking medications) or may need aid in making decisions regarding such matters as management of finances, e.g., estate planning, making a will, paying bills. Foster care provides them with the necessary short-term or long-term assistance to continue to live in a community-based setting and may prevent premature institutionalization.

- *Supportive services.* A variety of programs, funded by local, state, and national government agencies, provide older people who live in their own homes with day-to-day services, such as companions, legal and tax advice, and transportation (Eliopoulos 1979a; Ebersole and Hess 1990; Gress and Bahr 1984).

Critics of the present health care delivery sytem have begun to analyze its services and the gaps in these services for older clients. Because of an inefficient system, older persons are often admitted to institutions when in reality they could remain in their own homes and environments for many years if the proper services were available to them. With the passage of the Omnibus Budget Reconciliation Act (OBRA) of 1987, a preadmission screening and annual residents review (PASARR) is a regulation that applies to all older persons prior to admission to a nursing home or after admission to determine their eligibility for federally funded care. This procedure, when enforced, limits access to long-term care facilities to only those older adults who meet the criteria for admission. Older persons with mental retardation, mental illness, or chronic illnesses manageable outside skilled nursing facilities are ineligible for federal financing of institutional care, e.g., Medicare or Medicaid. Older persons, like others, are not eager to withdraw from society, from the lifestyles they have known—the environment that is familiar to them, the friends of long standing, the church that is the center of their lives, or the physicians and dentists who have long taken care of their needs—and move to an environment foreign to them in many ways. As more information becomes available, newer and more efficient aspects of a health care delivery system and programs to benefit older adults are being projected for the next fifty years. It is useful to examine some of these changes and how they will affect health professionals, primarily nurses who will be involved in these more creative approaches to health care and innovative settings.

CHANGES IN THE HEALTH CARE DELIVERY SYSTEM FOR OLDER ADULTS

In 1975 the ANA was requested by the United States Senate Special Committee on Aging, Subcommittee on Long-Term Care (ANA 1975) to prepare a document on long-term care. This study was concerned with the care of older adults, particularly in long-term care settings where "skilled" nursing care is delivered. At six hearings, nurses from around the country presented testimony regarding the quantity and quality of care received by older residents in these institutions. From these data, recommendations were formulated and submitted to the special senate committee chairman, Senator Frank E. Moss. These recommendations have been and continue to be used by the Congress in discussing innovation and creativity in the humane treatment of the older people of our nation.

Recommendations of the Senate Subcommittee on Long-Term Care:*

I. A national policy on care of the aging should be developed within which should be provision for care of the elderly in any setting, their right to quality care, and the right of the elderly to decision making in regard to their own care. The national policy on care of the aging should be built on the fact that the aged are vital, dynamic persons who have made and who continue to make contributions to society.

II. Because of high costs of essential health care services, coupled with the present provision of fragmented, uncoordinated, and incomplete health services to the aged, a plan for national health insurance should be developed to ensure that health care is provided for all citizens, guaranteeing coverage for the full range of comprehensive health services. The national health insurance plan should clearly recognize the distinctions between health care and medical care and provide options in utilization of health care services.

---

*These recommendations were published by the ANA and are reprinted with permission. American Nurses' Association: *Nursing and Long-Term Care: Toward Quality Care for the Aging: A Report from the Committee on Skilled Nursing Care.* Kansas City, MO: ANA, 1975, pp. ix–xx.

III. In considering options or alternatives for care, the Committee on Skilled Nursing Care recommends that a range of health and supportive services be made available to all elderly citizens. Thus, whether a person chooses to live in his own home and have services brought to him, to go to the services in a day care setting, or to move to a nursing home, he would have assurance that the needed services would be available.

IV. The word "skilled" should be deleted from the phrase, "skilled nursing care" as it currently exists in the federal standards and as the term is generally applied in actual practice, because it is not measurable nor can it be defined when related to the needs of a patient.

V. Because quality health care will depend primarily upon the competency of the persons providing direct care, all professional persons and workers involved in long-term health care in any setting should be taught at the educational levels of the individuals in the depth and detail each can understand and use. Preparation in gerontological nursing should be within an open educational system which promotes career mobility. The educational program of registered nurses at all levels should be developed and strengthened to correct specific deficiencies in the area of gerontological nursing (ANA 1975).

Because of these recommendations the improvement of care for older adults has become a focal point in the deliberations of congressional leaders. Bills that include older persons and their needs are being introduced at a greater rate. However, the formulation of public policy is a slow process. Seeking solutions to complex problems becomes a tremendous task; equal usage of resources based on human rights for older persons is essential. Conferences on social policy project such questions as: what age category should be focused on initially—the 60-year-olds or frail older adults in their 90s? How can we finance the increasing cost of institutionalization for older adults? Do the nonprofit nursing homes meet the needs of older adults better than those of a proprietary nature? Would it be better to change the policy regarding payment of hospital costs by Medicare and extend hospital coverage so that older adults would be in better condition when discharged, thus eliminating an intermediate stop at the nursing home before being placed in their own homes? How has the Prospective Payment System (PPS) program of discharge affected the well-being of older persons? Many such questions challenge legislators and medical and nursing personnel on the need for change in the health care delivery system.

The Omnibus Budget Reconciliation Act (OBRA) of 1987, 1989, and implemented effectively on October 1, 1990 projected major legislative changes to upgrade care of older adults in long-term care facilities for nursing home reform. This legislation identified regulations for the operation of nursing homes that have as their main focus the well-being of each older resident admitted for care. These changes were directed toward the rights of the older adult to high-quality care and services guaranteed them under federal law in Medicare- and/or Medicaid-funded facilities. Some of the areas included: nurse's aide training, preadmission screening and annual resident review (PASARR), disclosure of information on quality assessment and assurance committees, and a fourteen-day period for completion of the Resident Assessment Inventory. The Resident Assessment Inventory requires coordination by a licensed nurse and includes a nursing assessment section as well as all supportive services. Areas included are: physical therapy, occupational therapy, dietary, pharmacy, physicians, chaplain; responsibility of nursing homes for services provided for the mentally ill and mentally retarded residents; resident's right to refuse intrafacility transfers to a Medicare-distinct part of the facility; resident access to clinical records; inclusion of state notice of rights and a facility notice of rights to be posted in each facility; nurse staffing requirements (OBRA 1989).

A major regulation of OBRA is the completion of the MDS—Minimum Data Set Resident Assessment Inventory. This provides complete data on all residents, their preferences, health lifestyle practices, and care needs including physical therapy, occupational therapy, and other support services that allow each resident to enjoy a quality of life with an optimum level of functioning based on each person's health status and functional capacity. The completion of the form for each resident is coordinated by the licensed nurse who signs the form when all sections of the form have been filled in by the appropriate individual in each of the supportive services. Once completed, a copy is placed in the resident's chart and used as the basis for nursing care plans. A copy of the completed form is sent to the state agency on aging for data compilation on residents within the state, which in turn sends the compiled data to the Health Care Financing Agency (HCFA). This governmental agency is charged with pricing services to nursing homes for Medicare/Medicaid reimbursement more in keeping with the required care needs of older residents. This project, titled Multi-State Case Mix and Quality Demonstration Project, is currently executed on an experimental basis in five states (Kansas, Mississippi, North Dakota, Wyoming, and Nebraska). If it is successful, new reimbursement schedules will be placed on a national basis with all fifty states participating in a new payment formula (personal conversation, B. Cornelius, Project Director, MDST, January 17, 1992). This is a major breakthrough for gerontological nursing and nurses who may be able to better meet the needs of older, more acutely ill residents of nursing homes.

NURSING AND DELIVERY OF HEALTH CARE

Innovation and creativity in nursing settings come in small or minute progressive steps when the attitude and change are systematic. Havighurst (1977) noted that the nursing profession is in a key position to initiate such change since the care of most older adults falls under its jurisdiction. Such a change, for example, has been instituted by a gerontological nursing specialist, who holds a master's degree, in a large health care facility for institutionalized older adults in Kansas City, Missouri. This nurse assumed the position of nursing service director and immediately adopted a model of nursing practice based on Maslow's hierarchy of needs and assumed the philosophic position that all older persons are worthy of respect and dignity regardless of their mental and physical status. As a result of education in the tenets of her practice, her staff made outstanding progress in the rehabilitation of older persons, many of whom had been withdrawn and autistic for years. Through her efforts they once again enjoyed a quality of life that enabled them to be fully functioning human beings.

By obtaining positions on health planning boards such as the Health Systems Agency, nurses have participated in the review of service programs for older adults. Continued lobbying efforts and political activism by professional nurses bring the unique health needs of older citizens to the attention of legislators and policymakers. More emphasis on a delivery system built on the concept of community services enables nurses, many of whom believe it is most beneficial to interact with clients in their own homes, to use a wellness-oriented rather than an illness-oriented concept as a guide in coordinating medical care, nursing care, and the home environment.

Specifically, if nurses wish to bring about a systematic change in the care of older adults, the concept of health in older adults must be redefined (Mallick 1979; Gress and Bahr 1984; Ebersole and Hess 1985; Ebersole and Hess 1990). To measure the efficacy of interventions of nursing care for older adults, more specific factors contributing to health status allow for more accurate analysis of that level of health by the professional. Nurses have used a broad definition of health utilizing such terms as high-level wellness, self-care, and well-being as a guiding principle in their work; this definition gives little information as to what the term really means. Consequently, one of the most innovative means of achieving a systematic change in the health care delivery system is through the educational and research efforts of professionals who wish to have an impact on the health care of older people. These efforts culminate in more detailed health assessment and nursing intervention plans that aim at promoting the wellness of older persons.

NURSING EDUCATION AND THE CARE OF OLDER ADULTS

More attention needs to be given to the topic of gerontology in the curricula of both undergraduate and graduate nursing programs in order to prepare nurses to care for the large number of older adults in the population. This educational aspect is vital to the progress of the profession as well as to the improvement of institutional and community-based care of the older population of the nation.

It is important to include the topic of aging, especially in its biologic, psychosocial, and spiritual aspects, in nursing curricula. Various authors (Bahr 1986; Ebersole and Hess 1990) suggest that the health care delivery system for older adults will not change substantially until nursing personnel are educated about the aging process. Peabody (1977) noted that the nursing profession would be unprepared *(1)* if the federal government were to pass legislation in the near future to upgrade care in facilities to which older adults are admitted and *(2)* if nurse practitioners needed to staff the facilities in a new and creative way were not available because of a lack of proper education. The late Senator John Heinz had recommended a professional nurse staffing requirement for nursing homes to improve the quality of care in the nation's nursing homes. However, this legislative bill did not address the qualifications necessary in terms of preparation in gerontological nursing. The field of gerontological nursing has not been a popular career choice among nurses, probably because of their generally negative attitude toward older adults, a reflection of the attitudes of the larger society. A major thrust to provide more content in gerontological nursing is needed in baccalaureate programs in nursing. This level of education should provide the basic knowledge and skills in nursing, including nursing of the older adult, needed to prepare the generalist for practice in gerontological nursing (Partnership of Gerontological Nursing Practice and Education, Old Dominion University, February 1, 1992).

Attitudes of Nurses toward Older Adults

In American society it is difficult to accept the idea that people can continue to live productive lives after retirement, especially for one who has had little experience with retired persons over age 70 who are indeed productive, positive toward life, active, and involved. This perhaps is the best approach to attitude change—reversal of one's experience. Since nursing deals with the human being and is based on interacting with that person, the attitude held by the nurse is important. Attitude is the basis for behavior. The behavior exhibited by the nurse, then, can be traced to the attitude held in any given circumstance or toward any particular person. Hatton (1977) in her research study on attitudes, concluded that nursing care and its quality reflect the attitude held by the nurse. In her research she observed two hours of

nursing care given by seven registered nurses in a long-term care facility. In addition, each nurse completed the Kogan's Old People Attitude Scale. The students' behavior patterns were then categorized—they demonstrated many negative responses toward the aging residents that correlated with the attitudes held by the nurses (Hatton 1977). Similar results were obtained by Taylor and Harned (1978) in their study of nurses' attitudes toward older persons. The authors suggested implications that nurses should undertake self-analysis regarding their prejudicial attitudes before assessing their older clients. This self-knowledge helps nurses change their attitudes and leads to a more positive approach to older adults and their care.

Gomez, Otto, Blattstein, and Gomez (1985) investigated the impact of a three-week, eight-hour-per-week clinical experience of caring for ill older adults in long-term care institutions by baccalaureate students taking their first clinical course. These researchers discovered that there was a positive attitude toward the older adults by beginning baccalaureate nursing students after a three-week clinical experience with the ill older adults in nursing homes. They also found that older students held more positive attitudes toward older adults than did the younger students. In analyzing the relationship among the nurses' educational levels, ages, and the extent to which they worked with older adults compared to their attitudes, Brower (1985) found a definite trend for nurses educated in institutions of higher learning to have more positive attitudes toward the aged. A critical need, according to Brower (1985), is for more specialized educational programs in gerontological nursing to aid faculty who teach in schools of nursing to become more knowledgeable regarding gerontology and gerontological nursing.

In 1989 the Southern Regional Education Board (SREB) was awarded a three-year Nursing Special Projects Grant from the Division of Nursing, *Faculty Preparation for Teaching Gerontological Nursing* (D10NU24299). (SREB's affiliated organization, the Southern Council on Collegiate Education for Nursing (SCCEN), was responsible for project implementation.) A major project objective was to provide comprehensive continuing education programs to improve faculty practice in gerontological nursing. Targeted to nursing faculty with little or no formal

Table 1–1 Workshop Objectives: Faculty Preparation for Teaching Gerontological Nursing (SREB)

- Differentiating between the normal aging process and health problems associated with aging
- Recognizing the diverse physical and psychosocial responses of older adults to common health problems
- Describing ways in which nurses can promote successful aging
- Recognizing the importance of preparing nurses who use an holistic approach to older clients in preventive care, acute care, and long-term care
- Describing the curricular and research implications of the current scope of gerontological nursing content and practice

preparation in gerontological nursing, the project sponsored a series of one-week workshops that followed a master curriculum plan and included clinical observation experiences with well and ill older adults to achieve workshop objectives, Table 1-1.

Spaces in the 1990 workshops, pilot-tested at Georgia State University in Atlanta, quickly filled and a waiting list was maintained. The 1991 and 1992 workshops were held at eight regional sites: University of Alabama at Birmingham; University of Arkansas for Medical Sciences, Little Rock; University of South Florida, Tampa; Georgia State University, Atlanta; University of Mississippi Medical Center, Jackson; Clemson University, Clemson, South Carolina; University of Texas at Houston Health Science Center; and Virginia Commonwealth University/Medical College of Virginia, Richmond. Over 225 persons attended the 1991 workshops. Overall, almost 500 faculty participated in 42 workshops. Unfortunately, not all of these workshops were filled to capacity.

Participants in all workshops designed a project to meet a priority need in gerontological nursing in their school or community to be implemented within six months of workshop completion. Final reports of these projects have been published (Yurchuck 1992).

This approach of teaching gerontological nursing content to faculty responsible for curricular improvements is important to ensure the exposure of nursing students in associate degree and baccalaureate degree programs to current information about aging and care of older adults in all settings (Yurchuck 1992). With this positive opportunity to learn more

about aging and many age- and health-related issues, it is anticipated that there will be an improvement in the attitude of faculty toward gerontological nursing that will affect curricular decisions in baccalaureate programs in nursing. The beneficiaries of such decisions are the nursing students who will be providers of care to older persons in the future.

Meyer, Hassanein, and Bahr (1978) found in their research that nurses who worked directly with older clients held more negative attitudes toward them than nurses who worked with other clients such as young children in a specialized hospital setting. The authors used the Tuckman-Lorge Attitude Toward Old People test as the principal instrument for data collection. Meyer et al. concluded that nursing students should have more positive educational experiences with older adults; the students would then avoid a stereotyped attitude toward them. Consequently their image of gerontological nursing would be upgraded.

Changing the Attitudes of Nurses toward Older Adults

In attempting to change the attitudes of nursing students, Chamberland et al. (1978) initiated an educational experience in which the first encounter with an older person was with a client who was relatively well and in the client's own home. Students who took part in the educational program were taught about the normal physiologic and psychologic processes of aging, with emphasis on wellness and the normal aging process. The students learned to assess the strengths of older persons as well as the problems of illness and chronicity of conditions. Students also learned about behavior modification, the importance of stimulation of the senses, and reality orientation therapy. The students were then given a careful introduction to the clinical experience in a nursing home or another health care setting. Counseling and monitoring of the experience helped the students void major pitfalls. To evaluate the nursing students' attitudes, the Tuckman-Lorge Attitude Toward Old People test was administered as a pretest and posttest. An analysis of the data revealed that before the curriculum change the students had a negative attitude toward older persons. The authors hoped that the change in the curriculum and the learning experience would promote a more positive attitude in the students in the future.

Expanding Knowledge through Research

As a more positive attitude is acquired regarding gerontology with the inclusion of the subject of aging in the curriculum of educational programs on the undergraduate and graduate levels, more research is being geared toward understanding the complexity of the aging process. The American Academy of Nursing at its 1985 Scientific Session addressed the issue of gerontological nursing research needs in its publication conference *Setting the Agenda for the Year 2000: Knowledge Development in Nursing* (ANA 1986). Major clinical problems identified as needing research included incontinence, confusion, pain, restlessness, fatigue, immobility-induced disability, pressure ulcers, sensory deprivation or overstimulation, and infections in immunosuppressed hosts (ANA 1986). Many of these nursing clinical problems are now under study by the National Center for Nursing Research (NCNR) and the Agency for Health Care Research and Policy (AHCPR). Current re-

search is reported in such documents as the *Handbook of Aging and the Social Sciences, Handbook of the Biology of Aging, Handbook of the Psychology of Aging, Research in Aging* (a magazine that focuses on studies of social gerontology), *The Gerontologist*, and the *Journal of the American Geriatrics Society.** Annual meetings of gerontologists representing the disciplines of nursing, medicine, allied health, and the biologic and behavioral sciences are held to report new data and share current knowledge on the aging process and the behavior of older citizens. The Council of Gerontological Nursing of the ANA presents new clinical data on aging based on research and the applicability of this knowledge in clinical practice through regional and national forums. In addition, The National Gerontological Nursing Association was established in 1985 for nurses engaged in the care of aging persons in a variety of settings. This organization holds a national educational and research conference annually. Its first conference was held in September 1986 in Washington, DC. Eight hundred fifty nurses from the 50 states and Puerto Rico attended. The author was the national program chairperson for the first conference, the 1987 conference in Chicago, Illinois, the 1988 conference in New Orleans (which attracted twelve hundred nurse gerontologists with participants from many states, including Alaska and Hawaii, as well as Puerto Rico and the Philippines), as well as the 1989 and 1990 conferences in Los Angeles and Washington, DC respectively. The conferences continue on an annual basis.

Graduate Programs in Gerontological Nursing

The Division of Nursing of the United States Department of Health and Human Services funded a number of programs for advanced education of

* Birren, E. and K.W. Schaie, eds. *Handbook of the Psychology of Aging*. New York: Van Nostrand Reinhold Co., 1976.
Finch, C.E. and L. Hayflick, eds. *Handbook of the Biology of Aging*. New York: Van Nostrand Reinhold Co., 1976.
The Gerontologist. Gerontological Society, 1835 K St., NW, Washington, DC.
Journal of the American Geriatrics Society. The American Geriatrics Society, Inc., New York, N.Y.

gerontological clinical nurse specialists/practitioners. These programs were integrated into the graduate nursing education programs leading to a master's degree in nursing. Such programs address the issue of specialized preparation for gerontological nursing. A variety of avenues have been opened to those who wish to pursue such educational preparation, e.g., a sequence of courses giving an in-depth concentration in gerontological nursing, and a master's degree in gerontological nursing. It is gratifying that opportunities for such educational preparation of professional nurses are increasingly available in many regions of the United States. Currently there are 33 programs awarding graduate degrees in gerontological nursing in the United States (ANA 1992).

Not only are professional nurse educators spearheading the educational movement for the inclusion of gerontological nursing content in nursing curricula to upgrade the care of older adults, but others are becoming involved in the effort. Legislative action, such as that initiated in Kansas (1983) after strong lobbying efforts by a citizens' group, is contributing to changes in nursing education curricula. A resolution was passed by the state legislature requiring that curricula in state-supported schools for health care practitioners should include content that would prepare these practitioners to meet the unique health care needs of older persons. This resolution is to be enforced by withholding state funding from those Kansas educational institutions that do not satisfactorily meet the requirements after one year. With universities and community citizen groups joining forces, there should be evidence of better-prepared professionals and an upgrading of clinical practice and care.

GERONTOLOGICAL NURSING PRACTICE: ITS EXPANSION

The specialty of gerontological nursing practice is an expanding field of nursing. Since 1961, when the Division of Geriatric Nursing was established in the ANA, it has steadily grown in importance. As evidence of this growth, the first national conference on gerontological nursing, sponsored by the *Journal of Gerontological Nursing* publishers, was held in Miami in 1979 and attracted over 300 professional nurse gerontologists. This group demonstrated that this specialty had come of age and had moved forward to defining its functions, its scope, and its contributions to promoting and maintaining the health of older people. Four main components have been selected as the framework of professionalism for this newly recognized nursing discipline.

1. The definitions of terms to support the philosophic dimension of the discipline of gerontological nursing

2. The development of the *Standards and Scope of Gerontological Nursing Practice*, published by the Council of Gerontological Nursing of the ANA

3. The certification of gerontological nurses/clinical specialists/nurse practitioners as recognition of their excellence in practice

4. Selected nursing theories applicable in gerontological clinical settings to provide a melding of the theoretical and clinical components of care

Definitions

Since 1961, definitions that describe the scope of this new specialty area have emerged. This approach has marked much interest among nurses themselves. The following definitions are generally accepted:

- *Geriatrics*—the area of study related to the diseases of older adults

- *Gerontology*—the preferred term for the normal aging process. It encompasses the total phenomenon of aging, including the biologic, psychosocial, and spiritual aspects of the older individual

- *Gerontological nursing*—that branch of nursing "concerned with assessment of the health needs of older adults, planning and implementing health care to meet these needs, and evaluating the effectiveness of such care. . . . Gerontological nursing strives to identify and use the strengths of older adults and assists them to use those strengths to maximize independence" (ANA 1976)

- *Gerontic*—pertaining to old age

- *Gerontic nursing*—refers to nursing care of older adults; perhaps a more appropriate term than either *geriatric* or *gerontological nursing* (Gunter and Estes 1979)

Standards of Gerontological Nursing Practice

A sign of recognition for the emergence of a nursing specialty is the use of standards of care to guide the nursing practice of the specialty group. All professionals evaluate their contributions to the clientele they attempt to assist by their special knowledge and expertise. Professional nursing now recognizes that it needs measurable objectives to achieve quality care for its clients. Such guides ensure a professional approach to serving older adults who require a high level of knowledge and skill from those involved in their health care. The ANA *Standards of Gerontological Nursing Practice* (1976a) provided the initial guidelines for nursing practice in this field.

The ANA Council of Gerontological Nursing established a task force in 1987 to revise and update the 1976 Standards of Gerontological Nursing Practice. The revised statements were published in 1987. The author was one of three members of the task force to write this document following consultation with gerontological nurses throughout the nation who critiqued and gave suggestions for the revisions. A booklet containing the revised *Standards and Scope of Gerontological Nursing Practice* is available from the American Nurses' Association, Council of Gerontological Nursing, Washington, DC.

There are eleven standards, complete with a rationale, structure criteria, process criteria, and outcome criteria for each standard. Each standard is presented here (American Nurses' Association, 1988, pp. 13–18.*

Standard I. Organization of Gerontological Nursing Services. All gerontological nursing services are planned, organized, and directed by a nurse executive. The nurse executive has baccalaureate or master's preparation and has experience in gerontological nursing and administration of long-term care services or acute care services for older clients.

Standard II. Theory. The nurse participates in the generation and testing of theory as a basis for clinical decisions. The nurse uses theoretical concepts to guide the effective practice of gerontological nursing.

Standard III. Data Collection. The health status of the older person is regularly assessed in a comprehensive, accurate, and systematic manner. The information obtained during the health assessment is accessible to and shared with appropriate members of the interdisciplinary health care team, including the older person and the family.

Standard IV. Nursing Diagnosis. The nurse uses health assessment data to determine nursing diagnoses.

Standard V. Planning and Continuity of Care. The nurse develops the plan of care in conjunction with the older person and appropriate others. Mutual goals, priorities, nursing approaches, and measures in the care plan address the therapeutic, preventive, restorative, and rehabilitative needs of the older person. The care plan helps the older person attain and maintain the highest level of health, well-being, and quality of life achievable, as well as a peaceful death. The plan of care facilitates continuity of care over time as the client moves to various care settings, and is revised as necessary.

Standard VI. Intervention. The nurse, guided by the plan of care, intervenes to provide care to restore the older person's functional capabilities and to prevent complications and excess disability. Nursing interventions are derived from nursing diagnoses and are based on gerontological nursing theory.

Standard VII. Evaluation. The nurse continually evaluates the client's and family's responses to interventions in order to determine progress toward goal attainment and to revise the data base, nursing diagnoses, and plan of care.

Standard VIII. Interdisciplinary Collaboration. The nurse collaborates with other members of the health care team in the various settings in which care is given to the older person. The team meets regularly to evaluate the effectiveness of the care plan for the

---

*Reprinted with permission from *Standards and Scope of Gerontological Nursing Practice.* © 1987, American Nurses Association, Washington, DC.

client and family and to adjust the plan of care to accommodate changing needs.

Standard IX. Research. The nurse participates in research designed to generate an organized body of gerontological nursing knowledge, disseminates research findings, and uses them in practice.

Standard X. Ethics. The nurse uses the Code for Nurses established by the American Nurses' Association as a guide for ethical decision making in practice.

Standard XI. Professional Development. The nurse assumes responsibility for professional development and contributes to the professional growth of interdisciplinary team members. The nurse participates in peer review and other means of evaluation to assure the quality of nursing practice.

Certification of Gerontological Nurses

In 1973 the ANA's Division on Nursing Practice inaugurated its certification program for the purpose of providing a vehicle for recognition of personal excellence in nursing. Three levels of certification of examinations are available to the gerontological nurse through the American Nurses' Association Council of Gerontological Nursing: the Gerontological Nursing Generalist Examination, the Gerontological Nurse Practitioner Examination, and the Gerontological Clinical Nurse Specialist Examination. The latter two examinations require a master's degree in nursing for eligibility to take the examination. The generalist test requires a B.S.N. as of 1992. The process for certification in gerontological nursing includes an application fee, determination of eligibility based on licensure and gerontological nursing practice, and a comprehensive examination. The examination is administered on an annual basis at eighty different sites and may be retaken an unlimited number of times if necessary. If the nurse meets the criteria and is certified, reevaluation every five years is required to determine continuance of relevant and excellent nursing practice (American Nurses' Credentialing Center 1992). Recertification requirements for the Gerontological Clinical Specialist requires:

1. Experience
   a) Fifteen hundred hours of gerontological nursing practice

2. Education
   a) Option 1: Sit for and successfully pass the written certification.
   b) Option 2: Continuing Education (a minimum of two of the following categories or double any one single category):

   Category 1: seventy-five contact hours of continuing education

   Category 2: five academic semester credit hours or six quarter-hour credits

   Category 3: Participation as a presenter/lecturer in five academic semester courses (or six academic quarter courses)

   Category 4: Participation as a presenter/lecturer in five continuing education offerings/presentations

   Category 5: Evidence of publication of one article, book chapter, or research project

Each nurse to be recertified must meet the practice requirement and complete either option (American Nurses Credentialing Center Brochure 1992).

Selected Nursing Theories

Nursing theories provide a frame of reference for the individual nurse practitioner. More emphasis is being placed on the utilization of a nursing theory to formulate a model of practice that would aid in the evaluation of the outcomes of nursing action to differentiate the practice of nursing.

Many theories are emerging that remain untested in all possible clinical settings, but are important contributions in providing a basis for nursing practice. Three theories that are applicable to older persons in clinical settings are presented here.

Orem's Self-Care Theory. The self-care theory is one of the most prominent theories in nursing today (Orem 1971). The theory advances the concept that the nurse should not dictate health care judgments and practices and impose these on older clients. Rather the professional nurse, through personal knowledge and skill in interviewing and assessing the health care status, interprets the data provided by the client and projects with the client a care plan that is realistic, attainable, and measurable from the client's perspective. In using the self-care practices of the client, health care assumes a more integrated approach based on the client's cultural beliefs, health practices, and environmental aspects, fitting easily into the clients' lifestyle. Gerontological nursing promotes wellness of older adults. Consequently the self-care theory provides an excellent base of operations.

Roy's Adaptation Theory. Roy's adaptation theory (Roy 1974) describes a person's life as a positive or negative series of adaptations to the internal and external environments. There are four modes of adaptation: physiologic needs, self-concept, role function, and interdependence relations during health and illness. When people are aware of the stressors in their lives, they can adjust accordingly; their lives are then healthier. The gerontological nurse practitioner knows what events may be stressful (i.e., by referring to the Holmes and Rahe scale) and can assist older persons through nursing assessment and anticipatory guidance. The goal of the adaptation model and theory is thus to avoid pitfalls that may be harmful to older adults by planning care based on a knowledge of potential problem areas. Perkins (1987) demonstrated that Roy's adaptation theory is applicable to gerontological nursing when the interdependence mode of the theory was tested with family caregivers and the frail elderly. Significant findings indicated that if an affectional bond was present between the caregiver and the frail elderly person, strong interdependence was found. If obligation for responsibility of caregiving was indicated, a lesser degree of interdependence was found.

Neuman's Health Care Systems Theory. Neuman's health care systems theory stresses the importance of the total-person approach to patient problems (Neuman 1974) in raising the level of health through nursing action. This task is accomplished by identifying stress factors in a person's life and reducing them through appropriate interventions. These stressors can be interpersonal, intrapersonal, and extrapersonal. Each of these realms must be explored in the patient assessment by the professional nurse, who, using this inclusive data, plans care on a comprehensive basis. Holistic health is total health, according to Neuman. This theory is directly applicable to older clients who may have symptoms of illness but whose primary concern is financial.

Until the professional nurse helps resolve the priority issue, financial or otherwise, in the client's life, any direct nursing care to achieve a higher level of wellness and optimum functioning for older persons will be futile.

These theories demonstrate how models for nursing practice may be implemented in clinical settings where older adults are the major consumers of nursing care. By the application of such theories to nursing practice, problems and solutions are being identified more scientifically so that the quality of nursing practice is improved. However, as noted by Strumpf (1978), much remains to be learned by nurse researchers. There is a need to develop and test theories of aging that include and describe not only the interaction of humans with the environment but also the best methods of carrying out nursing actions based on this perception.

GERONTOLOGICAL NURSING ROLES

In the United States there are two major established roles for the gerontological nurse: the gerontological nurse practitioner and the gerontological clinical nurse specialist. Table 1-2 demonstrates the commonalities of knowledge and skills for these two roles and specified knowledge and skills peculiar to each major role.

Gerontological Clinical Nurse Specialist

Gerontological clinical nurse specialists are prepared at the graduate level (ANA 1991). The master's program in gerontological nursing provides advanced knowledge and skills in nursing to prepare the gerontological nurse specialist who assumes leadership in gerontological nursing. The curriculum may include courses in gerontological theory, nursing practice, and nursing research with electives in administration, consultation, and education (ANA 1991; Lee and Cosby 1987). The clinical nurse specialist is an expert in clinical practice who may be an educator, consultant, researcher, or administrator (ANA 1991). The complexity of care for older adults demands specialized education with a sound theoretical basis and a supervised clinical practicum to promote clinical judgments that are accurate and scientifically based on concepts of physiology, sociology, psychology, and nursing. As more qualified nursing specialists

Table 1–2 The Commonalities and Specifics of Two Gerontological Nursing Roles

Commonalities

Knowledge base of aging:

    Physiologic (normal and abnormal)

    Psychosocial

    Cultural

Knowledge and skill in:

    Nursing process

    Coordination and leadership

    Communication

Family dynamics theory

Teaching

Quality assurance

Business, management, and marketing

Research

Ability to work in a multidisciplinary

    environment

Professional development

Specifics

Gerontological nurse practitioner:

    Primary care

    Ambulatory clinics

    Long-term care facilities

Maintenance of care

    Continuity

Coordination

Case management

Patient advocacy

Setting

    Ambulatory clinics

    Long-term care facilities

    Independent practice

Gerontological clinical nurse specialist:

Direct patient care

    Acute hospital

    Home care

Consultation

Coordination

Discharge planning

    (case management)

Patient advocacy

Setting

    Hospitals

    Outreach programs

    Independent consultant

(Ebersole and Hess 1990)

become available, the clinical practice of gerontological nursing can grow to meet the challenges of care of older adults (Bahr 1986).

How has the gradual increase in the number of prepared clinical nurse specialists influenced the practice of gerontological nursing? Primarily, the emphasis is now on goals for older clients. Norton (1977) has noted that the essential component of nursing care for older clients is the anticipated resolution of problems presented by them, thus eliminating the negative orientation to care; that is, every problem observed in the older client in a clinical setting has a solution that becomes the projected goal of the nursing care. The plan

of care is based on the five elements of the nursing process: *(1)* assessment, *(2)* making the nursing diagnoses, *(3)* planning, *(4)* implementing the nursing care plan, and *(5)* evaluating the outcomes of the plan and the nursing care. Through this problem-solving approach a total health care plan can be implemented (Yura and Walsh 1988).

The expanding scope of the practice of the gerontological clinical nurse specialist is seen in the increasing insight into the caring process for each client as reflected in the nurse-client relationship. Each older person, as a result of a unique historical evolution of beliefs, life experiences, health practices, and habits, presents a challenge to the nurse. As the nurse acquires greater professional knowledge of the complexity of human beings and the individuality of each client, he or she gains awareness of the functions of the role in fulfilling the client's needs. No one protocol of role functioning can be applied to all older clients. Each client calls for a unique plan of care. The expansion of the nursing role, therefore, arises from the application of the nurse's knowledge, skill, and expertise to the unique conditions of each older person's life and symptoms, complaints, signs, or cues exhibited. The nurse's role lies partially in ferreting out, through skillful interviewing techniques, the true nature of the difficulty, rather than in accepting without question the initial complaints which may disguise the real reason for seeking health care.

Gerontological Nurse Practitioner

In addition to the clinical nurse specialist in gerontological nursing, the gerontological nurse practitioner role has been established within the past ten years. This role, based on the concept of the pediatric nurse practitioner model by Dr. Loretta Ford in the early 1970s, emerged in collaboration with physicians whose clientele were mainly the aging persons within a community. In more recent years the continuing education programs that prepared the gerontological nurse practitioner were, through the efforts of the nurse practitioners, transferred into institutions of higher education. Within the last five years most of the gerontological nurse practitioners are prepared in master's programs with a primary care nursing focus. These gerontological nurse practitioners serve in many clinical settings, including nursing homes, home health care agencies, hospice programs, community health agencies, hospitals, and private practice. Currently there is discussion within the American Nurses' Association's various Councils of Practice regarding the future retention of the term nurse practitioner because all professional nurses function within that role upon completion of a formal educational program in nursing. The trend appears to be the elimination of the title but integration of the role into that of the clinical specialist (ANA 1987) or advance practice (ANA 1992).

The State of the Art

The state of the art of gerontological nursing is revealed in the efforts of these nursing specialists to change custodial care, so common in many institutions where older adults are housed, to individualized care of each older person. By educating the technical and professional staff in care of older adults, the clinical nurse specialist/nurse practitioner serves as instructor to the caregivers and advocate for older clients. By basing the practice on a philosophy of aging and nursing care, the nursing specialist acts as a role model for the professional care of older adults. The holistic care model responds to human needs on all levels.

The goal of gerontological nursing care is to help older clients realize their highest potential through functioning as fully as possible. This challenge is one that each gerontological clinical nurse specialist must accept in order to perfect the art of nursing in the specialty field of gerontological nursing.

Expanding the scope of gerontological nursing practice requires the acquisition of specific competencies through formal and informal study to implement the ANA *Standards and Scope of Gerontological Nursing Practice* (1987). Each standard demands a high level of performance in which the nurse must continue to acquire knowledge, skill, and expertise in working with the aging person. This level of competency and commitment to excellence will lay the foundation for the future of gerontological nursing.

TRENDS IN GERONTOLOGICAL NURSING

The future will produce gradual change because of various factors and their interaction. Society's attitudes will greatly influence the future of older adults. If human life is revered and held sacred, the future will be bright for this growing segment of the population. An important trend for gerontological nursing is achievement of quality of life for all older persons. In projecting future trends, Gaitz and Samorajski (1985) reported that the aging population will gain from new knowledge in the neurosciences, which will help discover the relationships of brain function with conditions such as Alzheimer's disease, other dementias, brain tumors, and brain lesions. Progress

Table 1–3 Nursing's Specific Responses to the Aging Society

Practice
   Certification program for nurse practitioners/specialists in gerontic nursing
   Robert Wood Johnson teaching/nursing home projects (11 funded sites)
   Council on Gerontological Nursing in American Nurses' Association
   Mountain States Geriatric Nurse Practitioner Program, Boise, Idaho
   Establishment of National Gerontological Nursing Association

Education
   Annual National Conference of Gerontological Nursing for nursing personnel caring for elderly
   Professional journals on gerontological nursing (*Journal of Gerontological Nursing*; *Geriatric Nursing*)
   Short-term institutes (continuing education)
   Certificate programs in gerontological nursing in colleges and university settings
   Master's in Nursing programs in gerontological nursing preparing clinical specialists/practitioners

Planned Responses

Practice
   Revision of the Standards and Scope of Gerontological Nursing Practice (1987)
   Senator Heinz proposed legislation for upgraded R.N. staffing in nursing homes
   Upgrading of certification/recertification of nurses in long-term care facilities by American Nurses'
      Association
   Models of gerontological nursing practice based on nursing theories
   More attention addressed to mental health needs of older residents of nursing homes and long-term
      care settings

Education
   Utilization of the Standards and Scope of Gerontological Nursing Practice in nursing educational
      programs
   American Nurses' Association and National Gerontological Nursing Association lobbying for
      case-mix reimbursement
   National League for Nursing recommendation for incorporation of gerontological content in B.S.N.
      programs for accreditation of nursing programs
   Theory building of gerontological nursing in increasing number of doctoral programs in
      gerontological nursing
   Increased research studies in gerontological nursing issues to improve nursing practice in care
      of elderly

Source: Bahr, R.T. Nursing's specific responses to the aging society. *J Allied Health* 1987; 16(4):342. Edited by L. A. Selker. Used with permission.

in psychopharmacology, immunology, and biology will have a major effect on treatment modalities for older adults. With more advanced knowledge of the psychological, sociological, and spiritual dimensions of health care, more opportunities will be able to provide for a meaningful and purposeful existence in the later years.

Overcoming the handicaps of aging in the twenty-first century is the major agenda for those involved in geriatric medicine and gerontological nursing. Long-term care will be influenced greatly by new knowledge brought to the field by researchers in the biological sciences, social sciences, and humanities (Wahlstedt and Blaser 1984).

Frail older persons, the fastest growing population segment in the 1990s, will continue to challenge gerontological nursing. The demand for increased numbers of professional nurses will increase as the acuity level of frail older adults (mostly age 85 and older) requires more intensive patient care in long-term care facilities by registered nurses prepared in gerontological nursing (Selker 1987; Bahr 1987). Nursing's Specific Responses to the Aging Society are shown in Table 1-3.

RESEARCH AND PROFESSIONAL ACTIVITIES: MAJOR THRUSTS IN THE TWENTY-FIRST CENTURY

Research on the aging process will influence professional nursing generally and gerontological nursing specifically in future years. Many research projects are giving insights into the prolongation of life through such approaches as

- *Transplantation of organs*—Worn-out tissue may be replaced, resulting in a "new" and vibrant body structure.

- *Regeneration*—Reactivation of cells and genes to renew body tissue occurs.

- *Lipofuscin buildup delay or prevention*—This process would slow down aging by eliminating the cell debris that interferes with normal function.

- *Restriction of diet*—Better nutrition of the young and middle-aged will lead to a prolonged and vigorous old age.

- *Lowering of body temperature*—According to some researchers a lowered body temperature may prolong life in humans (Baines 1991).

Research findings raise moral and professional questions that society must answer if all people are to live meaningful, high-quality lives. What is being done to ensure a bright future for older adults?

Professional nursing groups are seeking ways to influence society through such efforts as presentation of testimony at hearings conducted on the local, state, and national levels, so as to influence decisions to improve conditions and treatment of older adults in institutions and in the community. Workshops and in-service education for professional nurse groups and nonprofessional groups are aimed at changing the attitudes of these groups regarding older people and their care. Emphasizing the positive elements of the aging process and consciousness-raising of societal members is another goal. It is important to emphasize positive strengths in realms of physical, psychologic, and spiritual matters rather than the health problems and to ensure that older adults have the opportunity to express their individuality instead of merely doing what is comfortable for others. To allow an older person to be himself or herself, to make decisions, and to continue the lifestyle he or she has known is the greatest contribution that gerontological nursing can make to older adults of today and tomorrow.

One approach is to assist families to view the older person with respect. The family may also be helped to understand the older member's need for comfortable, dignified living arrangements. The gerontological clinical nurse specialist will often be the health professional, in both institutional and community settings, who assists the older person in making choices that are feasible, realistic, and economically sound. The family may benefit from consultation with the gerontological clinical nurse specialist and gain insight into the needs of the older person and the way to meet those needs most effectively.

As inflationary costs continue to spiral, institutionalization of older adults will become a greater financial burden for the family. Officials of regional government agencies are considering the possibility of establishing neighborhood network systems that would offer comprehensive health care facilities and supportive services in a given geographic region. Such neighborhood systems would make it possible for more older adults to remain in their homes, allowing them to live independently in familiar surroundings. In addition, government agencies concerned with the aging population may provide salary subsidies for family members who care for older adults in their homes (Ertel 1979; Selby and Schecter 1982).

Another major thrust for the future care of older adults is greater emphasis on an interdisciplinary team approach. Older people require more kinds of care than one professional group alone can provide. The care and support of older adults are ideally suited to an interdisciplinary approach.

Long-term care facilities will continue to be an important part of the comprehensive health care system. In the future, it is to be hoped that administrators of such facilities will base their staffing policies on the needs of older clients in residence rather than on the minimum legal requirements. By providing a more homelike atmosphere for older adults living in long-term care facilities, gerontological nursing may make one of its most important contributions to the well-being of the older people of our nation.

The future of gerontological nursing is bright if society will develop an attitude, expressed in appropriate programs, that will allow older adults to live life fully each day. This is the challenge to gerontological nursing and its continuing expansion in the twenty-first century to fulfill the roles of educator, innovator, and advocate—a demanding but rewarding outcome of professionalism.

SUMMARY

Gerontological nursing has had a turbulent history because of the attitudes of society toward older adults. There has been slow progress through the years in this field, but more visibility and acceptance of nursing care of this age group are now evident. This change will help lay the groundwork for the practice of gerontological nursing in the 21st century. The discussion of the historical evolution of gerontological nursing practice has demonstrated how ageism in our society and in the profession itself has influenced practice settings and the types of personnel employed to care for older adults in community agencies, institutions, and other health care settings.

At present it is implied that older adults are often outside the present health care system. Few physicians are specially trained in geriatric medicine. Thus the type of medical regimen prescribed for older clients is often adversely affected. As a result, misdiagnoses occur, treatment modalities and medications prescribed for the conditions unique to older adults are mismanaged, and difficulties arise in completing medical treatment because of federal regulations that operate against the interests of older adults in terms of their hospital-stay and long-term-care-stay insurance coverage.

Also discussed were the types of health maintenance services available to older adults living in their own homes that allow them access to the health care delivery system, demonstrating that they can function if enough services are within their reach, geographically and financially. These circumstances have implications for nursing education.

Gerontological nursing is a specialty that demands highly skilled, knowledgeable clinical specialists educated at the graduate level. This level of preparation is more available as the role of the gerontological nurse expands. Because of legislative and consumer pressures on colleges and universities, the topic of the aging process will be included in the curricula of health professional programs to meet the health needs of the ever-increasing aging population.

Along with the educational component the expansion of clinical practice for the gerontological nurse was encouraged. The role of the gerontological nurse will continue to grow in stature and importance, particularly in community settings where the majority of older adults will continue to be located.

Trends point to the improvement of conditions for the aging population. Professional nurses, educated in this emerging specialty area of gerontological nursing, will be the key health professionals who will be able to say with pride, "We care for older adults—they are precious persons!"

STUDY QUESTIONS _____

1. How did the specialty of gerontological nursing evolve since Florence Nightingale's time?

2. What is meant by the word *ageism*? From your experience is this term applicable to your impression of older adults?

3. Why do the demographics of 1991 show such an increase in the aging population in America? What accounts for such an increase?

4. What types of health care delivery are currently available to older adults in America?

5. What role has nursing played in providing health care to older adults who are institutionalized or homebound?

6. How do attitudes held by nurses affect nursing care provided for older adults?

7. Discuss the *Standards and Scope of Gerontological Nursing Practice* and identify how the gerontological clinical nurse specialist utilizes the standards in providing care for the older person.

8. Identify the three nursing theorists who have contributed to the nurse's understanding of health care needs of older adults.

9. Describe the expanded roles of the clinical nurse specialist and nurse practitioner in gerontological nursing and give examples of each role.

10. Discuss the evolution of nursing science through research activities for the 21st century in terms of care for older adults.

REFERENCES _____

American Association of Retired Persons and Administration on Aging. 1991. *A Profile of Older Americans.* Washington, DC: US Department of Health and Health Services, 1990.

American Nurses' Association. 1975. *Nursing and Long-Term Care: Toward Quality Care for the Aging: A Report from the Committee on Skilled Nursing Care.* Kansas City, MO: ANA Division of Nursing Practice.

American Nurses' Association. 1976a. *Definitions of Nursing Practitioners.* Kansas City, MO: ANA Division of Nursing Practice.

American Nurses' Association. 1976b. *Standards of Gerontological Nursing Practice.* Kansas City, MO: ANA Division of Nursing Practice.

American Nurses' Association. 1986. *The Role of the Clinical Nurse Specialist.* Kansas City, MO: ANA.

American Nurses' Association. 1987b. *The Scope of Nursing Practice.* (Pub. No. NP-72). Kansas City, MO: ANA.

American Nurses' Association. 1987a. *Standards and Scope of Gerontological Nursing Practice.* Kansas City, MO: ANA Division of Nursing Practice.

American Nurses' Association. 1991a. *Facts About Nursing.* Kansas City, MO: ANA.

American Nurses' Association. 1991b. *A Statement on the Scope of Gerontological Nursing Practice.* Kansas City, MO: ANA Division of Nursing Practice.

American Nurses' Credentialing Center. 1992. *Recertification Catalog.* Washington, DC: ANA.

ANA, Council of Gerontological Nursing. Telephone conversation with N. Barr, ANA Staff Specialist, January 21, 1992.

Bahr, R.T. 1986. Professional and public education initiatives: Addressing health and related needs of elderly persons. *Community Based Initiatives in Long-Term Care.* New York: National League for Nursing.

Bahr, R.T. 1987. Nursing's specific responses to the aging society. *J. Allied Health* 16(4):342.

Bahr, R.T. 1992. Message of chairperson. *Oasis* 8(4).

Baines, E.B. 1991. *Perspectives on Gerontological Nursing.* Newbury Park, CA: Sage Publications, Inc.

Brower, T. 1985. Do nurses stereotype the aged? *Journal of Gerontological Nursing* 11(1):17-20, 26-28.

Butler, R. 1974. Successful aging and the role of the life review. *Journal of the American Geriatrics Society* 22:553.

Chamberland G., B. Rawls, C. Powell, and M. Roberts. 1978. Improving students' attitudes toward aging. *Journal of Gerontological Nursing* 4(1): 44-45.

Cornelius, B., Project Director. *Multi-State Case Mix and Quality Demonstration Project.* Personal conversation, January 17, 1992.

Ebersole, P. and P. Hess. 1985. *Toward Healthy Aging,* 2d ed. St. Louis: C.V. Mosby.

Ebersole, P. and P. Hess. 1990. *Toward Healthy Aging,* 3d ed. St. Louis: C.V. Mosby.

Eliopoulos, C. 1979. The gerontological nurse specialist. In *Current Practice in Gerontological Nursing,* edited by A. Reinhardt and M. Quinn, St. Louis: C.V. Mosby.

Eliopoulos, C., ed. 1979a. Services for the aged. In *Gerontological Nursing.* New York: Harper and Row.

Ertel, P. 1979. *Special Conference on Aging and the Future Trends.* Kansas City, KS: Graduate Nursing Program, Gerontological Nursing Project, University of Kansas School of Nursing, October 1979.

Gaitz, C.M. and T. Samorajski. 1985. Epilogue. In *Aging 2000: Our Health Care Destiny.* Vol. 1, Biomedical Issues. New York: Springer-Verlag.

Gomez, G.E., D. Otto, A. Blattstein and E.A. Gomez. 1985. Beginning students can change attitudes about the aged. *Journal of Gerontological Nursing* 11(1):6-13.

Gress, L. and R.T. Bahr. 1984. *The Aging Person: A Holistic Perspective.* St. Louis: C.V. Mosby.

Gunter, L. and C. Estes. 1979. *Education for Gerontic Nursing.* New York: Springer.

Hatton, J. 1977. Nurse's attitude toward the aged: relationship to nursing care. *Journal of Gerontological Nursing* 3(3):21–26.

Havighurst, R. 1977. Perspectives on health care for the elderly. *Journal of Gerontological Nursing* 3(2):21–24.

Kalish, R.A. 1979. The new ageism and failure models: A polemic. *Gerontologist* 19(4):398–402.

Kelly, L.Y. 1981. *Dimensions of Nursing.* New York: Macmillan.

Lee, C.A. 1987. Thrusts of Florence Nightingale in the social context of the 19th century. *The Kansas City Nurse* 62(2):3–4.

Lee, J.L. and M. Cosby. 1987. Gerontologic education: In search of a core curriculum. *Journal of Gerontological Nursing* 13(7):12–17.

Malleck, M.J. 1979. Defining health: The step "before the nursing assessment. *Journal of Gerontological Nursing* 5(3):30–33.

Meyer, M.A., R. Hassanein and R.T. Bahr. 1978. A comparison of attitudes toward the aged help by professional nurses. *Image* 12(3):62–66.

Neuman, B. 1974. The Betty Neuman health care systems approach: A total person approach to patient problems. In *Conceptual Models for Nursing Practice,* edited by J. Riehl and C. Roy. Conceptual Models for Nursing Practice. New York: Appleton-Century-Crofts.

Norton, D. 1977. Geriatric nursing—What it is and what it is not. *Nursing Times* 10:1622.

Nursing's Agenda for Health Care Reform. Washington, DC: ANA, NLN, AACN, 1991.

OBRA, 1989. *Long-Term Care Administration Subscriber Digest,* December 1989, no. 1:1.

Orem, D. 1971. *Nursing Concepts of Practice.* New York: McGraw-Hill.

Peabody, C. 1977. Implications for nursing service for major national health insurance proposals. *Journal of Gerontological Nursing* 3(2):37–41.

Perkins, I. 1987. An analysis of relationships among interdependence in family caregivers and the elderly, caregiver burden, and adaptation of homebound frail elderly. Doctoral Diss. The Catholic University of America School of Nursing, Washington, DC.

Roy, C. 1974. The Roy adaptation model. *Conceptual Models for Nursing Practice,* edited by J. Riehl and C. Roy. New York: Appleton-Century-Crofts.

Selby, P. and M. Schecter. 1982. *Aging 2000: A Challenge for Society.* Boston: MTP Press.

Selker, L.G., ed. 1987. Nursing. *Journal of Allied Health* 16(4):340–342.

Siegel, J.S. and C.M. Taeuber. 1986. Demographic dimensions of an aging population. *Our Aging Society, Paradox and Promise,* edited by A. Pifer and L. Bronte. New York: Norton.

Strumpf, N. 1978. Aging—A progressive phenomenon. *Journal of Gerontological Nursing* 4(2):17–21.

Taylor, K, and T. Harned. 1978. Attitudes toward old people: A study of nurses who care for the elderly. *Journal of Gerontological Nursing* 4(5):43–47.

Tedrow, J.L. 1979. The law and the elderly. *Current Practice in Gerontological Nursing,* edited by A. Reinhardt and M. Quinn. St. Louis: C.V. Mosby.

United Nations population division. 1982. *Aging 2000: A Challenge for Society,* edited by P. Selby and M. Schecter. Boston: MTP Press.

Wahlstedt, P. and W. Blaser. 1984. The long-term care continuum. *The Kansas Nurse* 59(11):3–4. Yura, H. and M. Walsh. 1988. *The Nursing Process: Assessing, Planning, Implementing, Evaluating,* 5th ed. Norwalk, CT: Appleton-Century-Crofts.

Yurchuck, R. 1992. *Presenting 1992 Workshops.* (A brochure.) Atlanta, GA: Southern Collegiate Council on Education in Nursing, Southern Regional Education Board.

Part 2

Changes of Aging

2 Developmental Changes

Allene Jones

CHAPTER OUTLINE

FOCUS

The primary focus of this chapter is to discuss the developmental theories and changes that occur in later middle age and old age and to identify related nursing interventions appropriate to each developmental stage.

OBJECTIVES

1. Differentiate between the changes of middle age and old age.

2. Discuss the theoretical views on later middle age and old age.

3. State the developmental tasks of later middle age and old age.

4. Apply selected nursing interventions from the developmental theories on later middle age and old age.

5. Analyze the effects of specific physical and psychological changes of sexual development in later middle age and old age.

6. Discuss the effects of aging on the family-life cycle.

Developmental tasks are important to all stages of the life cycle and vary with each stage. Developmental tasks are concerned with learning and meeting basic human needs. When their learning is hindered and their basic human needs are not met, people experience unhappiness and may be described by others as maladjusted.

To discuss the developmental tasks of the latter part of middle age intelligently, it is important to define *middle age*. It is frequently described as *matu-*

rity, or the *climacteric*, a time in one's life when the major responsibility of childrearing is over, when one is comfortable with one's self, and as a time for preparation for retirement (Rogers 1979). How each person feels about his or her own middle age is important. For some, later middle age is the prime of life; for others, it is a time of great upheaval and despair. One's view of middle age is in part a result of one's philosophy of life. For purposes of discussion, middle age is considered to be between 45 and 64 years (Rogers 1979), and later middle age is from 55 to 64. Neugarten and Havighurst (1979) have categorized people in the 55-to-75 age group as the *young-old* and people in the 75-and-older group as the *old-old*.

THEORETICAL VIEWS OF LATER MIDDLE AGE

According to Stevens-Long (1979) and a review of other literature, until recently, less has been written about middle age than all the other stages of growth and development. The theories of Erikson, Peck, Havighurst, Freud, and others are pertinent to a discussion of the later part of middle age.

Erik Erikson's Theory

Erik Erikson, a psychoanalyst, has postulated eight stages of development in the life cycle and has termed them the *eight stages of man.* Erikson's seventh stage of development—generativity versus stagnation—is analogous to middle age. Erikson stated that an individual who manages the previous stages of development successfully has a much better chance of managing the succeeding stages of development. Erikson viewed generativity to be synonymous with productivity and creativity. He viewed this stage as a time when the individual must make a choice between the preoccupation with one's own needs and comfort and those of others. He viewed generativity as primarily concerned with guiding the younger generation. For Erikson, generativity is concerned with ego expansion, which includes selflessness, productivity, and creativity. Thus, a generative person is able to meet his or her own needs and also the needs of the future generation.

The middle-aged person who exhibits generativity in a mature manner becomes involved in a variety of community activities that are designed to make the world a better place in which to live. The generative person can achieve a balance between activities performed in the community and those at home. In performing altruistic activities, the generative person is able to persevere. It is the true concern for others that enables the generative person to persevere.

The generative person is less self-centered than the adolescent or inexperienced young adult. He/she has many life experiences to draw on, is able to use these experiences to help solve the problems of others as well as his/her own. The mature middle-ager is able to get along with others, thus making problem solving less difficult.

The generative individual accepts the normal bodily changes that take place during this stage. He/she is not always looking back to an earlier stage of development when physical attractiveness dominated. This individual has no need to compete with the younger generation in terms of dress and behavior. The truly generative individual accepts physical changes but does not hasten to improve personal looks.

The person who accomplishes the developmental tasks of this stage

1. exhibits a positive view of life in general.

2. can accept personal weaknesses as well as strengths.

3. does not exhibit an overwhelming sense of guilt if he/she does not live up to his/her ideal self.

4. knows when to hold on and when to let go.

5. continues to strive for self-actualization.

6. values himself/herself as a helping person.

7. is self-directed rather than other directed.

8. can balance work with play.

9. can tolerate reasonable amounts of stress and anxiety.

10. knows the importance of developing a philosophy of life and a code of ethics.

11. does not dread the next stage of development.

A person who does not achieve the developmental tasks of generativity enters the stage of stagnation or self-absorption, the other end of the continuum. The individual who is in the stage of stagnation or self-absorption will regress to an earlier stage of growth and development, e.g., adolescence. Unlike the generative person, the stagnant or self-absorbed person hates his/her aging body. He/she is self-centered, rebellious, withdrawn, and hard to get along with.

Some individuals who are in the stage of self-absorption and stagnation tend to take on the characteristics of this stage too readily. Once they have reached middle age, they consider themselves old. They lose the zest for living. Many become depressed and exhibit a defeatist attitude toward life in general. They feel that since they have reached the magic time of middle age, they have nothing worthwhile to offer to others. Many are too busy feeling sorry for themselves.

A person who has entered the stage of stagnation or self-absorption becomes stagnated, self-absorbed, and depressed. These people exhibit pseudointimacy, regression, and childlike behavior. They tend to view middle age, especially the latter part of middle age, as something to avoid or fear. They do not see themselves as having much, if anything, to give to others, especially to future generations. Erikson believed that the individual who has not successfully accomplished the developmental tasks of this stage will have difficulty in accomplishing the next and final stage of development, i.e., *ego integrity versus despair* (Craig 1976; Erikson 1963; Erikson 1968; Murray and Zentner 1989). Although Erikson has received considerable praise for this theory of developmental tasks for middle age, not all theorists agree with his approach. For example, psychologist Robert Peck (Craig 1976; Peck 1968; Stevens-Long 1979; Vander Zanden 1978) considered Erikson's tasks for the last two stages of development too global and nonspecific. Peck thought that Erikson placed too much emphasis on the first six stages of life and not enough on the last two stages. To correct this imbalance, Peck attempted to expand on Erikson's developmental tasks of middle age and conceived the following four patterns.

Robert Peck's Theory

Valuing Wisdom versus Valuing Physical Powers. Peck stated that this first pattern is important because as one ages, there is a loss of physical stamina, strength, and attractiveness. With the loss of physical prowess, a person must find other means of coping with life. One way is to use one's wisdom or mental energies. A person is expected to use past life experiences to arrive at alternative solutions to the problems of everyday living. The person who fails to value and use wisdom instead of physical powers tends to become bitter and disgusted with himself or herself and life in general. Such people have little to offer future generations. They fail to achieve self-actualization and they experience problems in accomplishing the tasks of old age.

Socializing versus Sexualizing. In this developmental pattern, one is confronted with the climacteric, which may be accompanied by a change in sexual activity. For women there is the inability to produce offspring. For the woman who has achieved femininity primarily through her ability to give birth, a real crisis may result when she is no longer able to conceive. A similar pattern may also result for men when their sexual prowess begins to wane. Peck has suggested that these women and men value sexual intimacy more than companionship. Thus a comfortable balance must be reached between socializing and sexualizing. People who fail to achieve this balance are frequently frustrated and depressed because they still view themselves and their mates primarily as sex objects rather than unique personalities who are sources of comfort and companionship. The same people, in order to maintain the sex-object image, frequently have extramarital affairs. These people act sexually, ignoring opportunities to develop their communication or socializing abilities.

Cathectic Flexibility versus Cathectic Impoverishment. Cathectic flexibility refers to the ability to transfer one's emotional investments from one person to another, from one group to another, and from one activity to another. As people age, new contacts have to be made because of children leaving home, the death of family members and old friends, and retirements. People who are emotionally flexible receive a great deal of pleasure in forming new personal relationships and in new activities, even though they miss the old ones. The person who is suffering from cathectic impoverishment has great difficulty in establishing new contacts and becoming involved in new activities. Instead, he or she tends to withdraw and becomes depressed or highly anxious. Such a person views life as dull and unrewarding.

Mental Flexibility versus Mental Rigidity. The person who is mentally flexible is able to change with the times and welcomes new ideas while maintaining a positive attitude toward life. One who suffers from mental rigidity, however, has a mind closed to new ideas and techniques and insists upon doing things in a rigid and unchanging way. Such a rigid person will obviously experience rejection by others, feel alienated, and experience anxiety and depression. Equally important, the mentally rigid person fails to grow emotionally and usually has the difficulty in accomplishing the developmental tasks of old age.

Comparison of Peck's and Erikson's Theories. Peck's expansion of Erickson's developmental tasks for middle age provides a greater understanding of middle age, because Peck stresses the biologic as well as the psychosocial aspects. Erikson emphasizes the psychosocial aspects more and the biologic less. Obviously, it is necessary to adjust to both the psychosocial and biologic changes encountered in later middle age to perform the tasks for this stage of development successfully.

Robert Havighurst's Theory

According to Kaluger and Kaluger (1979), Robert Havighurst has been primarily concerned with human development in Western societies. Havighurst stated that certain developmental tasks arise at each age level; the nature of these tasks varies from culture to culture. Havighurst (1974, 2) defined a developmental task as "one that arises at or about a certain period in the life of the individual, successful achievement of which leads to his happiness and to success with later tasks, while failure leads to unhappiness in the individual, disapproval by the society and difficulty with later tasks."

Havighurst (1974) described the developmental tasks of middle age as biologic, sociologic, and psychologic in origin. Thus each person experiences internal changes as well as external changes such as environmental pressures (for example, retirement and reduced income).

Assisting Teenage Children in Becoming Healthy and Responsible Adults. Havighurst (1974) described seven developmental tasks of middle age. The first task is to assist teenage children in becoming responsible and healthy adults. Many parents do not face this task in later middle age, having been in their 20s when their children were born. However, many children are born to parents who are in their late 30s and

early 40s; these older parents find themselves responsible for their teenage children during the latter part of middle age. In fact, some men become new fathers in the latter part of middle age and even in old age.

Havighurst stated that parents should aid their teenage children in achieving independence. He also stated that it is important for parents to serve as good role models to help their teenage children become good parents, homemakers, providers, and citizens. To accomplish these tasks, parents must be willing to listen to and try to understand the problems faced by their teenage children. Parents must not be oversolicitous, overpunitive, or overprotective of their teenagers. Finally, parents must not only guide and protect their teenagers but also allow them a reasonable amount of freedom.

Achieving Civic and Social Responsibility. The second developmental task is to achieve social and civic responsibility. Havighurst stated that the middle-aged group must assume civic and social responsibilities, since they are at the peak of their influence.

Both sexes, especially members of the upper and middle socioeconomic classes, enjoy political, civic, and social activities. The working class shows less interest in the social and civic welfare of the community. However, as the level of education increases for members of the working class, so does their interest in social and civic affairs.

Reaching and Maintaining Satisfactory Performance in One's Occupation. Havighurst's third task for middle age is reaching and maintaining satisfactory performance in one's occupation. Men and women who have held satisfactory jobs all their adult lives usually reach their peak in status and income at this time. This situation is particularly true of professional people.

Many women, however, after raising a family, may return to the work force or join it for the first time. Some men, especially those who are able to retire early, start a new job or career. Thus, if a person changes jobs or career during this stage, it is to his or her advantage to remain as flexible as possible.

Developing Adult Leisure Time Activities. Developing adult leisure time activities is Havighurst's fourth task of middle age. People at this stage of development usually find that they have more leisure time because they are less absorbed in advancing their careers. Also, they find that they need a different, less strenuous kind of leisure experience. The more versatile and flexible a person is, the easier it is for her or him to find new leisure activities that are satisfying.

Relating to One's Spouse as a Person. The fifth developmental task of middle age, according to Havighurst, is to relate to one's spouse as a person. When motherhood for women and work or career for men become secondary, the middle-aged couple has more time for each other. Both husband and wife need to understand the physical and psychologic changes they are undergoing and the needs that accompany these changes. For example, the husband must understand the physical and especially the psychologic changes and problems that accompany menopause and the postmenopausal state. At this time the husband should let his wife know that he still sees her as attractive and appealing. He should maintain his physical appearance as well.

The wife also needs to understand and help her husband cope with some of the physical and psychologic changes that he is likely to experience during the latter part of this stage. She too needs to reinforce his physical and psychologic attributes. She should make a special effort to maintain her physical appearance. Most of all, husband and wife need to communicate with each other openly and honestly.

Accepting and Adjusting to the Physiologic Changes of Middle Age. To accept and adjust to the physiologic changes of middle age is Havighurst's sixth task. The physiologic changes become obvious during this stage of development and require an adjustment for both sexes.

The following biologic changes may occur, although some do not occur until a later age: *(1)* loss of skin elasticity, accompanied by wrinkling and dryness, *(2)* decrease in muscular strength, *(3)* diminishing neuromuscular skills, *(4)* presbyopia, *(5)* accumulation of fat around the midline, *(6)* stiff hair in nose, ears, and eyelashes of men, and *(7)* menopause in women. Normally, menopause occurs between ages 45 and 55. Many women experience the growth of hair on the upper lip and chin.

These physiologic changes require a psychologic adjustment by both sexes. For men the greatest adjustment appears to be to the loss of muscular strength and waning sexual potency. Women must adjust to menopause and their own perceived decrease in physical attractiveness. Not all women react negatively, however; some are able to accept these physiologic changes quite gracefully. Adjustment to these changes is culturally determined. For example, aging is viewed with dignity and respect in some cultures, whereas in others it is viewed with dread and disgust.

To a limited extent a person's knowledge of the physiology of aging aids in his or her adjustment to the physiologic changes that take place during middle age. Diversional activities also can help during this period of adjustment.

Adjusting to Aging Parents. The seventh and final task of middle age, according to Havighurst, is adjusting to aging parents. The middle-aged adult (about 55 years) often finds himself or herself in the middle of a three-generation family, in which he or she is responsible for aging parents as well as for teenage children. Such a person may be expected to supplement the income of a parent or parents, provide a place of residence for them, and make important decisions regarding their well-being and safety. For example, if the aging parents are no longer able to maintain a separate place of residence, the middle-aged child might be faced with having the parent live with him or her or selecting a nursing home or similar type of custodial residence. Such decisions are difficult for both the middle-aged person and his or her aging parents.

Socioeconomic status appears to be a factor in resolving the conflicts between older aging parents and their child or children. Older members of the upper socioeconomic class, because of their economic independence and involvement in civic and social functions, usually remain independent longer than those in the middle and lower socioeconomic classes. In the middle class the major problem is often the unresolved parent-child conflict rather than finances. This conflict is more obvious if the parents and child attempt to live together.

There appears to be less conflict between the parents and child among working-class people. Less hostility is noted between the two generations sharing the same residence. In many cases the aging parents accept the responsibility of caring for their grandchildren and the home while their middle-aged children work.

Sigmund Freud's Theory

The problem of the developmental tasks of later middle age was also considered by Sigmund Freud. Before Freud's concepts are discussed, it might be useful to compare Freud's psychosexual theory of human development with Erikson's psychosocial theory.

First, Freud believed that personality development had five psychosexual stages: the oral, the anal, the phallic, the latency, and the genital (Craig 1976). Because he felt that the first three stages were most important in personality development, Freud analyzed these stages in greater detail. He postulated that as a person entered each stage, certain conflicts had to be resolved. If these conflicts were not resolved adequately, the person was said to be *fixated* and would have greater difficulty in resolving the conflicts at the next stage. Despite Freud's great contribution to the understanding of personality development, critics complain that he failed to develop adequately his concept of the adolescent and adult stages of human development (Vander Zaden 1978).

Erikson, a stage theorist like Freud, vividly described the progress of a person through the life cycle in his discussion of the eight stages of man. Erikson's psychosocial theory is built on Freud's psychosexual theory, but Erikson's theory includes more of the social, psychologic, and environmental factors that are important to personality development (Sutterly and Donnelly 1973). It is beyond the scope of this chapter to give a thorough comparison of Freud's and Erikson's theories of personality development. In general, Erikson's theory presents more details of each part of the life cycle; it is more optimistic and more acceptable to most personality theorists than Freud's theory.

As stated earlier, Freud did not describe in detail the developmental tasks people must undertake during later middle age. He stated that an important task for the adult, however, was to love and work in harmony. If a person has a major conflict in these two areas, his or her chances of accomplishing the developmental tasks as described by others will be difficult and sometimes impossible.

Basically, Freud believed that if a person had suffered severe conflicts and anxieties in early childhood with little or no opportunity for their resolution, the chances for a successful adulthood for that person would be reduced. He also believed that the failure to

resolve conflicts and anxieties usually led to the overuse of defense mechanisms, lessening the person's chance of leading a happy and successful life. Also, the longer these defense mechanisms were overused to lower a person's anxiety level, the more difficult it would be for the person to behave in normal fashion. According to Vander Zanden (1978), Freud viewed adulthood as a reflection of childhood, especially of the first six years.

DEVELOPMENTAL TASKS OF LATER MIDDLE AGE

Now that the theories of Erikson, Peck, Havighurst, and Freud have been introduced, a comprehensive review of the developmental tasks of later middle age is appropriate. The developmental tasks of later middle age fall into two broad categories: *(1)* adjusting to physical and physiologic changes, and *(2)* adjusting to changes in the family life cycle.

Adjusting to Physical and Physiologic Changes

Many physical changes that affect self-concept and self-image are experienced with age. According to Stevens-Long (1979), a slight decrease in height may occur, the result of osteoporosis. There is usually a loss in visual and auditory acuity because of degenerative changes in the eyes and inner ear. These changes tend to be greater in old age. Degenerative changes in the inner ear are usually caused by prolonged exposure to noxious agents such as loud noises. Psychomotor and reaction time may slow down as a result of such factors as the general health of the person, past and present experiences, and the type of environment in which the individual has worked. See chapter 3 for a complete discussion of physiologic changes.

The first developmental task concerns the climacteric and changes in sexuality (the sexual response cycle in particular), with emphasis on cause and effect.

The terms *climacteric*, or *change of life*, and *menopause* are sometimes used interchangeably. According to Kaluger and Kaluger (1979), the climacteric in the male is called the *andropause*, and the climacteric in the female is called the *menopause*. The term *climacteric* is derived from two Greek words meaning "rung of ladder" and "a critical time." The term *change of life*, commonly applied to middle age, indicates a change from one phase to another for both men and women. The *menopause* refers to cessation of menstruation. According to Weideger (1976), the time and manifestations of andropause are not as sharply defined as those of menopause. It can be said that during the climacteric period both sexes experience a decline in the level and activity of the gonadal hormones that affect the body physiologically and psychologically.

Female Climacteric. In discussing the female climacteric, two important questions are often asked: *(1)* when does the menopause occur and *(2)* why does it occur? The first question is less difficult to answer than the second.

Age at Menopause. Kaluger and Kaluger (1979, 417) reported the following findings in a study of the cessation of menstruation of 903 women. It was found that the average age for the complete cessation of menstruation was 49.2 years. The other findings were "only 3.5% of the cases occurred before the age of 40 years, 20% occurred between 40 and 44 years, 44% occurred between 45 and 49 years, 30% occurred between 50 and 54 years, and only 1.5% occurred at the ages 55, 56, or 57 years." It is evident that there is wide variation in the age at which menopause occurs. The findings from this study also show that some women past the age of 55 experience symptoms of the menopause. The authors also stated that the menopause is usually completed sometime between two and four years. They observed that the menopausal pattern of the daughter is usually similar to that of the mother.

Weg (1987) and Stenchener (1991) stated that a review of the literature over the various periods reveals that most women experience menopause around 50 years of age. Weg (1987) concluded that "the multiple factors studied—socioeconomic conditions, race, marital status, income, geography, parity, height, and skinfold thickens—appear to have little influence on age at menopause." Both authors agree that women who are heavy smokers and those who live at high altitudes can expect to experience menopause at an earlier age.

Causes of Menopause. Why does menopause occur? According to Stenchener (1991), "menopause is a physiologic condition that is best described as a failure of the ovarian follicle to develop, mature, and produce estrogen." He stated that the "actual reason for this is unknown but could be related to an aging brain, hypothalamus, and pituitary gland." Weg (1987) stated the most commonly stated cause of menopause is ovarian failure. Both of these authors speculated that menopause may be related to the loss of ova in an aging ovary. This decreased ovarian function usually does not occur rapidly (Strauss 1978). According to Ambron and Brodzinsky (1979), the decline in the production of the ovarian hormones estrogen and progesterone usually begins in the late 30s and early 40s. The results of this lack of ovarian response are the inability to become pregnant, the cessation of menstruation, and the failure to produce estrogen and progesterone. Regardless of the reason, when the ovaries fail to respond to follicle stimulating hormone produced by the pituitary gland, the ova fail to mature and ovaries cease to produce adequate estrogen.

Symptoms of Menopause. The disturbances in hormonal balance mentioned above produce a number of symptoms commonly associated with menopause. The first of these symptoms involves at least one of the following changes in menstrual patter (Kaluger and Kaluger 1979):

1. A gradual lessening in the amount of flow, but with no irregularity

2. Irregularity in rhythm with skipped periods

3. Irregularity in rhythm and amount of flow

4. An abrupt cessation of menstruation

The other common symptoms of menopause are hot flushes (flashes), headaches, dizziness, and heart palpitations (Stenchener 1991). Some women experience anxiety, depression, irritability, insomnia, excessive desire for sleep, and pains in breast, chest, and neck (McCary 1978). According to Kaluger and Kaluger (1979), the decrease in the levels of ovarian hormones causes internal changes, such as the decrease in the size of the uterus and ovaries, a decrease in the size and length of the fallopian tubes, shortening and thinning of the vaginal canal, reduction in vaginal secretions, and a change in the hormonal content of the urine. Other internal changes that occur but have nothing to do with reproduction are a decrease in size of the spleen and lymphatic glands, changes in the intestinal wall (which usually result in constipation), and urinary incontinence. The authors also describe external symptoms associated with the menopause, such as a decrease in the size and firmness of the breasts; a tendency to gain weight, especially around the midline; thinning of hair on the scalp, axillae, and external genitalia; growth of hair on the upper lip; loss of labia firmness; flabby muscles of the upper arm and legs; and dry and itchy skin, especially after bathing.

Hot flashes, one of the most common and most uncomfortable symptoms, are thought to be due to the effect of the hormonal imbalance on the nervous and vascular systems. This hormonal imbalance affects the diameter of the blood vessels by causing abrupt dilation or contraction of the blood vessels. When there is abrupt dilation, a hot flush results, and when there is abrupt contraction, a cold flash results. How often hot flushes occur varies, but they can occur several times a day and last from one second to several minutes. It is believed "that the more hot flushes a woman experiences during the menopause the less likelihood there usually is that other troublesome conditions will develop" (McCary 1978, 83). The reason for this phenomenon is unknown.

Other Conditions Associated with Menopause. Associated with the menopause are other conditions of a more serious nature. For example, estrogen deficiency is associated with atherosclerosis, which can be a contributing factor in heart disease. Before menopause, heart disease is less common among women then among men of comparable age. Once women have passed through menopause, however, their rate of heart disease is almost equal to that of men.

The other condition associated with estrogen deficiency is osteoporosis. In this condition the bones become brittle, porous, and more subject to fracture following injury. A condition known as dowager's hump (kyphosis) may result from the compression of the cervical vertebrae. Because of osteoporosis, complaints of back pain are not uncommon among postmenopausal women.

Estrogen replacement therapy (ERT) is prescribed by some physicians to reduce menopausal or postmenopausal symptoms. Some physicians, however, are skeptical of ERT because of its possible role in causing uterine cancer and strokes. In any case, ERT is effective in some cases of menopausal syndrome and ineffective in others. In addition to ERT,

tranquilizers and counseling can help alleviate some of the distressing symptoms of menopause (Carnago 1987).

The Climacteric and the Sexual Response Cycle in Women. Changes in the reproductive systems may affect sexual response cycles in relatively minor ways. The sexual response cycle is divided into four phases: excitement, plateau, orgasmic, and resolution.

According to Ebersole and Hess (1990), Fogel and Lauver (1990), Pengelley (1974) and Woods (1979), the sexual response cycle of older women differs from that of younger women in the following ways.

Excitement Phase. In the excitement phase the older woman experiences a decrease in the amount of vaginal lubrication, and it takes longer for vaginal lubrication to occur than in the younger woman. The changes are thought to be a result of thinning of the muscles of the vaginal wall. There is also a decrease in the expansion of the inner two thirds of the vagina both in depth and breadth. This decrease in expansion of the vagina is again a result of muscle atrophy of the vaginal wall. Women who remain sexually active throughout their lives or those who are undergoing ERT experience less difficulty with vaginal lubrication and expansion. There is no significant difference in clitoral size or response between older women and younger women, although there are distinct changes in the labia minora and labia majora. Vasocongestion is reduced in the labia minora, and the labia majora exhibit less flattening separation and elevation. Sometimes these changes in the labia majora may be absent. The changes in the labia are thought to be due to a decrease in tissue elasticity. There is also a decrease in the deposition of fat in the labia majora and mons area. Changes in the uterus, such as elevation, occur more slowly, are less intense, or may not occur at all. Vasocongestion of the breasts is also decreased, especially in pendulous breasts. Last, the sex flush and heightened muscle tension commonly observed in the younger woman are reduced in the older woman.

Plateau Phase. During the plateau phase of sexual response there is a reduction in vasocongestion and there may be continued expansion of the inner two thirds of the vagina. The labia minora exhibit less intense change in color than those of the younger woman. The uterus exhibits less intense elevation. In the breasts there is less areola engorgement. A decrease in clitoral engorgement during this phase occurs after the woman reaches the age of 60 or 70. Other than the above changes, the plateau phase is much the same in older women as in younger women. In some cases the intensity may be slightly less than that of the younger woman.

Orgasmic Phase. Only two changes are noteworthy during the orgasmic phase in older women. In the postmenopausal woman the number of vaginal orgasmic platform contractions, or vaginal throbbing, is often reduced. Painful contractions of the uterus are also experienced by some older women. Otherwise the orgasmic phase for the older woman is similar to that of the younger woman, a satisfying and enjoyable experience.

Resolution Phase. In general the resolution phase is more rapid for the older woman than for the younger woman. Especially noticeable is the rapid return of the clitoris and vagina to their normal sizes. The loss of nipple erection, however, is less rapid for the older woman than for the younger woman.

In summary, sexual stimulation and enjoyment will vary from woman to woman, depending on their attitudes toward sex and aging. In general the older woman responds to sexual stimulation less rapidly than the younger woman, and the response may not be quite as vigorous. Despite these two relatively minor losses, sex should be enjoyable for the older woman.

Male Climacteric. Unlike women, men do not experience menopause, but the climacteric does produce noticeable changes in the male reproductive system that can affect a man's behavior and sexuality.

As in older women, older men show a decrease in the level of gonadal hormone, in this case, testosterone. Accompanying this decline in the testosterone level is a slight decline in sperm production (Ambron and Brodzinsky 1979). Stevens-Long (1979, 229) stated that there is approximately a 30% decline in sperm production "between the ages 25 or 30 and age 60 . . . ," and another 20% decrease occurs between the ages of 60 and 80. From these figures it is obvious that the decrease in sperm production is a result of the degeneration of the testicles.

The climacteric is not as dramatic in men as in women. The age at which the effects of the decrease in testosterone are observed varies from man to man but is usually between 55 and 65 years. This reduction in the level of testosterone produces bodily changes. Ambron and Brodzinsky (1979) stated that men, like women, may experience such changes as a tendency toward weight gain and an increased susceptibility to atherosclerosis and osteoporosis.

Physiologic Changes during Male Climacteric. In addition to the decrease in testosterone and decrease in sperm production, other changes in the reproductive system of the man have been described by McCary (1978). The testicles decrease in size and firmness and lose their ability to elevate during intercourse to the same degree as when the man was younger. There is a gradual deterioration of the seminiferous tubules, resulting in decreased sperm production. Enlargement of the prostate gland is common, and its contractions are less forceful during intercourse. Ejaculation decreases in force. The seminal fluid decreases in volume and viscosity. Orgasm is slower in starting and may not last as long as in a younger man. It takes longer for the older man to achieve an erection, but he can maintain the erection longer than a younger man. The frequency and intensity of erections also decrease. It may take several hours to have another erection.

Stevens-Long (1979) noted other changes: there may be fibrosis and sclerosis of the penis, and degeneration of the veins and arteries in the penis may be a factor in the decrease in the ability to achieve an erection.

Since men do not experience menopause, they seldom or never have the same symptoms as women. According to Stevens-Long (1979), however, if there is an abrupt decline in testicular functioning in middle age, men experience some of the same troublesome symptoms reported by women, such as hot and cold flashes, nervousness, dizziness, and tachycardia. It seems, then, that the degree to which a man experiences physiologic and psychologic symptoms during the climacteric depends on his body's level of male hormone and his attitude toward sexuality. Positive attitudes and beliefs about sexuality in later middle age are perhaps the most important factors in maintaining a satisfying sexual life.

The Climacteric and the Sexual Response Cycle in Men. The man also exhibits changes in the four phases of the sexual response cycle. According to Ebersole and Hess (1990), Fogel and Lauver (1990), Pengelley (1974), and Woods (1979), the sexual response of the older man differs from that of the younger man in the following ways.

Excitement Phase. It takes the older man two or three times longer to achieve an erection than the younger man, and the older man is able to maintain the erection longer than the younger man. In the scrotum there is less vasocongestion and "tensing" of the scrotal sac. The testes fail to elevate fully. They exhibit less contraction of the cremasteric musculature, and they rarely exhibit an increase in size due to vasocongestion.

Plateau Phase. The penis may not become fully erect until late in the plateau phase, and the preejaculatory emission may or may not exist. If it does exist, it is usually diminished. This phase can be prolonged because the man has better control of the demand for ejaculation. The degree of testicular elevation is reduced, and testicular vasocongestion is reduced or absent.

Orgasmic Phase. Generally the orgasmic period is shorter and less intense in the older man than in the younger man but is nevertheless enjoyable. In this phase the force of ejaculation is decreased from the twelve to fourteen inches observed in the younger man to six to twelve inches. Penile contractions occur at about the same frequency as in the younger man, but there are fewer contractions. The amount and viscosity of the semen are also decreased.

Resolution Phase. In this phase the loss of erection and testicular descent is more rapid, whereas the decrease of scrotal vasocongestion is slower for the older man than for the younger man. It also takes the older man longer to achieve another erection.

Masters and Johnson (1968) discussed six factors that affect sexuality in the older man.

1. Monotony in a sexual relationship
2. Male concern with economic pursuit
3. Mental or physical fatigue
4. Overindulgence in food and drink
5. Physical and mental infirmities
6. Fear of failure

These factors tend to reduce sexual performance and enjoyment. The older man should strive to avoid them.

In summary, both the older man and woman should continue to enjoy sex. They must keep in mind that although the frequency and vigor of sexual intercourse may decrease as they grow older, sex can and should still be enjoyable.

Age-Related Dysfunctions of the Reproductive System. According to Spence (1988), there are age-related dysfunctions that can affect the sexual response in the aging individual. These dysfunctions can occur at any age but are seen most often in the aging individual. For the female these dysfunctions include atrophic vaginitis, prolapse of the uterus, and cancer of the uterus, ovary, and breast. Benign prostatic hypertrophy, cancer of the prostate gland, and impotence are common dysfunctions in the male. Impotence, probably the most disturbing, can result from a variety of causes, such as diabetes, prostate surgery, disorders of the vascular or nervous system, and medications such as antihypertensive drugs. Fortunately the man can receive treatment for impotence by the use of vasodilators and penile implants. These penile implants can be of two types: the flexible rod or inflatable cylinder that is surgically implanted. Both of these devices provide for the necessary penile rigidity for sexual intercourse.

ADJUSTING TO CHANGES IN THE FAMILY-LIFE CYCLE

In this broad developmental task, the middle-aged couple must come to grips with problems such as coping with adolescent children, letting go of the children, adjusting to postparental life (which may include grandparenthood), maintaining a satisfactory career or job until retirement, adjusting to one's aging parents, and—the last phase—the aging family. This last phase has its own host of tasks, such as adjusting to retirement, reduced income, and the possibility of widowhood (especially for the woman); preparing for old age; and facing the idea of one's own death.

DEVELOPMENTAL TASKS OF OLD AGE

The developmental tasks of old age are similar to those of later middle age, but they differ in degree.

For example, physical and physiologic changes become more obvious and more incapacitating in the aged person. Also, the changes in the family-life cycle become more significant to the person with increasing age.

The developmental tasks associated with the physical and physiologic changes of old age include adjusting to changes in the sense organs, changes in physical stature and appearance, changes in homeostasis, and changes in reserve functional ability (Hayter 1974). These physical and physiologic changes further impair health and sexual functioning. As a person ages, the sense organs lose their acuity and predispose the aged person to sensory deprivation and possible trauma.

Changes in the musculoskeletal system are primarily responsible for changes in physical stature and appearance. For example, osteoporosis of the vertebral column coupled with weakened muscles gives rise to the stooped appearance of the aged, especially of the old-old.

Most organ systems are directly or indirectly concerned with homeostasis and reserve functional ability. Aging reduces the effectiveness of all the organ systems, but some are affected more than others. Impaired homeostasis and decreased functional reserve ability can lead to a decrease in the effectiveness of the aged individual's physical and psychologic functioning. Functional reserve is the ability of the body to meet greater demand than is usually placed on it.

THEORETICAL VIEWS OF OLD AGE

Erik Erikson's Theory

The person who has successfully completed Erikson's seventh stage of development—generativity versus stagnation—is now ready for Erikson's eighth and final stage of development—integrity versus despair. For Erikson this stage begins at 65 and ends at death. Erikson's description of this stage is rather general and without a clear and detailed description of *integrity.* Although Erikson's description of this stage is rather general, it is still critical in the life of an individual.

Integrity refers to the ability to view one's past life experiences in a positive manner, despite the mistakes along the way. Integrity involves the virtues of renunciation and wisdom. Renunciation involves the abandonment of unobtainable goals and the acceptance of life for what it has been and now is. Individuals exhibiting the virtue of renunciation are not always in the process of looking back and blaming themselves for past mistakes. Wisdom involves the passing on of one's accumulated knowledge, mature judgment, and experiences to the future generation. Thus, a person who possesses integrity at this stage of development exhibits maturity, characterized by acceptance of one's past lifestyle, serenity, and the willingness to continue to self-actualize and accept death. The individual who self-actualizes in this stage of development exhibits a desire to reach new goals, to learn about himself/herself and his/her world. The desired goals should be obtainable and realistic. An individual who is in the stage of integrity is a joy to be around because of his/her wisdom and positive view of life.

Despair, the negative aspect of the continuum, is characterized by exhibiting disgust with one's past life, the setting of unrealistic and unobtainable goals, and a morbid fear of death. An individual experiencing despair is usually avoided by others because of the tendency to dwell on the past and presentation of a negative view of life. Individuals who are in a state of despair have little wisdom to offer to future generations because they are too absorbed in reviewing their past mistakes. Such individuals are often unable to assess their past and present strengths because they are overly concerned with their weaknesses (Craig 1976; Erikson 1968). According to Murray and Zentner (1993), individuals in the state of despair feel that "life has been too short and futile. The person wants another chance to redo life" (675). These individuals are critical of others and project their own feelings of disgust and inadequacy onto them. Thus people who exhibit despair are often shunned by others because of their negativism. This avoidance by others only increases a sense of despair. The person experiencing despair might react by continuing to reach out to others in a negative manner or by withdrawing and becoming reclusive. Such a person will usually remain in despair unless intervention is undertaken by others. The following is an example of a person in despair.

Mr. K, a 75-year-old retired office supervisor for

the federal government, was admitted to a local psychiatric hospital because of a gradual change in his behavior after retirement at age 65. He was the father of four grown children who were married and living away from home with families of their own. His wife also was retired.

Upon admission, Mr. K was found to be quite negative in his approach to others, and he preferred to stay to himself. His family, especially his wife, described him as being a very hard worker who spent very little time with his family. He was very critical of himself for not being able to live up to his unrealistic and often unobtainable goals. Not only was he overly concerned with his own past mistakes and weaknesses, he was just as critical of the past mistakes and weaknesses of others, especially those of his nuclear family. Mr. K was given a thorough physical examination to make sure that there were no physical causes for his gradual change in behavior. His physical examination revealed no such causes.

Despite his negative attitude Mr. K's family was very concerned about his well-being and did everything in their power to aid in his recovery. When first approached by the psychiatric team, Mr. K was very resistant to receiving help. He was usually absorbed in his past life and had great difficulty forgiving himself for past mistakes. He would often say, "If I had not retired, I would be all right today." He did not talk much about dying, but his conversations revealed that he did not have a healthy attitude toward death.

After several months of group and individual therapy Mr. K became less reclusive and negativistic. At the time of release from the hospital he was beginning to spend more time with his family and with the patients on his unit. He was looking forward to going fishing with his grandchildren.

Six months after his dismissal from the hospital, Mr. K returned for an evaluation on an outpatient basis. He was smiling and responding to the health team in an appropriate manner. He stated that he was really enjoying life, especially his retirement and his family. This example serves to emphasize several important points regarding despair.

- Despair can be very painful from an emotional perspective for both the client and the family.

- Despair can and is often precipitated by events such as retirement.

- Despair can be relieved by concerned others and appropriate interventions.

Robert Peck's Theory

Ego Differentiation versus Work-Role Preoccupation. In discussing ego differentiation and the preoccupation with the work role, Peck's main concern is the value a person places on job and, to a certain extent, family. If a person achieves ego integrity chiefly through the job, what happens to that person's ego integrity after retirement? Will such a person be able to find other activities that result in a sense of continued value to self and society or will the loss of the job result in a sense of uselessness and loss of ego identity?

When children leave home, will the woman begin to feel useless and experience a loss of ego identity? To avoid crises related to retirement and to children leaving home, Peck has suggested that a person needs to develop valued alternatives and activities before retirement and old age to use his or her leisure time in the most effective way.

Body Transcendence versus Body Preoccupation. In this second dimension Peck is concerned with the older adult who allows the normal aches, pains, and decreases in physical health and recuperative powers to dominate his or her life. Peck believes that the person who exhibits body transcendence will be able to enjoy life to its fullest extent despite minor physical discomforts. The person who is preoccupied with physical discomforts, however, will fail to enjoy life at this stage, which should be characterized by sharing with others in a satisfying manner or using the creative abilities developed through past experience. The person who indulges in body preoccupation frequently alienates others, thus decreasing the opportunity for achieving happiness.

Ego Transcendence versus Ego Preoccupation. In this third and final dimension Peck is concerned with the person who is able to devote energies to the welfare of future generations and avoid becoming overly concerned with his or her own death. A person who exhibits ego transcendence has usually lived a generous and unselfish life. This person's philosophy of life includes a healthy acceptance of death; he or she realizes that death is an inevitable end of living. People should not become overly concerned with their own deaths, however. The ego-transcending person becomes actively involved with activities that make the world a better place in which to live for familial and cultural descendants. By assuming such an active role, a person can leave a legacy to be admired and emulated by others.

The person who exhibits ego preoccupation approaches and lives through this stage of life in a selfish and despondent manner. Because of a preoccupation with personal needs and death this person is unable to care about and give of self to younger generations in a meaningful and satisfying manner. Also, this type of person may spend much time in loneliness; others will avoid him or her because of such a negative and self-centered attitude.

Robert Havighurst's Theory

In his theory of the developmental tasks of old age Havighurst (1974) referred to old age as *later maturity*, with an age span from 65 to death. He also stated that the fundamental difference between the tasks of middle age and later maturity is *disengagement*. That is, the adult during later maturity disengages from some of the more active roles occupied in middle age. This disengagement leaves the person open to become involved or to continue involvement in other roles. These other roles include those of grandparents, citizen, club member, or friend.

Havighurst (1974) described six developmental tasks for later maturity.

Adjusting to Decreasing Physical Strength and Health. The first task is adjusting to decreasing physical strength and health. According to Havighurst, biologic aging is the result of a decrease in the functioning of cells and cellular systems. For example, the cells are unable to rid themselves of noxious substances, cellular nutrition is impaired, and there is a decrease in the cell's ability to repair itself.

Hardest hit by the biologic aging process are the cardiovascular, renal, and musculoskeletal systems. Impairment of the cardiovascular and musculoskeletal systems may interfere with a person's mobility; such a loss of mobility may have a negative effect on emotional well-being. Thus a person may have to adjust to invalidism or semi-invalidism. The longer a person is free of chronic crippling diseases, the slower the aging process. Under these conditions, life may be more enjoyable during this stage of development.

Adjusting to Retirement and Reduced Income. The second developmental task of later maturity is to adjust to retirement and reduced income. How a person adjusts to retirement depends on what the job has meant to that person. If the person has achieved a sense of worthiness mainly through an occupation, he or she is likely to suffer ego disintegration after retirement. Early retirement before the age of 60 is particularly hard on such a person. However, some people welcome early retirement. They look forward to other activities and lead happy lives.

Reduced income can be a serious problem for some older people. Sometimes a reduced income prevents people from continued membership and involvement in certain clubs and organizations. Travel and lifestyle may also be severely restricted by reduced income. The degree to which a person will suffer from reduced income depends on the activities he or she is forced to eliminate and how important these activities are to the person.

Adjusting to Death of Spouse. Havighurst's third developmental task for later maturity is the adjustment to the death of one's spouse. Women are more affected by the death of a spouse than men, simply because they live longer.

The loss of one's spouse during later maturity might cause a person to change the place of residence, to learn new skills, to seek a new mate, and to otherwise cope with the loneliness brought on by the loss. How much a person will suffer from the death of a spouse depends on the emotional ties between the two, the availability of helpful family members and friends, and how dependent the person was on the spouse for solving the problems of everyday living. Some older women are totally dependent on the husband in business matters. Men tend to be more dependent on their wives for cooking and housekeeping chores. The need to acquire a new skill or perform a new task because of the loss of a spouse comes at a time when learning new skills and ways of coping is the hardest.

Establishing an Explicit Affiliation with One's Age Group. Establishing an explicit affiliation with one's age group is Havighurst's fourth developmental task for later maturity. An affiliation with one's own age group is biologically, psychologically, and sociologically determined to a certain extent.

Biologic aging causes older people to slow down, making it more difficult for them to keep up with the activities of the middle-aged group. From a psychologic perspective one is forced to look at the concept of rewards and punishments. Sometimes older people are rewarded internally and externally for continuing the activities peculiar to middle age. Conversely older people may be punished internally and externally if they are no longer able to keep up with these same activities. Internal rewards result when the older person experiences a sense of achievement for being able to continue to participate in activities of the middle-aged group. External rewards result when he or she is accepted by this group. The reverse is true for punishment. Older people may be unable to perform the activities of middle age not only because of biologic slowing down but also because of reduced income or other drawbacks. They may be shunned by the middle-aged group because they are not able to "keep up" with them.

It can be psychologically rewarding for a person to associate with his or her own age group. There is less need for competition, companionship is less difficult to find, and one can find prestige in organizations closed to the middle-aged group. Unfortunately some people may feel a sense of failure or punishment when they are more or less forced to associate with their own age group. This is particularly true of those people who have a negative view of aging and are unable to appreciate its positive aspects.

Adjusting and Adapting Social Roles in a Flexible Way. The fifth developmental task of later maturity for Havighurst is to adjust and adapt to new social roles. According to Havighurst, most older people receive great satisfaction and happiness by compensating for the loss of roles of middle age through a program that is flexible. Havighurst (1974, 113) also states that the ability to expand "family roles, develop and expand roles of community activity, cultivate new activities, and maintain a balanced slow-down of activity, generally leads to satisfactory patterns of living."

Establishing Satisfactory Physical Living Arrangements. Havighurst's sixth and final developmental task of later maturity is to establish satisfactory physical living arrangements. The biologic, psychologic, and sociologic changes associated with aging often necessitate a change in living arrangements.

Biologic Needs. Most older people, especially the old-old and those suffering from chronic debilitating diseases, such as heart disease and joint diseases, are no longer able to function in homes that require excessive physical exertion. For example, a person with arthritis or heart disease may be forced to move from an upstairs apartment because of the inability to climb stairs.

Psychologic Needs. According to Havighurst (1974, 114), studies have revealed that the "principal [psychologic] values that older people look for in housing are . . . quietness, privacy, independence of action, nearness to relatives and friends, cheapness, closeness to transportation lines and communal institutional libraries, shops, movies, churches, etc."

Sociologic Needs. Most people during later middle age live as couples and maintain homes in much the same manner as they did in their early 60s. If they are unable to do so, however, women tend to move in with their children more often than do men.

Since the 1950s, older people have begun to seek living arrangements in warmer climates. Also, a relatively small number of older people now seek housing communities that consist mostly of older people. However, Havighurst has stated that housing designed especially for older adults as part of three-generational residential areas and communal-type housing appears to be the most satisfactory type of dwelling for older people during later maturity.

Sigmund Freud's Theory

Freud's developmental tasks of old age are similar to those of middle age. According to Freud, the ability to love is still important for people entering old age, but greater emphasis should be given to the old person's ability to cope with death and dying rather than to work.

NURSING INTERVENTIONS FOR LATER MIDDLE AGE

Nurses should have an adequate understanding of the developmental tasks for people throughout the life cycle. The nurse who possesses an adequate understanding of developmental tasks is in a much better position to assess, plan, and evaluate nursing care; to know what to look for in patients of various age groups; to predict the outcomes of intervention; and to be effective as a teacher.

The nurse can use the knowledge of developmental tasks to help people other than patients. For example, the nurse is often consulted by the family and friends in various age groups regarding problems related to the developmental tasks of clients. The nurse who is able is to give the correct information or to refer such people to an appropriate source is in effect practicing primary prevention, a much-needed service.

Attitude of the Nurse

Nurses must assess their own attitudes toward middle age as well as toward the person who is coping with the developmental tasks of middle age. The nurse who has a negative view of middle age will communicate this attitude to the middle-aged patient. Sometimes the nurse has unrealistic expectations of the middle-aged patient. The nurse who lacks adequate knowledge of the developmental tasks of middle age may consciously or unconsciously expect people to master these tasks with no outward sign of emotion or conflict. The nurse's age can also be a factor in helping people cope with the developmental tasks of middle age. For example, young nurses may have a negative view of middle age and difficulty in understanding the problems faced by the middle-aged person; whereas nurses who are middle-aged themselves may be expected to show a more positive and understanding attitude toward these clients.

Helping Clients Adjust to Physical and Physiologic Changes

In helping a client adjust to physical and physiologic changes, the nurse must first of all find out what the physical change means to the client. The nurse should concentrate on listening and giving needed information but should avoid giving false reassurance.

Physical illnesses and unexpected emotional stresses can interfere with a person's normal method of coping with developmental tasks. In assessing the effect of a particular illness on a patient, the nurse should first find out from the patient how the illness or stress has affected his or her life. The family can also be helpful to the nurse in the assessment process. If the nurse fails to understand the patient's perception of his or her problem, the plan of care might be inappropriate.

In many cases, an illness or crisis can seriously interfere with the patient's ability to cope with such roles as provider, homemaker, parent, and husband or wife. The nurse should be alert for cues that indicate the patient is having problems in these areas. The patient who can talk about problems openly and freely in a nonjudgmental atmosphere will experience less anxiety and waste little energy on defense mechanisms such as denial, rationalization, repression, and projection to hide thoughts, feelings, and needs. The more nurses know about and understand the patient's problems, the better they will be able to help patients assess their situations and make plans for the future.

Helping Clients Adjust to Changes in Sexuality

The nurse often encounters patients, family members, and friends who are having problems coping with the climacteric. Since the climacteric involves sexuality, the nurse should assess his or her own attitudes about sexuality in general and sexual activity in the middle-aged group in particular. To be more effective in helping the individual deal with sexual concerns, the nurse needs an adequate knowledge base. According to Woods (1979), this knowledge base should include an understanding of the anatomic, physiologic and sociologic aspects of human sexuality. The nurse should also understand how the climacteric affects the sexual response cycle in both men and women and how the menopause differs from the andropause.

Adjusting to Changes in the Sexual Response Cycle

Of concern to many men and women are the changes that are noticed in the sexual response cycle. For example, a man might be concerned about the decrease in the frequency of erection, in the force of ejaculation, in the volume and viscosity of semen, and in sexual desire. These changes are also observed by the mate. These changes are usually of great concern to the man who has achieved his sense of masculinity and self-esteem chiefly through his sexual prowess. The nurse must emphasize that the changes are normal, so as to alleviate the client's anxieties and fears of failure, which can give rise to impotency. Once these fears and anxieties are removed, however, the man's sexual functioning will be normal for his age.

The postmenopausal woman usually notices that at times she experiences pain on penetration during intercourse. The man usually notices that occasionally penetration is more difficult. Once the couple understands why it takes longer for vaginal lubrication to occur in the woman past the age of menopause and the need for extended foreplay, the problem is usually resolved. Older women should be informed that water-soluble lubricants may relieve the pain and discomfort and allow sexual activity to continue. Without the nurse's intervention the conditions that cause the pain might continue, so that the woman may lose interest in sexual activity and avoid it whenever possible. This avoidance of sexual intimacy can have a negative effect on the marital relationship. Stereotyped attitudes of family members and health professionals may dictate the sexual expression of older couples more than the couple's own wishes.

The nurse can also be of help to a woman who is experiencing difficulty during menopause. First, the nurse should acquaint the patient with the normal changes that occur at this time. By supplying correct information about the menopause, the nurse can dispel many of its associated myths.

Adjusting to Changes in the Prostate Gland

Enlargement of the prostate gland is not uncommon in the middle-aged man. According to Carter (1987), the cause of benign prostatic hypertrophy (BPH, or prostatism) is not adequately understood. Nevertheless the symptoms can be troublesome to men and interfere with their sexual performance. Common symptoms associated with BPH are difficulty in starting the stream, a smaller stream, frequent urination, nocturia, and in severe cases a failure or inability to urinate. The failure to empty the bladder completely can result in

infection. Stagnant urine provides a good medium for bacterial growth. Sometimes the man does not understand his condition and may be too embarrassed to see a physician unless there is total obstruction. When the obstruction becomes serious, a prostatectomy is performed.

A prostatectomy may be emotionally upsetting to some men and their mates. The man often feels that he will lose his potency. The nurse can dispel this belief by assuring him that, in most cases, he will again be able to enjoy sex. The nurse might want to discuss with the patient and his mate the possibility of a dry orgasm (retrograde ejaculation), the reason for its occurrence, and its lack of harmful effects. McCary (1978) has stated that 80% of men who have undergone a prostatectomy will experience a dry orgasm. In retrograde ejaculation the semen is discharged into the bladder instead of the urethra. According to McCary, the condition results from a contraction of the compressor muscles located just below the prostate gland. Normally these glands are relaxed during ejaculation, allowing the passage of semen to the urethra. When these muscles are contracted, the semen is forced into the bladder (the muscles of the bladder are relaxed, allowing for the backward flow of urine). The semen is then expelled along with the urine at the first voiding after ejaculation. According to McCary, diabetes with its resulting neuropathy can also cause retrograde ejaculation.

The nurse can also teach the patient and his or her mate about the effects of drugs on sexual desire. Some drugs, such as tranquilizers and antihypertensive agents, will decrease libido. McCary (1978, 182) stated that some tranquilizers may inhibit "the ejaculatory centers" without "affecting the neural network involved in the organs." Some men and women refrain from taking antihypertensive drugs because they fear a loss of their sexual potency. The risk of having a stroke is less anxiety producing for them than being unable to perform sexually in a satisfactory manner. The nurse who understands these factors can be more understanding of and helpful to patients who have problems with sexuality.

Helping the Client Adjust to Changes in the Life Cycle

The nurse often encounters middle-aged people who are having difficulty in coping with changes in the family cycles. Some of these problems include coping with adolescent children, adjusting to the children leaving home (the empty-nest syndrome), adjusting to retirement accompanied by reduced income, maintaining a happy marriage, coping with widowhood or divorce, coping with grandparenthood, and adjusting to aging parents. It is beyond the scope of this chapter to discuss the role of the nurse in each of these situations. In general, the nurse can be a good listener and help the person assess the situation and plan for change.

Helping the Client Adjust to the Loss of a Spouse

Many middle-aged widows and widowers need help in coping with the stresses caused by the death of the spouse. Ebersole and Hess (1990) discussed crisis interventions that could be utilized by nurses for the newly bereaved. Nurses are in a unique position to help the bereaved. Dysfunctional grieving can have negative effects on both widows and widowers. According to Valente and Sellers (1990), "the elderly widows and widowers living alone are particularly vulnerable to alcohol abuse and suicide." Mental and physical illnesses are also high among this group. Farrell (1990) stated that there are more widows than widowers because "women still outlive men by about two to one." With this information in mind, the nurse should make a special attempt to help the newly widowed person cope with the bereavement so that he or she can again lead a happy life.

Many widows and widowers face the problem of fulfilling their sexual needs. Although some persons have no objection to engaging in extramarital sex, others are not willing to do so. Fulfilling sexual needs may entail deciding whether or not to marry again. The nurse is often consulted by middle-aged people facing this dilemma. The nurse can help them first by listening and second by suggesting methods to relieve sexual tension that are congruent with each one's moral beliefs. One common method of relieving sexual tension is masturbation. Some middle-aged people believe that masturbation is harmful to the body in general and to the mind in particular. Some also believe that masturbation is sinful, which poses a larger problem. Based on sociocultural and religious beliefs, the individual can decide whether or not he or she wants to use masturbation as a means

of relieving sexual tension. In general, widows appear to have more difficulty in fulfilling their sexual needs than widowers.

The problems accompanying divorce are similar to those of widowhood; the major difference is that the former mate is still alive. For religious reasons, the divorced person may experience conflicts about remarriage. The divorced woman, like the widow, faces a shortage of men in her own age group to date or marry. Some resolve this conflict by dating younger men. Others, unable to find a suitable mate, withdraw and lead a single life, which may be happy or unhappy. People coping with problems caused by divorce will often consult a nurse for aid in solving these problems.

The person who has never married may find this stage of life depressing and lonely because of the loss of family and friends. Some are afraid to marry at this time of life because they fear they will be unable to adjust to living with a member of the opposite sex.

Grandmother-Client Example. As previously stated, grandparenthood can be a source of joy to the middle-aged person, but it can also be a source of despair. Here is an example of how grandparenthood became a source of despair for a middle-aged couple. This case also depicts the role of the nurse in helping to relieve this despair.

Mrs. X, a woman in her middle 50s, lived with her husband and had assumed sole care of her four grandchildren, who ranged in age from 1 to 5 years. A nursing student was assigned this family. The four children were the identified recipients of care. After several unsuccessful attempts to get Mrs. X to take her grandchildren to the clinic for their immunizations, the nursing student became discouraged, as had the community health nurse who had been caring for this family.

The nursing student and the nursing instructor conferred on goals for the family. First, it was decided that the needs of the grandmother had not been considered, since all the nurse's attention had been focused on the children. As a result of this discussion, during several visits to the family, attention was centered on the grandmother, Mrs. X.

From these visits, the nursing student learned that the grandmother was having conflicts about keeping her grandchildren. In addition, Mrs. X was experiencing some uncomfortable side effects of menopause. To compound the problem, the grandfather resented his wife's assumption of the responsibility for the grandchildren; marital conflict resulted.

On each visit, the grandmother, under no pressure from the nurse, revealed more about her predicament. The problem seemed to stem from the fact that each of Mrs. X's three daughters, the mothers of the four grandchildren, had become pregnant before marriage but all had eventually married the fathers of the children. The grandmother stated that the premarital pregnancies of her three daughters had hurt her very much, but most of all, "I felt guilty because I felt a failure as a mother. I guess that is why I keep the children, so that they can have some happiness." She also stated that two of her daughters were pregnant again and that she was keeping the first children so that the daughters would really enjoy their second pregnancies, since the first ones had been so traumatic.

On the next-to-last visit, the grandmother complimented the nursing student on showing deep concern about her needs. She stated that she knew her grandchildren needed their immunizations but that she did not wish to take them to the clinic on the bus. In a serious manner, she remarked, "I guess I just resent having to be a mother at my age." During these visits the nursing student assumed the role of listener, concentrating primarily on feelings and answering only questions relevant to the situation, and avoided giving advice.

On the last visit the grandmother told the student, "I have made the decision to let my daughters assume the care of their children and I do not feel guilty." The nursing student talked with Mrs. X about the feelings that accompanied her decision and found that the grandmother was greatly relieved. Mrs. X also said that her husband was pleased with the decision and that now they could plan their lives so that both of them would be happy.

Regretfully no follow-up on this case was possible, since the semester was ending. This example, however, serves to emphasize several important points for nursing.

1. It is important to consider the needs of people. In this case, the previous nurse had failed to consider the needs of the middle-aged grandmother.

2. Listening is important.

3. Grandparenthood, if inappropriately assumed, may prevent the middle-aged person from dealing with developmental tasks.

4. Nursing care can be effective in resolving the emotional trauma that results from the failure to accomplish developmental tasks.

NURSING INTERVENTIONS FOR OLD AGE

The developmental tasks of old age are similar to those of later middle age, but they differ in degree. Knowing that the physiological and psychological changes become more pronounced and incapacitating in old age, the nurse should be prepared to help clients and their families adjust to and cope with these changes. As with later middle age, the nurse should have an adequate understanding of the developmental tasks of old age. Nurses who do not possess this knowledge tend to be less effective in their nursing interventions. It is extremely important for nurses to assess their own attitudes toward old age. It is difficult to intervene in a positive manner if one has a negative and hopeless attitude toward old age. This is extremely important because nurses will be caring for an increasing number of patients in this age group both inside and outside of the hospital.

During old age the client usually experiences a further decrease in physical strength and health. The nurse, according to Walker (1991), should include interventions geared towards health and health education in all plans of care for the older adult in a variety of settings. Health promotion and health education are two important factors that tend to prevent the older person from having illnesses commonly seen during this stage of growth and development. Keeping the older person as healthy as possible prevents needless hospitalizations, dependence on others, and financial problems. Phipps and Kelley-Hayes (1991) stated that "Older adults utilize short-stay hospitals more frequently and for longer periods of time than any other age group." Hospitalizations and acute illness are more difficult for the older adult to cope with. They are more prone to develop complications, many of which may be life threatening.

The nurse should also be concerned about the economics of aging or the financial aspects of aging. Brock (1991) discussed the "Economics of Aging" from quite a pertinent and practical perspective. She stated that with modern technology more people are living longer, especially the old-old (75+ years). Many of the old-old have distinct disadvantages of having more illnesses, being poorer, and being more dependent on others than the young-old (55-75 years). Those who are 85 and older are the fastest growing group of those who are 65 and older. Except for the wealthy many older people live on a reduced fixed income that is inadequate to keep up with inflation. Thus many old-old people find themselves at or below the poverty level. Being at or below the poverty level predisposes poor older people to inadequate health care, poor housing, and inadequate diets. Poor older people, especially minorities, often are not aware of resources available to them. With this information in mind a major intervention for the nurse is to first make a thorough assessment of the client and his/her environment, and secondly to inform the client and family of the financial resources available to them. After older clients have been introduced to the available financial resources, the nurse should be available to assist them in utilizing these services. The nurse should also remember that some of the poor refuse to accept assistance of any kind because they do not want to be put in a position of being dependent on others.

A drastic change in roles often accompanies aging, especially in the old-old. This change in roles can cause anxiety and depression. Most older persons have been accustomed to being in charge of their lives, but now because of changes beyond their control, they are forced into being more dependent on others. The nurse is usually in a strategic position to help them adjust to their new roles. Without help, these individuals can become withdrawn, depressed, and often suicidal.

Carp (1991) stated that the house and neighborhood where the older adult lives are necessary for the well-being of the older adult. It is within the home and the environment that the adults meet the basic needs of everyday living. She further stated that older adults usually "live in ordinary houses and apartments in their communities" (186) and own their own homes. They also live in a variety of rented facilities, such as apartments, congregate housing, and institutions.

Some of the houses where older adults live are not safe. Depending on their health older people might no longer be able to care for themselves or their living facilities. They sometimes have to live with friends or relatives or be institutionalized. As the older adult increases in age, so does the need for institutionalization. It is important to keep the older adult in the home as long as possible, but not to the point of endangering his or her life. The nurse, along with other health team members, can be instrumental in finding a suitable living arrangement for the older adult who is no longer able to live alone.

From this brief discussion of nursing interventions of individuals of old age, it is obvious that the nurse needs to be knowledgeable about the developmental tasks and changes that occur within this age group. Nurses are in a key position to help the older adult live as happy and productive a life as possible by early identification of potential problems and planning for the prevention of their occurrence.

In summary, providing nursing care for older people can be exciting and rewarding for the nurse, provided that the nurse *(1)* assesses his or her own attitude toward old age, *(2)* is aware of his or her strengths and limitations in giving care to these people, and *(3)* is able to help these people assess their own strengths and limitations during this phase of the life cycle.

SUMMARY

The developmental tasks of later middle age and old age as proposed by Erikson, Peck, Havighurst, and Freud have been discussed. Of these theorists, Havighurst has presented the most comprehensive view of developmental tasks. It is important that the nurse consider both physical and psychological changes and how they affect people throughout these last two stages of development.

A review of the literature for this chapter has revealed a need for more research regarding the developmental tasks of single people in later middle age and old age. In summary, nurses should strive to understand their older patients' needs and current behavior in terms of developmental tasks and family-life cycle.

STUDY QUESTIONS

1. Describe the theoretical views of later middle age.

2. Describe the theoretical views of old age.

3. Identify the developmental tasks of later middle age.

4. Identify the developmental tasks of old age.

5. Describe common physiologic and psychologic changes that affect the development process in old age.

6. State symptoms associated with the menopause and andropause.

7. Compare the sexual response cycle of the younger adult with that of the older adult.

8. State nursing interventions that can help the aging individual adjust to the changes associated with the aging process.

9. Describe how the attitude of the nurse can affect the aging individual's ability to cope with the developmental tasks of aging.

10. State nursing interventions that can be utilized with the aging individual who has to adjust to living alone.

REFERENCES

Ambron, S.R. and D. Brodzinsky. 1979. *Lifespan Human Development*. New York: Holt, Rinehart and Winston.

Brock, A.M. 1991. Economics of aging. In *Perspectives on Gerontological Nursing,* edited by E.M. Baines. Newbury Park, CA: Sage Publications, Inc.

Carnago, L.C. 1987. Female reproductive problems. In *Medical-Surgical Nursing,* 2d ed., edited by S.M. Lewis and I.C. Collier. New York: McGraw-Hill.

Carp, F.M. 1991. Living environments of older adults. In *Perspectives on Gerontological Nursing,* edited by E.M. Baines. Newbury Park, CA: Sage Publications, Inc.

Carter, M.A. 1987. Male reproductive problems. In *Medical-Surgical Nursing,* 2d ed., edited by S.M. Lewis and I.C. Collier. New York: McGraw-Hill.

Craig, C.J. 1976. *Human Development*. Englewood Cliffs, NJ: Prentice-Hall.

Ebersole, P. and P. Hess. 1990. *Toward Healthy Aging: Human Needs and Nursing Response,* 3d ed. St. Louis: C.V. Mosby.

Erikson, E. 1963. *Childhood and Society*. New York: Norton.

Erikson, E. 1968. Generativity vs. stagnation. In *Middle Age and Aging,* edited by B.L. Neugarten. Chicago: The University of Chicago Press.

Farrell, J. 1990. *Nursing Care of the Older Person*. Philadelphia: J.B. Lippincott.

Fogel, C.I. and D. Lauver. 1990. *Sexual Health Promotion*. Philadelphia: W.B. Saunders Co.

Havighurst. R.J. 1974. *Development Tasks and Education,* 3d ed. New York: David McKay.

Hayter, J. 1974. Biologic changes of aging. *Nursing Forum* 8(3):289–307.

Kaluger, G. and M.F. Kaluger. 1979. *Human Development: The Span of Life*. St. Louis: C.V. Mosby.

Masters, W. and V. Johnson. 1968. Human sexual response: The aging female and the aging male. In *Middle Age and Aging,* edited by B. Neugarten. Chicago: The University of Chicago Press.

McCary, J.L. 1978. *McCary's Human Sexuality*, 3d ed. New York: Nostrand.

Murray, R.B. and J.P. Zentner. 1993. *Nursing Assessment and Health Promotion Strategies Through the Life Span,* 5th ed. East Norwalk, CT: Appleton & Lange.

Murray, R.B. and J.P. Zentner. 1989. *Nursing Assessment and Health Promotion Strategies Through the Life Span,* 4th ed. Norwalk, CT: Appleton & Lange.

Neugarten, B.L. and R.J. Havighurst. 1979. Aging and the future. In *Dimensions of Aging: Readings,* edited by J. Hendricks and C.D. Hendricks. Cambridge, MA: Winthrop.

Peck, R. 1968. Psychological developments in the second half of life. In *Middle Age and Aging,* edited by B.L. Neugarten. Chicago: The University of Chicago Press.

Pengelley, E.T. 1974. *Sex and Human Life*. Reading, MA: Addison-Wesley.

Phipps, M.A. and M.T. Kelly-Hayes. 1991. Rehabilitation of older adults. In *Perspectives on Gerontological Nursing,* edited by E.M. Baines. Newbury Park, CA: Sage Publications, Inc.

Rogers, D. 1979. *The Adult Years: An Introduction to Aging*. Englewood Cliffs, NJ: Prentice-Hall.

Spence, A.P. 1989. *Biology of Human Aging*. Englewood Cliffs, NJ: Prentice-Hall.

Stenchener, M.A. 1991. Hormone replacement. In *Caring for the Older Woman,* edited by M.A. Stenchener and G.A. Aagaard. New York: Elsevier.

Stevens-Long, J. 1979. *Adult Life: Development Processes*. Palo Alto, CA: Mayfield.

Strauss, D. 1978. The climacterium and the crisis of middle age. In *Understanding Human Behavior in Health and Illness,* edited by R.L. Simmons and H. Pardes. Baltimore: Williams and Wilkins.

Sutterly, D.C. and G.F. Donnelly. 1973. *Perspectives in Human Development: Nursing Throughout the Life Cycle*. Philadelphia: J.B. Lippincott.

Valente, S.M. and J.R. Sellers. 1990. Effective coping. In *Nursing Care in An Aging Society,* edited by D.M. Corr and C.A. Corr. New York: Springer Publishing Co.

Vander Zanden, J.W. 1978. *Human Development*. New York: Knopf.

Walker, S.N. 1991. Wellness and aging. In *Perspectives on Gerontological Nursing,* edited by E.M. Baines. Newbury Park, CA: Sage Publications.

Weg, R.B. Demography. 1987. In *Menopause: Physiology and Pharmacology,* edited by D.R. Mishell. Chicago: Year Book Medical Publishers, Inc.

Weideger, P.A. 1976. *Menstruation and Menopause: The Physiology and Psychology, the Myth and the Reality*. New York: Knopf.

Woods, N.F. 1979. *Human Sexuality: In Health and Illness,* 2d ed. St. Louis: C.V. Mosby.

3 Physiologic Changes

Laura Talbot

CHAPTER OUTLINE

FOCUS

The primary focus of this chapter is to present theories of biologic aging and common physiologic changes seen in the older adult. Specific nursing interventions are needed to assist the older adult to cope with these age-related changes.

OBJECTIVES

1. State the two major theoretical categories of biologic aging.
2. Discuss age-related changes associated with the integumentary system.
3. Describe methods that the older person can use to compensate for the age-related sensory-neurological changes that occur.
4. Explain the relationship between nutrition and muscle/bone integrity in the older person.
5. Summarize the pathological cardiovascular conditions seen in the older person.
6. Identify the single factor that retards the loss of lung function in the aging adult.
7. Compare and contrast the incidence and symptoms of problems of the gastrointestinal tract of the older adult to those of the younger adult.
8. Discuss the hormonal changes seen in the older adult.
9. Describe the age-related changes that predispose the older adult to urinary incontinence.

Because more people are living to old age than ever before and more is being learned about changes in body functioning with aging, chronologic age is not a reliable indicator of organ system functioning. There is great variability in the rate of physiologic aging among people and among the organ systems of any one person.

Rapidity of aging depends on a person's heredity, lifelong dietary patterns, the amount of habitual exercise, past illnesses, the presence of one or more chronic illnesses, and the stresses experienced throughout life. Some generalizations can be made regarding changes attributed specifically to aging. These generalized changes include

- a decrease in the rate of mitosis in tissue composed of cells that regenerate, for example, epithelial tissue

- a deterioration of more specialized nondividing cells, particularly neurons and skeletal muscle cells, leading to a decreased functional capacity

- changes in connective tissue leading to increased rigidity and loss of elasticity, producing change in organ systems

Aside from individual differences, there is a general loss of *reserve functional capacity* in all organ systems with old age. Body systems ordinarily maintain homeostasis, but when they are under stress, a longer time is required to adjust and return the body to a state of homeostasis.

THEORIES OF BIOLOGIC AGING

Many theories have been proposed to determine why people age. None has been able to explain satisfactorily all aging processes or why people age at different rates. Each person also shows differences in the rate that aging occurs (Kain, Reilly, and Schultz 1990). A list of generally accepted theories of physiologic aging follows (Norwood 1990; Cristofalo 1990)

1. Wear-and-tear theories of aging:
   a) Free radical theory—free radicals are unpaired electrons that are formed by radiation as enzymatic reactions. The free radicals then react with lipids, proteins, and other substances and disrupt normal chemical bonds or membranes (Norwood 1990).
   b) Lipofuscin accumulation—lipofuscin is thought to result from the breakdown of mitochondria or lyposomes. It increases as a person ages but has not been clearly linked to problems (Norwood 1990).
   c) Cross-linkage—this theory states that changes in aging occur when macromolecules are linked by a hydrogen bond or by other means. DNA may be damaged and result in cell death. Cross-linking in collagen is thought to decrease elasticity and permeability (Cristofalo 1990).

2. Genetic programming theories:
   a) Finite doubling potential theory states the control for aging is found in the nucleus of the cell. Cells are postulated to be able to reproduce themselves a limited number of times. This limited ability to divide has been shown to occur in the laboratory, but whether the same is true within the living body is not yet known (Cristofalo 1990).
   b) The immunologic theory of aging states that the immune system produces fewer antibodies with age, and as a person ages, more instances of autoimmune problems occur (Cristofalo 1990). Atrophy of the thymus gland occurs before the decrease in the immune system.
   c) The neuroendocrine theory states that all losses in the neurologic system and the endocrine system lead to the other changes seen with aging.

None of the above theories is accepted widely, and it is still thought that the primary reason why aging occurs has not yet been determined. It is apparent from the list of theories of aging that although scientists are not in agreement about the basic cause of aging, much is known concerning the effects of aging on different organ systems. Nurses should be aware of this information in order to provide quality care to aging patients. It is important to remember, as stated earlier, that no two people age at the same rate and that different organ systems show great variations in aging in each individual (Kain 1990).

Because the rate of aging is so individual, nurses should evaluate older clients carefully to identify their individual capabilities and needs when planning nursing care or helping clients meet their own needs for health maintenance.

MAJOR CHANGES AND PATHOLOGIC CONDITIONS IN ORGAN SYSTEMS AND RELATED NURSING IMPLICATIONS

Changes in Integument

Several changes occur in the skin and its appendages—hair and nails—with aging. Well-known changes are the graying of hair and wrinkling of the skin that lead to feelings of loss of self-esteem in many people in American society because these changes are so obvious to others (Balin 1990).

Skin. Wrinkling is caused by the loss of subcutaneous fat and water in the epidermal layers and exposure to the sun over many years. There are also fewer elastic fibers, resulting in reduced skin turgor, so that pinching the skin is no longer a valid indication of the state of hydration in an older person. The condition of the tongue may be a better indicator of dehydration than the skin. Sebaceous glands produce less sebum in the aging person, so the skin may feel dry and scaly and may itch. This condition can be partially overcome by the use of tepid rather than hot water and less soap or an oily soap in bathing. An emollient lotion can be applied after the bath. With the thinning of the epidermis, the skin is easily injured and healing is slow if the blood flow to the dermis is impaired, as it frequently is.

Nails. The nails of older clients may be thick and easily split (Balin 1990). It is imperative that nails be soaked in warm water before being cut or shaped to prevent splintering and to avoid possible trauma leading to infection. The condition of an older client's toenails may help to indicate whether the person is capable of living alone and caring for personal hygienic needs. An older client should be encouraged to seek professional care for the feet from a podiatrist at periodic intervals to prevent trauma, especially if the client has a severe visual deficit, vascular problems, and diabetes, or if the client's body is no longer flexible enough to allow him or her to care for the feet.

Benign Changes. Older people develop brown, pigmented areas called lentigo senilis on the dorsum of the hands, arms, and face. Lay people sometimes refer to these areas as liver spots or age spots. These areas are harmless but may result in a feeling of self-consciousness on the part of the person who develops them.

Keratoses frequently occur on the exposed skin of the older person. Senile and actinic keratoses are identified by raised areas that appear scaly and may bleed at the edges. There may be an area of inflammation around the border of the lesion. The lesions are unsightly and may become malignant, so they should be seen by a physician, particularly if any change in character of a keratosis is noted. Seborrheic keratoses are yellowish-to-brownish wartlike areas and are usually covered with an oily scale. These lesions are more common in persons with oily skin and do not usually become malignant (Balin 1990).

Cancer. Older people exposed to the sun or other irritants for long intervals are susceptible to the development of skin cancer on the exposed surfaces of the skin. Cancer of the skin can be of either the basal cell or squamous cell type. Basal cell tumors grow slowly and rarely metastasize, but they are locally invasive. Early medical treatment is essential. Squamous cell carcinoma may begin as a lesion with central ulceration or with increased keratinization. Squamous cell carcinoma will metastasize to regional lymph nodes if not treated early. Since many skin lesions in the elderly appear similar early in their occurrence, medical advice should be obtained soon after a lesion is noted (Balin 1990).

Nursing Interventions. Nursing actions, in addition to those already stated, include care in shifting the position of a very old person to prevent shearing forces from causing a tear in the skin. This disruption of the epidermis on the back or over a bony prominence may progress to a pressure ulcer. Pruritus may be a problem for older persons because of excessively dry skin. If warm baths and the use of superfatted soap do not relieve the pruritus and no obvious skin pathology is present, then the individual needs to be assessed for the presence of systemic disorders that may cause pruritus. Some diseases that may cause pruritus are diabetes mellitus, hyperthyroidism, renal failure, and hepatic failure (Balin 1990).

Neurologic Changes

There is much discussion among biologists concerning the neurologic changes that occur with the normal aging process. Most research has been conducted with animals and may or may not apply to human beings.

The brain has great reserve capacity. However, in very aged people there is a decrease in the size and weight of the brain, with some decrease in the number of functioning neurons, especially in the substantia nigra, striatum, and dorsal nucleus of the vagus nerve (Poirier and Finch 1990). It should be noted that no real correlation has been drawn between brain size and functioning (Poirier and Finch 1990). Nurses should evaluate the ability of each client to respond to the environment in deciding whether there are several pathologic conditions or none. It is generally conceded that nerve transmission is slower in older people. Nerve conduction velocity is reduced, so that by the age of 70 there is somewhat slower voluntary movement, slower decision making, and a slowed startle response.

Thought processes, reasoning, learning, and memory are now thought to be retained in normal aging, however. Thus it behooves nurses to treat older people as intelligent adults who are capable of comprehending events unless they have a pathologic condition superimposed upon the aging process. However, a longer reaction time should be allowed for them to respond to requests (Poirier and Finch 1990).

There seems to be a consensus among biologists that the number of neurons decreases with age. There is a depletion of dopamine and some of the enzymes in the brain of aging persons (Poirier and Finch 1990). Older people who appear to have reduced response to environmental stimuli increase their ability to respond spontaneously and appropriately when in an environment of consistent stimulation.

There appears to be a consistent increase in the amount of the pigment lipofuscin in the cytoplasm of neurons in older people, but there is no consensus whether this pigment is harmful to neuronal activity.

The total amount of daily sleep declines with age, as does the time spent in stage IV and rapid eye movement (REM) sleep (Haponik 1990). As a result the older person may awaken with a feeling of inadequate sleep. Many people resort to hypnotic drugs as they get older; such use leads to other problems that are discussed in the chapter on medications. A nap during the day may interfere with an older person's sleep at night. The nurse should identify the part of the night during which the person sleeps best and help to direct the time of retiring to suit individual sleep patterns. Some older people find that spending more time sleeping will compensate for changing sleep patterns. For some older people a later bedtime, a change from a light to a heavier evening meal, or both will enhance sleep and the person will sleep longer in the morning. A light snack at 5:00 p.m. with no bedtime snack may cause older people to awaken early because of hunger.

Because of the interrelated and neurologic changes, older people may be susceptible to either heatstroke or hypothermia, depending on the environmental temperature. Very old people who develop hypothermia do not shiver to increase body heat; vasoconstriction of peripheral vessels does not occur as in a young person. So the elderly person who feels cold may have skin that is pink rather than blue or pale (Abrass 1990). Because of the reduction in the functioning of the sweat glands and skin capillaries, the very old person cannot dissipate heat from the body and is predisposed to heatstroke if subjected to high environmental temperatures. Using this knowledge, nurses should educate older people about the necessity of protecting themselves from direct exposure to the sun during periods of very hot weather. Conversely, during periods of very cold weather, older people need to be protected from developing hypothermia. Because of the loss of subcutaneous fat, the reduction in vasoconstriction, and the inability to increase body metabolism enough to increase heat production, older people are more susceptible than the young to exposure to cold. Older people should be encouraged to wear more layers of clothing and to wear materials that prevent loss of body heat, particularly wool garments or newer synthetics that trap body heat. Adequate covering for the feet and legs is especially important because there is less heat near the floor. Old people should be encouraged to participate in activities that increase the body's heat production and to maintain adequate nutrition for body metabolism to provide heat.

Pathologic Conditions of the Neurologic System.

Stroke. Cerebrovascular disease is the third leading cause of death in North America, with 85 percent occurring in those over 65 years of age (Power and Hachinski 1990). In addition and perhaps more important for many people is the number of older people who suffer incapacitating strokes and live with the residual effects of decreased mobility, altered speech, loss of control of bladder and bowel, and loss of independence. Of particular importance to nurses is the need to know the signs and symptoms that indicate transient ischemic attacks. The most common sign is a neurologic deficit that lasts only a few seconds or a few minutes, with full recovery of function (Power and Hachinski 1990). The deficit may be loss of speech, weakness, paresthesia or paralysis, altered vision, memory dysfunction, or a combination of these defects. The majority of people who experience a transient ischemic attack can be treated successfully, and most can be prevented from experiencing a cerebrovascular accident. Nurses must be able to recognize the early warning signs and promote preventive habits.

After a stroke many older people do not receive the rehabilitation that younger people receive. Too often they become bedridden or are lifted bodily from bed to chair when, with a little time and education, the older person could accomplish the transfer from bed to chair alone or learn to walk with a walker or cane. Constant efforts by all nurses are required to assist an older person in returning to maximum independence. Such effort is more than rewarded by the psychologic, sociologic, and financial benefits to the person, family, and society. Too often the stroke victim is placed in an institution for long-term care where the health provider is least prepared, inadequately supervised, and neither motivated nor educated to help the person regain what function is possible. In the long run less care is required when the person is assisted in regaining whatever function remains. Nurses must establish ongoing in-service education, formal or informal, for nursing assistants who care for the elderly, wherever they are employed.

Parkinson's Disease. Parkinson's disease is one of the most frequently occurring movement disorders of older people (Cote and Henly 1990). This syndrome is characterized by rhythmic tremors of fingers, feet, lips, and head with progressive rigidity of the facial and trunk muscles. When the joints are passively moved, one may feel a cogwheel roughness of motion. There is flexion of the trunk and extremities. Facial muscles become fixed in a masklike expression, and speech may be slow and difficult to understand. Nurses should be alert to early signs of the disorder, so as to encourage medical care as well as to educate the patient, family, or other care providers concerning the effects of drug therapy.

Safety must be stressed, since walking is difficult and falls occur easily. The person with Parkinson's disease may have a shuffling gait, with the body leaning forward and a propulsive movement. Swallowing may be affected, so someone must be present during mealtimes to prevent choking. Food must be of the kind that is easily chewed and swallowed. Drug therapy may affect the person's appetite, making supervision of nutrition even more important. The drugs used in the treatment of Parkinson's disease have multiple side effects; the client and family should know about them. To counteract these side effects, a second drug may be added to the treatment regimen. Parkinson's is a chronic, usually progressive disease that requires continuing re-evaluation of the needs of the client. Nurses should help these clients cope with progressive deficits, body image change, adjust-

ments in lifestyle, and in increasing dependence on others.

Sensory Changes

Some sensory change begin in early middle age. They are progressive and are apt to cause limitation of activity in later years. All the sensory organs show some degree of altered function by the age of 70 and older. In general the changes in sensory function with aging include a higher sensory threshold and a decrease in sensory acuity (Perlmutter and Hall 1985).

The sensation of pain may be diminished in older people. Therefore it may be more difficult to evaluate acute pain because of poor localization of pain. Pain may be referred from the site of origin. The autonomic response to pain may not occur in the elderly individual so that rapid pulse, elevated blood pressure, pallor, and nausea may be absent (Payne and Pasternak 1990). However, every person exhibits learned behaviors in response to pain, and older people may have experienced chronic discomfort for such a long time that they fail to respond to a new stimulus. Also, with extreme aging, the inflammatory response is often reduced or delayed, resulting in a decreased stimulus for pain. The pain associated with myocardial infarction described by most older people is different in location and intensity from the pain experienced by young adults with the same condition. Such pain may not be intense because the older person has developed collateral circulation, and the amount of necrosis is actually less in the aging heart. The distention of the colon associated with progressive cancer may be significant before an older person complains of discomfort. The nurse must use a combination of assessment skills to detect the presence of pain in the elderly, since the usual signs and symptoms are often not present.

Tactile Sensation. Since the sense of touch may be decreased in an older person, a firmer touch may be needed to elicit a response. Many older clients respond to touch; perhaps it indicates a special sense of caring by another person. Nurses should be mindful of this fact and use a hand on the shoulder or a handclasp to establish contact and provide support.

The sense of balance is precarious in many very old people, particularly when they try to hurry. Apparently the coordination of muscular activity for bodily movement requires a longer interval for processing than in younger people. Older people should be reminded to sit up slowly, stand firmly, and be sure of their balance before walking.

Vestibular and Kinesthetic Senses. The response to both vestibular and kinesthetic stimuli is reduced in very old people. Vestibular sense receptors are located in muscles and tendons and relay signals to the central nervous system concerning joint motion and body position in space. Since both these senses help maintain equilibrium, coordination, and body position, a diminution in their effectiveness produces a general unsteadiness, a lack of coordination in movements, and an increase in the amount of body sway in the older person. Since a longer time is required for stimuli to reach the central nervous system and be interpreted and for messages then to be sent to the periphery, there is a great need for older people to move slowly, have a wide stance, and perhaps use a cane for support when walking. When balance is precarious in older people, they should be encouraged to walk slowly, to refrain from rapid body or head turning to maintain balance and prevent falls, and to walk with a wider stance than in youth. Older people should be instructed not to make rapid changes in direction, since such movements also may cause loss of balance.

Visual Changes. A decrease in visual accommodation begins in the 30s and progresses with aging, so that presbyopia, or an inability to change the shape of the lens for near vision, affects most people 45–50 years old, making glasses necessary for reading fine print. The size of the pupil decreases with aging, necessitating a brighter light for vision. Sensitivity to glare also increases with age due to changes in the opacity of the lens (Blair 1990); therefore, for reading, older people should have a bright but diffused light. Color discrimination decreases with the yellowing of the lens in the aging process (Perlmutter and Hall 1985). The blue-greens and violet are difficult to see because the yellow lens screens out these colors. The yellow, orange, and red hues remain more clearly visible. Sharp contrasts in color, such as pairing yellow and black, provide an effective medium for visual discrimination. The colors mentioned above serve as a valuable medium for orientation to a setting. These different colors can be used to provide highly visible landmarks for older patients in hospitals and nursing homes. Because of the reduced color discrimination, older people often wear clashing colors and need guidance in selecting clothing. As vision decreases, depth perception is altered. Because of these changes, some method of determining where the steps of a staircase begin and end and the edge of each step becomes important. A narrow strip of red or yellow at the edge of each step will help an older person avoid a misstep and be aware of the absence of steps.

Older people need a longer time to focus on near objects. The inability to focus quickly and the lessened ability to adapt to light-dark changes contribute to accidents that happen when an older person moves from a lighted area to a dark area, especially if there are stairs to be negotiated. Older people should be encouraged to allow time for their vision to adapt before they begin to move in a dark area. Hand rails are necessary on stairs to prevent falls from poor vision as well as poor balance.

Another change in the eyes that accompanies aging is arcus senilis, or the accumulation of a lipid substance in the outer rim of the cornea. This appears as a greyish or white circle at the edge of the cornea. Such a change usually does not affect vision.

The lacrimal glands produce fewer tears, resulting in a dry, irritated cornea that can be relieved by eyedrops of the methylcellulose variety. The very aged person may have entropion or ectropion of the eyelids, leading to more dryness or chronic irritation caused by the lashes rubbing the cornea or sclera. Minor surgical correction of entropion or ectropion will relieve this discomfort. Glasses must be free of scratches to prevent distortion of vision.

Hearing. Presbycusis, the progressive loss of hearing and sound discrimination with age, is related to changes in the organ of Corti, or the loss of nerve cells in the eighth cranial nerve, accompanied by the loss of perception of high tones. Presbycusis is more common in men than in women. Exposure to loud noises over a long period of time, such as loud music at concerts, the use of earphones with radios played at exaggerated volumes, and increased noise levels in the community or in homes, increases hearing losses, so that in middle and old age the deficits may be severe. Impacted cerumen also is a common occurrence in older individuals and may lead to the assumption that the person has a hearing loss. This cerumen may need to be removed by the physician or nurse. Drops may be recommended to soften the wax before removal. The ability to discriminate among higher frequencies is often impaired by the age of 50 and markedly declines after the age of 65. Most people who are described as "hard of hearing" suffer from a selective high-frequency loss rather than a generalized decrease in hearing acuity. Thus voices, horns, telephones, and doorbells are more easily heard by older people if they have a low tone and high intensity. Their decreased ability to identify high-frequency tones causes older people difficulty in discerning the subtle tones and pitches in human speech. The older person has increased difficulty in discriminating among sounds, particularly the consonants s, f, t, and g. Further, pitch discrimination and threshold may decrease, so that older persons have difficulty hearing accurately because of an impairment in their ability to filter words from interfering background noise.

Hearing loss progresses slowly and unevenly. Such loss may first be noticed when the older person complains that everyone seems to be mumbling. The increase in a person's threshold of hearing can be especially troublesome. The older person may have to increase the volume of sounds to a point that is intolerable to anyone with normal hearing who happens to be close by. Although an older person may hear little of a conversation held at a normal voice level, increasing the volume does little to help. The older person hears the higher level of sound as shouting, because of the impairment in hearing at the upper frequencies.

Taste Buds. It is believed by some that the number of taste buds decreases with age, but such a decrease has not been proven. There seems to be decreased taste sensation, which leads to a change in the type of foods preferred. Older people seem to like more spices, highly seasoned foods, or simply more sugar or salt in food so it can be tasted. In the Baltimore Longitudinal Study, Shock (1984) found that advanced age required a greater stimulus for salt and bitter, but no difference was found for the stimulus level for sour or sweet. These problems should be considered by people who prepare food for the elderly. Many very old people continue to taste sweets, however, and because high-carbohydrate foods are easier to chew, they tend to consume large amounts of sweets and neglect other types of foods.

Olfactory Nerves. The olfactory nerves are also thought to have fewer cells functioning in older people. Since the odor of foods stimulates salivation and hunger, a diminished sense of smell often contributes to a decreased appetite. A decreased sense of smell also leads to the inability to smell danger in the environment, such as leaking gas, stove burners that are not completely turned off, and spoiled food. The very old person living alone should develop the habits of checking all burners after use to be certain they are turned completely off and marking the date food is placed in the refrigerator to prevent eating spoiled food.

Disorders of the Senses

Cataracts. Cataracts are the most common eye disorder in the older age group (Rich 1990). Degenerative cataracts occur in both eyes but at different rates. There is a gradual diminution of vision. Some people with cataracts complain that bright lights, such as car lights approaching at night, are blinding or that they see wagon wheel spokes radiating from the light. When visual acuity is reduced enough to interfere with the person's daily activities, surgery is the treatment of choice.

Cataract surgery is usually performed as an ambulatory or same-day surgery procedure. Still, many older cataract patients require hospitalization for close observation of a pre-existing condition. Factors to consider in the decision to observe overnight are age, type of cataract, general health, pre-existing conditions, and type of operative procedure used.

Usually only one eye is operated on at a time; the eye that has less visual acuity is operated on first. With modern techniques of surgery and materials, such as atraumatic sutures and needles, the operating microscope, and Nd:YAG laser, the trauma of the surgery has been reduced. The restrictions placed on the patient after surgery are not as great as in the past. Immediately postoperatively the patient might complain of short periods of intermittent eye pain or discomfort. Analgesics are not usually required for the discomfort. Either the patient or a family member will be taught to instill eyedrops and cleanse the eye after the surgery. Only the operated eye is patched for one to two days. To prevent inadvertent damage to the eye, a metal or plastic eye guard is usually worn at night for five to six weeks until healing is complete.

Optical rehabilitation following cataract extraction consists of assisting the older adult to become adjusted to the substituted lens. There are three methods used to replace the lens: eyeglass correction, contact lenses, and intraocular lens implantation.

Eyeglass correction magnifies images 35 percent larger than before the cataract extraction. This requires the individual to make distance adjustments. Peripheral vision is distorted. Binocular vision is not possible until both eyes have been operated on. Double vision occurs with eyeglass correction if the unoperative eye has good vision.

Contact lenses result in 7 percent magnification without distortion of peripheral vision. Rehabilitation is directed toward assisting the individual in making adjustments for spatial orientation. The disadvantage for the older adult is the need for manual dexterity in maintaining and inserting the contact lens. For this reason the implanted intraocular lens (IOL) is a popular choice for this age group.

The implanted intraocular lens (IOL) does not magnify images or distort peripheral vision. Optical rehabilitation is faster. The IOL is implanted permanently, requiring no maintenance. The IOL may be implanted during the initial cataract extraction or at a later time, based on the surgeon's preference.

Glaucoma. Glaucoma is the most common eye disorder leading to blindness among older people. Glaucoma may be acute or chronic. In acute or narrow-angle glaucoma the angle between the iris and the cornea is narrow. With dilation of the pupil, the aqueous humor outflow becomes obstructed. This leads to an increase in intraoccular pressure (IOP). The eye appears red and the person complains of pain and blurred vision. Medical attention is sought because of the pain. Medical treatment is focused towards operative intervention to relieve the obstruction and reduce the IOP so as to prevent permanent damage to the optic nerve.

Chronic glaucoma (wide-angle glaucoma) has an insidious onset which does not cause pain. Unfortunately significant loss of peripheral field vision occurs before it is detected. For this reason it is recommended that all people over the age of 40 have annual evaluations of intraoccular pressure (IOP). Obstruction is caused by a lack of ability to filter aqueous humor. First-line medical treatment is pharmaceutical and laser therapy. Only if this is unsuccessful is surgical intervention warranted. Pharmaceutical intervention uses topical medications, such as miotics, long-acting parasympathomimetic drugs, levoepinephrine,

and beta-adrenergic blocking agents. Carbonic anhydrase inhibitors are used systemically when topical drugs are ineffective. Laser trabeculoplasty is another option for the treatment of glaucoma. Laser therapy has many advantages for the older adult. It can be done on an outpatient basis, using topical anesthesia. This makes it perfect for the high-risk operative patient. Since it is noninvasive and sterile, the procedure minimizes postoperative infection and pain.

Nursing responsibilities concerning glaucoma include encouraging yearly eye examinations with IOP screening for all older adults and, for the person with a diagnosis of glaucoma, encouraging the use of eyedrops as prescribed or ensuring the correct use of systemic carbonic anhydrase inhibitor.

Senile Macular Degeneration. Senile macular degeneration is another cause of visual loss in the very old person (Rich 1990), characterized by a slowly progressive loss of central vision. Peripheral vision is usually retained so that blindness is not complete. The sudden onset of loss of central vision caused by macular degeneration is due to hemorrhage of the choroidal vessels at the macula. Through the early use of laser beam therapy to produce photocoagulation, some people may retain some central vision. Since rapid loss of vision may also indicate acute glaucoma or retinal detachment—conditions that are treatable—any symptoms of rapid loss of vision should be referred to an ophthalmologist for diagnosis and treatment.

Vascular Disease. Vascular disease of the retina may occur when the older person has hypertension, atherosclerosis, or diabetes mellitus. Hemorrhage and exudate may be present in the retina of older people with vascular diseases and may lead to scarring and some permanent loss of vision. Diabetic retinopathy is one of the leading causes of blindness in people who have been diabetic for 20 to 30 years. Any change in vision, sudden redness of the eye, or pain in the eye should alert the nurse to the need for medical attention.

Disorders of the Vitreous Body. As aging progresses, the vitreous body sometimes becomes more liquid and shrinks away from the retina. As the vitreous body ages, the presence of opacities causes the *floaters* seen by many older people. If the floaters are accompanied by light flashes, medical attention is needed because retinal tears may be occurring. If no light flashes occur, the floaters are benign but annoying when they move into the visual field. Usually eye movements will cause the floaters to move out of the visual field (Rich 1990).

Musculoskeletal System

With advancing years there is a gradual loss of muscular strength and endurance because the muscle cells atrophy and because of the loss of lean muscle mass. There is a concomitant loss of elastic fibers in muscle tissue, leading to reduced flexibility and increased stiffness. Persons who remain physically active show less muscle atrophy and stiffness. Proper nutrition is essential to help reduce muscle atrophy. Many older people do not have enough protein, vitamins, and minerals in their diets to maintain muscle and bone integrity. Older people are subject to loss of both muscle and bone structure with time. Any teeth that can be retained should be, and partial plates should be fitted around the intact teeth. The presence of teeth helps prevent bone resorption in the jaw. Old people who have been edentulous for a long time may not be able to tolerate dentures (Felder 1990). Poor dental health or lack of all teeth interferes with mastication and swallowing.

Osteoporosis is a common manifestation of bone abnormality in older people and occurs more frequently and at an earlier age in women than in men. Both trabecular and cortical bones are affected by osteoporosis, but trabecular bone is more severely involved. In older people, resorption exceeds accretion of bone, resulting in a thinning of the vertebrae, long bones, and pelvic bones. Bone thinning increases the possibility of fracture resulting from weight bearing or stress. Vertebral osteoporosis leads to fracture and skeletal deformities of aging (kyphosis and scoliosis) as well as severe back pain or pressure on the spinal nerves. Vertebrae are particularly vulnerable to osteoporosis because of their high proportion of trabecular bone (Chestnut 1990).

Many chronic illnesses of older people, such as intestinal malabsorption, diabetes mellitus, and uremia, increase the rapidity with which osteoporosis occurs. Osteomalacia, the adult equivalent of rickets, is an abnormality of increased resorption of bone resulting from reduced absorption of calcium from the small intestines. Resorption occurs to maintain blood serum calcium levels, but there is concomitantly less

formation of new bone. Some research is underway with a hormonal form of vitamin D that increases calcium absorption and utilization even when the liver or renal enzyme systems are malfunctioning and unable to convert vitamin D into its active form (Chestnut 1990).

Active exercise and a nutritionally adequate diet are now thought to decrease the rapidity with which muscle mass and bone density decrease, so the older person should be encouraged to be as active as he or she is physically capable. Walking is a good exercise for the elderly, as is swimming, if neither is carried to excess. Walking has the added advantage of providing a change of environment and sensory stimuli. But the pace must be slow enough for safety and the person should stop and rest when tired. The older person should be reminded to stand as erect as possible while walking to help retain balance. Well-fitting supportive shoes should be worn. Postmenopausal women should consume dairy products to provide 1000 mg calcium daily or take calcium fortified with vitamin D (Chestnut 1990).

Disorders of the Musculoskeletal System

Arthritis. Aside from reduced muscle strength, arthritis in some form is probably the most common disorder of the musculoskeletal system in older people.

Osteoarthritis. Degenerative joint disease (osteoarthritis) is the most common type of arthritis and affects most people to some degree by age 75. It is characterized by joint cartilage deterioration accompanied by new bone formation, called spurs, at the joint surface (Ettinger and Davis 1990). There is increasing pain, made worse by movement of the joint, which is relieved by rest. There are no systemic manifestations. The joints affected are the weight-bearing joints (vertebrae, hips, knees, feet) and the fingers. Analgesics that have anti-inflammatory properties are frequently ordered for pain. The client should be encouraged to exercise affected joints, take frequent rest periods, and be alert for side effects of the drugs ordered. This type of arthritis does not usually lead to severe crippling but does produce discomfort.

Rheumatoid Arthritis. Rheumatoid arthritis occurs in all age groups including older persons and is now thought to be an autoimmune reaction characterized by inflammation in the synovial membranes lining the joints. There is hypertrophy of the synovial membrane with damage to the cartilage, bones, and tendons. This disease varies from mild to severe, with rapid crippling. It may have an insidious onset, characterized by fatigue, morning stiffness, and low-grade fever. The proximal interphalangeal and metacarpal joints of the hands, the cervical spine, the hips, the knees, and the feet are affected. Rheumatoid arthritis is usually progressive and crippling. For this reason early medical care is needed to minimize the pain and deformity. Treatment incudes anti-inflammatory drugs, physical therapy to maintain function, and, if crippling becomes extensive, surgical replacement of the joints. These patients may be taking drugs that have systemic side effects, to which nurses must be alert. Salicylates are given with meals to reduce gastric irritation. Both aspirin and glucocorticoid steroids may lead to gastric bleeding. If gold compounds are used, a pruritic rash may occur, and in some people, bone marrow depression occurs. Other side effects are ulceration of the mouth and nephritis. The steroids may mask infection, increase the blood glucose level, or precipitate diabetes mellitus. Nonsteroidal anti-inflammatory drugs are being used more frequently for older persons who have rheumatoid arthritis, and careful attention must be given to the side effects of these drugs. They cause gastric irritation, bleeding, nausea, and tinnitus (see chapter 9).

Fractures. Because of osteoporosis, fractures are common in older people. Those most at risk are postmenopausal, short, thin, white females who have a history of osteoporosis in the family, who drink and smoke, and who are over age 75. Fractures may occur in the thoracic and lumbar vertebrae, leading to pain and kyphosis and scoliosis with altered chest movement and impaired respiration. Fracture of the head of the femur often results in poor healing because of the decreased blood supply to the area. When the older person must be immobilized to treat a fracture of the hip, many complications may arise. Among the most common are pneumonia, pressure ulcers, and muscle wasting. When an older client is immobilized, care must be taken to ensure deep breathing and coughing to prevent respiratory complications. Skin care is also essential to prevent skin breakdown over pressure areas. Turning the older patient and sliding him or her across the sheet may cause skin trauma that heals poorly. Some of the new types of mattresses that al-

ternate pressure help to prevent skin breakdown but are not a substitute for turning and skin care.

Because of the altered balance and stance of many older people, a fall frequently results in a Colles' fracture of the wrist—the hand is extended to stop the fall and it then sustains the weight of the body. When a fall causes fracture of both a wrist and a hip, early mobilization with a walker is very difficult. Another person may be needed to help support the patient during his or her attempts to walk.

Cardiovascular Changes

As with other muscles, the cardiac muscle has increased amounts of collagen and fat with increasing age. There is much discussion concerning the specific causes of the declining functioning capacity of the heart with aging, but it is generally agreed that cardiac output declines with age (Murphy and De-Mots 1984). Cardiac output may be adequate for normal activity, but when undergoing vigorous exercise, stress, or illness, the heart of an older person cannot meet the additional demands placed on it. This is thought to be a factor in the rapidity with which older people tire. In aging, a greater percentage of the total cardiac output of blood is sent to the brain and coronary arteries, with the result that the skeletal muscles and viscera may receive inadequate blood supplies when there is increased demand for blood flow. Consistent exercise throughout one's lifetime is felt to be the best and safest way to maintain an adequate cardiac output throughout old age. With vigorous exercise the maximum heart rate of the older person is consistently less than the maximum heart rate attained by a young person and requires a longer time to return to its usual rate (Wenger 1990). The valves of the older person's heart become more rigid and may compromise cardiac function, and any pre-existing valvular heart disease tends to become more pronounced with age, further compromising cardiac output.

The vascular system of older Americans typically shows some degree of atherosclerosis affecting the aorta, coronary arteries, and carotid arteries. The changes associated with atherosclerosis reduce the distensibility and elasticity of the large arteries and limit, to the degree of the pathologic condition, the ability to increase the amount of blood available to vital organs. The effect is greatest when tissue demands increase because the diseased arteries make the work load of the heart greater. Neither the heart nor the arteries can respond to the increased need to the degree possible in young people. Therefore anything that greatly increases the need for blood, e.g., fever, vasodilation, strenuous exercise, or any stress, can produce angina or syncope because the heart or brain becomes hypoxic. The aged heart has problems with arrhythmia, which can also reduce the amount of blood flow available to tissues and cause further cardiac or cerebral problems.

Pathologic Cardiovascular Conditions. Older people are subject to all the cardiovascular abnormalities the young experience, from congenital defects to hypertensive heart disease, endocarditis, valvular heart disease, myocardial infarction, and congestive heart failure. However, with increasing age, the incidence of cardiac disorders, particularly atherosclerosis, increases.

Hypertension. Hypertension has been shown to be a significant abnormality in the older population. There is a controversy regarding the point at which an older person should be considered hypertensive and treated. Usually treatment is recommended for people over 65 when, after several blood pressure checks, their systolic pressure is above 16 mm Hg and the diastolic pressure is above 9 mm Hg. A diastolic reading of 90 mm Hg on three or more occasions indicates the need for treatment (Frohlich 1990). Some physicians now believe that high blood pressure should be lowered slowly, because rapid lowering may precipitate decreased cerebral, myocardial, and renal blood flow and produce additional pathologic conditions (Applegate 1990). Sodium restriction, weight loss, or both may be advised for older persons whose blood pressure is slightly elevated. If this does not reduce the pressure, then drug therapy may be instituted. If several drugs are used to control blood pressure, the patient, family, and nurses must be alert for possible drug reactions, particularly electrolyte depletion. If the drugs used to treat hypertension reduce the sympathetic nervous system effect on peripheral vessels, the client should learn to rise from a recumbent position slowly and to sit on the side of the bed until the blood pressure can adjust to the upright position before the patient begins to walk.

Ischemic Heart Disease. Ischemic heart disease, manifested by such disorders as acute myocardial infarction, congestive heart failure, arrhythmias, or angina pectoris, is the most frequently occurring pathologic condition of the heart in people over 60 years of age. Some of these disorders are discussed next.

Acute Myocardial Infarction. Acute myocardial infarction in the elderly may cause the same symptoms as in a younger person, or the pain may be less severe and signs of congestive failure such as shortness of breath may be the first symptoms seen. When examined, many older people are found to have had prior myocardial infarctions but had not experienced the substernal pain typically associated with this condition. Dyspnea—after activity or at rest—may be the symptom described by an older person who has had a myocardial infarction (Irvine 1990). There is an increase in the mortality of the older population with myocardial infarctions. Sinus arrhythmias also occur more often in the older population after a myocardial infarction. Since the older person has a significant reduction in lung vital capacity and muscle tone, it is important that the older patient maintain some degree of mobility and independence even during the acute phase of care to prevent any great loss of function during convalescence. For example, by using a bedside commode rather than a bedpan the older patient can maintain muscle strength as well as a sense of self-worth and dignity. The nurse should encourage the physician in charge to initiate these measures. Sometimes, however, the greatest amount of activity that can be permitted will be passive range of motion until the most acute phase has subsided. The nurse must consider how the aging process complicates nursing care. The enforced rest may require the use of stool softeners to prevent straining while having a bowel movement. Passive exercise will be needed to prevent further loss of muscle tone and flexibility. If severe pain is present, the dose of the analgesic may need to be reduced to prevent respiratory depression. When nitrates are administered to prevent or treat angina, careful observation of blood pressure is required. If propranolol (Inderal) is being given, the nurse should observe for a slowed heart rate and decrease in cardiac output, which may be manifested by a reduced urinary output or dyspnea. The calcium-channel blockers such as verapamil hydrochloride (Calan, Isoptin) or diltiazem (Cardizem) may also cause a drop in blood pressure, especially orthostatic hypotension (Elster 1987). As the person recovers from myocardial infarction, activity should be interspersed with rest to maintain the activity level allowed.

Congestive Heart Failure. Congestive heart failure frequently causes severe fatigue, especially with activity, because the skeletal muscles receive a decreased percentage of blood; the heart and brain receive more. However, if the pumping action is extremely depressed, there may be changes in behavior, such as irritability, poor memory, and restlessness, since even the blood flow to the cerebrum is reduced, resulting in hypoxia. The pulse rate may not increase as significantly as in the younger person, and the client with mental confusion may not be able to express his or her increasing dyspnea. When any condition occurs that requires a greater cardiac output, such as hyperthyroidism, infection, or stress, the nurse must be alert for early signs of impending pump failure. Congestive heart failure in older patients may be accompanied by Cheyne-Stokes respirations and by atrial fibrillation. Nurses should be alert to the possibility of either of these events and should document their occurrence and inform the physician. Other symptoms that might indicate the occurrence of congestive heart failure include minor changes in respiration, irregularities of the pulse, a slight rise in the pulse rate with no activity, fatigue, increasing dyspnea, dependent edema, irritability, and a decreased appetite. Rest is essential during the acute phase of pump failure, especially for the elderly. During convalescence, rest interspersed with activity is essential (Elster 1987). When assessing the heart rate of the elderly person for congestive heart failure, one should check the apical beat for rate and regularity. When atrial fibrillation is present, the pulse is usually rapid and irregular (Elster 1987). The person should be observed for jugular vein distention, which indicates right-side heart failure.

Arrhythmia. Any of the arrhythmias that produce a rapid heart rate are not well tolerated by the elderly who have decreased functional capacity. Therefore the physician should be notified of a change in rate or character of the pulse. Monitoring is essential because critical arrhythmias may occur. The heart rate should be counted at the apex.

Conduction Defects. Conduction defects are frequently present in older clients and may appear as a slowed conduction at the atrioventricular (AV) node with a first-degree heart block or as a complete heart block with a very slow heart rate. A heart rate of 30 or 40 beats per minute does not provide adequate blood flow to the tissues, especially to cerebral tissue when the patient is in an upright position. As a result, syncope may occur and the person may be restricted to bed. A pacemaker is frequently the treatment for this condition and usually allows the client to continue normal activities.

When the blood flow to the area of the sinoatrial node is decreased, sinoatrial dysfunction may be produced, along with feelings of faintness or dizziness or even seizures. Since the body's own normal pacemaker is no longer functioning regularly, other areas of the atrial cardiac muscle or the conduction system take over the role of pacemaker, leading to irregular pulse patterns. This condition may also be treated by the surgical insertion of an artificial pacemaker that produces a regular ventricular beat (Elster 1987).

Atherosclerosis. Atherosclerosis of the arterial tree of the lower extremities is common in older people. Few older people who have this condition complain of pain and discomfort because of reduced circulation. However, disease of the arteries of the lower extremities may produce pain with activity or rest, pale skin color, and eventually ulcerations or infections of the lower extremities. Blood clots may develop in the lower extremities when there is a rapid reduction of blood flow. An early sign of arterial clotting is severe pain. Other early signs are changes in skin temperature and color and the absence of pulses below the level of the arterial obstruction. Any of these symptoms should alert the nurse to the need for rapid medical care. Diabetes mellitus increases the incidence of vascular occlusions, peripheral neuropathy, and infections of the lower extremities. These lesions demand prompt medical attention in order to avoid gangrene and the possibility of amputation.

Thrombophlebitis. The incidence of thrombophlebitis increases with age (Walker and Love 1987). This condition is often the result of immobilization that is frequently necessary after the trauma of surgery. Care must be taken to prevent thrombosis, since it may not be detected until an embolus occurs. Exercise of the lower extremities soon after surgery, a position in bed that does not obstruct the iliac veins, and early ambulation are all essential to protect the older patient from thrombophlebitis after surgery. Thrombosis of deep veins is suspected when a vein is firm to the touch, tender, and warm. The temperature may be slightly elevated. Medical attention is necessary to prevent an embolus, which could be fatal. Bed rest is recommended until the patient is seen by a physician.

Other Interventions. Nurses should grasp all opportunities to teach the older client and family some general principles that will help the client keep the heart and blood vessels as healthy as possible. Older people should know the principles of a proper diet, particularly the need for proteins and vitamins, and the need to lower salt, cholesterol, and fat intake. Other factors in maintaining a healthy cardiovascular system include moderate regular exercise, such as walking, that does not produce pain or dyspnea. The necessity of consulting a physician before beginning an exercise program should be stressed. Any physical activity should be started slowly enough to build an exercise tolerance gradually and prevent undue fatigue or dyspnea. Any older person with cardiac problems should know that periods of activity must be interspersed with periods of rest and that an activity must be stopped before dyspnea occurs.

Respiratory Changes

The changes in the respiratory systems of older people are similar to those in other systems. There is generally a decreased functional reserve capacity. Drugs often produce a significant negative effect on respiration in the elderly, so that breathing is very slow and shallow. Hypoventilation is ineffective for maximal gas exchange. Pulmonary tissue in the older person has an altered level of function because of loss of elasticity, leading to some degree of hyperinflation of the lung. Bony changes in the thorax and vertebrae further reduce the ability of the lungs to distend. Therefore, if any circumstance occurs that demands greater oxygen consumption, the lungs are not able to respond appropriately. The poor response is also partly due to impaired cardiac function. During the aging process there is a larger portion of dead air space in the respiratory tree, so that even if the respiratory rate increases with need, the ventilation/perfusion ratio is decreased, resulting in less gas exchange. Lung vital capacity is reduced with aging, so that the amount of air that can be forcibly exhaled decreases. With the gradual decline in respiratory muscle structure and function, there is a corresponding decrease in strength for breathing and/or coughing. In older persons the vital capacity is reduced primarily due to the increase in the residual volume of air. Residual volume is the amount of air remaining in the lung at the end of a forced exhalation. The exchange of oxygen-carbon dioxide in the alveoli and capillaries decreases with the aging process. Persons who exercise consistently have less decrease in lung function. The major decrease in lung function occurs when the older person has to have maximal breathing for a period of time (Shock 1984).

The respiratory system usually is able to meet the needs of a normal older person, but when illness or stress precipitates a need for increased respiratory function, the reserve capacity may be inadequate to meet the need. For most people the reserve capacity is greater if the person has remained active throughout life.

Respiratory Disorders. Chronic bronchitis and emphysema are both more common among the elderly than among the younger population. Chronic bronchitis produces some degree of hypoxemia caused by ventilation/perfusion abnormalities due to mucus-plugged airways, so that blood flows through areas of little or no air exchange. Chronic hypoxemia eventually leads to pulmonary hypertension and cor pulmonale, or right-sided heart failure. Emphysema produces a breakdown of alveolar walls. Its most common symptom is dyspnea after exertion, leading to increasing disability. Chronic bronchitis and emphysema frequently occur together. As these diseases progress, they lead to further reduction of vital capacity, increased residual lung volume, reduced gas exchange, and frequent infection (Morris 1990). Nurses can assist clients with chronic respiratory disease by helping them understand their disease, preventing infections, and supervising or teaching breathing exercises that consist of slow breathing with the abdomen relaxed during inhalation and contracted during exhalation. Many patients can exhale more efficiently through pursed lips, which helps prevent small airway collapse during exhalation, thereby increasing the diffusion of gases. The physician may recommend increasing amounts of exercise, particularly walking, which nurses can assist with or teach the patient and family members. A supply of oxygen may be needed so that the client can walk. Many of these clients are able to increase their exercise tolerance. They can then carry on the activities of daily living and are generally more independent and happier.

Older clients should also be taught ways of reducing recurrent infection. They should learn to take adequate nutrition, avoid others with upper respiratory infections, and contact the physician when an infection first appears. Fluid intake that is adequate to keep sputum thin enough to be expectorated is also important.

Older persons who have obstructive lung disease or emphysema have air trapped in the lung periphery at the end of exhalation. Many have bronchodilators ordered to improve ventilation. The xanthine derivatives aminophylline and theophylline are frequently ordered as timed-release tablets (Morris 1990). These drugs may have interactions with other drugs such as erythromycin and cimetidine (Tagamet) and increase the action of theophylline (Skidmore-Roth 1988). The patient should be observed for gastrointestinal symptoms, irritability, headache, muscle twitching, and tachycardia.

Gastrointestinal Changes

The salivary glands secrete less ptyalin and amylase as age advances, the saliva becomes more alkaline, and the bony structure of the mouth begins to shrink. Many older people have missing or decayed teeth, making eating difficult and less pleasurable than in younger years. Because of changes in the smooth muscle of the digestive tract and reduced stimuli to the autonomic nervous system, peristalsis is slowed from the esophagus to the colon in very old persons. There is delayed emptying of the esophagus and the stomach, causing a feeling of fullness (Perlmutter and Hall 1985). With the shrinking of the gastric mucosa, there is a decrease in the stomach secretions pepsinogen and hydrochloric acid, delaying digestion. In addition, many older persons show a decrease in the intrinsic factor, leading to pernicious anemia.

There is also a slight decrease in the amount of pancreatic enzymes with aging, which further decreases digestion and the absorption of nutrients. Bile tends to be thicker and the gallbladder empties slowly. Thus digestion is slowed but remains fairly adequate until an advanced age. In spite of reduced peristalsis, reduced abdominal muscular strength,

and inadequate exercise, most older people have a daily bowel movement. Some older persons may have problems related to relaxation of the anal sphincters because of cold environments, anal ulcers, or hemorrhoids which lead to constipation (Cheskin and Schuster 1990).

Pathologic Conditions of the Gastrointestinal Tract. The gastrointestinal tract of the older person is subject to the same diseases as that of young adults, but the incidence and symptoms may vary.

Disorders of the Esophagus. Disorders of the esophagus are most marked in the very old. There is an increase in the nonrhythmic, nonperistaltic wave contractions of the esophagus of some older people. This may be accompanied by achalasia, or failure of the esophageal sphincter to relax and open until sufficient food is swallowed and exerts pressure on the sphincter. The esophagus becomes distended, and there is a feeling of dysphagia, leading to decreased food intake and weight loss in some old adults.

These symptoms may also be present in people with cancer of the esophagus, which increases in incidence with age. An older person with this combination of complaints should be referred for medical care (Nelson and Castell 1990a, p. 350).

Hiatal Hernia. The incidence of hiatal hernia increases rapidly as aging progresses, but many produce no symptoms. Attention is demanded when there is obvious discomfort or regurgitation and aspiration of gastric content, leading to pneumonitis. People with known hiatal hernias should be instructed regarding diet, avoidance of bedtime snacks, and avoidance of a reclining position for one hour after meals. There may be a need to elevate the head of the bed on blocks. If esophagitis occurs, the client must be taught the correct use of antacids. Some antacids tend to produce constipation and some cause diarrhea. Cimetidine (Tagamet) has an increased half-life in older people and the usual adult dose may cause confusion, drowsiness, or dizziness (Avon and Gurwitz 1990).

Ulcers. The ratio of gastric to duodenal ulcers increases with age (Deters 1987). The increasing use of drugs that are gastric irritants by the elderly in addition to the decrease in their gastric mucus production may account for part of the increase. The gastric mucosa atrophies with age and the secretion of hydrochloric acid and pepsinogen decreases, leading to a feeling of gastric fullness or discomfort after eating. Because of the lack of the intrinsic factor in the stomachs of some older people, there is an increase in the incidence of pernicious anemia. The anemia may lead to complaints of fatigue, increased pulse rate, and peripheral neuropathy. When an older person has any of these complaints, the stool should be examined for evidence of bleeding. Medical attention should also be sought to rule out a diagnosis of cancer of the stomach; this group of symptoms is nonspecific, and the rate of stomach cancer increases with age. When an older person complains of gastric pain or occult blood in the stool, medical attention should be sought. Bleeding ulcers lead to iron deficiency, anemia, pallor, and weakness. If the treatment is antacids, they can lead to constipation or diarrhea. The patient should also be observed for the toxic effects of cimetidine (Tagamet).

Obstructions. There may be reduced absorption of nutrients in the small bowel, but the condition that occurs most frequently is obstruction due to adhesions, strangulated hernia, or ischemia of the bowel.

Ischemia. Ischemia results from herniation or occlusion of the superior mesenteric artery, with resulting necrosis of the small bowel. Ischemia of the bowel can also occur when there is a rapid decrease in blood pressure from any cause, with reduced flow to the mesenteric artery. Early warning signs may be a periumbilical, colicky pain; tachycardia; hypotension; confusion; and agitation. Medical care should be sought early to reduce mortality and morbidity (Nelson and Castell 1990a, p. 355).

Cholelithiasis. Cholelithiasis in the gallbladder or bile duct is very common in the elderly but may be symptom-free unless cholecystitis occurs or unless the biliary ducts are obstructed. Cholecystitis produces pain in the upper right quadrant, fever, anorexia, and nausea and vomiting. Any or all of these symptoms may be very mild in the older person, so nurses should be alert for any changes that occur.

Cancer. The incidence of cancer of the rectum, sigmoid, and colon increases with age. The first sign may be obstruction of the colon, unless bleeding with anemia has produced earlier signs. Obstruction may be complete before the symptoms are detected. Complaints of constipation, incontinence, abdominal cramping, or anemia must be heeded and further assessments made. Many drugs prescribed for the elderly produce constipation, and the person may

not heed other early warning signs of a pathologic condition.

Endocrine Changes

There seems to be no general decrease in hormone secretions with aging with the exception of estrogen and testosterone. It appears that there is a lack of response to some hormones and even an increase in the secretion of some hormones, notably antidiuretic hormone. Although growth hormones continue to be secreted, less of the hormone is secreted in the elderly than in younger people in response to a stimulus such as a low blood sugar level.

There is some evidence that the hormones cortisol and thyroxin are not degraded as rapidly in older people as in the young, so that the negative feedback mechanisms cause a decline in secretions (Perlmutter and Hall 1985). There are two theories that attempt to explain the increasing incidence of diabetes mellitus with aging. One states that there are specific cell membrane receptors for insulin on tissue cells and that the number of these receptors declines with age. According to the other theory the aging body produces antibodies against insulin. Regardless of what future research reveals, older people generally show fairly normal fasting blood sugar levels but cannot respond to a glucose load. A glucose tolerance test will reveal glucose levels that are high and remain so longer than in young adult nondiabetic subjects. Since older people exhibit delayed responses in other areas of homeostasis control, it is not surprising that the complex mechanism for maintaining their blood glucose levels and glucose metabolism is slowed or inadequate.

In women, after menopause and the resulting decrease in estrogen levels, there are changes in breast tissue that result in less glandular tissue, reduced elasticity, and more connective tissue and fat. These changes lead to the sagging seen in older women's breast tissue, but the size of the breast may not change, since the glandular tissue is replaced by fat.

The uterus becomes smaller after menopause, and in very old age it is about one-half the size of the young adult uterus. The fallopian tubes also decrease in size and, with the decline in estrogen levels, become less motile. The vulva and external genitalia shrink with aging because of a loss of subcutaneous fat.

In men, a gradual decline in the secretion of testosterone from young adulthood to old age is assumed to occur, although there is no abrupt decline in hormone secretion or in spermatogenesis. With aging there is an increased incidence of benign prostatic hypertrophy and consequent difficulty starting the voiding stream. Cancer of the prostate occurs frequently in older men, so any indication of prostate enlargement should be referred for medical care.

Disorders of the Endocrine System

Hypothyroidism and Hyperthyroidism. Both hypothyroidism and hyperthyroidism occur in older adults, but their signs and symptoms may not be typical (Gregerman 1990). Hypothyroidism is more frequent. Among the initial complaints are mental and physical slowing, intolerance to cold, apathy, and coarseness and puffiness of the skin about the eyes. These symptoms may be mistaken for the signs of aging itself, but early treatment can correct them and prevent later signs of myxedema. Thyrotoxicosis in the older person causes different complaints than in young people. Weakness and apathy, which mimic depression, along with weight loss and congestive heart failure with atrial fibrillation, are common. Since the heart cannot tolerate this stress for long periods, early medical attention is vital (Gregerman 1990). Many older persons who have hyperthyroidism may have normal thyroid function test results (Gregerman 1990) and are found to have nodular goiter. Nurses and other caregivers need to be alert to the possibility of thyroid disease and suggest medical attention when these signs and symptoms are present. Therapy for hyperthyroidism is usually with radioactive iodide (I131). The person needs close observation for four to six weeks after treatment since that period is required to destroy the thyroid. Congestive heart failure may be a serious problem during this time. Beta blockers (propranolol) may be ordered during the period until the heart rate is reduced and cardiac decompensation is not present. Propranolol may further depress cardiac contractility, so cardiac function must be assessed frequently.

Diabetes. Diabetes increases in frequency in the older age group. Some diabetes specialists suggest that the higher blood glucose level observed in glucose tolerance tests should be considered normal for older people; treatment should be insti-

tuted only if plasma glucose levels are elevated as much as 10 mg/dl per decade after age 50 when checked two hours after a glucose load is given. Some physicians consider a fasting blood sugar level of 140 mg/dl as diagnostic of diabetes. Shock (1984) found that in older individuals the blood sugar rose higher than in young or middle-aged persons and stayed elevated much longer. He also noted that obese individuals who had not been diagnosed as diabetic had the same resistance to insulin as did maturity-onset diabetics. Urinary glucose is not as accurate as blood glucose measurement because urinary glucose lags behind blood sugar approximately two hours. For this reason capillary blood and the glucometer are used to control diabetes when insulin is needed. Older people often show a fairly normal fasting blood sugar level but an abnormal response to the glucose tolerance test. If the trend toward considering a higher blood sugar to be normal in the elderly continues, fewer older people will probably be diagnosed as diabetic. Diabetes is an important pathologic entity in the elderly because of the vascular abnormalities and neuropathy and retinopathy that accompany it and lead to visual defects with blindness, severe renal disease, and peripheral vascular problems.

Nurses should educate the older person with diabetes, the family, and other helpers concerning the significance of diet, exercise, and the use of either insulin or an oral hypoglycemic agent in the control of the disease. If renal function is decreased, the excretion of both insulin and the oral medications is slowed, increasing the risk of hypoglycemic reactions. The symptoms of hypoglycemia due to oral hypoglycemics may be bizarre. For example, one older woman developed hypoglycemia suddenly and demonstrated unusual behavior with vulgar language and rage at family members. A decrease in her dosage of tolbutamide from 0.5 g three times daily to 0.5 g twice daily eliminated the hypoglycemia, and she returned to normal, fairly placid behavior.

Because of its many manifestations and the different drugs used in its control, diabetes may be difficult to manage in the older person. The diabetic diet prescription must take into account the patient's usual dietary habits, the state of the teeth, and the ability of the older person to cope with a radical change of lifestyle. Frequent reinforcement of instructions regarding urine testing, foot care, diet, exercise, and medications will help the older person maintain better control of diabetes. People who have been diabetic for many years will need to be retaught, since aging affects what they were taught in the past. Written instructions for medicines and diet make them easier to follow. Foot care for the older diabetic is essential to prevent infections or ulcers that can lead to gangrene and eventual amputations. Persons who have had diabetes for 20 years or more need to be reminded to see an ophthalmologist to detect any retinal problems.

When vision is limited and insulin is required, assistive devices are available to help the person manage his or her own injections. Arrangements can be made for a community health nurse to prepare the syringes with the prescribed amount of insulin and leave them for the patient to administer. The American Diabetes Association can provide information on other helpful ideas for the older diabetic at home.

Sexual Changes

Refer to chapter 2 for a complete discussion of sexual changes and related interventions.

Genitourinary Changes

The number of nephron units of the kidney decreases during the aging process, but this decrease does not account for the primary age-related changes of renal function unless the person is severely stressed. There is also a gradual degenerative change in the remaining nephron units. The renal blood flow gradually decreases—about 6% per decade after the age of 30—and is accompanied by a proportional decrease in glomerular filtration. By the age of 70 or 80 the filtration rate is approximately one half of the rate at age 30 (Shock 1984; Anderson 1990).

Because of decreased filtration, there is a decrease in the clearance of substances normally excreted in the urine. Some of the substances that show an increase with advanced age are blood urea nitrogen, creatinine, and uric acid. Also, with decreased glomerular filtration, drugs previously excreted in the urine may remain in the bloodstream and produce toxic levels (see chapter 9). The tubule cells decline in their reabsorption and selective secretion abilities, which can lead to loss of water and electrolytes. Steroids such as glucocorticoids and sex hormones that

were formerly excreted in the urine are also retained. The function of the kidneys is usually adequate until some event occurs that demands a rapid change, e.g., an event that precipitates acidosis, alkalosis, dehydration or electrolyte imbalance.

Because of a reduced response to antidiuretic hormones in older people, there is a decreased ability to concentrate urine. The total quantity of extracellular fluid remains fairly constant, but the intracellular fluid compartment decreases. The composition of body fluids remains relatively normal. In the aging individual the renal system is inefficient in its ability to regain normal fluid and electrolyte balance after a rapid loss of fluids. The renal tubules of older people are not as responsive to an increased acid or base load as those of a younger person. The tubules are not as active in secreting ammonia to be converted to ammonium chloride that aids in the removal of excess hydrogen ions from body fluids. Therefore acidosis is not corrected as quickly as in a young person. The mechanism for correcting alkalosis is also less effective and requires a much longer time than in the young person. The kidney also requires a longer time to correct electrolyte disturbances (Shock 1984).

During the aging process the ureters and bladder tend to lose some muscle tone and the bladder loses enough tone to result in incomplete emptying, increasing the risk of retention and cystitis. Usually bladder capacity decreases with age, and since the kidneys no longer concentrate urine well, frequent urination and nocturia result. Many older women, particularly those who are multiparous, experience incontinence because of the relaxation of the pelvic muscles with or without the presence of a cystocele. Incontinence is embarrassing in our society. Older women should be reminded that the external urethral sphincter is controlled by the pelvic muscles and should be taught to contract these muscles (Kegel exercises) several times throughout the day to strengthen their external urethral control.

Older men experience frequency of urination because of hypertrophy of the prostate and decreased bladder capacity. Both men and women may avoid shopping trips or visiting because of frequent or urgent urination or the fear of incontinence. Frequent rest stops and an understanding of their hesitation to state their need for relief should be anticipated by family, associates, and nurses.

Many older people also restrict their fluid intake to prevent frequent micturition. They need clear, concise explanations of the hazards of dehydration that can result from this restriction and should be encouraged to take at least 2,000 ml of liquids in 24 hours unless contraindicated.

Genitourinary Disorders

Urinary Incontinence. Urinary incontinence is not a normal part of the aging process. It is a symptom with an underlying cause. Still, age-related changes to the genitourinary system can predispose the older adult to incontinent episodes. Pharmacologic and pathologic insults to the older adult can trigger transient incontinent episodes, which if left unchecked, can lead to the misconception that incontinence is part of the aging process and untreatable.

Treatment of incontinence focuses on finding the underlying pathology through urodynamic testing and a complete physical examination. Once the cause is identified, the goal of the practitioner is to restore continence. If incontinence persists, the focus will be directed toward assisting the individual to modify the environment and utilize available resources so that activities of daily living can be carried out with minimal disruption. For example, an older person who suffers a stroke may have irreparable damage to the neurological system which innervates the urinary system. Incontinence may be a result. Since a cure may not be possible, managing incontinence through modifying the environment would be the management approach.

Many older people who develop an acute illness and are bedridden will develop a problem related to continence. The person who is aware of the problem may feel a loss of self-worth. Efforts should be directed toward establishing urinary control as the person recovers from the illness. Environmental factors can also play a vital part in achieving continence. A common situation is the nurse's delayed response to an older patient's request for assistance to the bathroom. Older people may not have the ability to hold their urine for an extended period of time. When the sensation of urinary urgency occurs, action needs to be taken right away. Nursing care should be focused on finding a means of restoring continence, because success can mean the difference between home care and institutionalization for the older person.

Prostate Pathology. The primary pathologic condition of the genitourinary tract in the older male population is found in the prostate gland, where either benign prostatic hyperplasia (BPH) or prostate cancer may occur. A high-fat diet is thought to play a part in the etiology of both conditions. Few symptoms, if any, occur until there is some obstruction to the outflow of urine from the bladder. Obstructive changes in voiding patterns are nocturia, urinary incontinence, an increase in the frequency of urination, or a decrease in the force of the stream of urine. BPH tends to have a slower onset of obstructive symptoms, whereas prostatic cancer occurs more rapidly. The older man with obstructive symptoms should be quickly referred for a medical evaluation. In both cases, prompt medical intervention can prevent secondary complications and permanent disability.

Immunologic System Changes

Research is being pursued to learn more about the immune system in humans. Two views are held concerning changes in this system as people age. One theory that is widely accepted is that the very old have a delayed or inadequate response of the immune system to infectious agents, so that infections in the very old, as in children, are more likely to be fatal than they are in younger adulthood.

The second theory that seems to be recognized by the scientific community holds that as people age, there is an increase in the production of antibodies that fail to recognize the person's own tissue and cause an increasing incidence of autoimmune diseases (Burns and Goodwin 1990; Shock 1984). Shock (1984) stated that the T lymphocytes are decreased in number and in their ability to function as efficiently as in young individuals. This is thought to be due to the involution of the thymus gland.

In addition to having a delayed immune response to infections, older adults have a delayed or inadequate response to the stress of an infection, so there is a real hazard for the older person who develops conditions such as pneumonia or cholecystitis. The altered inflammatory response leads to altered signs and symptoms, such as little or no fever, less pain sensation, and minimal leukocytosis, that, unaltered, would alert both a younger adult and the physician to a medical problem. Nurses should have a high index of suspicion when early warning signs of illness are present in very old people. More research is needed concerning the differences in the responses of older people to social as well as physiologic stress. Nurses must be particularly alert in assessing early changes in homeostasis maintenance mechanisms in older people and should refer the person for medical attention when stressful situations occur.

In the older person the total blood volume is about the same as in a young person of comparable size and sex. However, the older individual may not be able to redistribute blood volume when anemia, blood loss, or congestive heart failure is present. The veins in the feet and legs may be enlarged and have loss of elasticity (Lipschitz 1990b). Hemoglobin values vary greatly in individuals of the same age and sex with aging, but this is thought to be due to disease rather than aging alone. However, Lee and Walsh (1990) stated that bone marrow studies show a decrease in erythropoietic function in the older person. There is a decrease in the formation of leukocytes as one ages, so the ability to respond effectively to infection is decreased. Iron deficiency anemia is common due to poor nutrition or blood loss.

Hematologic Changes

Anemia. Iron deficiency anemia is one of the most common types of anemia in older clients. The incidence is greater among the institutionalized than among the elderly living in private homes (Lipschitz 1990a). Older people in institutions tend to have several chronic illnesses that cause anemia; more attention must be given to the nutrition of these clients.

The most common cause of anemia may be blood loss caused by drugs, the presence of peptic ulcer, or cancer of the gastrointestinal system.

Pernicious anemia occurs more often among the elderly and presents a picture of anemia and the signs and symptoms of peripheral neuropathy. Nurses should be alert to this possibility and encourage early medical diagnosis and treatment, so that the neuropathy can be reversed. Folic acid deficiency anemia is common among the elderly who must survive on reduced financial means, because this substance is obtained primarily from fresh fruit and vegetables. Folic acid deficiency may be accompanied by deficiency of vitamin C, since it is found in similar foods. Increasing dyspnea, fatigue, and anginal pain are the early symptoms of anemia. People who show signs and symptoms of anemia should always be referred for medical attention, since these signs and symptoms may be a result of bleeding from other causes that need prompt attention. Severe anemia can lead to congestive heart failure, because the heart cannot respond to the need for increased blood flow.

Leukemia and Other Immunologic Changes. There is an increase in the incidence of chronic lymphocytic leukemia in people over the age of 60. Some experts believe this increase reflects an altered immune reaction of the elderly. In fact, some authors suggest the altered immunologic system may account for the rising rate of cancer as people age (Lee and Walsh 1990). In addition, the thymus and the lymphatics undergo decrease in size and function with aging. Research in hematologic and immunologic changes in aging is just beginning and much remains to be discovered in these areas.

SUMMARY

Chronologic age is not a good indicator of physiologic age or of organ system functioning. The rate of age changes varies among people and among organ systems in each person. As a general rule the client who is 75 years or older is expected to show the greatest accumulation of age change and is considered very old.

There is a decrease in the reserve capacity in all organ systems with aging. Body systems have greater difficulty maintaining homeostasis when they undergo illness or social or psychologic stresses. The organ systems require a longer time to respond to the stress and return to a state of equilibrium. In the very

old client the reserve capacity may not be great enough to restore equilibrium, and death may result from a situation that would be a minor problem in a young adult, e.g. diarrhea with severe fluid and electrolyte loss.

In addition to physiologic losses older clients are apt to experience multiple chronic illnesses that require several drugs for treatment, thereby increasing the risks of adverse effects of drug interactions. Symptoms of illness in older people are often nonspecific and easily ignored because of the general belief that the symptoms result from the aging process. Age alters the response to disease by causing a slower and lower level of response; for example, there is often little if any temperature rise with infection. Pain perception is usually decreased in the elderly and therefore its protective function is lost.

Summary of Nursing Implications

Nurses, indeed all health providers, must divest themselves of the stereotypes they hold of older people and consider each client as an individual with unique capabilities and needs. Nursing actions to meet the needs of older people should be based on a specific data base for each individual, just as for young adults.

Some generalizations about care can be made, however. Older people should be encouraged to be as active and independent as their physical condition allows so as to maintain whatever level of functional capacity is present. The speed of activities should be well paced. Rest should be encouraged before fatigue occurs. Explanations or instructions for the elderly should be clear and given in a relaxed manner. Enough time should be allowed for a response. If detailed explanations are needed, reinforcement is helpful. Nurses should encourage an adequate fluid intake, since the sensation of thirst may be reduced and the ability to concentrate urine may be decreased. Nurses should always be aware that older clients often show minimal signs and symptoms of serious physical problems. Careful attention should be given to early changes in behavior and other aspects of the physical and psychosocial assessment.

STUDY QUESTIONS

1. Analyze two theories of biologic aging.

2. Why are older individuals susceptible to hypothermia and hyperthermia?

3. Evaluate two safety measures that may prevent accidents related to stairs when older persons have developed cataracts.

4. How can a middle-aged individual prevent the development of osteoporosis?

5. What are the major changes in cardiac functioning in the very old individual?

6. Define transient ischemic attacks. What significance do these attacks have?

7. What is the advantage of the intraocular lens when cataract surgery is performed? What is a major problem after the lens implant for some people?

8. What is the major cause of central vision loss in older adults?

9. How may symptoms of a myocardial infarction differ in older adults from those that occur in younger adults?

10. What symptoms may indicate congestive heart failure in an older adult?

11. Why may syncope occur when an older person assumes the upright position?

12. Describe the symptoms that indicate progressive obstruction of the arteries of the lower extremities.

13. Why might the dose of oral antidiabetic medicine need to be reduced for the older person who has diabetes?

14. How many symptoms of hypoglycemia differ from those usually seen after insulin administration when the older person is taking oral hypoglycemics?

REFERENCES

Abrass, I. 1990. Disorders of temperature regulation. In *Principles of Geriatric Medicine and Gerontology*, 2d ed., edited by W.R. Hazzard, R. Anders, E. Bierman and J. Blass. New York: McGraw-Hill.

Anderson, S. 1990. Nephrology/fluid and electrolyte disorders. In *Geriatric Medicine*, 2d ed., edited by C. Cassel, D. Riesenberg, L. Sorensen and J. Walsh. New York: Springer-Verlag.

Applegate, W. 1990. Hypertension. In *Principles of Geriatric Medicine and Gerontology*, 2d ed., edited by W.R. Hazzard, R. Anders, E. Bierman, and J. Blass. New York: McGraw-Hill.

Avon, J. and J. Gurwitz. 1990. Principles of pharmacology. In *Geriatric Medicine*, 2d ed., edited by C. Cassel, D. Riesenberg, L. Sorensen, and J. Walsh. New York: McGraw-Hill.

Balin, A. 1990. Aging of human skin. In *Principles of Geriatric Medicine and Gerontology*, 2d ed., edited by W.R. Hazzard, R. Anders, E. Bierman and J. Blass. New York: McGraw-Hill.

Blair, K. 1990. Aging: Physiological aspects and clinical implications. *Nurse Practitioner* 15(2): 14–28.

Burns, E. and J. Goodwin. 1990. Immunology and infectious disease. In *Geriatric Medicine,* 2d ed., edited by C. Cassel, D. Riesenberg, L. Sorensen and J. Walsh. New York: Springer-Verlag.

Cheskin, L. and M. Schuster. 1990. Constipation. In *Principles of Geriatric Medicine and Gerontology,* 2d ed., edited by W.R. Hazzard, R. Anders, E. Bierman and J. Blass. New York: McGraw-Hill.

Chestnut, C.H. 1990. Osteoporosis. In *Principles of Geriatric Medicine and Gerontology,* 2d ed., edited by W.R. Hazzard, R. Anders, E. Bierman and J. Blass. New York: McGraw-Hill.

Cote, L. and M. Henly. 1990. Parkinson's disease. In *Principles of Geriatric Medicine and Gerontology,* 2d ed., edited by W.R. Hazzard, R. Anders, E. Bierman and J. Blass. New York: McGraw-Hill.

Cristofolo, V. 1990. Biological mechanisms of aging: An overview. In *Principles of Geriatric Medicine and Gerontology,* 2d ed., edited by W.R. Hazzard, R. Anders, E. Bierman and J. Blass. New York: McGraw-Hill.

Deters, B. 1987. Nursing role in management: Problems of digestion. In *Medical-Surgical Nursing,* 2d ed., edited by S. Lewis and I. Collier. New York: McGraw-Hill.

Elster, S.E. 1987. Coronary artery disease and congestive heart failure. In *Medical-Surgical Nursing,* 2d ed., edited by S. Lewis and I. Collier. New York: McGraw-Hill.

Ettinger, W. and M. Davis. 1990. Osteoarthritis. In *Principles of Geriatric Medicine and Gerontology,* 2d ed., edited by W.R. Hazzard, R. Anders, E. Bierman and J. Blass. New York: McGraw-Hill.

Felder, R. 1990. Oral diseases. In *Geriatric Medicine,* 2d ed, edited by C. Cassel, D. Riesenberg, L. Sorensen and J. Walsh. New York: Springer-Verlag.

Frohlich, E. 1990. Hypertension. In *Geriatric Medicine,* 2d ed, edited by C. Cassel, D. Riesenberg, L. Sorensen and J. Walsh. New York: Springer-Verlag.

Gregerman, R.I. 1990. Thyroid diseases. In *Principles of Geriatric Medicine and Gerontology,* 2d ed., edited by W.R. Hazzard, R. Anders, E. Bierman and J. Blass. New York: McGraw-Hill.

Haponik, E. 1990. Disordered sleep in the elderly. In *Principles of Geriatric Medicine and Gerontology,* 2d ed., edited by W.R. Hazzard, R. Anders, E. Bierman and J. Blass. New York: McGraw-Hill.

Irvine, P.W. 1990. Patterns of disease: The challenge of multiple illness. In *Principles of Geriatric Medicine and Gerontology,* 2d ed., edited by W.R. Hazzard, R. Anders, E. Bierman and J. Blass. New York: McGraw-Hill.

Kain, C., N. Reilly and E. Schultz. 1990. The older adult: A comparative assessment. *Nursing Clinics of North America* 25(4):833–848.

Lee, M. and J. Walsh. 1990. Hematology. In *Geriatric Medicine,* 2d ed, edited by C. Cassel, D. Riesenberg, L. Sorensen and J. Walsh. New York: Springer-Verlag.

Lipschitz, D. 1990a. Anemia in the elderly. In *Principles of Geriatric Medicine and Gerontology,* 2nd ed., edited by W.R. Hazzard, R. Anders, E. Bierman and J. Blass. New York: McGraw-Hill.

Lipschitz, D. 1990b. Aging of the hematopoietic system. In *Principles of Geriatric Medicine and Gerontology,* 2d ed., edited by W.R. Hazzard, R. Anders, E. Bierman and J. Blass. New York: McGraw-Hill.

Morris, J.F. 1990. Pulmonary diseases. In *Geriatric Medicine,* 2d ed, edited by C. Cassel, D. Riesenberg, L. Sorensen and J. Walsh. New York: Springer-Verlag.

Nelson, J. and D. Castell. 1990b. Gastroenterology. In *Geriatric Medicine,* 2d ed, edited by C. Cassel, D. Riesenberg, L. Sorensen and J. Walsh. New York: Springer-Verlag.

Nelson, J. and D. Castell. 1990. Aging of the gastrointestinal system. In *Principles of Geriatric Medicine and Gerontology,* 2d ed., edited by W.R. Hazzard, R. Anders, E. Bierman and J. Blass. New York: McGraw-Hill.

Norwood, T. 1990. Cellular aging. In *Geriatric Medicine,* 2d ed, edited by C. Cassel, D. Riesenberg, L. Sorensen and J. Walsh. New York: Springer-Verlag.

Payne, R. and G. Pasternak. 1990. Pain and pain management. In *Geriatric Medicine,* 2d ed, edited by C. Cassel, D. Riesenberg, L. Sorensen and J. Walsh. New York: Springer-Verlag.

Perlmutter, M. and E. Hall. 1985. *Adult Development and Aging.* New York: John Wiley and Sons.

Poirier, J. and C. Finch. 1990. Neurochemistry of the aging human brain. In *Principles of Geriatric Medicine and Gerontology,* 2d ed., edited by W.R.

Hazzard, R. Anders, E. Bierman and J. Blass. New York: McGraw-Hill.

Power, C. and V. Hachinski. 1990. Stroke in the elderly. In *Principles of Geriatric Medicine and Gerontology,* 2d ed., edited by W.R. Hazzard, R. Anders, E. Bierman and J. Blass. New York: McGraw-Hill.

Rich, L.F. 1990. Ophthalmology. In *Geriatric Medicine,* 2d ed, edited by C. Cassel, D. Riesenberg, L. Sorensen and J. Walsh. New York: Springer-Verlag.

Shock, N.W. 1984. Energy metabolism, caloric intake and physical activity of the aging. In *Normal Human Aging: The Baltimore Longitudinal Study of Aging*, edited by N. Shock. Washington, DC: NIH Publication.

Skidmore-Roth, L. 1988. *Mosby's Nursing Drug Reference*. St. Louis: C.V. Mosby Company.

Walker, S.N. and C.W. Love. 1987. Nursing role in management: Postoperative client. In *Medical-Surgical Nursing,* 2d ed., edited by S. Lewis and I. Collier. New York: McGraw-Hill.

Wenger, N. 1990. Cardiovascular disease. In *Geriatric Medicine,* 2d ed, edited by C. Cassel, D. Riesenberg, L. Sorensen and J. Walsh. New York: Springer-Verlag.

4 Psychosocial Changes

Kathy Ryals Simpson
Jeanette Lancaster

CHAPTER OUTLINE

FOCUS

Several major social theories of aging are presented in this chapter. Some of the psychosocial changes of aging relate to social role changes, reaction time, performance, sensory acuity, intelligence, learning, problem solving, memory, motivation, attitudes, interests, values, self-concept, and personality. Understanding these common changes is important when caring for older adults.

OBJECTIVES

1. Analyze five social theories of aging.

2. Identify common social role changes in later life.

3. Evaluate the reasons for myths related to older adults.

4. Discuss cognitive changes that occur during the aging process.

5. Explain how intelligence, learning, problem solving, and memory change in old age.

6. Evaluate whether or not personality changes as one ages.

7. Discuss how the environment affects the older person's psychosocial functioning.

8. Devise nursing interventions appropriate for the psychosocial changes in older persons.

Since the 1950s, social and technologic changes have occurred at a faster pace than ever before in recorded history. Possibly the older population is affected by rapid change more than people at any other stage in the developmental cycle. Although modern medical advances have significantly increased the life span of the American citizen, change, stress, increased urbanization, and rapid technologic advances have taken their toll on older people. Psychosocial changes associated with older adulthood can present challenging and demanding tasks. Because of these changes, older people must adapt to new and often stress-producing situations at a time in life when the capacity for adaptability and adjustment is already diminished. Continuous exposure to circumstances that require adjustment as well as the cumulative effect of multiple stress situations over an extended period of time may militate against effective psychosocial adjustment.

There is widespread debate concerning the causes of psychosocial changes in older adults. Some researchers contend that the physiologic alterations that occur during the aging process, such as the decreased supply of oxygen to the cells caused by the arteriosclerotic narrowing of vessels, lead to perceptual and behavioral changes. Other researchers stated that behavioral changes may result from an inability to cope with multiple losses sustained as a result of the aging process (Brocklehurst 1985; Hampton 1992).

Despite the fact that some psychosocial changes occur as one grows older, for most adults aging is a positive experience and a rewarding part of the life cycle. Because aging is considered extremely complex and variable, it must be discussed with a multidisciplinary perspective. This perspective helps incorporate the influence of physiological, social, emotional, and environmental factors on aging and helps one focus on the uniqueness of the individual person.

MULTIDISCIPLINARY VIEW OF AGING

Because aging is a highly complex and variable process, it must be viewed from many different perspectives to explain behavioral changes. Birren and Cunningham (1985) stated that people age along three dimensions: biologic, psychologic, and social. Biologic aging refers to physical changes and is often viewed as the extent to which individuals have "used up" their biologic potential. A person's psychologic age is defined by the level of adaptive capacities that are operational. The capacity to adapt to the environment depends on the accuracy as well as the speed of perception, memory, learning, and reasoning ability; self-image; motivation; and drives. A person's social age can be defined by the different social roles that are assumed.

To be able to age successfully along these three dimensions requires constant adaptation to the environment. In general each person must fulfill basic needs:

- physiologic parameters, such as oxygen, food, fluid, temperature, rest, sleep, and elimination

- safety

- a sense of individuality and a recognition of one's own worth

- a sense of belonging and being valued by others

- a feeling of purpose

- a sense that life is worthwhile

These basic needs are often particularly difficult for the older person to attain because of physiologic deficits, the status of the elderly in society, and the presence of myths that stereotype the aging process. Physiologic deficits are relative to specific cognitive aspects of psychosocial aging such as thinking, memory, and reasoning that affect psychosocial adaptation. Status, social values, and myths influence the public's view of aging.

SOCIAL THEORIES OF AGING

A number of social theories have been developed to investigate the phenomenon of aging. Cummings (1976) proposed that normal aging is a "mutual withdrawal" between the aging individual and society and postulated that this *disengagement* is a universal phenomenon that occurs in all cultures.

The *activity* theory was developed in opposition to the disengagement theory and implies that adjustment to aging is the ability to maintain the activity level of middle age (Atchley 1991). The older person continues middle-aged roles or develops "useful" new roles in order to remain socially and psychologically fit (Berghorn et al. 1978). A longitudinal study conducted by Duke University researchers seems to confirm this theory as it demonstrated that when activities remain high or increase, life satisfaction remains high or increases (Palmore 1969).

The *continuity* theory, which does not share a developmental perspective, was built on the assumption that people wish to maintain a familiar pattern of living throughout life. However, a person could decide to modify these patterns in any direction (Berghorn et al. 1978). In other words the active young person is more apt to become an active old person, and the shy, withdrawn young person is more apt to become a disengaged elderly person. Atchley pointed out that this theory also encompasses the complex interrelationships between biologic and psychologic changes.

Another theory to be discussed is that of aging as a subculture. Rose (1976) projected that significant trends of American society favor conditions under which the older population may develop a subculture, although all older people will not participate. A subculture develops when any group within a society interacts with its own members more than it interacts with people outside the group. This type of selective interaction occurs when either one of two sets of circumstances is present. According to Rose, one set of circumstances is "that the members have a positive affinity for each other on some basis," and the other is that "the members are excluded from interactions with other groups in the population to some significant extent" (48–49). Both sets of circumstances are true for many of the elderly in this society. The trend toward age-segregated housing tends to intensify these circumstances.

One of the more recent social theories proposed by Lawton (1982) is that of the interrelationship of the person with the environment. This theory looks at the demand from the environment that is most advantageous for the older person's functioning level. The environment has a much greater impact as a person's functioning level declines (Miller 1990).

These various theories demonstrate the difficulty encountered in studying any human phenomenon or in working with any one person. The interrelationship of numerous variables makes it almost imperative that any study dealing with human behavior be multivariable. The nurse is consistently reminded of the social, physical, emotional, and psychologic problems that arise while working with older people. No other age group offers the nurse such challenges, frustrations, and rewards.

AGING: STATUS AND ROLE CHANGES

The attainment of a sense of purpose during the later stages of life is often difficult for the aging person. Certain life events frequently occur during this developmental phase. For example, retirement and subsequent economic penalties for earning more than a minimal amount while receiving retirement benefits can decrease self-esteem and generate a high degree of stress (Neuhs 1990). Moreover, the older person's sense of purpose and worth may be damaged by the ostracism to which one is subjected by younger members of society. The young feel threatened by the inevitability of aging and its apparent obstacles to meeting goals. Younger people seem not to realize that goals can be modified successfully as physiologic resources change with age.

Additionally, loss of friends or spouse due to death can significantly alter the older person's position and status in society. Dependency, depression, economic difficulties, and changes in relationships with married children and other friends can be a result of widowhood (Porcino 1985; Miller 1990).

Relocation, another common life event for older individuals, can also significantly affect psychosocial adjustment. Even when relocation is desirable, stress is experienced and individuals can have difficulties with social status and self-worth (Ebersole 1990).

Snyder, Pyrek, and Smith (1976, 491) contended that the mental impairment and subsequent alterations in behavior observed in older adults are the result of a "complex and interacting relationship of biological, psychological, social, and environmental factors." They stated that the behaviors ascribed to older adults can be traced to two sets of circumstances. First, because society expects older people to show decreased physiologic and psychologic functioning, the subsequent behavior evidenced by the elderly may be due to their acceptance of the socially assigned role. Second, older people respond inappropriately to environmental cues because of impaired hearing and sight rather than diminished intelligence. Appropriate behavioral responses depend largely on accurate interpretation of environmental stimuli.

In planning nursing measures, the likelihood of faulty perception by older people must be considered. Actions such as verifying with patients what was heard or seen can reduce the incidence of behavior that is an inappropriate response to a stimulus.

Also, nurses should constantly seek to maintain optimal functioning among older adults by counteracting the common misconception that people who have reached the age of 65 years automatically become inept. It is important for nurses to expect the older person to be able to perform a variety of activities. All too often, health care institutions encourage more dependency than is indicated by the older person's physical or psychologic status. Patients should be allowed and encouraged to do for themselves all that they are capable of doing. The key is careful assessment to determine each patient's maximum capability.

The diminishing opportunities to make decisions, to choose how and by whom they will be taken care of, and the lack of options as to the services they will use promote a sense of isolation among older people. As they become less active, older adults tend to feel apathetic and useless because they are so seldom called upon to be of help and service to others. Nursing practice must accept the challenge to keep older people as active and responsible for themselves as possible.

Myths Related to Aging

It is especially important to understand the psychosocial changes that occur during the aging process, because many of these changes are greatly exaggerated by mythical beliefs. Most of the myths, stereotypes, and prejudices that surround the concept of aging deal with psychosocial adaptation, e.g., the supposed mental rigidity of old age, declining intelligence, lack of a capacity to learn and profit from one's own experiences, and an overall impression that all older people are "senile."

Myths and stereotypes about aging are particularly rampant in language and humor. Terms like "old coot," "old goat," "dirty old man," "silly old biddy," as well as adages such as "you can't teach an old dog new tricks" influence thinking about this age group.

The very word *aging* elicits a complex set of images, including grey and thinning hair, wrinkles, stooped posture, slow gait, and forgetfulness (French 1990). One firmly held myth states that older persons are resistant to change and cannot learn new concepts (Butler and Lewis 1982).

Stereotypic images of aging are detrimental both to the people who hold these views and to those subjected to them, in that they increase both the alienation between the generations and the societal fear of growing old (Butler and Lewis 1982). The attitudes that nurses hold toward older adults often influence the performance level of patients.

Social Value

Although some changes are part of the physiologic aging process, many others can be prevented by modifying the environment as well as by strengthening the coping capacity of the person. The interaction between physical and psychosocial changes should not be underestimated. Many older people appear mentally inept because of physiologic deficits that appear as psychologic impairments. For example, *sensory blurring* due to diminished acuity in the perception of environmental stimuli results in decreased sensitivity to light, noise, odor, and pain. Older people may appear withdrawn when in actuality they have not seen, heard, smelled, or felt the stimulus.

Since the American public has an image of aging that includes psychosocial impairment, the role expectations of both older people and those who interact with them perpetuate this image. The social climate in which older people behave has an appreciable effect on their performance. Several aspects of the environment influence the behavior of the elderly, so that it becomes a self-fulfilling prophesy. These people are expected to have difficulty remembering, thinking, and taking care of themselves generally, so they become inclined to live up to the role expectations of those around them (Labouvie-Vief 1985; French 1990).

Socially accepted standards of everyday performance are lowered dramatically as retirement approaches. Even more important, reinforcement of and rewards for successful role performance decrease once a person is no longer sought out for advice and responded to as a sexually attractive person. Nursing research has a fertile field in the whole area of social demands and societal recognition in relation to factors such as self-esteem and anxiety.

Stress

Stress affects the quality of an individual's interaction with the environment by impairing the person's ability to perceive cues accurately and respond appropriately. High levels of stress tend to make it difficult to see all aspects of a situation clearly. Excessive stress can accelerate the aging process because "it may lead to physical disease which manifests as or interacts with aging to increase degeneration" (Eisdorfer and Wilkie 1977, 251).

Stress occurs as a result of demands, either internal or external, placed on the individual that tax or exceed available resources (Whitbourne 1985). The stimuli that elicit a stress response are often unfamiliar, unexpected, and rapidly changing. Also, whether any given stimulus is perceived as stressful depends on the environmental context in which it occurs. That is, a person's resources, such as past experiences in handling stress, support systems, perceptual acuity, intelligence, and ability to think clearly and logically, as well as personality and general state of health, influence the amount of stress perceived. Frequently observed sources of stress for older adults include rapid changes that require an immediate reaction, changes in lifestyle resulting from retirement or physical incapacity, acute or chronic illness, loss of loved ones, financial hardships, and a generalized lack of purpose in life (Ebersole and Hess 1990).

Behavioral responses to stress include erratic performance rates, malcoordination, increased errors, fatigue, and repetitive behavioral actions. Specifically, stress is suggested as a key precipitating factor in problem drinking and drug abuse among older adults. Loneliness, isolation, and the feelings aroused by the loss of capabilities, people, and objects all cause a stress reaction. Older persons, like people in all stages of the life cycle, often use drugs in an attempt to cope with stress. The most common form of drug dependence in older persons is alcoholism. See chapter 10 for further discussion of alcohol abuse in older adults.

In general, the more physiologically disabled an older person is, or the greater the perception of his or her lowered social status, the more susceptible that person will be to stresses and assaults from the external environment. While a concerted societal effort is necessary to offset the environmental stressors for the aging population, nurses who work in the community as well as those who work in institutional settings must meet a special challenge to prevent these undue stresses on older adults. For example, community health nurses have the opportunity to educate families and other caregivers in ways to diminish the impact of stressors on the older person. Relatives may be unaware that older persons are often less able to process rapid sensory stimulation.

COGNITIVE/PSYCHOSOCIAL CHANGES DURING THE AGING PROCESS

It is important to remember that although certain behavioral patterns are common to the aging process, there are also wide individual differences in the psychosocial concomitants of this developmental stage. Social status, religious beliefs, and cultural, economic, educational, and intellectual differences influence psychosocial adaptation. One of the most important functions of any organism is the ability to interact with both its internal and external environments. Effective interaction with the environment depends largely on the ability to receive accurate information from sensory receptors located at specific nerve endings in the eyes, ears, skin, and muscles.

The principal point to keep in mind when discussing psychosocial changes that occur with aging is the marked variability among individuals. Aging is a highly individual process that results in great diversity among older persons. Thus generalizations about changes in psychosocial function with aging are extremely difficult to make. Significant changes in personality do not occur with normal aging. Changes that do occur in behavioral patterns frequently are the result of physical, socioeconomic, or cultural factors (Shock 1984).

Reaction Time

With aging comes a general slowing of a person's response to sensory stimuli. The mechanism that accounts for this slowing of reaction time is poorly understood. One approach is to explain reaction time in terms of systems theory. In this framework, sensory input commences the process. The information is then processed: understanding the content of the information, integrating this understanding into the person's mind, making a decision about it, sending signals that activate muscles, and then executing actions to produce sensory system output. Psychomotor performance is affected by a weakness at any point in this chain of events. In working with older people, it is important to accept their slower pace and help them appreciate the need to proceed at a slower speed to avoid both physical injuries and the psychologic impact of feeling inadequate.

Generally, reaction time slows with age, but it is important to note that there is an increase in variability among individuals in their speed of performance with advancing age (Welford 1984). Reaction time is affected not only by the stimulus itself but by the interrelationships of perception, memory, movement, and choice. Other factors that influence reaction time include motivation, familiarity with the task, amount of extraneous stimulation that distracts from understanding the primary stimulus, and the degree of comfort the person feels in the surroundings.

It is helpful to simplify the context in which a reaction by the older person is expected. For example, if a person is being taught a new procedure or task, environmental distractions, such as noise from radios, television, or conversations, should be minimized or totally avoided. Also, new material is most easily learned in a familiar setting where the client has only to respond to the teaching-learning activity and is not distracted by an unfamiliar environment. The pace of any teaching experience should be geared to the client's rate of absorption of the information. The person must hear, comprehend, process, and react to the incoming stimuli. Processing and the subsequent reaction are more efficient when incoming information is limited in quantity and when a minimal amount of entirely new information is introduced at any given time. It is important to assess whether learning has occurred through astute observation of the client's reaction and to pace the next step in the teaching-learning activity. Facial expressions such as frowns, grimaces, or quiet mumblings may indicate that the client is having difficulty in learning at the pace at which information is being given.

Performance Capacities

Although one of the most prominent characteristics of aging is an overall slowing down of performance, this feature is not limited to the population over 65 years of age. A professional football player is old after 30 years of age; parents react more slowly than their young children. Thus slowing down actually begins early in life; it merely becomes exaggerated and thereby more noticeable in the older population.

Declining performance has several causes. It involves a decreasing efficiency in the sensory processes; the central nervous system processes stimuli less efficiently, resulting in a slower response time. Not only is processing time increased in the older person, but efficiency and ultimately accuracy are also affected. Processed information received from the environment is poorer both in quality and intensity. In facing complex tasks, the older person tends to work more slowly and carefully and may divide the task into smaller units that can be dealt with in a sequential fashion. In planning nursing actions, older adults need to alter the pace of task completion. Hurrying an older person causes frustration and subsequent ineffectiveness in performance.

Perception refers to a person's ability to receive a stimulus as well as to register and process the information (Weinberg 1976). People are not passive receivers of information, but they actively organize and process the information received as stimuli from the environment and subsequently discharge information back into the environment in response. Perceptual activity occurs at the psychologic points of contact between a person and the internal and external environments. "Sensory, cognitive, motor, conceptual and affective processes are all linked with one another in any given perceptual act" (Weinberg 1976, 8). Changes in perception influence behavior more directly than do changes in sensation. While structural and sensory changes can be adjusted or adapted to, the way in which the central nervous system organizes incoming data is considerably more fixed.

Perception is the way in which verbal and nonverbal communication and other environmental stimuli are intellectually comprehended, experienced through the senses, and understood by the recipient. Each person receives information from the environment based on a unique frame of reference that is determined by past experiences, capabilities, quality of the sense organs, attitudes, biases, and cultural, religious, and social beliefs. In nursing interventions the clarity of the older person's perception of the event should be carefully assessed. The nurse might receive either verbal or nonverbal cues indicating that the older person has perceived the situation quite differently from the way it was meant or the way it actually occurred. The nurse must consistently be alert for the reactions of fear, doubt, skepticism, or hurt that are signals of the client's perceptual inaccuracy. If there seem to be any ambiguities in meaning, the nurse should ask the patient what he or she heard or thought had happened. If the patient's perception differs from that of the nurse, it is helpful to review the situation to clarify this misperception.

Older people commonly fear the unknown. They tend to be anxious in the face of new situations because they are not sure they can assess the situation accurately and react in socially acceptable ways. Nurses must be constantly watchful for signs of fear and anxiety, because each of these emotions interferes with performance by altering the perception of and concentration on the present event.

Sensory Acuity

Although alterations in sensory acuity are physiologic in nature, they influence the psychosocial mechanisms that help maintain homeostasis by reducing or distorting the information available for processing by the person. Cognitive aspects of functioning such as thinking, intelligence, problem-solving ability, communication, and, to some degree, self-image are influenced by the quality of sensory acuity and can greatly alter psychosocial adaptation. Decisions and subsequent actions that are based on a less-than-comprehensive store of information are generally either doomed to failure or have less-than-optimally productive outcomes. When people make decisions based on incomplete information, they may be subject to criticism from the people around them; such criticism may reinforce an already poor self-image. Refer to chapters 3 and 6 for more detail on sensory changes.

Intelligence

Intelligence is difficult to define and to measure. Some say it is the ability to "communicate, understand, care for oneself" (Eisdorfer 1977, 212). It is also described as "a person's capacity to acquire and utilize information for the purpose of reaching some appropriate goal" (Eisdorfer 1977, 212). One difficulty in measuring intelligence is that the "slice of life" being observed may not be typical of the person's ordinary behavior.

Age and Intelligence

Measured intelligence has been shown to be a function of many independent factors, both endogenous and exogenous, with cohort effects and health status probably of greater significance than chronologic age (Woods and Britton 1985). The average physically and mentally healthy older person does not usually show signs of decreased intelligence. Rather, decreased mental functioning is related to health status, especially to vascular diseases that affect the cerebral cortex and diminish the brain's capacity to store information (Schawnkhaus 1991).

Presently there are no completely satisfactory ways of assessing normal aging changes in cognitive function. The main concern is to distinguish between changes that reflect a maturational process and those that are attributed to environmental or cohort influences (Woods and Britton 1985).

In general two types of study methodologies have yielded discrepant results. Cross-sectional measurements compare different age segments in the population simultaneously. The major criticism of this method is that it compares differences between groups of people rather than examining changes in one group of individuals over time (longitudinal study). Since it is impossible to match subjects accurately in each group, cross-sectional research is generally considered less valid than longitudinal studies. One weakness of longitudinal studies is the extremely high attrition rate seen in the older population. Individuals who do persevere and are available for frequent retesting over a long period may differ from their general age group on factors such as motivation and health status (Birren and Cunningham 1985).

Intelligence Tests

Intelligence tests were originally developed to be used with school-age populations. Early intelligence testing for the adult population used unidimensional measures and suggested a peak in intellectual performance during the mid- to late 20s, with a progressive and steady decline into old age. Advances in research have challenged these findings, and the greatest need has been to develop valid and reliable tests specifically suited for the older population (Woods and Britton 1985). Many factors must be considered in evaluating the results of intelligence tests given to an older population. First, the administration technique may need to be modified for this population. The older person's attitude toward the test may affect the results, since people in this age group often approach the test with less confidence and more apprehension than younger people. Frequently an older person views the testing situation as a measure of memory and begins to worry about test performance, becomes anxious and tense, and subsequently may "block" on many questions that would present no difficulty under less stressful conditions.

A number of factors besides anxiety and fear of poor performance may interfere with accurate test results; among them are fatigue, short attention span, hearing difficulties, and visual impairment. Moreover, the slower response time of older persons may make it necessary to decelerate the testing format, repeat instructions, allow frequent rest periods, and provide opportunities for questions and clarification. Older people also tend to perform more efficiently when they are not timed; time limits increase stress and may lead an older test subject to withhold answers. Another factor may be that older individuals attempt to cope with physical and social changes brought on by the aging process and do not choose to expend energy on psychometric tests that are not useful to their current situation (Woods and Britton 1985).

In general, decline in most cognitive abilities does not begin until age 65 or later. These declines are generally on measurements of speed performance, problem-solving abilities, or organizational skills (Labouvie-Vief 1985). Individual differences account for a large variability in intellectual change. Verbal abilities, vocabulary, and comprehension remain in accord with those of younger individuals well into the seventh decade (Woods and Britton 1985).

The accuracy of any one test for an aging population is open to debate. The Wechsler Adult Intelligence Scale (WAIS) is the most popular tool available for assessing age-related changes in intelligence. An age factor has been incorporated into the WAIS score to make scores between old and young persons comparable. Despite this correction factor older people tend to score lower than younger people. Critics of the WAIS claim that the test is biased—it measures a knowledge of material currently being taught in the educational system.

Nurses can develop new techniques for providing care for older clients by using the information gained from the performance of this age group on intelligence tests. The setting, timing, type of test, and procedure in administering the test can be evaluated to establish a workable format for intelligence testing in this population. For example, older patients perform more thoroughly and have better command of their cognitive processes when they do not perceive a time limitation. Deadlines, time parameters, and a general feeling of being rushed interfere with the older person's effective functioning. It is helpful for nurses to convey the feeling that they have patience and that there are no deadlines when they work with older persons.

Although in reality many nurse-patient situations are characterized by a lack of time, the nurse should keep such pressures from affecting the client's performance. Also, since older persons become fatigued more easily than young ones, scheduling of activities is critical. Morning hours for procedures, treatments, and activities are the most desirable, although certainly not everything of importance can be accomplished in the morning. Rest periods can be built into the day's activities so that the client can replenish energy and proceed with tasks and activities later in the day. Nursing research can address the variables that affect the measurement of intelligence in the older population.

Learning

It is exceedingly difficult to assess whether learning capacities are directly affected by aging because of the number and complexity of the interrelations evident in the learning process. Health, reaction time, and motivation influence a person's ability to learn, as does the older person's hesitancy to become involved in too many "new things" at once. According to Arenberg (1983, 42), evidence suggests that "performance in memory and learning decline in late life even on tests where speed is not a factor." Small increments of age-related decline in learning occur even in healthy, well-educated individuals. These declines, however, occur very late in life with a wide margin for individual variability. Differences in learning capacity are frequently thought to be due to external factors, such as motivation, attitudes, perception, and situational components.

Older people learn better when they can pace learning so as to monitor both the rate and amount of incoming stimuli. They tend to be cautious and hesitant in new learning situations and commit omission errors rather than performance errors, reflecting a need to be certain of the outcome of their activities before acting. Further, older people are motivated to learn and become engaged in activities that they find meaningful; they tend not to do well in learning tasks they judge to be irrelevant or unnecessary.

Kim and Grier (1981) studied whether slowing the pace of medication teaching would decrease the number of response errors and increase the gain from pretest to posttest. Their results indicated that slowing the pace of speaking from 159 to 106 words did significantly increase the gain derived from the instruction and decreased the number of errors in responding to questions during the instruction. In a later study on response time and health care learning of older patients, Kim (1986) found that older people being given nutrition instruction responded more effectively to self-paced learning situations than to either slow- or fast-paced response conditions.

Rendon et al. (1986) encouraged nurses when teaching older clients to remember not only to take into account possible changes in vision and hearing, but also to provide a nondistracting environment and to present learning experiences in a calm way. The nurse needs to convey optimistic expectancy and create an environment in which the client feels capable of suc-

cess, free to take risks, and ready to learn new tasks.

Organizational skills tend to decline in older age, which can greatly affect one's ability to learn new concepts. Presentation rate can also affect the ability of the older individual to learn. Major deficits in learning can be observed in the older population if the presented material is given rapidly. Arenberg (1983) suggests that research should be directed toward development of mnemonics and other learning tools designed specifically for the learning deficits of the older population.

The whole subject of learning among older persons offers a rich arena for nursing research. Further, the outcome of any research on learning among an older population would provide valuable data to be used in directing patient care of this population. For example, research is needed to determine the conditions under which learning takes place most effectively in the older population. Older people find themselves facing many new learning situations in dealing with the health problems they encounter in old age. After cerebrovascular accidents, patients must often relearn many basic skills, long taken for granted. It is important to know the most effective method for teaching such patients. It seems probable that a slow pace, much repetition, minimal stress, and a great deal of support and encouragement provide the most effective stimuli for relearning. Yet little research has been done to confirm these theories.

It is also important to determine if learning among the elderly is influenced by each person's basic personality. Do extroverts learn more readily and with less stress than quieter, more introverted people? Or is the reverse true? Also, is learning among older people in any way related to self-esteem? It seems probable that self-confident people feel less threatened in a situation that requires new learning, since their self-concept may be less affected by failure in the learning experience than that of people with a more fragile self-view.

Problem Solving

An older person attacks a problem differently from a younger one in that, instead of progressing rapidly from start to finish, the older person tends to refer back to previous experiences in search of solutions to the current problem. People in this older age group adopt a literal rather than a hypothetical approach to problem solving. If they cannot draw on past experience for solutions to current problems, the situation presents an overwhelming challenge. It is believed that older people have increasing difficulty in problem solving because of their inefficiency in organizing complex material, in their short-term memory, and in making fine discriminations among multiple stimuli.

The elderly are more cautious in problem-solving situations, thus taking more time for these tasks. They are less willing to take risks and less likely to change strategies even when their responses are incorrect (Reese and Rodeheaver 1985). Problems tend to be solved by using solutions that previously were successful in similar situations. Additionally, information overload affects the ability of older individuals to perform complex problem solving; therefore, directions for learning should be guided carefully (Arenberg 1983).

Nursing actions should reflect a careful assessment of each client's ability to solve problems. If the client seems overwhelmed by stimuli in a complex situation, the nurse can break the problem down into small, manageable parts and assist the client in handling each part in sequence until the client has dealt with the entire problem. The nurse may also offer alternative routes to solving the problem. The older person many be better equipped intellectually to select from a limited number of alternatives than to devise his or her own solution to a problem that may first seem exceedingly complex and frightening. The nurse should try to convey the feeling that "I will see you through this task [problem-solving]." With this kind of support, older people may be better able to use their own resources.

Memory

Studies have shown that age-related changes in memory do occur, but decline in function is highly variable and, in general, results in minimal impairment. Memory is usually divided into immediate, recent, and remote categories (La Rue 1982). Immediate memory involves recollection over a period of a few seconds and is frequently tested by asking patients to repeat a string of digits. This function is rarely impaired significantly by aging. Remote memory is defined as recall of items learned many years earlier. This function also remains unimpaired

in the normal elderly. Recent memory, which is recall of items presented more than a few minutes earlier, is generally reduced in older people. Also, this memory function may decline due to physiologic or psychologic influences. In a person with mild impairment of recent memory who is able to function normally in daily life, a physiologic stress such as hypoxemia, or even a psychologic stress such as death of a loved one, can result in severe loss of memory capacity. Finally, the elderly often have difficulty transferring data from immediate or short-term memory to long-term memory for later retrieval.

Remote memory is involved in reminiscing. Contrary to popular opinion, empirical studies have demonstrated that older persons do not engage in thinking about the past appreciably more than they think about the present. However, reminiscing can be a valuable source of information for completing a nursing assessment of an older person. As discussed in the section on personality, older people are not greatly different in personality, habits, emotions, and values than when they were younger. By encouraging an older person to talk about past experiences, interests, and worries, as well as previously successful ways of coping, valuable information may be gained upon which to base nursing actions.

It is often less threatening to talk about emotionally charged topics by reminiscing than by talking about them in the present tense. For example, a discussion about losses that occurred at an earlier stage of life could easily lead to a discussion about current losses and the subsequent feelings of depression, anger, guilt, or fear. Also, a description of previously enjoyed activities can either lead to an elaboration of how these activities might be modified for current use or to alternative activities that might provide similar gratification. Not only does reminiscing provide information about the older person, it often contributes to a feeling of self-worth as the person reveals things accomplished in the past (Butler and Lewis 1982).

Regarding remote memory, people tend to remember best those things that were particularly important to them. Such items, laid down in youth when neuronal functioning is at its peak efficiency and frequently used over the years, are more likely to be preserved.

Older people typically consult health providers

about their failing memory, particularly their difficulty in remembering names of people, especially new acquaintances. An older person may state, "I can remember clearly what happened when I was a kid, but for the life of me I can't remember what I did last Thursday." Other older people forget events momentarily but later have good recall. These occurrences are described as "benign senescent forgetfulness" and are nearly universal among older populations (Miller 1990). The older individual should be assured that these changes are normal and do not progress to severe memory deficits.

Suggestions for assisting older adults to effectively utilize their memory functions include slowing the pace of new learning, providing opportunities for the learner to practice the new activity, and repeating demonstrations of the new activity. Such a step-by-step exercise for learning is particularly useful in teaching treatment techniques or self-medication procedures. For example, if the nurse is teaching a newly diagnosed diabetic how to self-administer insulin, the demonstration should be carried out slowly, with preciseness of action. The nurse should ask the older person to "walk through" the procedure verbally—after a careful nursing demonstration—to determine the level of comprehension at this stage of the teaching-learning session. If the verbal step-by-step description of the activity is accurate, the patient could then demonstrate to the nurse the insulin-injection procedure. If inaccuracies are detected through the verbal technique, the nurse should repeat the procedure and again move from a verbal trial to demonstration. Visual tools, including posters, handouts, and other audiovisual materials may augment learning by enhancing memory. These should be designed with large block letters and appropriate yellow-orange colors with attention given to decrease glare (Jinks and Baker 1986).

The pace of presentation of any teaching-learning activity must be slower than the nurse might use with other population groups. Older learners usually require more time to comprehend materials presented due to a decline in the use of organizational strategies (Craik and Rabinowitz 1985). Thus if material is grouped or categorized and presented in an organized fashion, learning is enhanced. Because recent memory is more likely to be impaired than remote memory, the nurse can provide the patient with clues that will nudge the memory without calling attention to the forgetfulness. For example, if the older person is attempting to remember the date of a past appointment, the nurse might verbally "walk" the patient through the activities of the past few days in order to stimulate recall of the specific events. Also, it is important to avoid putting the older person "on the spot" by pressing for answers to specific questions that the client has forgotten. It is particularly crucial to avoid emphasizing the client's memory deficits in front of other people; such public exposure may have a devastating impact on the client's feelings of self-esteem.

Motivation

Motivational changes that occur during the aging process can greatly affect the performance of older people. Recent literature suggests that older individuals are most deficient in learning tasks that are not meaningful to their situation, and least deficient or not deficient at all in learning meaningful tasks related to everyday life (Ebersole and Hess 1990). This means that older individuals are better motivated to achieve when the goal is made explicit and has meaning for them. The older person is also frequently motivated by a fear of failure as shown by taking less risks and being cautious when making decisions.

Older people should be allowed to pace their own activities and should be encouraged and supported but not coerced into activities that seem repugnant or fearful to them. Many older people hesitate to try a new activity. Encouragement, an offer to do the activity with the client, and support throughout the attempt are all helpful, but the crucial point is to assess accurately where encouragement stops and coercion begins. When the client seems genuinely fearful of the new activity—most often because of a fear of failure and subsequent embarrassment—and if a discussion of the fear and hesitation does not alleviate the client's fears, another activity should be considered.

Attitudes, Interests, and Values

Attitudes, values, and interests tend to remain fairly constant throughout the life cycle. Differences observed in the older population are not necessarily due to aging but to cultural variations between this generation and the current younger population.

Differences in values, interests, and attitudes are much more likely to be influenced by social class, occupation, geographic region, religious background, and ethnic characteristics. Consider the person who is currently over 65 years of age. This person has seen enormous social and technologic changes and has lived through two world wars as well as the harshness of a national depression. A person in this age group may especially value security, a home of his or her own, and the comfort of knowing that a warm meal will be provided daily. Younger people who have always had these needs met may take them for granted.

It is not easy to change attitudes or values. In general, change is most readily accomplished in knowledge, followed by attitudinal change and lastly by behavioral changes. Thus teaching-learning activities directed toward providing new information rather than toward altering attitudes and beliefs might be most effective. It is important to respect the attitudes and beliefs of clients, different as they may be from one's own. Of equal importance is the challenge to try to understand the values and beliefs that underlie the decisions upon which the behaviors of older persons are formed. Such understanding comes from observation, questioning, and astute listening both to what the person says and to what is obviously omitted from conversation.

Self-Concept

The self-concept or self-image consists of what a person thinks and feels about self. These attitudes and opinions form an abstraction recognized as *me*. The self-image includes physical and psychosocial appraisals. Each person has both positive and negative assessments of self as a physical being as well as an emotional and interactional person.

The self-image of the older person is determined by a combination of factors, including interactions with significant others during early growth and developmental stages, past experiences, and the nature of current interactions. The significance of a positive feeling of self-worth should not be underestimated. Adler (1924) emphasized this point in his early writings, when he stated that low self-esteem represents the central problem of mentally ill persons. Adler viewed humans as social animals whose life task is primarily one of finding a place in the social group.

A sense of belonging and being valued is essential to social and emotional well-being. Not belonging to any group represents for most people a lonely existence.

According to Labenne and Green (1969), what people believe about themselves is related to their interpretation of the reactions of others. No one can ever know exactly how others see him or her; one infers how others think and feel by evaluating their behavior toward one. Self-concept then depends to some extent on what people think others think about them.

A positive self-concept is one of the greatest assets a person can have. People who think well of themselves have more resources for coping with problems of everyday living, since self-esteem has a profound effect on thinking processes, emotions, desires, values, goals, and behavior.

Self-esteem is related to the social self according to two sets of information available to people: task-specific self-esteem and socially influenced self-esteem (Korman 1970). A person attains task-specific self-esteem by a feeling of success, a sense of accomplishment in a given activity. Older people are seldom afforded opportunities to complete a task because a younger person can do it faster, with less effort, and less methodically. Also, the older person may be unfamiliar with the items necessary for task completion, because these might have been developed since the older person routinely performed the task. Nursing intervention to promote task-specific self-esteem begins by providing the older person with an opportunity to complete a meaningful task, by making certain that all the necessary tools and materials are readily available, and that directions, if any, are clearly explained or easily readable.

Socially influenced self-esteem refers to how well an individual meets the expectations of others. When others think a person is competent in a particular role (such as friend, relative, citizen, or group member) and communicates that evaluation to the person, socially influenced self-esteem is high. All too often older people are forced by social pressure into a "sick role." They are expected by society to be incompetent, inadequate, and useless (Labouvie-Vief 1985).

Older people often experience alterations in self-concept because of acute or chronic illness; changes in their physical, social, or economic environment; the death of a spouse or pet; or even the temporary loss of an appliance such as eyeglasses or a hearing aid (Harris 1986). Interventions to increase self-esteem include adding a pet, which can provide unconditional acceptance to the person; encouraging the older person to become a community volunteer, such as in a hospital, with children through work in day-care centers, or as foster grandparents; and through special employment, such as in retail stores offering part-time opportunities for older adults.

It is incumbent upon nurses working with older people to support a positive self-concept. If a patient suffers from low self-esteem and feelings of worthlessness, nursing efforts should be directed at motivating the older person toward gaining a positive self-view through experiences that encourage the older person to feel capable and valued. Both task-specific and socially influenced self-esteem nursing interventions can serve a motivating function. Attention should be focused on providing an environment in which older persons can socialize with other people who have similar interests and in which they can experience the positive reinforcement of accomplishment.

For example, in the hospital or nursing home older people can be encouraged to spend time with others who have similar hobbies or past career interests, who are from the same geographic area, or who are from similar ethnic or religious backgrounds. This certainly does not mean that older people only enjoy the companionship of others in the same age group. Their interests and attitudes may be more compatible with people who are considerably younger. Thus the nurse who uses an accurate assessment of individual client differences can help increase socially influenced self-esteem by introducing patients to compatible groups of people. In nursing homes the choice of age group is generally limited, but this does not negate the importance of helping older people meet others with similar interests.

Older people who live in their own homes can be interviewed to ascertain their interests, their favorite groups (past as well as present), and their church or club affiliations, so as to encourage their current involvement or introduce them to new areas for social interaction. Some older people have little interest in activities outside their homes. In this instance the nurse can encourage the patient and others who live in the home to expect the older person to contribute to the maintenance of the household. Such daily involvement reinforces older people's feelings that they are needed and valued members of the family. For example, one older woman had worked in a laundry during her earlier years. When she moved in with her daughter's family, she assumed the responsibility for the family laundry. She laundered many items by hand that clearly could have been cleaned more efficiently in the washing machine. It was often difficult for the daughter to stand by and watch her mother "slave" over the laundry, yet the mother obviously believed that no machine could do as satisfactory a job as she could by hand. She felt that she was an invaluable asset to the family.

Personality

Personality is one of the most difficult psychologic variables to measure, define, and categorize (Shock 1984). Personality is a product of a person's heredity and environment and constitutes the person's own unique way of perceiving, thinking, acting, and feeling. Many of the concepts previously discussed—such as motivation, self-esteem, attitudes, and values—are integral components of inner personality; whereas its outward dimensions are determined by the characteristics each person presents to the world.

Personality and aging are interrelated in a variety of ways. In general an individual's personality is a key variable in determining reactions to aging. Personal losses and the need to adapt are inherent aspects of aging. How well people cope with the losses, crises, and the many changes that accompany advancing age is related to how well they coped during earlier developmental stages. Although some personality characteristics may change through aging, it has been shown that major personality traits remain relatively stable over time (Schulz 1985). How a person copes at any given time is more similar to his or her own personality patterns than to those of peers of the same age.

Behavioral responses may become more exaggerated and obvious in older people, but they bear a resemblance to each person's previous mode of coping. Older people face the heightened stressors of diminishing biologic resources and the simultaneous losses of friends, family, or income that influence their coping patterns. Because of their diminished abilities in reaction time, learning capability, and perception, many older people become introverted and conservative. Fearing their inability to complete a task or activity with their usual skill, they hesitate to become involved, thus avoiding possible failure.

Thus although personality in general remains the same, the impact of multiple stressors and psychosocial changes cannot be overestimated. An older person may seem fearful and anxious out of proportion to the situation. Nursing action should be directed toward assessing past coping mechanisms and then determining the total scope of the current stress situation. If a person reacted to crises during middle age by crying, he or she will probably respond similarly during the older years. However, it is still important to determine exactly what the stressors are. Earlier coping mechanisms may not prove sufficient in the face of cumulative stressors. The nurse is responsible to discover how the older client handled stress in previous years by asking directly or talking with family and friends and also by looking at the total impact of the stressors on the person.

ENVIRONMENTAL IMPAIRMENT IN OLDER ADULTS

The declining efficiency of the senses in older adults creates an overall effect that is much subtler and often more difficult to deal with than with the result of each specific sensory deficit. Older people are simply less aware of what is going on both within and around them than they once were. At any specific time most younger and middle-aged people are aware of a specific task, such as reading a book, as well as a variety of distractions in their environment, such as the radio, other people talking, the telephone, or television. People older than 60 years have fewer resources available to deal with environmental stimuli, since they must focus most of their attention on the primary task at hand. With aging, one's field of awareness narrows and the periphery fades, making it difficult to be aware of more than the focal stimulus.

Each person's environment is formed by the physical surroundings, rules, and other people nearby. For people with diminished physical or mental capacity the type and quality of the environment is important. With declining visual and auditory capabilities and impaired reaction time, new environmental situations create special challenges often accompanied by stress and anxiety.

An understanding of the older person's lack of adaptability to the environment helps explain the often-noted tendency of the elderly to appear preoccupied. Their attention is focused almost totally on the task at hand to the exclusion of all other environmental stimuli. Thus older people appear forgetful and rigid in their behavior, when in truth it is not so much that their mental processes are crippled as they just have less energy available to focus on subtle environmental cues.

Because of the decline of sensory and perceptual functions with advancing age fewer environmental stimuli are intercepted, with a consequent risk of maladaptive behavior that is simply due to diminished cues to assist in the determination of situationally relevant actions (Weinstein and Ventry 1982). Faulty perception of the surroundings may elicit inappropriate and poorly timed cues to the stimuli and may precipitate behavior that appears to result from disordered thinking. For example, an older patient may not be able to discriminate between a urinal and a water pitcher, since both items have a similar shape and are usually of the same or a similar color. Also, a male patient who awakens in the middle of the night in a hospital or nursing home may mistake a white porcelain water fountain for a urinal in the bathroom. Such behavior could easily be classified as "senility" rather than a misperception caused by poor vision.

Special attention must be given to the environment of older patients in hospitals and nursing homes to help them maintain optimal functioning and mental health. Each person needs some personal space, such as a cabinet, closet, night stand, or favorite chair. Older people need to participate in deciding how the space will be arranged, e.g., where the chair and night stand will be placed. Such participation in decision making helps to offset such detrimental effects of institutionalization as a feeling of powerlessness. Patients also need to keep a few personal items nearby to make the setting seem more familiar and comfortable.

Lighting is especially important for optimal visual acuity as well as for safety. Light can affect mood, orientation, and functional ability. Although fluorescent lighting is efficient and has a low operating cost, it tends to cause glare and eyestrain. It is often difficult to provide satisfactory lighting in institutional settings, since many rooms have multiple uses, such as for meals, crafts, and social events. Often overhead lighting can be supplemented by table lamps during social events.

NURSING INTERVENTIONS THAT PROMOTE PSYCHOSOCIAL ADAPTATION

To promote positive psychosocial adaptation for the older client, it is crucial for the nurse to counteract the stereotypes and myths that abound regarding the older person. It is important to give older people the opportunity to be productive and to take care of themselves as well as others, lest psychologic decline become a self-fulfilling prophecy. For example, when people are expected to be unable to care for themselves or anyone else, they begin to live up to these expectations and do only what seems mandated by their role as an "older person." The nurse should evaluate the capabilities and particular interests of each older person carefully and give each one responsibilities that are meaningful and in keeping with his or her ability.

Careful interviewing can elicit a wealth of information about the person's past interests, work patterns, hobbies, and choices of social outlets. Such preferences do not tend to change with age; rather, the actual involvement in the preferred activities may decline quantitatively. The nurse can use this information to involve the client in responsible activities in the hospital, home, or community setting. For example, if the client had previously been an avid jigsaw puzzles fan, the nurse could provide puzzles whose pieces are of a size consistent with the person's visual ability. After a puzzle has been assembled, the older person could glue it together to form a wall hanging that might be used as a gift for another person or as a decoration in the hospital, home, or agency.

The nurse can generally make alterations in the environment so as to increase the sensory acuity and perception of older adults. Lack of sensory acuity causes alienation from the environment. Older people often have difficulty reading fine print, doing handiwork, or assembling projects that have minute parts. Darkness also tends to reduce visual acuity and increase confusion. A night light is particularly helpful in maintaining orientation to the environment.

Healthy mental functioning is defined as the ability to respond to stimuli appropriately in terms of both content and emotional reaction on an ongoing basis. It is essential in working with an older population to recognize that to demonstrate appropriate behavior, older people must be able to interpret and understand the stimuli received from the environment. Sensory decline, especially vision and hearing losses, contributes significantly to a decrease in perception to stimuli and can cause inappropriate responses (Hampton 1991). Hearing loss due to degeneration of the central and peripheral auditory mechanisms as well as increased rigidity of the basilar membrane often leads to personality changes. Behavior such as suspiciousness, irritability, and paranoid thinking may result from defective hearing; the older person may hear mumblings instead of distinct speech. Inaudible messages may be interpreted as "they are always talking about me." The person may become fearful and withdraw further from the environment. Few older people have the courage to confront those who seem to be mumbling for fear of ostracism and possible rejection.

It is important to orient the patient carefully to new activities or expectations. In addition it is essential that the nurse listen carefully to the older person and the family to pick up cues as to the degree of comprehension. In giving instructions and support, the use of touch is helpful.

The cognitive and emotional needs of older adults can be met in a variety of ways. Clear, concise communication, demonstrations, and written instructions increase understanding of current procedures and events. Before any procedure is taught, the purpose of and necessity for the procedure should be explained in understandable language. Instructions should be given in small units for easy assimilation, and practice opportunities should be incorporated into any teaching-learning situation. It is necessary to give the older person ample time to respond and to ask questions. All contacts with the older person should reflect respect and encouragement for client independence.

The older person's self-esteem and feelings of competence can be supported by encouraging the person to maintain as much control as possible over his or her own life and to participate, whenever opportunities are available, in decision making. It is important to assess the client's competency continuously and carefully, so that he or she can make accurate choices. The older person should not be given more information than needed; the implication is that the older person is inadequate or incompetent.

As role relationships change with aging, self-esteem can decrease. When such societal roles as parent, spouse, worker, and housekeeper shrink, older people often assume a new role characterized by ambiguity. There is not a clear-cut and easily definable social role for "retiree" or "older person."

Since the social role at this developmental stage is blurred and the elderly cannot rely on past experiences to help determine current expectations, they become especially dependent on external cues to maintain a feeling of worth and as a gauge for role conformity. These cues often imply that the older person is indeed not valued. Society tends to expect older people to be cranky, slow, inept, and hard of hearing. Nurses often reinforce such worthless feelings by doing things for patients that they could do themselves with little or no help. Many older people can bathe themselves, keep their homes or hospital space clean, and feed themselves. Unfortunately, the older person is often rewarded by smiles and praise for meeting the social role expectations of dependency and being "sick." How often have nurses said to an older person, "Now Mr. Jones don't do that yourself, let me help you," or even worse, "Let me do that for you"? A principle of mental health nursing holds that nurses should never do for patients what they can do for themselves. This principle can be applied to people of all ages but is especially relevant in providing care for the older adult. The nurse should not take away from any patient the right to feel competent and able to perform as many tasks as possible.

SUMMARY

The aging adult can be described as an organism slowly undergoing changes in physical resources, whose behavior is a function of the ability to adapt available resources to ever-pressing environmental demands. The changes in behavior during this phase of the developmental sequence are the responses of a less energetic, physically inefficient, although highly experienced organism attempting to cope with a world that is continually changing.

Psychosocial changes that occur in accord with the aging process are multifactorial and vary greatly among individuals. Health status, motivation, multiplicity of losses, and coping skills can contribute to behavioral changes in older adults. Additionally, societal expectations of dependency and worthlessness can lead to lowered self-esteem and eventual inadequate psychosocial adaptation.

Because of decreased efficiency in sensory processing abilities, impairments in memory (especially recent memory), and diminishing physical resources and capabilities, the older person's basic motivational stance is often geared toward simplicity of activity. Frequently the older person adopts a preference for simplicity to conserve energy by avoiding any unnecessary arousals. Also, because of diminished perceptual and sensory acuity older people prefer simplicity and familiarity, which reinforce their coping capacities and do not continually call attention to deficits. The ability to perform tasks and meet the expectations of one's social group supports self-esteem and is another reason for the preference for simplicity, economy of effort, and familiarity.

Several behavioral manifestations in the older person reflect preferences for simplicity. The first is to avoid new, complicated, or novel situations or ideas; in so doing, the person appears restrained, cautious, with narrow interests. Second, the older person may remain totally preoccupied with repeating such old, familiar behavioral patterns as performing rituals or reminiscing about the past. Such repetitive behavior tends to bring success, since the older person is totally in control. A third form of preference for simplicity involves adding structure to an essentially unstructured situation. This may be seen in the addition of unnecessary rules or absolute thinking about a subject when a number of possible variations actually exist. Nurses working with older people should appreciate their need for simplicity and realize that it assists the older client in structuring life so as to maintain maximal competence.

The personality structure of the individual seems to be the single most influential determinant in coping with aging. Personality refers to each person's unique way of perceiving and responding to life events and includes both inner and outer dimensions. Inner aspects include self-esteem, moods, values, and reactions to people and events; whereas outer aspects are essentially the face one presents to the world, be it cranky, sad, or happy. While basic personality structure certainly is an important influence in adaptation to aging, nursing interventions can reinforce the inner dimension and thereby alter its outer appearance.

The nursing actions listed here reinforce the positive aspects of inner personality functioning.

1. Avoid hurrying an older person; hurrying tends to lead to faulty performance and subsequent feelings of failure.

2. Explain all procedures slowly and carefully before asking a patient to cooperate; understanding tends to increase compliance and cooperation.

3. Maintain a calm environment; confusion and extraneous stimuli interfere with performance by overloading a system that is already working at capacity.

4. Maintain a set routine; pattern and order give the older person a sense of familiarity and certainty.

5. Talk to older people as though you expect them to understand. Use clear, concise language appropriate to their intelligence and educational level; keep in mind that there is no firm evidence that intelligence automatically decreases with age.

6. Encourage self-care; doing for a patient what he or she can do for himself or herself decreases feelings of competence and worth and increases the likelihood that the person will lose these abilities.

7. Address the older patient in a friendly manner and by the patient's choice of name; addressing an older person by a given name without being asked to do so undermines the person's feelings of competence and self-esteem.

8. Give clear, direct instructions, and use visual aids in large, bold print when appropriate (Jinks and Baker 1986).

9. Identify meaningful roles for older adults by acknowledging contributions and involvement in productive tasks.

STUDY QUESTIONS

1. Explain why it is important to understand the diversity of the older population when discussing psychosocial changes in the older adult.

2. Discuss five social theories of aging.

3. Discuss the major myths related to aging.

4. Relate ageism to psychosocial changes.

5. Explain why society's view of aging can perpetuate psychologic decline in older individuals.

6. Why is physical health an important factor to consider when assessing an older person's psychosocial status?

7. Describe some of the problems associated with current methods of testing intellectual ability in the older population.

8. Discuss two sensory changes that occur frequently with aging and that can affect the way older individuals respond to their environment.

9. Define *benign senescent forgetfulness* and explain what information should be given to the patient with this diagnosis.

10. Explain why reminiscing can frequently be an important tool for nurses to utilize in assessing older adults.

11. Describe five nursing interventions that may be useful in promoting psychosocial adaptation in the older person.

REFERENCES

Adler, A. 1924. *The Practice and Theory of Individual Psychology*. London: Kegal Paul.

Arenberg, D. 1983. Memory and learning do decline late in life. In *Aging: A Challenge to Science and Society*. Vol. 3, Behavioral Sciences and Conclusions, edited by J.E. Birren, J.A. Munnichs, H. Thomas, and M. Morois. Oxford: Oxford University Press.

Atchley, R.C. 1991. *Social Forces and Aging: An Introduction to Social Gerontology* 6th ed. Belmont, CA: Wadsworth.

Berghorn, F.J., D. Scharer, G. Steers, et al. 1978. *The Urban Elderly—A Study of Life Satisfaction.* New York: Universe Books.

Birren, J. and W. Cunningham. 1985. Research on the psychology of aging: Principles, concepts, and theory. In *Handbook of the Psychology of Aging*, edited by J.E. Birren and K.W. Schaie. New York: Van Nostrand Reinhold.

Brocklehurst, J., ed. 1985. *Textbook of Geriatric Medicine and Gerontology.* New York: Churchill Livingstone.

Butler, R. and M. Lewis 1982. *Aging and Mental Health*, 3d ed. St. Louis: C.V. Mosby.

Craik, F., and J. Rabinowitz. 1985. The effects of presentation rate and encoding takes on age-related memory deficits. *J Geront* 40(3):309–15.

Cummings, E. 1976. Further thoughts on the theory of disengagement. In *Aging in America*, edited by C. Kary and B. Manard. Van Nuys, CA: Alfred Publishing Co.

Ebersole, P. and P. Hess. 1990. *Toward Healthy Aging: Human Need and Nursing Response.* St. Louis: C.V. Mosby.

Eisdorfer, C. 1977. Intelligence and cognition in the aged. In *Behavior and Adaptation in Late Life.* 2d ed., edited by Busse, E.W. and R. Pfeiffer. Boston: Little, Brown and Co.

Eisdorfer, C. and F. Wilkie. 1977. Stress, disease, aging, and behavior. In *Handbook of the Psychology of Aging*, edited by J.E. Birren and K.W. Schaie. New York: Van Nostrand Reinhold.

French, S. 1990. Ageism. *Physiotherapy* 76 (3):178–82.

Hampton, J. 1991. *The Biology of Human Aging.* San Luis Obispo, CA: William Brown Publishers.

Harris, M. 1986. Helping the person with an altered self-image. *Geriatric Nursing* 7(2):90–92.

Jinks, M. and D. Baker. 1986. Addressing senior audiences. *Am Pharm* NS26(4):28–33.

Kim, K. 1986. Response time and health care learning of elderly patients. *Research in Nursing and Health* 9:233–39.

Kim, K.K. and M.R. Grier. 1981. Pacing effects of medication instruction for the elderly. *Journal of Gerontological Nursing* 7(8):464–68.

Korman, A.K. 1970. Toward an hypothesis of work behavior. *J Appl Psychol* 54(1):31–41.

Labenne, W. and B. Green. 1969. *Educational Implications of Self-Concept Theory.* Santa Monica, CA: Goodyear.

Labouvie-Vief, G. 1985. Intelligence and cognition. In *Handbook of the Psychology of Aging*, edited by J.E. Birren and K.W. Schaie. New York: Van Nostrand Reinhold.

La Rue, A. 1982. Memory loss and aging. *Psychiatr Clin North Am* 5(1):89–103.

Lawton, M. 1982. Competence, environmental press and the adaptation of older people. In *Aging and the Environment: Theoretical Approaches*, edited by M. Lawton, P. Windley, and T. Byerts. New York: Springer Publishing Co.

Miller, C. 1990. *Nursing Care of Older Adults: Theory and Practice.* Glenview, IL: Scott, Foresman, and Co.

Neuhs, H. 1990. Predictors of adjustment in retirement of women. In *Pre-retirement Planning for Women: Program Design and Research*, edited by C. Hays and J. Deren. New York: Springer Publishing Co.

Palmore, E. 1969. Sociological aspects of aging. In *Behavior and Adaptation in Later Life*, edited by E. Busse and E. Pfeiffer. Boston: Little, Brown and Co.

Porcino, J. 1985. Psychological aspects of aging in women. *Women and Health* 10(2/3):115–22.

Reese, H. and D. Rodeheaver. 1985. Problem solving and complex decision making. In *Handbook of the Psychology of Aging*, edited by J.E. Birren and K.W. Schaie. New York: Van Nostrand Reinhold.

Rendon, D.C., D.K. Vaid, E.D. Gioiella, and M.J. Tranzillo. 1986. The right to know: The right to be taught. *Journal of Gerontological Nursing* 12(12):33–37.

Rose, A. 1976. The subculture of the aging: A framework for research in social gerontology. In *Aging in America*, edited by C. Kary and B. Manard. Van Nuys, CA: Alfred Publishing Co.

Schulz, R. 1985. Emotion and affect. In *Handbook of the Psychology of Aging*, edited by J.E. Birren and K.W. Schaie. New York: Van Nostrand Reinhold.

Schwankhaus, J., F. Murphy, and J. Kurtzke. 1991. The aging brain. *Internal Medicine World Report* 6(19):11–15.

Shock, N. 1984. *Normal Human Aging: The Baltimore Longitudinal Study of Aging* (NIH Publication No. 84-2450). Washington, DC: United States Government Printing Office.

Snyder, L.H., J. Pyrek, and K.D Smith. 1976. Vision and mental function of the elderly. *Gerontologist* 16(6):491–95.

Weinberg, J. 1976. On adding insight to injury. *Gerontologist* 16(1):4–10.

Weinstein, B., and I. Ventry. 1982. Hearing impairment and social isolation in the elderly. J Speech Hear Res 25:592–99.

Welford, A. 1984. Between bodily changes and performance: Some possible reasons for slowing with age. *Exp Aging Res* 10(2):73–85.

Whitbourne, S. 1985. The psychological construction of the life span. In *Handbook of the Psychology of Aging*, edited by J.E. Birren and K.W. Schaie. New York: Van Nostrand Reinhold.

Woods, R., and P. Britton. 1985. Cognitive loss in old age—Myth or fact? In *Clinical Psychology with the Elderly*, edited by R.T. Woods and P.G. Britton. Rockville, MD: Aspen.

Part 3

ASSESSMENT AND RELATED INTERVENTIONS

5 HEALTH PROMOTION

Kathleen Ryan Fletcher

CHAPTER OUTLINE

FOCUS

Health is a criterion for successful aging. Certain beliefs and behaviors influence health and healthy change. This chapter will explore health promotion, disease protective client behaviors, as well as common detrimental behaviors that affect physical, psychosocial, and spiritual well-being. The nurse's role is important in facilitating clients' well-being within these domains.

OBJECTIVES

1. Discuss the efficacy of health promotion and disease protective measures as applied to an older population.

2. Describe health as a criterion for successful aging.

3. Explore beliefs and values that influence health and healthy change.

4. List federal initiatives that have generated interest in preventive health care.

5. Describe the constituents of physical, psychosocial, and spiritual well-being.

6. Provide examples of health promotion and disease protective behaviors within the physical, psychosocial, and spiritual domains.

7. Illustrate behaviors that may jeopardize well-being.

8. Detail the role of the gerontological nurse in the area of health promotion and disease prevention with older adults.

HEALTH PROMOTION

No one disputes the merits of disease prevention and health promotion in general. Controversy arises when asked to consider the efficacy of these measures when applied to the older population. Increasing evidence suggests that making better lifestyle choices does influence health and longevity even when changes are made later in life. Health promotion involves the development of behaviors that improve the body's ability to function and enable the individual to adapt to a changing environment. Disease prevention involves actions to reduce or eliminate exposure to risks that might increase the chances that an individual or group will incur disease, disability, or premature death (Gilford 1988).

In 1900 a newborn could expect to live to be about 47 years of age. Today the average life expectancy at birth is around 75 years. The nearly thirty-year gain in longevity since the turn of the century was an unprecedented one. Demographers speculate that the gains will continue with considerably less momentum into the next millennium.

The future perspective for an older adult today appears promising. Those 65 and older can expect to live another 17 years. The individual who reaches age 85 can expect to live another 5 years. The older one lives to be, the more likely that one will live longer. Unfortunately the quantity of added time has not translated into quality. Examining the issue more closely, one might note that for the 65-year-old, only about twelve of those additional years are likely to be healthy ones, Figure 5-1.

Most of the diseases that affect older adults are lifestyle diseases. The three major causes of disability and death for those over age 65 are heart disease, cancer, and stroke. All of these conditions have been strongly linked to the behaviors of smoking, poor diet, lack of exercise, and stress. Less frequent but still significant causes of illness include influenza, pneumonia, arteriosclerosis, injuries, pulmonary disease, diabetes, and renal disease. Lifestyle behaviors often precipitate or contribute to these conditions. These disease processes have been extensively studied, yet until recently researchers examining and evaluating the effectiveness of health promotion programs on reducing the risk factors have excluded people over age 60.

The health care system has traditionally expended a disproportionate amount of time, energy, and resources focused on the diagnosis and treatment of existing diseases. In the medical community, prevention

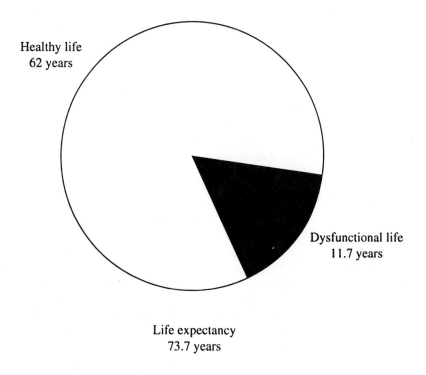

Healthy life
62 years

Dysfunctional life
11.7 years

Life expectancy
73.7 years

Figure 5–1   Years of healthy life as a proportion of life expectancy. U.S. population (1980)

Source: National Vital Statistics System and National Health Interview Survey (CDC) in *Healthy People 2000 Summary Report,* U.S. Department of Health and Human Services, Public Health Service, Boston Jones & Bartlett Publishers, 1992, p. 45

of disease has received more attention in the past few years, yet little research or clinical activity has directly addressed the older population (Lavizzo-Mourey, Day, Diserens, and Grisso 1989). Nurses have been in the forefront of health care reform in requesting a restructuring of health care services. They seek a better balance between the prevailing orientation toward illness and cure and a new commitment to wellness and care (National League for Nursing 1991). Many nurses do not perceive older people as a population that could benefit from health promotion (Kleinman 1986).

Nurses as a whole have recognized that the definition of health as the absence of disease is no longer a valid one and have accepted a more holistic orientation. The major goal of the health promotion/disease prevention approach is to identify the health problems for which preventive efforts can result in improvements in health status (Gilford 1988). Gerontological nurses need to embrace this goal with strength and enthusiasm. The time is critical and the environment is conducive.

HEALTH AND SUCCESSFUL AGING

What is successful aging and is health a necessary prerequisite? The definition of aging itself is elusive. Biologically it has been defined by some as a unidirectional programmed process of physical deterioration. Most professionals prefer to take a broader, more positive view by defining it as the sum total of all changes that occur in a living organism with the passage of time.

Conceptualizations of successful aging and of the parameters of measurement have been attempted by various disciplines over the years. In the psychosocial domain life satisfaction has been the most frequently studied dimension. Neugarten, Havighurst, and Tobin (1961), in some very early attempts to measure life satisfaction, identified the qualities of the successful older adult as zest, fortitude, resolve, enthusiasm, and optimism.

In the mid-1980s the scientists, motivated by some of the longitudinal study results, became dissatisfied with the concept of normal aging (Echevarria, Ross, Bezon, and Flow 1991). Researchers in the biological realm are now investigating the distinction between usual aging and successful aging, hoping to explore how nutrition, exercise, and stress manage-

ment interventions may influence the aging process (Rowe and Kahn 1987).

Although health is a significant factor, it may not be a prerequisite for aging successfully. With nearly 90 percent of those over age 65 suffering from chronic disease, it would appear that few individuals would even be considered candidates for mastery. Many of us know those with multiple chronic disease and significant impairment who embody a strong "but other than that" philosophy. Dr. Seuss's Everyman (1986), when having completed a battery of tests was informed that "you're in pretty good shape for the shape you are in." Perhaps it is the adaptation and adjustment to disease that is most important.

Clark and Anderson (1967) proposed that successful aging was dependent on the accomplishment of adaptive tasks, accepting one's situation and using it positively. There is no consensus on what constitutes successful aging. There appears to be as many theories as there are older persons.

HEALTH VALUES AND BELIEFS

Before it can be determined what value a person places on health, it is important to consider what health means to that individual. Self-perception of health should top the list of any assessment protocol for older adults. There are individuals who appear to be healthy, yet who constantly verbalize concern over their health status. There are other individuals with multiple complex problems who consider themselves to be healthy as long as these problems are manageable in daily life. Older people whose perception of their health state is poor are six times more likely to die than those who perceive their health as excellent (Idler and Kasl 1991).

Nursing literature is filled with clinical examples and research endeavors on the issue of noncompliance. If clients do not perceive their health to be at risk or compromised, then acceptance of nurses' advice is unlikely. The concept of noncompliance may become obsolete in a health model that focuses on client autonomy and self-choice.

The Health Belief Model (HBM) addresses four areas of beliefs that influence the adoption and maintenance of behavior change (Janz and Becker 1984). These beliefs include perceived susceptibility, perceived severity, perceived benefit, and perceived barriers.

Good health is not a strong motivator for change. Most of us prefer to believe that we are not vulnerable to poor health. We are often impelled to change when we feel ill and wish to feel better. The individual who feels well must experience the threat to future health. The older adult may not recognize the need for seeking help even if he or she is symptomatic. The person may not feel well but attributes the aches and pains to the aging process and may not believe these symptoms are changeable.

In making a choice, the individual considers the severity of the problems. The physical and social consequences of action and inaction are weighed by the individual. The threat may be clear, yet the person may not believe that a certain action will alleviate it. The perceived benefit is weighed against the potential risks, side effects, and costs. The analysis of the studies using the HBM demonstrated that the strongest influence on behavior change was the perceived barriers (Janz and Becker 1984).

Although the Health Belief Model has been tested extensively to identify the relationship of beliefs to health action in a variety of settings, it is a psychosocial model with limitations. It has not been applied to illness behaviors in later life or among those with complex health problems (Binstock and George 1990). Not all behaviors can be explained on the basis of beliefs. Some behaviors may be cultural habits, some actions are taken for social acceptance, some desired actions are doomed because of inadequate finances. Health insurance still does not reimburse for many health promotive assessments. The risks for a hazardous work or living environment may be recognized. However, the individual may not be in a position to change in order to achieve a higher level of health.

Recognition that a behavior is harmful might exist, yet the obstacles to change may be insurmountable. Access to the needed information may be limited, the individual may lack the skill and savvy to negotiate the morass of health services, and social supports for making and maintaining the change may be nonexistent. The supportive social environment may be the most important factor in changing behaviors that contribute to many leading health threats (United States Department of Health and Human Services 1991). The nurse's role in health education is a critical one and a thorough assessment of the beliefs, values, and influencing factors that determine healthy or nonhealthy behaviors need to be examined.

Studies do show that older adults are more prevention-minded than younger and middle-aged persons (Prohaska, Leventhal, Leventhal, and Keller 1985). Karp (1988) speculates that around the 50th birthday, people begin to consider their mortality and pay more attention to their health. What better opportunity could exist? Confucius noted that when the student is ready, the teacher appears. The gerontological nurse needs to be prepared; there is a growing number of older students waiting.

Prevention: Initiatives and Levels

Federal initiatives have generated a growing interest in health promotion and disease prevention by emphasizing that these measures are essential to improving the health of the nation (United States Department of Health, Education, and Welfare 1979; United States Preventive Services Task Force 1989; United States Department of Health and Human Services 1980). The initiatives all emphasize the role of the clinician and identify interventions to be taken by the professional.

The model that is used in these documents is that of levels of prevention with all the directives focusing on the first two levels. Primary prevention includes those measures taken to render a population or individual at risk for a target condition less vulnerable to it. The client is asymptomatic and lacks clinical evidence of the specific disease. The client may or may not be healthy. Secondary prevention addresses those interventions taken to detect disease early. The client remains asymptomatic yet is at risk and may have a disease that is not yet clinically apparent. Tertiary prevention deals with the diseased and symptomatic client. The clinician's activities are focused on reducing the duration and severity of the disease and preventing sequelae.

These levels of prevention are useful in considering risk and presence of acute conditions, but have limited applicability when contemplating chronic disease. Here the focus becomes disability prevention rather than disease prevention. The goal may be to reduce pain and help the individual adjust to the chronic condition. The clinician is usually trying to prevent, maintain, and modify loss of function as a result of physical, mental, or social impairment (Institute of Medicine 1990).

In a wellness model the individual assumes responsibility for his or her own health with the clinician's role primarily being that of facilitator. Table 5-1 illustrates client behaviors consistent with the previously defined levels of prevention and adds a fourth dimension that addresses chronicity.

DOMAINS OF WELL-BEING

Health concerns in the aged are multidimensional in nature and may surface in the physical, psychosocial, or spiritual domain. Pender's differentiations between health protection and health promotion serve as the framework for client behaviors and clinician intervention (Pender 1987). It is recognized that the distinctions are not always clear and that there is considerable overlap.

Physical Well-Being

Health is multifaceted. Although much attention has been focused on physical diseases, only recently has the promotion of physical well-being been addressed by health professionals. Physical systems all decline with aging, at different rates within one individual, and the processes vary considerably between individuals. Can actions be taken to modify or delay deterioration and prolong a physically functional state of well-being? Will a well-balanced moderate diet, a regular exercise program, and adequate sleep and rest make a difference in physical health? Both researchers and clients are answering these questions in the affirmative.

Pender makes a distinction between two modes of healthy behaviors (Pender 1987). Health promotion behaviors are proactive and seek to enhance a positive health state and to expand the health potential. Health protective or preventive behaviors are disease-specific and are often a response to a perceived threat to health. Certain behaviors, such as

Table 5–1   Levels of Prevention and Clients' Behavior

Level	Client Condition	Client Behavior
Primary	No disease Risk factors	Minimize stressors Risk-factors reduction Strengthen defenses
Secondary	Preclinical No symptoms	Periodic health exam Alert to early warning signs
Tertiary	Symptoms present	Seek counsel and guidance of clinician Take appropriate rehabilitative/restorative action
Quaternary	Chronic symptoms present	Main functional capacity Minimize pain Symptom control Adaptive/coping response

smoking and multiple drug usage, have been proven to be particularly damaging to physical well-being.

Exercise. Exercise is an intervention that will help maintain and enhance functional ability as chronological age increases (Blair, Kohl, Paffenberger, Clark, Cooper, and Gibbons 1989). Physiologically, exercise in older adults has a demonstrated effect on reducing declines in the respiratory, cardiovascular, and musculoskeletal systems (Schilke 1991). Functional fitness components shown to improve include cardiorespiratory endurance, muscle strength and endurance, agility, flexibility, and balance (Hopkins, Murrah, Hoeger, and Rhodes 1990). Psychological advantages for exercise performers have been documented to include stress reduction, sleep enhancement, positive mood states, improved self-image, and better cognitive functioning.

Over 60 percent of those over age 65 report getting no form of regular exercise. An exercise goal established for older Americans was an attempt to get at least 50 percent of them participating in physical activity three or more times/week for thirty minutes at a time (United States Department of Health and Human Services 1980). Dishman (1989), noted that we missed goal achievement by over 40 percent. Reluctance to exercise may stem from an overrating of the amount of daily activity that constitutes adequate exercise, an overestimation of health risks, and a perception that exercise is for the young (O'Brien and Vertinsky 1991; Johnson-Pawlson and Koshes 1985). The sedentary alternative results in a decrease in physical ability, decreased functional capacity, and a diminished sense of well-being (Fitzgerald 1985).

Prior to an exercise prescription, a detailed assessment is in order. A fitness evaluation should determine if there are health problems that contraindicate an exercise regimen. A comprehensive history and physical examination need to be conducted, as well as a determination of aerobic capacity and an evaluation of body composition, flexibility, and strength. A stress test is somewhat controversial but is indicated in those with existing coronary artery disease or risk factors for heart disease. The test should be considered in those who have previously been sedentary. The assessment should include barriers to exercise, e.g., personal lethargy, anxieties about health, fear of pain, incontinence or injury, and lack of facilities or transportation. Time, energy, and commitment to

regular exercise may be overwhelming to individuals unless a community program provides older participants with creative and self-paced participation opportunities (O'Brien and Vertinsky 1991). Motivation is a critical factor with dropout rates of 50 percent even for programs that involve short periods. The importance of a social support network has a strong association with continued efforts.

Recommended health-promoting behaviors include aerobic exercises—those that use the large muscle groups for exercise and including swimming, brisk walking, and cycling. An exercise prescription for older adults includes three days a week for twenty to thirty minutes, at 60–75 percent of the individual's maximal heart rate (mhr) that has been adjusted for older adults by subtracting age from the absolute mhr of 220 (Schilke 1991). A more moderate approach may be indicated, since this rate may be too great an expectation for many older people.

Health protective benefits have been noted with even lower-intensity exercise behaviors. These have been shown to improve flexibility and balance and minimize age-related bone loss (Morey, Cowper, Feussner, DiPasquale, Crowley, Samsa, and Sullivan 1991). Exercise facilitates weight maintenance, improves bone mineral content, and reduces fracture risk. Regular physical activity combats hypokinesis, the disease of inactivity.

Risk-taking behaviors include attempting to do too much too soon. Begin with warm-ups—stretching decreases risk of injury and probability of dysarrhythmia. Cool-downs take longer with older adults (over ten minutes) to allow circulatory adaptation. Clients should gradually work up to avoid overdoing it. They should stop if they become breathless, if the heart pounds after ten minutes, or if joint pains last over two hours or persist. The clients should stop immediately if they experience dizziness, chest pain or pressure, or fainting (Simpson 1986).

Nutrition. Favorable nutritional status throughout life can increase life expectancy (Institute of Medicine 1990). It has been estimated that 30 percent of noninstitutionalized older persons have a deficit in at least one important dietary nutrient. The highest risk is among those persons living alone in high rise housing or rural areas, females, alcoholics, and those with inadequate incomes (Forciea 1989). Most common dietary inadequacies are found in the total caloric intake, protein, water, the B vitamins, thiamine, folate, vitamins C and D, and calcium (Gupta, Dworkin, and Gambert 1988).

Estimating the prevalence of nutritional disorders has been difficult especially among those most advanced in years. The two National Health and Nutrition Examination Surveys conducted by the National Center for Health Statistics in the early and late 1970s did not collect data on individuals over 74 years of age (Murphy, Davis, Neuhaus, and Lein 1990). There are no RDAs established specifically for this group. The 1989 RDA standards are inclusive of all persons over age 50.

Total energy requirements decline with age primarily as a result of a decrease in physical activity, but also because the basal metabolic rate slows over time. Most older persons adjust total calories accordingly but not always appropriately. The caloric composition and distribution among protein, fat, and carbohydrate categories along with the assurance of adequate intake of essential nutrients are most important.

Although there is a documented decline in lean body mass with age, the dietary intake should remain consistent at 1g/kg of body weight or 12–14 percent of the total energy intake. Dietary protein intake needs to be high enough to minimize the age-related loss of skeletal muscle (Carter 1991).

Sufficient fat—at least 10 percent and no more than 30 percent—is required to allow an adequate intake of fat-soluble vitamins and the essential fatty acids. The fats should primarily be unsaturated ones. The remaining energy intake—about 60 percent—should come in the form of complex carbohydrates rather than the simple type. There is no absolute established here, but in the absence of carbohydrates fatty acids are incompletely oxidized leading to ketosis, which may cause lethargy and depression (Carter 1991).

Nutritional assessment includes more than just intake of nutrients. A comprehensive assessment includes checking the adequacy of intake, eating patterns, eating function, food supply, food storage

Table 5–2   Signs and Symptoms of Nutritional Deficiencies

Nutritional Deficiencies	Signs and Symptoms
Protein-calorie malnutrition	Low body weight, decreased subcutaneous fat, pallor and fatigue, temporal wasting, dermatitis, and edema
Vitamin deficiency:	
B1 (Thiamin)	Anorexia, malaise, leg weakness, burning feet syndrome, sluggish or absent reflexes, palpitations, heart failure
B2 (Riboflavin)	Cheilosis, angular stomatitis, misty vision with burning eyes, excessive hair loss
B3 (Niacin)	Depression and mood changes, irritability and forgetfulness, peripheral neuropathy, altered reflexes, spinal ataxia, easily fatigued
Folic Acid	Anorexia, irritability, forgetfulness, paranoid behavior
C (Ascorbic Acid)	Loss of energy, spontaneous bruising, arthralgia, gingivitis, bleeding gums

Nutritional Deficiencies	Signs and Symptoms
A	Poor night vision, dermatitis
B12	Glossitis, neurologic changes
Mineral deficiency:	
Calcium/phosphorus	Aches and pains, repeated fractures
Zinc	Loss of taste and smell, excessive hair loss, impaired night vision, poor wound healing, anorexia
Fluoride	Dental caries

Adapted from K. Gupta, B. Dworkin and S. Gambert. 1988. Common nutritional disorders in the elderly: Typical manifestations. *Geriatrics* 43(Feb):87–97

and preparation, use of dietary supplements, physical activity, smoking, alcohol, medications, and socio-economic conditions. A clinical nutritional assessment examines the signs and symptoms of deficiencies (Table 5-2); takes anthropometric measurements, such as weight, stature, and skinfolds; and at times may include hematological and biochemical analysis.

Nutritional guidance should focus on maintaining adequate energy intakes with the selection of foods from the high nutrient density types. Nutritional programs must target the most vulnerable groups including women, the oldest-old (85 years and up), persons in poor health, persons on weight loss diets, and those with inadequate money for food (Murphy et al. 1990).

Health-promoting behaviors include assuring that caloric intake is adjusted for age, level of activity, and the decreases in metabolic rate and muscle mass. A properly balanced diet assures that protein sources are adequate but not excessive, that fat is confined to less than 30 percent of the total caloric intake, and that complex carbohydrates are the largest percentage of a diet that includes few refined carbohydrates. Oral health is essential to reducing dental decay and periodontal disease that can alter dietary intake. Exercise is important to preserve lean body mass, increase the resting metabolic rate, and increase energy expenditure.

Health-protecting behaviors include maintaining weight (or reducing/gaining as needed). Higher body weight increases the risk of heart disease and diabetes and puts greater pressure on joints. Lower body weight causes higher risk for hip fracture.

Nutritional composition should include a moderate cholesterol intake (300 mg/day or less) with elevations causing increases in heart disease and deficiencies, increases in cancers and hemorrhagic strokes. Fiber intake is optimal at a level of 25–35 g/day since colonic cancer is lower in those with higher fiber content. Adequate fiber from a variety of sources including fruits, vegetables, legumes, and grains is effective in decreasing the symptoms of constipation and diverticulosis. Fluid intake maintained at 2 liters/day helps preserve bodily functions and prevent dehydration. Although the requirement for calcium intake is controversial, the RDAs suggest a minimum of 800 mg/day to prevent osteoporosis.

There are several risk-taking behaviors to assess and address in this group. One is fast weight loss. In a diet with less than 1200 calories intake per day, an older person is unable to meet the RDAs. Obesity is a common problem among the population as a whole as well as the older age group. Those who are 40 percent or more above their ideal body weight suffer an increased risk for carcinoma. Obesity aggravates the problems of diabetes, hypertension, and osteoporosis, as well as having a negative impact on the individual's functional ability.

High alcohol intake is particularly risky in that it advances nutrient deficiencies (especially thiamine and niacin) and damages organs and tissues essential to nutrient absorption and utilization. The alcoholic has less appetite and ability to eat.

Drug usage increases the risk of drug nutrient interaction. Drugs can alter the appetite and the senses of taste and smell and cause gastrointestinal side effects. Nutritional supplements are rarely considered as drugs by the client and are often overlooked during the assessment by the health professional. Many older adults take vitamin and mineral supplements that can potentiate side effects when used with other drugs. Some vitamins are toxic when taken in larger doses. In excess, vitamin E can lead to liver damage, vitamin C can interfere with B12 absorption and increase renal calculi, and high doses of vitamin D with calcium can promote hypercalcemia (Gupta et al. 1988).

Poor oral health has a profound impact on the adequacy of nutrition, and nutritional intake has a significant impact on healthy teeth. Teeth (or well-fitting dentures) are required to chew properly. Diets that are high in sticky, fermentable carbohydrates increase the risk of dental caries.

Sleep. Sleep is a restorative process, a time for cell growth and repair. Little is known about the benefits of sleep; considerably more is known about what happens with the lack of sleep. Sleep deprivation results in increased irritability, a heightened pain sensitivity, decreased daytime alertness, and lethargy. The average person will spend about one-third of a lifetime asleep. However, the amount of time needed for this process varies considerably—some individuals need four hours of sleep a night, others need twelve.

Nearly one-half of all older adults have difficulty sleeping. The most common complaint is insomnia (difficulty falling asleep, staying asleep, waking too early), although hypersomnia also occurs with more frequency in this age group. Sleep changes that are influenced by the aging process can be compounded by sleep fragmentation—disturbances occurring with certain pathological and iatrogenic conditions, Table 5-3.

Table 5–3   Sleep Disturbances in Older Adults

Influences	Potential Effect
Physiological	Increased number of awakenings Less deep sleep Decrease in total sleep time
Pathological	Nocturia Sleep apnea Periodic leg movements Pain Gastric secretions
Iatrogenic	Medications (such as beta blockers, tricyclic antidepressants, diuretics, antiParkinson's drugs
Psychological	Dementia Depression Bereavement Anxiety Relocation

Sleep assessment involves eliciting the sleep history, bedtime routines, and description of the sleeping environment. Sleep patterns should be identified and examined for the number of awakenings; the time taken to fall asleep; total time slept; and the number, length, and time of naps (Schirmer 1983). A sleep log that is completed immediately upon awakening may be a useful adjunct. The practitioner should attempt to detect physical or psychological symptoms that may potentiate sleep disturbance.

Health-promoting behaviors include maintaining regular routines and habits. Regular times for going to bed and for getting up are sleep supportive. Johnson's study (1991) confirmed that consistent presleep activities can enhance sleep. A warm and quiet environment with a supportive, comfortable bed can facilitate the sleep process. The presleep mood is important and relaxation techniques such as meditation, muscle tension/release exercises, stretching exercises, and prayer may help reduce tension and provide comfort. Tryptophan, an ingredient in milk, increases the level of brain serotonin and may be sleep inducive. Naps have not been demonstrated to affect nighttime sleep pattern and they can have a therapeutic effect (Hayden 1985). Sleep restriction—confining the time spent in bed to time asleep only—has been shown to reduce insomnia (Friedman, Bliwise, Yesavage, and Salom 1991). Exercise during the day may promote nighttime sleep.

Sleep-protective behaviors are important for those with underlying conditions that potentially interfere with sleep. Giving an analgesic just prior to bed may prevent the awakening from pain; taking the diuretic earlier in the day or giving the antiParkinson's or antidepressant drug at bedtime may improve sleep as well as the disorder.

Risky behaviors include taking stimulants or experiencing stimulating activities just prior to sleep. This might include eating a heavy meal, drinking caffeine or alcohol, smoking, exercising, or having an emotionally arousing experience. Older adults are the highest consumers of sleep medications; estimates that around 15 percent of noninstitutionalized and about 35 percent of those in institutions use them (Morgan 1987). The short-acting benzodiazepines have replaced the more habit-forming barbiturates as the treatment of choice. But most of these drugs loose sleep-promoting properties within 3–14 days (Morgan 1987). Rebound insomnia occurs when they are discontinued. Because older adults excrete them less efficiently, they can have a hangover effect and the residual drug may impact on daytime behavior.

The periodic health examination. The annual physical examination with routine screening diagnostics may not always be appropriate in the asymptomatic individual. Because of the physiological and psychological changes with aging, the prevalence of disease at different ages, and the natural history of disease some screening activities might be appropriately scheduled at regular intervals for older persons (Gallo, Reichel, and Anderson 1988). The periodic health examination provides the clinician the opportunity to determine the client's perception of health status, assess the client's multidimensional level of well-being, detect early signs of disease, and reinforce positive promoting and protecting behaviors. Educating the client about those actions that might further promote health status and those that are detrimental to it is imperative. If the periodic exam is done in the home, it further permits the clinic to evaluate the social context in which the client resides and any hazards in the environment. Preventive services should not be limited to the periodic examination but rather incorporated into the episodic visit as well. Any time the client accesses the health care system, even a cursory review of systems can facilitate the search for unreported illness; the process may provide some potential teachable moments.

The frequency and the content of the periodic health evaluation need to be individualized. Older people are not a homogeneous group. The priority for health promotion and disease prevention may be quite different for each older person. The frail, old woman with end-stage lung disease and debilitating arthritis may not achieve the benefit of an uncomfortable Pap smear. However, for the healthy, independently functioning woman it may make a significant difference in mortality. All individuals, regardless of age and state of health, have an optimal level of well-being. Preventive services must be established for each person. The leading causes of morbidity and mortality in the age group cohort can help to establish a priority. Guidelines based on such a prioritized method have been established by the United States Preventive Services Task Force (1989), Table 5-4.

Table 5–4   Guidelines for Health Evaluation—Ages 65 and Over

Leading Causes of Death

Heart disease

Cerebrovascular disease

Obstructive lung disease

Pneumonia/influenza

Lung cancer

Colorectal cancer

SCREENING

History

Prior symptoms of transient ischemic attack

Dietary intake

Physical activity

Tobacco/alcohol/drug use

Functional status at home

Physical Exam

Height and weight

Blood pressure

Visual acuity

Hearing and hearing aids

Clinical breast exam[1]

HIGH-RISK GROUPS

Auscultation for carotid bruits *(HR1)*

Complete skin exam *(HR2)*

Complete oral cavity exam *(HR3)*

COUNSELING

Diet and Exercise

Fat (especially fat), cholesterol, complex carbohydrates, fiber, sodium, calcium[3]

Caloric balance

Selection of exercise program

Substance Use

Tobacco cessation

Alcohol and other drugs:

Limiting alcohol consumption

Driving/other dangerous activities while under the influence

Treatment for abuse

Injury Prevention

Prevention of falls

Safety belts

Smoke detector

OTHER PREVENTIVE SERVICES

Immunizations

Tetanus-diptheria (TD booster)[5]

Influenza vaccine[1]

Pneumococcal vaccine

HIGH-RISK GROUPS

Hepatitis B vaccine *(HR16)*

This list of preventive services is not exhaustive. It reflects only those topics reviewed by the United States Preventive Services Task Force. Clinicians may wish to add other preventive services on a routine basis and after considering the patient's ongoing medical history and other individual circumstances.* Examples of target conditions not specifically examined by the Task Force include:

• Chronic obstructive pulmonary disease

• Hepatobiliary disease

• Bladder cancer

SCREENING	COUNSELING	OTHER PREVENTIVE SERVICES
Palpation of thyroid nodules (HR4)	No smoking near bedding or upholstery	• Endometrial disease
Laboratory/Diagnostic Procedures	Monitor water heater temperature	• Travel-related illness
Nonfasting total blood cholesterol	Safety helmet	• Prescription-drug abuse
Dipstick urinalysis	**HIGH-RISK GROUPS**	• Occupational illness and injuries
Mammogram[2]	Prevention of childhood injuries (HR12)	
Thyroid function tests3		**Remain alert for:**
HIGH-RISK GROUPS	**Dental Health**	• Depression symptoms
Fasting plasma glucose (HR5)	Regular dental visits, tooth brushing,	• Suicide risk factors (HR11)
Tuberculin skin test (PPD) (HR6)	flossing	• Abnormal bereavement
Electrocardiogram (HR7)		• Changes in cognitive function
Papanicolaou smear[4] (HR8)	**Other Primary Preventive Measures**	• Medications that increase risk of falls
Fecal occult blood/Sigmoidoscopy (HR9)	Glaucoma testing by eye specialist	• Signs of physical abuse or neglect
Fecal occult blood/Colonoscopy (HR10)	**HIGH-RISK GROUPS**	• Malignant skin lesions
	Discussion of estrogen replacement	• Peripheral arterial disease
	therapy (HR13)	• Tooth decay, gingivitis, loose teeth
	Discussion of aspirin therapy (HR14)	
	Skin protection from ultraviolet light	
	(HR15)	

*The recommended schedule applies only to the periodic visit itself. The frequency of the individual preventive services listed in this table is left to clinical discretion, except as indicated in other footnotes.

[1] Annually.   [2] Every 1–2 years for women until age 75, unless pathology detected.   [3] For women.   [4] Every 1–3 years.   [5] Every 10 years.

HIGH-RISK CATEGORIES

HR1 Persons with risk factors for cerebrovascular or cardiovascular disease (e.g., hypertension, smoking, CAD, atrial fibrillation, diabetes); persons with neurologic symptoms (e.g., transient ischemic attacks) or a history of cerebrovascular disease

HR2 Persons with a family or personal history of skin cancer or clinical evidence of precursor lesions (e.g., dysplastic nevi, certain congenital nevi); persons with increased occupational or recreational exposure to sunlight

HR3 Persons with exposure to tobacco or excessive amounts of alcohol; persons with suspicious symptoms or lesions detected through self-examination

HR4 Persons with a history of upper-body irradiation

HR5 The markedly obese; persons with a family history of diabetes; women with a history of gestational diabetes

HR6 Household members of persons with tuberculosis or others at risk for close contact with the disease (e.g., staff of tuberculosis clinics, shelters for the homeless, nursing homes, substance-abuse treatment facilities, dialysis units, correctional institutions); recent immigrants or refugees from countries in which tuberculosis is common (e.g., Asia, Africa, Central and South America, Pacific Islands); migrant workers; residents of nursing homes; correctional institutions, or homeless shelters; persons with certain underlying medical disorders (e.g., HIV infection)

HR7 Men with two or more cardiac risk factors (high blood cholesterol, hypertension, cigarette smoking, diabetes mellitus, family history of CAD); men who would endanger public safety were they to experience sudden cardiac events (e.g., commercial airline pilots); sedentary or high-risk males planning to begin a vigorous exercise program

HR8 Women who have not had previously documented screenings in which smears have been consistently negative

HR9 Persons who have first-degree relatives with colorectal cancer; persons with a personal history of endometrial, ovarian, or breast cancer; persons with a previous diagnosis of inflammatory bowel disease, adenomatous polyps, or colorectal cancer

HR10 Persons with a family history of familial polyposis coli or cancer family syndrome

HR11 Recent divorce, separation, unemployment, depression, alcohol or other drug abuse, serious medical illnesses, living alone, or bereavement

HR12 Persons with children in the home or automobile

HR13 Women at increased risk for osteoporosis (e.g., Caucasian, low bone mineral content, bilateral oophorectomy before menopause or early menopause, slender build) and who are without known contraindications (e.g., history of undiagnosed vaginal bleeding, active liver disease, thromboembolic disorders, hormone-dependent cancer

HR14 Men who have risk factors for myocardial infarction (e.g., high blood cholesterol, smoking, diabetes mellitus, family history of early-onset CAD) and who lack a history of gastrointestinal or other bleeding problems, or other risk factors for bleeding or cerebral hemorrhage

HR15 Persons with increased exposure to sunlight

HR16 Homosexually active men, intravenous drug users, recipients of some blood products, or persons in health-related jobs with frequent exposure to blood or blood products

Source: United States Preventive Services Task Force. 1989. *Guide to Clinical Preventive Services:: An Assessment of the Effectiveness of 169 Interventions.* Baltimore, MD: Williams and Wilkins.

The periodic health evaluation can also be used to identify functional impairments and disability. Vision and hearing are both likely to decline with age, but the individual may not notice the decline. The annual vision screening by the clinician that checks near, distant, and side vision is simple to do. The hand-held audiometer provides an easy way to screen for hearing impairments.

The physical examination does have its limits in identifying how well a person may perform daily living tasks. For the healthy individual the physical examination may be adequate and sensitive. For the individual in whom functional impairment is suspected, a more thorough evaluation of activities of daily living and instrumental activities of daily living needs to be conducted.

The accidental death rate for those over age 65 is twice that of younger people (Young and Olson 1991). Consequently injury prevention needs to be addressed. Most accidents occur in the home; therefore a home safety determination is in order, Table 5-5.

Falls and burns are the major considerations in environmental safety. Most falls do not result in serious injury and therefore other injuries might remain undetected. The client is less likely to communicate this information voluntarily for fear that relocation to another environment may be considered. Burns are another problem. Smoke detectors should have loud sirens. Those with visual signals should be obtained for the hearing impaired. The batteries need to be replaced periodically to assure sensitivity. The decline in smell sensation can result in deficient awareness of smoke or hazardous environmental odors. The risk of immersion burns is higher in the older individual due to peripheral sensation decline. It is advanta-geous to lower the hot water temperature at the source or at least use a thermometer to check the level prior to bathing.

Regular vehicle seat-belt usage lessens the severity of injury and saves lives at all ages—the practice should be encouraged. Older adults are at higher risk of driving accidents due to changes in vision and diminished coordination.

Upon completion of the physical exam, screenings, and functional assessment, the administration of vaccines should be considered. The older adult with impaired immunological response and respiratory changes is more susceptible to pneumonia and influenza. The influenza vaccine is highly recommended for yearly administration to all those over age 65. Pneumococcal vaccine 23 valent should be given once with revaccination considered in those who received only the 14 valent vaccine (Institute of Medicine 1990). Tetanus vaccination should be given every ten years (Sims 1989).

High-Risk Behaviors. Certain behaviors are particularly damaging to the physical health of the older adult. Two of the more common ones are smoking and the use of multiple medications. Smoking is the single most important cause of premature death in the United States. It is an implicated factor in three leading causes of death in those over age 65 (Forciea 1989). There are 7 million smokers over age 60, with a particularly strong contingency among the urban poor (Remington 1985). Older adults represent a significant risk because they generally have smoked longer, smoked heavier, and often are more dependent on nicotine.

Smoking cessation is effective in reversing the damage done. Improvement in cerebral blood flow

Table 5–5 Home-Safety Evaluation

- Adequate lighting with minimal glare (for reading, night light, on stairs, entry way)
- Supportive handrails for stairs and bathroom
- Pathways clear of clutter and entanglement risk minimized
- Smoke detectors present and operational
- Hot water temperature regulated to 110–120 degrees/Fahrenheit
- Heating and cooling systems operating safely
- Kitchen safety assured

and increased pulmonary function has been demonstrated post smoking cessation (LaCroix 1991). The risk of coronary artery disease mortality declines (Hermanson, Omenn, Kronmal, and Gersh 1988), and although impact is slower, the risk of cancer also declines. In addition to quantity of life the quality of life may also improve. A recent contact with a 97-year-old by this author identified an individual who stopped smoking at age 92 because he wanted to feel better.

Stopping smoking may be more challenging to the older adult. The teachable moment may come when the client has an acute illness that is smoking related. Clinicians have preconceived ideas about the willingness of the older client and the effectiveness of withdrawal of the habit in later life. They are less likely to counsel the older adult than they are the younger adult.

Another habit of particular concern is multiple medication usage. Older adults consume the majority of drugs (both prescribed as well as over-the-counter) in this country. Nearly one-third of all their health expenditures are spent on drugs (Miller 1991). Many older persons who live independently take ten drugs a day (Stewart 1987). Compliance rates in older people are the same as with the younger group. Vestal (1984) acknowledges a form of intelligent noncompliance in which the older adult adjusts therapy to maximize the benefit and minimize the undesired effects of the drug.

Adverse drug reaction (ADR) increases as the number of medications increases and the margins for doing good and doing harm increasingly narrow with any therapeutic used in later life. ADR is an important cause of hospitalization, with over 19 percent being caused by medications available over the counter (Lavizzo-Mourey 1989). The most frequently used types of over-the-counter medications include laxatives, antacids, vitamins, and cold preparations (Boyd 1984). Guidelines for a preventive approach to therapeutics in the older age group include simplification of the regimen and education, Table 5-6.

Psychosocial Well-Being

Physical well-being is contingent upon psychosocial well-being. The environment, the social structure, and personal relationships play a critical role in development of psychosocial well-being. In later years many adjustments are necessary to assure continued health of the psyche. The older adult experiences several role changes, survives stressful life events, and strives to remain socially integrated in a time of flux.

Role changes. Roles define our relationship to the environment. This social structure helps give us definition. Self is a process of interaction between the individual and the surroundings. There are several dimensions of self. Self-concept is the cognitive part of self-perception—our views of ourselves as individuals. Self-esteem is the emotional component of self-perception and refers to the judgments that the individual makes about self (George 1990).

Does self-perception change with age or does it remain consistent? This remains unclear. However, what is more obvious is that older adults do use active strategies in an attempt to maintain self-concept. For an older person whose self-concept is based on social roles and others' expectations, role losses have a significant impact on that individual's self-esteem.

Social roles are those positions we assume in so-

Table 5–6   Strategies for Reducing the Risk of an Adverse Medication Reaction

- Simplify and individualize the regimen
- Review each visit all medications taken
- Look for potential interactions with medications and foods
- Take every opportunity to educate and inform about medication use
- Assess other factors associated with medication use: when taken, how taken, how and when refills are obtained, how containers are opened, how medications are stored

ciety for which there are certain expectations. When the work role is removed upon retirement, when the wife outlives her spouse, when the mother role is altered significantly with children living independently, rapid adjustments are required. Fortunately other roles are assumed or begin to take on greater significance. Grandparenting, volunteering, or leisure-time roles may be substituted. These generally have less status and therefore this exchange may have a negative impact on an older adult's self-esteem.

Older adults may become dependent on a societal definition of self. Cox (1988) described the labeling theory. He noted that an individual derives a concept of self from interaction with other people. With role loss and a loss of spouse and friends the older individual becomes dependent on external sources for self-identification. He/she eventually comes to accept the definition given and begins to identify with the roles and integrate them. This might be quite healthy, except that society may offer a negative label. The person particularly vulnerable is the individual with an uncertain self-concept.

Health-promoting behaviors used to facilitate role transition include anticipatory preparation. Knowing that one is about to make a change gives one time to adjust to the idea. Not all role changes can be anticipated and other strategies are used to facilitate adaptation.

Health-protective behaviors include using the past for validation. Some people look to the past to compensate for a lack of relatedness to the present (Tobin 1991). Some are able to sustain a positive image by identifying with an older-adult subculture (such as in a retirement community). The collective effort can provide some security and protection.

Role conflict and uncertainty do occur. Nurses with a focus on wellness can assist the client by encouraging anticipatory preparedness, helping the client with role identification, and encouraging the protective behaviors.

Life Transitions. As we grow older, we experience multiple changes that require us to respond and adapt. The event that is generally considered to be most stressful in life is loss of spouse. The majority of widowed Americans are women and this number will continue to grow. The average age of widowhood is 56, so a woman might expect to live an additional twenty years after the death of her spouse. This event leads to changes in lifestyle as well as daily activities.

Widowhood has been shown to have an impact on health and may precipitate death (Ferraro 1989). When the process of change has been a slower one, the individual has had time to prepare. Health-protective behaviors include enlisting the support of the social system, family, and friends who serve as a buffer.

Retirement is another life event that precipitates loss—loss of role and status in addition to loss of income. Much of who we are revolves around what we do—the work role providing us with a source of self-worth and identity. The worker who identifies with the work role strongly will feel the impact much greater than the individual whose sole reason for working is to make a living (McGoldrick 1989). Thirty percent of persons find retirement stressful. This has been associated with two predictor variables: inadequate finances and poor health (Bossde, Aldwin, Levenson, and Workman-Daniels 1991). In the past, ill health was the primary factor influencing the decision to leave the work force. The trend in the past thirty years has been towards early retirement. Less then 30 percent stay on past 65 years of age, and most of them work part-time (Cox 1988).

Health-promotion behavior when nearing retirement involves personal preparedness. Those individuals who voluntarily choose to retire adjust better than those who do not. They have more time to thoroughly assess their circumstances and prepare for the transition. Some individuals find it easier to phase themselves out of the work force. Once they are out of the work force, they establish contacts and continue relations with the work site.

Health-protective behaviors include using social supports as a buffer. Having a stable relationship with an individual who can serve as one's confidant is of major importance to successful adjustment. The employing agency can play a significant part in preparing the person for retirement, just as it prepared the individual for assuming the work role.

Those individuals at risk are those who do not choose to retire or who make the move abruptly. Lack of control and a disbelief in self-efficacy have been strongly linked to feelings of helplessness, passivity, and depression (McGoldrick 1989).

Life events are acute conditions that require adjustment. Chronic stressors may have an even greater impact on well-being. Lazarus and Folkman (1984) noted that daily hassles (more than life events) cause most stress.

Stress can be defined as body or mental tension. Excess stress can overtap resources. While mild stress can improve performance and efficiency, extreme stress impedes it. Physical and psychological health cannot be separated. There is a growing body of literature suggesting that when a person experiences multiple stresses, a serious illness will follow.

Health-promotion behaviors may include taking on some challenges and assuming some risks because a little stress is good. Health-protective behaviors include maintaining control or reattaining it as soon as possible. The individual who retains control over the situation is more likely to have a satisfactory outcome (McGoldrick 1989).

Defensive postures may be temporarily assumed in a protective manner. Some individuals project blame onto others thereby showing aggressive tendencies. Those who are nonpassive and mobile tend not to self-blame, a situation that may lead to depression (Tobin 1991). Aggressiveness is seen most often in circumstances where the individual has no control.

Some, in coping with change, need to perceive the change as ideal. This has been called magical coping or myth making. Positive mental health states may be accomplished not necessarily by an accurate appraisal of the situation but through a self-enhancing illusion (Tobin 1991).

High-risk situations occur when unexpected situations arise, when multiple stressors or events occur in a short period of time, or when the person loses control over the situation. Some common behavioral responses include loss of hope, loss of self-esteem, social isolation, loss of power to find alternatives, feelings of burden, and helpless withdrawal (Harper 1991). Tremendous amounts of emotional and physical energy are expended during grieving while adapting to change and during the recovery process.

In obtaining assessment data from older clients, especially those with complex physical problems, nurses sometimes forget to elicit or tease out the psychosocial concerns. Older adults suffer tremendous losses and fears associated with these events. They need buffers or mediators to facilitate a more healthful response.

The individual may use some behaviors to help get through a crisis. While these maybe adaptive ini-

tially, with prolonged reliance they become maladaptive. These may include repression (excluding from awareness), suppression (temporarily putting out of one's consciousness), denial (blocking out the event or feelings), counterphobia (being compelled to expose self to danger and confront it), projection (blaming others to minimize self-vulnerability), and reaction formation (rejecting real feelings and reinforcing opposite feelings to protect self from dangerous ones) (Harper 1991).

The nurse and other health care providers must recognize and understand the need to use defense mechanisms and not criticize the patient for their occasional use. The psychological treatment goal is one of obtaining insight and determining resolution possibilities with the client.

Social Integration. Older adults who perceive themselves as in control are less likely to experience depression as a result of stress (George 1990). The self as protagonist not only reacts to social structure but also shapes or creates it.

A considerable amount of time and energy is still required in daily life even without work participation. As a person ages biologically, attending to the physical demands of daily life (e.g., cooking, cleaning, and travel) takes more time (Ross 1990). Discretionary time does increase. Leisure is a defined activity chosen primarily for its own sake. It encompasses more than just filling time or busy time; it provides interaction with significant others. For many, leisure helps to define the self; in fact, it may be more of an expression of self than work was.

Some leisure activities are affiliative, some are solitary. For most older people leisure activities are primarily solitary, such as watching television, reading, or visiting with family and friends. Cultural differences exist. Ching-Sang's and Allen's (1991) work demonstrated how older black women frequently perform self-help practices and informal assistance to others. In mid-life, quiet and physical activities are balanced. In later years there is a reduction in physical exertion and activities are closer to the home base (Kelly, Steinkamp, and Kelly 1986).

Butler (1963) suggested that contemplation is a valuable form of leisure, that engaging in life review may afford the actor an opportunity to reintegrate self-concept and generate a sense of completeness. Reminiscing is a part of the life review process. Some people may have validating or positive appraisals; others have lamenting themes, such as regrets or rebukes over past events/behaviors (Kovach 1991).

A growing number of older adults are volunteering as a meaningful leisure-time experience. Older people still in the work force are more likely than retired ones to volunteer (Fischer, Mueller, and Cooper 1991). Frequently volunteerism is a pattern established earlier in life. Some studies show volunteers are less lonely and feel their work is vital to others. There is a growing number of volunteer networks, such as the Retired Senior Volunteer program (RSVP), foster grandparent programs, and senior companions. The focus within the community for these programs may be the church, senior center, or the Area Agency on Aging.

Older adults are more likely than younger people to vote and engage in other political activities (Jacobs 1990). The interest in politics grows with age. No substantive evidence shows fundamental cleavage to a particular political party. As older adults become more politically active, some concern has been raised about intergenerational equity.

Social integration appears to be a health promotive and protective activity for many. Disengagement may be appropriate for some individuals. Studies have shown, however, that the more active individual experiences more life satisfaction than the person who withdraws.

Nursing assessment involves determining the activities of interest and degree of satisfaction with involvement. The nurse needs also to identify the reasons for nonparticipation. For some older adults the transportation issue might be hindering them from involvement. Transportation options and ways of getting involved in the immediate community might be explored by the nurse. Older individuals might be encouraged to form advocacy groups to shape the future for themselves.

Evaluating the client's overall psychosocial well-being cannot be underemphasized. Older adults are not exempt from mental illness. Older adults use mental health services at about half the rate as the general population. Nurses are in a position to detect, evaluate, counsel, and refer individuals with problems. An evaluation of psychosocial functioning includes a mental status evaluation, an assessment of coping responses, and a determination of life satisfaction.

High-Risk Behaviors. Substance abuse occurs in older adults as well as younger groups. In many cases it is the prescription medication rather than the illicit drug that is taken. The most commonly abused chemical is alcohol. Surveys of use among older persons have revealed that there are two distinct groups of alcoholics: those who began to drink heavily before age 65 and those who begin in old age (Hooyman and Kiyak 1991). Those individuals who start drinking later may be reacting to age-related stressful events. The increase in leisure time and more social occasions to drink may also cause heavier intake. As a whole most older adults reduce their intake of alcohol because the desired effects are experienced with less of it.

Detection of the older alcoholic is more difficult. It becomes more of a hidden problem and is sometimes treated by family and clinician with a permissive attitude. Because the clinician is not inclined to look for it, the symptoms the client presents with may be attributed to other physical disorders and the disease is overlooked. Upon entry into a recovery program, detoxification for the older adult takes longer. The rate of relapse—about 40 percent—is consistent with the younger group.

The problem with excess alcohol is not simply that of serious organ damage. There are also other problems it may precipitate or reinforce. Alcohol may be taken in place of adequate nutrients, create safety issues from the increased potential for falls, and cause interaction with other medications the client may be taking. For the depressed patient, alcohol can exacerbate the problem. Alcohol can also interfere with sleep, impair memory, decrease muscle coordination, and disturb balance.

Nursing assessment involves being aware of the potential for alcohol abuse and then facilitating access to appropriate support services. A major preventive approach is targeting the susceptible 55- to 65-year-old population and redirecting them to more healthful coping strategies.

Spiritual Well-Being

Physical well-being refers to the health of the body systems; psychosocial well-being identifies one's relationship to self and to others. Spiritual well-being refers to one's relationship to a higher being. It is included here as a distinct domain, for as Hamner

(1990) noted, providing emotional support in a psychosocial context is not necessarily an efficacious way to respond to spiritual needs.

Spirituality is the human propensity to find meaning and purposefulness in life. This may or may not be expressed through participation in religious practices or by affiliating with a specific church. The desire for self-transcendence and increased awareness of the spiritual self seems to occur with more resolve in later life and particularly as the body, mind, and perhaps the soul show signs of failure. Religious coping behaviors were noted most frequently as the response to a stressful event (Koenig, George, and Siegler 1988; Mull, Cox, and Sullivan 1987).

In many cases as people age, they become less involved in organized religious activity and are more reliant on personal devotions. Perhaps the most influential factor is the decline in physical capacity that makes outings difficult.

With an uncertain future, perhaps the search to give life meaning and purpose takes on greater significance. Religion is not the only path to spiritual enlightenment. Some transcend self by being altruistic, seeing their needs within the context of others. Compassion may be a form of hope. Caring may not be confined to other persons; the opportunities for caring may also be found in caring for plants and animals.

Having a sense of the spiritual is obviously a contributor to well-being. Later in life, key sources of meaning in life may be compromised by the losses that occur. Faith may be questioned as one experiences suffering. As a person becomes physically less able to perform self-care, becomes socially less confident and integrated, and outlives the individuals with whom he/she was most intimate, doubts about being loved or the ability to love may arise. The spiritually intact, frail, debilitated individual is able to say, "Even though I can no longer bathe or toilet myself, I still have something vital to offer, I am worthy of dignity, respect and love" (Peterson 1985, 24).

Nurses working with older adults need to have an appreciation and understanding of the significance of the spiritual dimension. They further need to be able to assist the client in spiritual growth. Assessment instruments are not particularly useful here. The best approach is to be an active listener. Clues often emanate from older clients to the nurse who has the sense of transcendence. Nurses who feel connected with all

humans, who desire to give life, and are free to do so can be compassionate because they have the inner resources that enable them to draw upon their own spirit (Lane 1987).

Health-promotion behaviors involve moving towards self-transcendence. Self-transcendence refers broadly to a characteristic of developmental maturity whereby there is an expansion of self boundaries and an orientation towards broadened life perspectives and purposes (Reed 1991). There is a letting go to move forward. Transcending the physical boundaries may be accomplished through creative work, religious beliefs, being with nature, caring for others, or leaving a legacy (heir, documents). Potential nursing approaches may include encouraging meditation, self-reflection, visualization, religious expression, journal keeping, or volunteering.

Health-protective behaviors may involve reminiscing because memories can facilitate the health process. Attending church services and using the community as the supportive network can also protect well-being. The rituals may be stabilizing influences in a time of constant change. The nurse can be supportive by recognizing the significance of these behaviors and enabling attendance and participation. Protecting one's spiritual health requires a commitment of time alone or with others.

The nurse may not have achieved enlightenment but still can provide a great deal. The spiritual is nurtured through relationships. The nurse who becomes involved may allow exploration of the client's fears, hopes, and meanings. Nursing interventions are broad and varied. Treating all individuals with respect and dignity, trying to know the person, and becoming open to spiritual discussions can facilitate the client's well-being. Nurses cannot give people who are uncertain the prescription for meaning, purpose, hope, and love; but they can enable them to discover it for themselves.

ROLE OF THE GERONTOLOGICAL NURSE IN HEALTH PROMOTION

The goal of gerontological nursing care is to help older clients function as fully as possible by attaining their highest potential (Bahr 1987). The most recent update of the American Nurses' Association Standards and Scope of Gerontological Nursing Practice (1987) added the concepts of health promotion, health maintenance, disease prevention, and self-care to reflect the current nature of gerontological nursing practice. These concepts are not new ones. Florence Nightingale embodied these ideals. But as nurses responded to the technological advances in health care and became more affiliated with an illness model, the wellness orientation became somewhat obscured.

Nurses are beginning to identify more and more with a wellness focus. The issues are being addressed by nursing in the areas of practice, education, and research. Nurses are additionally recognizing the potential they have to contribute positively to the resolution of the health care dilemma. Central to the nursing ideal is the idea of promoting the health of all individuals.

Nursing Practice

Professional nurses have an established presence in primary care delivery of health-promotion and disease-preventive services. Nursing centers and clinics are opening. Using nursing models of health, professional nurses in these centers diagnose and treat human responses to actual and potential health problems. They also promote health and optimal functioning among target populations and communities (American Nurses' Association 1987).

A primary objective in the nursing of health promotion and disease prevention is to facilitate movement of the individual and community from a high health risk situation to a lowered health risk situation, Figure 5-2.

The primary approaches include assessment, goal setting, intervening, referring, educating, and evaluating. Assessment would include an identification of the client's current perception and state of physical, psychosocial, and spiritual well-being; a determination of promotive and protective behaviors; and a review of current behaviors and environmental circumstances that may be detrimental to health. Goals for improvements in well-being are established by the client. The emphasis is on self-care and autonomy. Nursing interventions may be identified

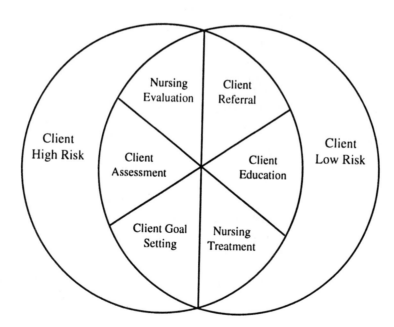

Figure 5–2   Nursing practice spproaches to health promotion and disease prevention

to resolve existing conditions that potentially impair well-being (for example, cutting toenails, removing cerumen from the ear canals). When problems or potential problems are identified that are not best accomplished by the nurse, the client is referred to appropriate community resources.

The nurse as educator enables and empowers the client to make informed decisions about health practices. Nursing has begun to focus on assisting the patient and family to develop self-care skills and coping abilities to promote a higher-level wellness (Spellbring 1991). Evaluating individual and community outcomes is another component of the practice role.

Nursing Education

Nursing texts are reflecting the change in nursing practice. Many include concepts for the promotion of health for individuals, families, and communities. Nursing educators are recognizing the growing role for nurses in this area. They are attempting to equip future nurses with the appropriate skills to function in the role of health facilitator as well as health provider.

Nursing Research

A review of gerontological nursing research reveals the absence of research on and a deficiency in nurses' orientation to health maintenance and/or promotion and disease prevention (Adams 1987). In view of the emerging role of nurses in this area the paucity of research work on which to build strategies is disconcerting. We can remain hopeful that new directions in practice will drive nursing research in health promotion and disease prevention.

SUMMARY

There is the desire of all of us for a healthy, longer life. Health, although not necessarily a prerequisite for successful aging, is an important component of it.

Many older adults have chronic diseases. The majority of these diseases are strongly linked to the lifestyle behaviors of smoking, poor diet, lack of exercise, alcohol intake, and stress. Lifestyle choices do influence health and longevity; even when better habits are elected later in life, they can result in health improvement. Older adults are more prevention-minded than younger adults. Health-promotive behaviors are proactive efforts; disease protective actions are reactive ones. Health beliefs and values do impact on choices and behaviors.

Health concerns are multidimensional and may surface in the physical, psychosocial, or spiritual domain. Physical well-being refers to the health of the body systems. Regular exercise, proper nutrition, and adequate sleep are health promotive. A periodic health examination may facilitate early disease detection and provide the clinician the opportunity to reinforce positive behaviors and identify and counsel the client about risky behaviors.

Psychosocial well-being involves one's relationship to self and others. The later years, a time of role changes and stressful life events, can result in role ambiguity and depression. Older adults who perceive themselves to be in control and those who remain socially integrated more often express life satisfaction.

Spiritual well-being refers to one's relationship to a higher being. Older persons often attribute their success in adjusting to change to a belief in God. They find solace in religious rituals. Spirituality is the human propensity to find meaning and purpose in life. Spiritual practices may also include creative work, being with nature, or caring for others.

The goal of gerontological nursing is to help clients function as fully as possible and achieve a maximal level of well-being. Nurses have addressed the issue of client wellness through practice, education, and research. Using models of health, clinics are opening in which professional nurses are diagnosing and treating health problems while promoting health and function. Nursing educators are teaching future nurses how to be health facilitators in addition to health providers. Gerontological nursing research in health promotion and disease prevention is greatly needed.

STUDY QUESTIONS

1. What constitutes successful aging? Is health a necessary prerequisite?

2. Discuss the efficacy of health-promotion and disease-preventive measures as applied to an older population.

3. Identify beliefs that influence the adoption and maintenance of behavior change.

4. List the levels of prevention. Give examples of client behaviors for each level.

5. Distinguish between health-promotive and disease-protective behaviors.

6. Analyze health promotion and health protective behaviors important to maintaining a high level of physical well-being.

7. How does anticipatory preparation reduce the stress associated with role changes and life events?

8. Detail some stress-management strategies used by older individuals.

9. Explain the concept of self-transcendence and how it can promote spiritual well-being.

10. What is the role of the gerontological nurse in health promotion and disease prevention in older adults?

REFERENCES

Adams, M. 1986. Aging: Gerontological nursing research. In *Annual Review of Nursing Research* 4:77–95, edited by H. Werley, J. Fitzpatrick, and R. Tauton.

American Nurses' Association. 1987. *The Nursing Center: Concepts and Design.* Kansas City, MO: American Nurses' Association.

American Nurses' Association. 1987. *Standards and Scope of Gerontological Nursing Practice.* Kansas City, MO: American Nurses' Association.

Andresen, G.P. 1988. A fresh look at assessing the elderly. *RN* 52(6):28–40.

Bahr, S.R.T. 1988. An overview of gerontological nursing. In *Nursing Care of the Older Adult*, edited by M. Hogstel. New York: John Wiley and Sons.

Binstock, R.H. and L.K. George. 1990. *Handbook of Aging and the Social Sciences*, 3d ed. San Diego: Academic Press.

Blair, S.N., H.W. Kohl, R.S. Paffenberger, D.B. Clark, K.H. Cooper, and L.W. Gibbons. 1989. Physical fitness and all cause mortality: A prospective study of healthy men and women. *Journal of the American Medical Association* 262:2395–2401.

Bossde, R., C.M. Aldwin, R.M. Levenson, and K. Workman-Daniels. 1991. How stressful is retirement? Findings from the normative aging study. *Journal of Gerontology* 46(1):9–14.

Boyd, J.R. 1984. Therapeutic dilemmas in the elderly. In *Current Geriatric Therapy*, edited by T. Covington and J. Walker. Philadelphia: Saunders.

Butler, R.N. 1963. The life review: An interpretation of reminiscence in the aged. *Psychiatry* 26:65–76.

Campbell, L.A. and B.L. Thompson 1990. Evaluating elderly patients: A critique of comprehensive functional assessment tools. *Nurse Practitioner*, 15(8), 11–12, 14–16, 18.

Carter, W.J. 1991. Macronutrient requirements for elderly persons. In *Geriatric Nutrition*, edited by R. Chernoff. Gaithersuburg, MD: Aspen.

Chin-Sang, V. and K.R. Allen. 1991. Leisure and the older black woman. *Journal of Gerontological Nursing* 17(1):30–34.

Clark, M. and B.G. Anderson. 1967. *Culture and Aging.* New York: Charles C. Thomas.

Cox, G. 1988. *Later Life: The Realities of Aging*, 2d ed. Englewood Cliffs, NJ: Prentice-Hall.

Dishman, R.K. 1989. Determinants of physical activity and exercise for persons 65 years of age and older. In *The Academy Papers: Physical Activity and Aging*, edited by W.W. Spirduso and H.M. Eckert. Champaign, IL: Human Kinetics.

Echevarria, K.H., V. Ross, J.F. Bezon, and J. Flow.

1991. A successful aging project: Pooling university and community resources. *Journal of Gerontological Nursing* 17(5):27–31.

Ferraro, K.F. 1989. Widowhood and health. In *Aging, Stress and Health*, edited by K.S. Markides and C.J. Cooper. New York: John Wiley and Sons.

Fischer, L.R., D.P. Mueller, and P.W. Cooper. 1991. Older volunteers: A discussion of the Minnesota senior study. *The Gerontologist* 31(2):183–94.

Fitzergald, P. 1985. Exercise for the elderly. In Symposium on medical aspects of exercise. *Medical Clinics of North America* 69(1):189–95.

Forciea, M.A. 1989. Nutrition, alcohol and tobacco in late life. In *Practicing Prevention for the Elderly*, edited by R. Lavizzo-Mourey, S.C. Day, D. Diserens, and J.A. Grisso. St. Louis, MO: C.V. Mosby.

Friedman, L., D.L. Bliwise, J.A. Yesavage, and S.R. Salom. 1991. A preliminary study comparing sleep restriction and relaxation treatments for insomnia in older adults. *Journal of Gerontology: Psychological Sciences* 46(1):1–8.

Gallo, J.J., W. Reichel, and L. Anderson. 1988. *Handbook of Geriatric Assessment*. Rockville, MD: Aspen.

Garner, B.C. 1989. Guide to changing lab values in elders. *Geriatric Nursing* 10(3): 144–145.

George, L. 1990. Social structure, social processes and social psychological states. In *Handbook of Aging and Social Sciences*, 3d ed., edited by R.H. Binstock, and L. George. San Diego: Academic Press.

Gilford, D.M., ed. 1988. *The Aging Population in the 21st Century: Statistics for Health Policy*. Washington, DC: National Academy Press.

Gupta, K., B. Dworkin, and S.R. Gambert. 1988. Common nutritional disorders in the elderly: Atypical manifestations. *Geriatrics* 43(2):87–97.

Hamner, M. 1990. Spiritual needs: A forgotten dimension of care? *Journal of Gerontological Nursing* 16(12):3–4.

Harper, M., ed. 1991. *Management and Care of the Elderly: Psychosocial Perspectives*. Newbury Park, CA: Sage Publications.

Hayden, J.H. 1985. To nap or not to nap? *Geriatric Nursing* (March/April):104–6.

Hermanson, B., G.S. Omenn, R.A. Kronmal, and B.J. Gersh. 1988. Beneficial six year outcome of smoking cessation in older men and women with coronary artery disease. *New England Journal of Medicine* 319:1365–69.

Hooyman, N.R., and H.A. Kiyak. 1991. *Sociology Gerontology: A Multidisciplinary Perspective*. 2d ed. Needham Heights, MA: Allyn and Bacon.

Hopkins, D.R., B. Murrah, W.W.K. Hoeger, and R.C. Rhodes. 1990. Effect of low impact aerobic dance on the functional fitness of elderly women. *The Gerontologist* 30(2):189–92.

Idler, E., and S. Kasl. 1991. Health perceptions and survival: Do global evaluations of health status really predict mortality? *Journal of Gerontology: Social Sciences* 46(2):55–65.

Institute of Medicine. 1990. *The Second Fifty Years: Promoting Health and Preventing Disability*. Washington, DC: National Academy Press.

Jacobs, B. 1990. Aging and politics. In *Handbook of Aging and the Social Sciences*, edited by R.H. Binstock and L. George. 3d ed., San Diego: Academic Press.

Janz, N., and M. Becker. 1984. The health belief model: A decade later. *Health Education Quarterly* 11(1):1–47.

Johnson, J. 1991. A comparative study of the bedtime routines and sleep of older adults. *Journal of Community Health Nursing* 8(3):129–36.

Johnson-Pawlson, J., and R. Koshes. 1985. Exercise is for everyone. *Geriatric Nursing* 6(6):322–25.

Karp, D.A. 1988. A decade of reminders: Changing age consciousness between fifty and sixty years old. *The Gerontologist* 28(6):727–38.

Kelly, J.R., M.W. Steinkamp, and J.R. Kelly. 1986. Later life leisure: How they play in Peoria. *The Gerontologist* 26(5):531–37.

Kleinman, L. 1986. A healthy aging America. *Journal of Gerontological Nursing* 12(11):3.

Koenig, H.G., L.K. George, and T.C. Siegler. 1988. The use of religion and other emotion-regulating coping strategies among older adults. *The Gerontologist* 28(3):303–10.

Kovach, C.R. 1991. Content analysis of reminiscences of elderly women. *Research in Nursing and Health* 14:287–95.

LaCroix, A.Z. 1991. Smoking and mortality among older men and women in three communities. *New England Journal of Medicine* 234:1619–25.

LaGodna, G. 1988. Psychiatric/mental health nursing of older adults. In *Adult Psychiatric Nurs-

ing, 3rd ed. J. Lancaster, ed. New York: Elsevier.

Lane, J.A. 1987. The care of the human spirit. *Journal of Professional Nursing* 3:332–37.

Lavizzo-Mourey, R. 1989. Preventing adverse drug reactions in the elderly. In *Practicing Prevention for the Elderly*, edited by R. Dax, S.C. Diserens, and J.A. Grisso. St. Louis, MO: C.V. Mosby.

Lavizzo-Mourey, R., S.C. Day, D. Diserens, and J.A. Grisso, eds. 1989. *Practicing Prevention for the Elderly*. Philadelphia: C.V. Mosby.

Lazarus, R.S., and S. Folkman. 1984. *Stress, Appraisal, and Coping*. New York: Springer.

Lekan-Rutledge, D. (1988). Functional assessment. In *Gerontological nursing concepts*, edited by M.A. Matteson and E.S. McConnell , (pp. 57-91). Philadelphia: Saunders

Linderborn, K.M. (1988). The need to assess dementia. *Journal of Gerontological Nursing 14*(1): 35–39.

Mayfield, P.M., M.L. Bond, M.A. Browning, and J.C. Evans 1980. *Health Assessment: A Modular Approach*. New York: McGraw-Hill, pp. 377–388.

McGoldrick, A.E. 1989. Stress, early retirement and health. In *Aging, Stress and Health*, edited by K.S. Markides and C.L. Cooper. New York: John Wiley and Sons.

Miller, M. 1991. Drug use and misuse among the elderly. In *Health, Illness and Disability in Later Life: Practice Issues and Interventions*, edited by R. Young and E.A. Olson. Newbury, CA: Sage Publications.

Morey, M., P. Cowper, J. Feussner, R.C. DiPasquale, G.M. Crowley, G.P. Samsa, and R.J. Sullivan. 1991. Two-year trends in physical performance following supervised exercise among community-dwelling older veterans. *Journal of the American Geriatrics Society* 39:986–92.

Morgan, K. 1987. *Sleep and Aging: A Research Based on Guide to Sleep in Later Life*. Baltimore, MD: The Johns Hopkins University Press.

Mull, C.S., C.L. Cox, and J.A. Sullivan. 1987. Religion's role in the health and well-being of well elders. *Public Health Nursing* 4(3):151–59.

Murphy, S., M. Davis, J. Neuhaus, and D. Lein. 1990. Factors influencing the dietary adequacy and energy intake of older Americans. *Journal of Nutrition Education* 22(6):284–309.

National League for Nursing. 1991. *Nursing's Agenda for Health Care Reform*. New York: National League for Nursing.

Neugarten, E.L., R. Havighurst, and S. Tobin. 1961. The measurement of life satisfaction. *Journal of Gerontology* 16:134–43.

O'Brien, S. and P.A. Vertinsky. 1991. Unfit survivors: Exercise as a resource for aging women. *The Gerontologist*. 31(3):347–57.

Pender, N. 1987. *Health Promotion in Nursing Practice*. 2d ed. Norwalk, CT: Appleton and Lange.

Peterson, E. 1985. The physical, the spiritual, can you meet all your patient's needs? *Journal of Gerontological Nursing* 11(10):23–27.

Prohaska, T.R., E.A. Leventhal, H. Leventhal, and M.L. Keller. 1985. Health practices and illness cognition in young, middle aged, and elderly adults. *Journal of Gerontology* 40(5):569–78.

Reed, P.G. 1991. Toward a nursing theory of self transcendence: Deductive reformulation using developmental theories. *Advances in Nursing Science* 13(4):64–77.

Remington, P.L. 1985. Current smoking trends in the United States. *Journal of the American Medical Association* 253:2975–78.

Ross, M.M. 1990. Time use in later life. *Journal of Advanced Nursing* 15:394–99.

Rowe, J.W., and R.C. Kahn. 1987. Human aging: Usual and successful. *Science* 237:143–49.

Schilke, J.M. 1991. Slowing the aging process with physical activity. *Journal of Gerontological Nursing* 17(6):4–8.

Schirmer, M. 1983. When sleep won't come. *Journal of Gerontological Nursing* 9(1):16–21.

Seuss, Dr. 1986. *You're Only Old Once*. New York: Random House.

Simpson, W.M. 1986. Exercise: Prescriptions for the elderly. *Geriatrics* 41(1):95–100.

Sims, R. 1989. Immunization in the elderly. In *Practicing Prevention for the Elderly*, edited by R. Lavizzo-Mourey, S.C Day, D. Diserens, and J.A. Grisso. St. Louis, MO: C.V. Mosby. 37–46.

Spellbring, A.M. 1991. Nursing's role in health promotion: An overview. *Nursing Clinics of North America* 26(4):805–14.

Spencer-Legler, M.A. 1988. The nursing process as a framework for psychiatric nursing. In *Adult psychiatric nursing*, 3rd ed., edited by J. Lancaster. New York: Elsevier.

Stewart, R. 1987. Drug use in the elderly. In *Therapeutics in the Elderly*, edited by J.C. Delafuente and R.B. Stewart. Baltimore, MD: Williams and Wilkins.

Tobin, S.S. 1991. *Personhood in Advanced Old Age: Implications for Practice*. New York: Springer Publishing.

United States Department of Health and Human Services. 1980. *Promoting Health/Preventing Disease: Objectives for the Nation*. Washington, DC: Public Health Service, United States Department of Health and Human Services.

United States Department of Health and Human Services. 1991. *Healthy People 2000: National Health Promotion and Disease Prevention Objectives*. DHHS publication no. (PHS) 91-50212.

United States Department of Health, Education and Welfare. 1979. *Healthy People: The Surgeon General's Report on Health Promotion and Disease Prevention*. DHEW publication no. (PHS) 79-55071.

United States Preventive Services Task Force. 1989. *Guide to Clinical Preventive Services: An Assessment of the Effectiveness of 169 Interventions*. Baltimore, MD: Williams and Wilkins.

Vestal, R. 1984. *Drug Therapy in the Elderly*. Boston: ADIS Health Science Press.

Young, R., and E.A. Olson. 1991. *Health, Illness and Disability in Later Life: Practice Issues and Interventions*. Newbury Park, CA: Sage Publications.

6 Health Assessment

Mira Kirk Nelson
Peggy Mayfield

CHAPTER OUTLINE

Focus
Objectives
Health History
  Identifying data
  Chief complaint
  History of present illness
  Past health history
  Family history
  Personal habits

Functional abilities
Review of physiologic systems
Patient profile
Mental status
Physical assessment
Laboratory tests
  Summary
  Study questions
  References

FOCUS

This chapter focuses on the comprehensive health assessment of older adults. There are two sections: Health History and Physical Assessment.

OBJECTIVES

1. Identify the major components of a comprehensive health history.
2. Discuss why it may be necessary to alter one's approach when taking a history of an older adult.
3. Describe the procedure for a functional assessment of an older adult.
4. Identify the importance of assessing the personal habits of an older adult.
5. Explain the purpose of including the review of systems in the health history.
6. Describe the components of a functional assessment.
7. Identify the major elements that are usually assessed in a mental status assessment.
8. Discuss alterations in the process that may be necessary during the physical assessment of an older adult.
9. Compare and contrast age-related benign skin lesions.
10. Describe the age-related physical changes in each of the following body systems: integumentary, vision, hearing, smell and taste, cardiovascular, respiratory, abdominal, musculoskeletal, neurologic, and genitourinary.

Health assessment is a process by which data about an individual's health are collected and analyzed. It must be carried out in a systematic manner to be sure that the information compiled gives a complete data base of the client's health and functional status. It is the first step in the nursing process and provides the basis upon which nursing care is planned and implemented. A complete and comprehensive health assessment uses an holistic approach, which includes the appraisal of the anatomic normality, status of the various body systems, the individual's ability to perform the activities of daily living, and the individual's functioning within the family and community.

The goal of a comprehensive health assessment is to compile a complete picture of an individual's strengths and weaknesses, functional abilities, and competency for self-care. With these data the nurse may attempt to enhance the quality of life for older adults and promote the highest possible wellness in their remaining years. A complete health assessment may take up to three or four hours to compile and may be extremely tiring for the older adult. Therefore it may be necessary to collect the information over several sessions. A partial health assessment may be done initially when time or client condition does not permit a complete health assessment. A partial assessment focuses on one problem area that is disrupting life at the present time, includes one or more systems that may be involved, and is used to analyze specific symptoms. At some later time, however, a comprehensive health assessment should be made. A comprehensive health assessment consists of a health history, functional assessment, mental status assessment, and a physical examination.

HEALTH HISTORY

A thorough health history is the first step in health assessment. The health history is best obtained through interviewing the client. However, when the physical or mental condition of the client makes this impossible, then a significant other person, along with previous health records, may be consulted.

There are many things to keep in mind when interviewing the older client. Always allow plenty of time for the interview, as older clients usually have a long history to tell and their reaction times may be slower as they reflect and respond to questions. The client will feel more at ease if both the client and nurse are seated comfortably in a quiet, private, well-lighted environment. When asking questions, use a well-modulated voice tone, speaking clearly and slowly while facing the client. To begin, use open-ended questions, such as "Tell me about . . .," which allows clients to use their own words. If clients tend to ramble from one subject to another, attempt to bring them back to the subject by refocusing strategies (see chapters 7 and 16). Assess mental status, vision, and hearing difficulties early in the interview because visual and hearing losses can distort exchange of information. Recent and remote memory can be validated by a family member or by testing (see page 123 and Hogstel 1991).

The major components of the health history are outlined in Table 6-1. A discussion of these components follows.

Identifying Data

Identifying data include name, address, phone number, birth date, race, gender, marital status, occupation

Table 6–1   Health History Outline

Identifying data

Chief complaint

History of present illness

Past health history

Family history

Personal habits

Functional abilities

Review of physiologic systems

Patient profile

Mental status

---

or retirement status, children or other family in the home, date of interview, informant, and a comment on the reliability of the informant.

Chief Complaint

The chief complaint, or why the client is seeking care, is a brief statement phrased in the client's own words and describes the most important symptom or problem. Careful questioning may be required to discover what the main concerns are for the client. Some problems are not easily identified (e.g., weight loss, depression, weakness) but will become clear with further patient questioning.

History of Present Illness

This is a general summary and symptom analysis, which includes a chronologic description of the primary problem, beginning from the time the client last considered himself or herself well. The following data should be included: date and mode of onset (gradual or sudden), precipitating factors, character of the complaint (location, quality, quantity, severity), frequency, duration, alleviating factors, associated factors, any treatment and its effect, the absence of symptoms in all physiologic systems that might be pertinent to the present symptoms, and whether or not the symptoms are interfering with activities of daily living.

Past Health History

Childhood Illnesses. A history of rubella, rubeola, mumps, chicken pox, rheumatic fever, scarlet fever, polio, or pertussis is sought.

Immunizations. The tetanus series, polio, pneumonia, and influenza immunizations are particularly important.

Allergies. Questions about asthma, hay fever, food idiosyncracies, eczema, drug reactions, serum reactions, and unusual reactions to immunizations should be asked.

Serious Accidents. Since falling is a problem for many older adults, inquire whether the client has experienced a fall recently and what its complications were. Accidents resulting in fractures or penetrating

wounds or those associated with unconsciousness are of particular interest. Dates of occurrence, treatment, and any complications should be noted.

Major Adult Illnesses. Include all illnesses that required a physician's attention, with dates of occurrence and treatment. Some examples are arthritis, pneumonia, tuberculosis and other chronic lung diseases, diabetes mellitus, cardiac or renal disease, hypertension, jaundice, nervous or seizure disorders, mental health problems, gastrointestinal dysfunction, cancer, thyroid disorder, and diseases of the eyes or ears.

Surgical Procedures. Gather information on the dates, location, name of physician performing, indications for, and any complications of surgical procedures.

Other Hospitalizations. Determine whether there were any other hospitalizations that were not discussed previously, e.g., for examinations or diagnostic tests. Include the dates, location, and results.

Obstetric History. Note the number of complete pregnancies and the outcome, number of incomplete pregnancies, and a summary of complications.

Environmental Hazards. Inquire about exposure to environmental hazards in the home and community, such as lead, arsenic, asbestos, chromium, poisonous gases, radiation, and intense noise. See further assessment of the environment in Appendices C and D.

Blood Transfusions. Include dates, reasons, and any reactions to blood transfusions.

Foreign Travel. Note the dates and location of any illness contracted during foreign travel.

Family History

Family members of concern are blood relatives: siblings, children, parents, maternal and paternal grandparents, aunts, and uncles. The general health and illnesses of family members, their ages, and, if deceased, the cause of death should be included. The following illnesses should be noted: cancer, diabetes mellitus, heart disease, hypertension, seizure disorders, mental illness, mental retardation, anemia, alcoholism, endocrine diseases, kidney disease, tuberculosis, stroke, arthritis, and headaches.

Personal Habits

Personal habits are actions that may affect the overall health of the individual, such as use of tobacco and alcohol.

Current Medications. Prescription and over-the-counter drugs, vitamins, home remedies, and street drugs should be noted. Medications are a critical area for the nurse to assess, because older adults often take several prescription medications for one or more chronic illnesses and may take a number of over-the-counter medications as well. The names of medications, by whom and when prescribed, dosage prescribed per day, amount taken per day, and any problems with compliance should be recorded. Compliance problems may include complicated or inconvenient dosage schedule, large number and variety of drugs, visual difficulty, unpleasant side effects, inability to afford drugs, difficulty in swallowing or administering the drug, inability to get to the pharmacy, belief by the client that the drug is ineffective, and client overdosing. It should be determined if the client takes any medications borrowed from others. It is helpful if clients bring all prescribed medicines with them because sometimes they are taking medications prescribed by more than one physician and are unaware of the names and purposes of drugs.

Caffeine. Determine the amount of caffeine consumed per day. Consider all sources, such as coffee, tea, soft drinks, and chocolate.

Alcohol. Determine the daily use of alcohol, including wine, beer, and mixed drinks; use when alone or in social situations; and/or use of alcohol with pills.

Tobacco. Determine the types of tobacco used, the frequency, and how many years the client has used these products.

Last Examination by a Health Care Provider. Note the date of the last physical examination.

Functional Abilities

Functional assessment is a systematic attempt to objectively measure performance in the areas of daily living, activities of daily living (ADL), instrumental activities of daily living (IADL), mental status, social status, and economic resources. Assessment of these functional areas attempts to uncover the potential source of disability, impairment, or needs of older people that can lead to improved diagnostic evaluation and selection of interventions. While social status and economic resources are important aspects of functional assessment, they are not included in the focus of this chapter (Campbell and Thompson 1990; Lekan-Rutledge 1988).

Ask the client to describe a typical day to give a brief overview of the daily pattern of living.

Work. Describe occupation or employment and the duration, as well as retirement concerns, such as reduced income, moving or selling of home, role change, time adjustment, or problems with spouse because of retirement.

Rest. Describe hours of sleep at night and whether it is continuous or interrupted; difficulty falling asleep or with early morning awakening; disturbing dreams; whether client feels rested after sleep; and naps during the day.

Play and Recreation. Describe the amount of time the client has for self that is free of responsibilities and the amount of laughter, fun, and humor enjoyed. List any hobbies enjoyed. Report actual time spent and describe activities.

Coping Style/Relaxation. Determine what the client does to relieve stress. Inquire if client knows any relaxation techniques and if he or she practices them regularly. Describe the techniques and duration of use.

Nutrition. List a sample of all intake for one day. Determine if salt added to food at the table and how many teaspoons of sugar the client uses in such foods as coffee, tea, or cereal. Show the client's weight gain or loss history by determining the average maximum and minimum weights during the past month, year, and five years. Describe any special diet, current appetite patterns, food preferences, amounts consumed at one time, hunger more marked at different times of day or night, and loss or gain of appetite recently or over the past year. Determine food consumption patterns, fluid intake, and who buys and prepares the food. If someone else buys and prepares the food, does the client like it? If the client purchases food, inquire about difficulty of access to the market. If the client prepares food at home, is preparation a problem (e.g., fatigue, eating alone, decreased vision, difficulty in use of refrigerator and stove)? Does the client have problems with chewing, swallowing, or choking? Is the client able to afford the food desired and needed?

Exercise. Describe the amount, type, and regularity of aerobic or anaerobic exercise practiced and the regularity. List any restrictions or problems encountered during exercise.

Other Health Assessments. Note the nurse/physician/clinic who provided the last examination and the findings, advice, and instructions. Include not only physical examinations, but also dental examinations, evaluation of vision (including tonometry), tests of hearing, electrocardiogram (ECG), chest Xray, Pap smears, mammograms, and proctoscopic examinations. Note the various health care practitioners used by the client.

Activities of Daily Living. This component deals with the ability of an individual to care for personal hygiene and live independently. A person may be independent in all areas, dependent in a few areas, or totally dependent in all areas. Inquire about all areas of living that seem appropriate at a given time. If help is needed to perform any of these activities, examine further the extent of help that is needed.

Dressing. Inquire if any assistance is needed in dressing, including fastening buttons or zippers and tying shoes.

Grooming. Determine ability to trim nails (feet and hands), shave, brush teeth, and brush hair.

Bathing. Inquire if any assistance is needed in bathing in tub or shower, such as preparing bath water, getting into or out of tub or shower, and washing all body parts.

Toileting. Determine if help is needed in using the toilet.

Mobility. Inquire if the client has difficulty in ambulating in the home, such as getting into and out of bed, lowering to or rising from a chair, walking, climbing stairs, reaching for items in cupboards, and opening doors.

Eating. Ask if any help is needed in eating, such as handling the utensils, cutting food, and putting food in mouth.

Instrumental Activities of Daily Living. These activities include the more complex and demanding skills of doing the laundry, using the telephone, housekeeping, transportation, food preparation, taking medicines properly, and managing money.

Laundry. Inquire as to the ability to do one's own laundry with machine or by hand.

Telephone. Determine ability to read numbers, dial the phone, hear the phone ring, and hear conversation over the phone.

Housekeeping. Inquire if any assistance is needed in performing housekeeping chores, such as making bed, cleaning house, washing dishes, and taking out trash.

Access to Community. Determine access to transportation, such as taking the bus or driving a car to shop, go to the doctor, and perform other necessary functions outside the home.

Food Preparation. Determine ability to plan, prepare, and serve adequate meals independently.

Medication. Determine ability to take medications in the right dose at the right time.

Managing Money. Determine ability to plan, budget, write checks or money orders, and exchange currency or coins. Includes ability to count and to open and post mail.

Review of Physiologic Systems

This review of symptoms includes the past and present status of each body system and serves to uncover any items that may have been missed previously.

General Health. This is the overall impression the client has about his or her general state of health. Question the client regarding fatigue patterns; difficulty going to sleep or staying asleep; exercise tolerance; episodes of weakness; fevers; sweats; frequency of colds, infections, and illnesses; and ability to care for own activities of daily living, such as self-care, dressing, grooming, and elimination. In-depth assessment may be used if the client has multiple complaints or disabilities, such as vision loss, limited energy, deficits in motor skill, mental difficulties, or arthritis.

Integumentary System

Skin. Inquire about lesions, rashes, pruritus, excessive dryness, sweating or odors, changes in pigmentation, ease of bruising, changes in texture or temperature, sun sensitivity, decreased sensation to pain or heat, and past skin diseases.

Hair. Ask about hair thinning, dulling, texture changes, brittleness, and breaking, as well as the use of dyes and permanents.

Nails. Inquire about changes in appearance and texture, brittleness, peeling, breaking, thickening, and difficulty in cutting toenails.

Head and Neck. Ask about the frequency of headaches, previous trauma, dizziness, syncope, pain or stiffness in neck, swelling or enlarged glands, and goiter or thyroid trouble.

Eyes. Inquire about use of glasses or contact lenses, disturbances in vision, pain, burning, itching, excessive or decreased tearing, diplopia, photophobia, history of eye disease (glaucoma, cataract, infection, etc.), difficulty with night vision, and whether vision changes interfere with activities of daily living. Learn the date of the last eye examination.

Ears. Ask about difficulty in hearing, use of a hearing aid, earache with colds or airplane flights, excessive cerumen, infection, vertigo, constant noise in ears, chronic itching, and whether there is interference with activities of daily living.

Nose and Sinuses. Inquire about chronic runny or stuffy nose, loss of smell, chronic drip from nose to throat, epistaxis, dryness or crusting, allergies, sneezing, pain, mouth breathing, and frequent use of nose drops.

Mouth and Throat. Inquire about frequent colds or sore throat, hoarseness, changes in voice, pain in mouth, dryness, lesions, bleeding gums, loose teeth, missing teeth, toothache, gum disease, dental decay, diminished taste, chewing difficulty, patterns of dental hygiene, and date of last dental examination. If the client has dentures, determine the wearing habits

(e.g., always, seldom, never, for appearance only, for meals only). Wearing problems, such as rubbing, looseness, clicking noises, or talking difficulty, should be determined. Ask about cleaning habits and any problems with care of the dentures.

Cardiovascular System.
Chest pain may be absent or reduced in older adults. The primary symptom of a problem may be dyspnea on exertion. Ask about the number of pillows used for sleep. Ask about chest pain, dyspnea on exertion and amount, palpitations, unusual breathing patterns, orthopnea, paroxysmal nocturnal dyspnea, episodes of confusion, cough, dizziness, syncope, edema, history of murmur, high or low blood pressure, previous ECG, and any cardiac and hypertension medications.

Also determine peripheral vascular difficulties of extremities, such as coldness or numbness, discoloration, varicosities, cramping, claudication, muscle pain, edema, other swelling, and thrombophlebitis. Ask if rings have become too tight.

Respiratory System.
Determine history of wheezing, bronchitis, or other breathing problems: painful breathing; chronic cough; sputum production (amount, color, time); hemoptysis; night sweats; exertional capacity; swelling of hands or ankles; numbness or tingling of arms or legs; leg cramps in bed, sitting still, or while walking; long-term exposure to industrial dust, coal dust, or asbestos; smoking; and dates of chest Xray and tuberculin test.

Breasts and Axillae.
Inquire about swelling, pain, or tenderness of breasts, changes in nipples; nipple discharge; lumps or dimples; lumps or tenderness in axillae; skin irritation; and frequency of breast self-examination. Ask the date of the last mammogram in women.

Gastrointestinal System.
Inquire about indigestion, heartburn, or food intolerance; difficulty in swallowing; abdominal pain; jaundice, excessive belching; bloating; flatulence; anorexia; nausea; vomiting; diarrhea; hemorrhoids; usual bowel habits and any changes; constipation; rectal bleeding, pain, or itching; hernia; abdominal mass; and use of digestive or evacuation aids.

Genitourinary System.
Assess carefully the client's voiding patterns in a twenty-four-hour period, noting

frequency, nocturia, and any recent changes. Note any problems in urinating, such as retention, straining to void, incomplete emptying of bladder, change in force of stream, hesitancy, dribbling, or incontinence with stress, sneezing, or coughing.

Ask about abnormal color or odor, polyuria, oliguria, dysuria, hematuria, albuminuria, pyuria, kidney disease or stones, urethral discharge, pain (renal, colic, suprapubic, lumbar, sacral, perianal, testicular), history of urinary tract infections, edema of face or hands, and cystoscopy. Determine any history of sexually transmitted disease.

Female Genitalia. Determine history of lumps, lesions, odor, pain, burning, vaginal itching, increased discharge, dyspareunia, number of pregnancies and complications, and date of last Pap smear. Obtain a menopausal history showing onset, course, last menstrual period, associated problems, bleeding since last menstrual period, and any severe menstrual problem. If sexually active, is the client satisfied with sexual activity?

Male Genitalia. Learn whether there is any history of prostate trouble, testicular pain, and change in size of scrotum. Determine the frequency of scrotum self-examination. Is the client able to achieve full erection, maintain erection to his satisfaction, and complete ejaculation? Is there pain before, during, or after erection?

Musculoskeletal System. Determine any history of injuries, fractures, dislocations, or whiplash. Ask about muscle twitching, cramping, weakness or pain with use, or coordination difficulties. Inquire about joint swelling, pain, redness, deformity, or stiffness (pronounced at certain times of the day or associated with activity or inactivity). If there is limitation of joint movement, specify which joints are involved. Inquire about backache. Ask about any pain in hands or feet and any difficulty the client has noticed in gait, such as weakness, balance, or fear of falling. Specify any equipment used such as cane, walker, bed board, special mattress, or prosthetic device. Inquire if musculoskeletal problems interfere with activities of daily living.

Neurologic System. Inquire about episodes of unconsciousness, seizures, twitching, sensory disturbances (paresthesia, hyperesthesia, diplopia), motor disturbances (paralysis, ataxia, paresis, tremor, weakness, loss of balance and coordination), and difficulty with cerebral function (memory, orientation, thought processes, mood changes, etc.)

Hematopoietic System. Ask about history of anemia, bleeding tendency, bruising, blood dyscrasia, radiation exposure, or excessive fatigue.

Endocrine System. Inquire about temperature intolerance (heat and cold), thyroid problems, goiter, sudden unexplained changes in height and weight, symptoms of diabetes, changes in secondary sex characteristics (voice, hair distribution, etc.), hormone therapy, anorexia, and weakness.

Patient Profile

The patient profile provides an outline of the psychosocial components, including past and current personal and family information. See chapter 7 for further information about psychosocial assessment.

Mental Status

A mental status examination is one component of the assessment of the neurologic system. It is included at the end of the history because the mental status examination should be done within the context of the interview. While talking with the client, assess the level of consciousness; general appearance; affect; and ability to pay attention, remember, understand, and speak. Note the use of vocabulary and general fund of information in the context of the cultural and educational background. The client's response to illness allows one to infer the client's use of judgment. If the client has unusual thoughts, beliefs, or perceptions, they should be explored as the subject arises. For many clients this limited information is enough. Those with documented or suspected brain dysfunction and those in whom family members or friends have observed behavioral symptoms need further specific assessment.

The process of mental status or psychological assessment of the older person may differ minimally from that used for younger adults. However, the tools used and the points emphasized need to be specifically designed for the older client.

There are several points to keep in mind.

- Select a familiar and comfortable setting free from noise or visual distraction.

- Determine early in the interview if sensory deficits are present.

- Begin the interview by introducing yourself and explaining the type of information you are seeking.

- Phrase questions by using words easily understood by the client.

- Begin with less personal information to help reduce initial anxiety.

- Observe for signs of fatigue.

- Listen carefully.

- End the assessment interview by summarizing the conversation (LaGodna 1988).

A sample of areas to assess in a mental status examination can be found in Table 6-2. A comprehensive mental status examination that includes components of the examination, areas to assess, and specific areas to observe can be found in Spencer-Legler (1988).

In some situations it is necessary to obtain more specific quantitative data about mental status in order to determine the degree of cognitive impairment. A description and evaluation of the following tools are found in Linderborn (1988):

- Mini-Mental State (MMS)

Table 6–2   Mental Status Assessment

Component of Examination	*Areas to Assess*
General appearance	Appearance in relation to age, clothing, hygiene, and grooming; cosmetics; odor; posture; facial expression; eye contact
Psychomotor behavior	Gait, handshake, movements, coordination, and rate of movement
Mood and affect	Appropriateness, range, and stability of affect; attitude toward nurse, specific mood observed, congruency of verbal and nonverbal expression
Anxiety level	Ranges from mild to panic
Speech	Flow, speed, intensity, volume, clarity, spontaneity, quantity
Intellectual performance	Attention and concentration, immediate, recent and remote memory, abstraction, insight, orientation (to person, place, time), judgment, fund of knowledge, perception
Thought patterns	Clarity, relevancy/logic, flow and content of thoughts
Level of consciousness	Responsive to stimuli
Impulse control	Good, fair, poor, uncertain

- Cognitive Capacity Screening Examination (CCSE)
- Short Portable Mental Status Questionnaire (SPMSQ)
- Philadelphia Geriatric Center Mental Status Questionnaire

Linderborn (1988) also provides a number of references for each of these tools if more specific information regarding their development and use is needed. See Hogstel (1991) for a simple tool that can be used to assess changes in mental status over time.

PHYSICAL ASSESSMENT

While performing a physical assessment on clients over the age of 70, the nurse must consider several important physical and psychologic factors. First of all, the client may not be accustomed to having a physical examination by a nurse. The examiner should therefore explain the role of the nurse, especially if the client has questions. The examiner should also briefly explain what special procedures will be performed, about how long the examination will last, and answer any questions the client has.

Older people often are especially apprehensive about having an examination of their eyes (because of the frequency and fear of cataracts), blood pressure (because of publicity about the dangers of high blood pressure), breasts (because of modesty and fear of cancer), and genital region (because of modesty and perhaps lack of recent sexual activity). These areas should be examined with special care, giving information and explanations to the client as needed to allay fear and anxiety.

Because the elderly are at higher risk for hypothermia than younger adults, the temperature of the room should be comfortably warm (68°–75° F), and the client should not be exposed any more than is needed. Many older clients also are very modest. The client may need assistance undressing, e.g., unbuttoning buttons and opening hooks and snaps, especially if osteoarthritis is present in the hands, wrists, and shoulders. A sturdy straight-backed chair with side arms should be near the examining table so the client can sit safely and comfortably while removing shoes, hose, and underwear.

Some older clients are prone to dizziness, decreased balance, and other proprioceptive problems, so it is important to assist them on and off the scale and examining table. The older client should never be left alone in the room while on the examining table. The client could momentarily forget where he or she is or not realize how high the table is and try to get off the table and fall to the floor. Many also are not able to stand on one foot or walk a straight line safely.

Special care should be taken with glasses, hearing devices, and dentures if they are removed. A complete oral examination is important, however, because of the common occurrence of ulcers under dentures that do not fit well.

While checking range of motion, joints should be moved slowly and carefully because of possible pain and discomfort due to osteoarthritis, osteoporosis, and joint stiffness. If the hip and knee joints are very stiff and painful, the vaginal and rectal examination may have to be performed in the lateral or Sim's position. While moving, turning, and positioning the old-old (age 85 and older), the nurse should take special care to prevent trauma to thin, fragile skin. Using the palms of the hands on joints rather than the fingers on soft tissue will prevent skin trauma.

Most examining tables are quite hard and cause discomfort to the thin, frail older person. The table could be covered with a folded blanket for comfort. Also, if the head of the table cannot be raised, one or more pillows may need to be added to facilitate breathing. Some older people cannot lie flat on their backs for even a few minutes. The basic techniques for performing a physical assessment of the older client are essentially the same as those used in assessing the younger adult client. The procedure for examination must be individualized, however, since no two clients are alike. The examination should be organized to minimize the need for changes in body position and to conserve the client's energy. If the client is weak or tires easily, a complete examination in one session may not be feasible. As many procedures as possible should be combined. For example, a partial musculoskeletal assessment can be made while the nurse observes the client walking into the examining room or moving from the chair to the examining table. Sometimes older people like to talk and tell stories about the past, so it is important that the examiner not allow his or her attention to be diverted while still listening to and being supportive of the client. Since older clients need additional time to respond or react to verbal stimuli and because their movements are slower, sufficient time must be allowed for the examination so that the client and the examiner do not feel rushed.

The form used for the physical assessment of the older client is an assessment guide developed for a younger adult with a column of age-related changes added. See Table 6-3. The focus is on physiologic changes related to the aging process. It is often difficult to differentiate changes that are pathologic from those that are due to the normal aging process. Findings that need referral or follow-up are marked with an asterisk. See chapter 3 for more information on physiologic changes. The form is concise and therefore incomplete, but it is intended to serve as a practical and usable guide that can be adapted for individual older clients. (*Text continues p. 140*)

Table 6–3   Physical Assessment Guide

Temp _____   Pulse _____   Resp _____   Height _____   Weight _____

Blood Pressure: Sitting _____   Standing _____   Supine _____

Physical Findings	*Age-Related Changes and Observations*
GENERAL OVERVIEW	
Normal posture, stature, gait	Stooped posture, slow gait
No involuntary movements	Slow movements
Articulates well; no speech impediments	Slowed response. Voice weak and high pitched
Facial appearance	
Neat and well groomed	
Nutritional status	
Well oriented	
Cooperative	
SKIN	
Color	
Temperature	Subnormal temperature readings are common
Texture	Thinning of skin, transparent, scaling
Good turgor	Decreased turgor, wrinkling, sagging, or drooping of skin, assess for dehydration on the abdomen or forehead
No lesions or rashes	Brown, pigmented spots (solar lentigenes, or "age spots" on backs of hands, arms, face)
	Cherry angiomas (small bright red papules)
	Seborrheic keratoses (raised, pigmented wart-like lesions, color ranging from yellow to brown or black), especially on the face and trunk
	Differentiate from actinic keratoses (raised, rough, tan to brown lesions), which may be malignant.*
	Cutaneous skin tags (acrochordons) on neck and upper chest (soft, flesh-colored, pedunculated)
	Vitiligo (hypopigmented areas)
	Other skin lesions may be malignant*

Note: * Indicates changes that may be pathologic and need referral or follow-up.

Physical Findings	*Age-Related Changes and Observations*
Skin *(continued)*	Assess and refer: changes in a wart or mole, such as an increase in size, variegated color, bleeding, irregular border; a new growth or lesion that has been present for three weeks and is reddened, shiny, translucent, rough, scaly, or ulcerated
No vascular or purpuric lesions	Red blotches on skin surfaces (senile purpura)
	Differentiate from elder abuse*
No reddened areas or pressure areas	Inspect for redness or tissue breakdown over pressure areas*
No varicosities	
No unusual odors	
No excessive dryness or oiliness	Dry, scaly skin
NAILS	
No cyanosis of nail beds	
Angle of base of nail approximately 160°; no clubbing	
Rapid capillary filling	
Nail plate semitransparent, convex, rectangular	Tough, brittle, thickened, and yellow, especially the toenails
	Longitudinal ridges, splitting
Nails trimmed	Inability to trim nails is a problem because of limited mobility, decreased vision, and strength.
HAIR	
Color	Graying to white
Texture	Fine
Amount	Thinning, balding, receding hairline (more common in men)
Distribution	Coarse facial hair on chin and upper lip of women. Increased hair in nostrils and ears of men. Sparse axillary and pubic hair. Reduced amount of hair on trunk and extremities.
No foreign material	
No lesions on scalp	
No dandruff or scaling of scalp	
HEAD AND FACE	
Normocephalic, symmetric	Sagging, loose tissue, especially below the eyes and chin
	Vertical wrinkling of perioral skin
No lumps or tenderness	
Facial nerve (N. VII):	
Symmetric, movement intact	

Physical Findings	*Age-Related Changes and Observations*
Head and Face *(continued)*	
Trigeminal nerve (N.V.):	
Motor and sensory; all three divisions intact	
Temporomandibular (TM) joint freely movable, no pain	
NECK	
Full range of motion (ROM)	Decreased flexibility
Spinal accessory (N. XI):	Diminished strength
Intact, strong	
Trachea in midline	
Thyroid: nonpalpable, no masses	
Salivary glands, nontender, not enlarged	
Carotid pulses 4+, equal	
Lymph nodes: no enlargement or tenderness; small, shotty nodes may be palpable	
Preauricular	
Postauricular	
Occipital	
Tonsillar	
Submindibular (submaxillary)	
Submental	
Anterior cervical	
Posterior cervical	
Supraclavicular	
Infraclavicular	
EYES	
Eyes, brows, and lids:	Eyes may appear sunken due to loss of periorbital fat
Good alignment, symmetric	
Lids: No lid lag, no inflammation	Entropion and ectropion; significant if cornea or sclera is dry or irritated.*
Sclera: White	
Conjunctiva: Pink, uninflamed	Dryness due to diminished tear production
Lacrimal glands: Nontender	Excessive tearing due to lacrimal duct stenosis
Iris: Round, intact	
Pupils equal, round, react to light and accommodation (PERRLA)	Pupil size diminished; impaired accommodation

Physical Findings	*Age-Related Changes and Observations*

Eyes *(continued)*

Normal visual fields (N. II)

Convergence within 5–8 cm

Diminished peripheral vision

Extraocular movements (EOM) intact, (N. III, IV, VI)

Diminished upward gaze

Visual acuity:

Diminished central vision

Corrected:

OD   OS

Presbyopia. Reading glasses usually needed. (Check near vision by having client read from a book held twelve to fourteen inches from face.)

Uncorrected:

OD   OS

Diminished color discrimination, especially blues, greens, and purples

Cornea: No irritation or opacities

Diminished lacrimal secretion may cause dryness or irritation. Arcus senilis, opaque white ring around periphery of cornea due to lipid deposits in cornea.

Corneal reflex intact (N.V)

Lens: No opacities

Senile cataracts. Yellowing and cloudiness of lens. (Examine with +12 to +15 diopter and slowly decrease positivity until retina is seen.)

Fundi:

Optic disks: Flat, yellow; margins clear

Physiologic cup flat

Arteries, veins, normal ratio

Inspect for diabetic and hypertensive retinopathy*

No AV nicking, hemorrhage, or exudate

Scleral brown spots

EARS

Symmetrical

Correct alignment with eyes

Auricle: No masses or tenderness

Auricle larger and more prominent

Pendulous lobes

Canal: No lesions or discharge; cerumen is present

Thickened cerumen, not to be confused with impacted cerumen*

Tympanic membrane: Clear, intact, good light reflex, all landmarks present

Thickened tympanic membrane

Auditory acuity (N. VII) normal to ticking watch or whisper

Diminished hearing, especially high-frequency sounds (presbycusis)

Physical Findings	*Age-Related Changes and Observations*

Ears *(continued)*
    Weber: Lateralizes equally
    Rinne: Air conduction (AC) is
        greater than bone conduction
        (BC)

NOSE AND SINUSES
    Mucosa and turbinates: Pink;   Nose appears larger and more prominent
        no discharge, polyps, or edema
    Septum: No deviation
    Patent bilaterally
    Sense of smell intact (N. I)   Diminished sense of smell
    Sinuses: Nontender
        Frontal
        Maxillary

MOUTH AND PHARNYX
    Lips: No lesions or edema   Observe closely for lesions on long-time pipe smokers
    Teeth and gums: In good repair,   Teeth darkened, may be worn down from use
        no obvious caries, no bleeding   Gums pale
        or edema
    No loose or broken teeth
    Wears dentures (Remove dentures
        during examination)
    Properly fitting dentures   Recession of gums may cause elongated teeth or ill-fitting dentures. Rule out periodontal disease.*

    No lesions under dentures
    No difficulty in swallowing   Diminished cough reflex and decreased ability to swallow
    Mucuous membrane: Pink; no   Fordyce granules (yellow papules) may be present on oral mucosa
        lesions
    No leukoplakia or erythroplasia   Leukoplakia and/or erythroplasia are precancerous.* Inspect buccal mucosa, tongue, and floor of mouth.

    Tonsils: Pink, no lesions,
        fasciculations, or asymmetry
        (N. XII)
    Gag reflex present (N. IX, X)   Diminished gag reflex
    Soft palate and uvula rise
        (N. IX, X)

Physical Findings	*Age-Related Changes and Observations*

THORAX AND LUNGS

Thorax symmetrical, no deformity — Bony changes in thorax (kyphosis); increased AP chest diameter with emphysema

Respiration: Regular rhythm — Weakness of respiratory muscles

Rate of respirations

Respiratory expansion symmetric

Diaphragmatic excursion 3–5 cm — Diminished chest expansion

Fremitus equal, bilateral

Lungs resonant

Limit requests for deep breaths
  and holding breath during
  examination

Breath sounds normal

  Vesicular: Inspiration is
    greater than expiration

  Bronchovesicular: Inspiration
    is equal to expiration

  Bronchial: Inspiration is less than
    expiration

  No rales, rhonchi, wheezes, or
    rubs

  No reduction of vital — Reduction of vital capacity
    capacity with match test
    (can blow out match held
    six inches from lips without
    pursing lips)

  Is able to evacuate 95 percent — Increase in residual volume (larger lung fields)
    of air from lungs in three
    seconds with forced
    respirations

BREASTS AND AXILLAE

  Size

  Symmetric

  Smooth contour, no dimpling — Breast tissue loose, atrophied, pendulous. Inspect for skin
    or flattening — irritation under pendulous breasts.* Include bimanual palpation of pendulous breasts. Refer any lumps.

  No masses or tenderness — Thickening of mammary ridge at lower part of breasts

  Nipples erect, no discharge — Nipples flatter, smaller

  No gynecomastia (male)

  Instructed in BSE

  Axillary lymph nodes: No
    enlargement or tenderness

Physical Findings	*Age-Related Changes and Observations*

Breasts and Axillae *(continued)*
    Lateral
    Central
    Pectoral (anterior)
    Subscapular (posterior)

HEART

Physical Findings	Age-Related Changes and Observations
Apical impulse left midclavicular, fifth interspace	
No thrills or abnormal pulsations	Slower heart rate
Regular sinus rhythm; rate	Arrhythmias are more common with age; they may or may not be significant.
Aortic-pulmonic: S_2 is greater than S_1, no murmurs or rubs	Stiffened valves, aortic lengthening, and sclerotic; changes may cause murmurs. Differentiation between benign and pathologic murmurs is difficult.*
Tricuspid-mitral: S_1 is greater than S_2, no murmurs or rubs, no S_3 or S_4	S_3 is pathologic. S_4 may be heard due to decreased left ventricular compliance, but may also be pathologic.

PERIPHERAL VASCULAR SYSTEM

Physical Findings	Age-Related Changes and Observations
Blood pressure in both arms lying and sitting are within normal limits for age	Increased systolic and diastolic blood pressure; may be pathologic*
Jugular venous pressure is less than 3 cm above sternal angle	Inspect with client reclining at 45° angle. Vary position if unable to detect jugular vein.
Carotid pulses: 4+ (on 0-to-4 scale), symmetric	Auscultate carotid arteries for bruits. Do not palpate both carotid arteries simultaneously.
Arms and hands; Skin and nail beds pink, smooth, warm, and dry	
No clubbing or edema	
Radial, ulnar, and brachial pulses 4+	Thickening, hardening, and loss of elasticity of vessels
Legs and feet: Skin and nail beds smooth, warm, and dry	Gradual pink or purple discoloration common on toes and feet
No pretibial, ankle, or hand edema	
No varicosities or ulceration	Superficial vessels tortuous and prominent
Homan's sign negative, no calf tenderness	
Femoral, popliteal, posterior tibial, and dorsalis pedis pulses 4+	Posterior tibial and dorsalis pedis pulses difficult to locate

Physical Findings	Age-Related Changes and Observations
Peripheral Vascular System *(continued)*	
Epitrochlear nodes nonpalpable, nontender	
ABDOMEN	
Skin: no scars, striae, rashes, lesions, or dilated veins	Sagging, rounded countour due to loss of muscle tone and increase in fat deposits
Umbilicus: Normal contour, no herniation; contour	
No distention, rigidity, or ascites	
Liver size within 6–12 cm, midclavicular	Liver size decreased. Liver may be 1–2 cm below right costal margin due to large lung field.
Normal aorta width, 2.5–4.0 cm	Aorta dilated
Bowel sounds present, no hyperactivity	
No bruits or friction rubs	
Light palpation: No masses or tenderness	Thinner abdominal wall
Deep palpation: No masses, tenderness, or rebound tenderness	
Liver, spleen, kidneys, nonpalpable, nontender	
Inguinal lymph nodes: Nonpalpable, nontender	
No inguinal or femoral herniation	
MUSCULOSKELETAL SYSTEM	
TM joint: No swelling, tenderness or crepitation	Reduced muscle and bone mass (osteoporosis)
Neck	
Full ROM	Diminished joint flexibility
No joint deformity, swelling, or tenderness	Degenerative joint changes
Normal muscle strength	Diminished muscle strength bilaterally, diminished muscle mass
Hands and wrists	
Full ROM	Diminished joint flexibility
No swelling, nodules, or bony enlargement	Heberden's nodules from osteoarthritis
No deformity or atrophy	
Muscle strength normal, symmetric	Diminished muscle strength bilaterally, diminished muscle mass, especially in dorsum of hand. Unilateral weakness needs referral.*

Physical Findings	*Age-Related Changes and Observations*
Musculoskeletal System *(continued)*	
Elbows	
Full ROM; no nodules, tenderness, or swelling	Diminished joint flexibility
Shoulders	
Full ROM	Diminished joint flexibility
No swelling, deformity, or atrophy	Degenerative joint changes
No tenderness or crepitation	
Normal muscle strength	Diminished muscle strength bilaterally, diminished muscle mass
Thorax	
No swelling or tenderness (costochondral junctions)	
Rib cage symmetric	
Ribs intact	
Clavicles intact	
Feet and ankles	
Full ROM	Diminished joint flexibility
No deformities or nodules	Heberden's nodules from osteoarthritis
No calluses, corns, or bony enlargement	
No tenderness or swelling/fluid	
Normal muscle strength	Diminished muscle strength bilaterally, diminished muscle mass
Knees and hips	
Full ROM	Diminished joint flexibility
Normal muscle strength	Diminished muscle strength bilaterally, diminished muscle mass
No deformity, crepitus, fluid, tenderness, atrophy, or bony enlargement	
Spine	
No scoliosis, lordosis, or kyphosis	Mild scoliosis, kyphosis, and stooped body posture are common
No tenderness or spasm of paravertebral and trapezius muscles	Diminished bone mass of vertebrae
No tenderness of spine	
Full ROM	Diminished joint flexibility

Physical Findings	*Age-Related Changes and Observations*
Musculoskeletal System *(continued)*	
No pain on straight-leg lifting	
Performs normal activities of daily living	Slowed movement, diminished sense of balance, diminished joint flexibility, diminished muscle strength
Sits	
Lies down	
Sits up	
Gets up	
Stands	
Walks/gait	
Bends over and retrieves objects	
Ties shoes	
NERVOUS SYSTEM	
Cranial nerves	
N. I: Correctly identifies odors	Diminished sense of smell
N. II: Normal visual fields	Diminished peripheral vision
Visual acuity corrected	Presbyopia; reading glasses usually needed
OD	Diminished color discrimination
OS	
Optic disks: Within normal limits	
N. III: PERRLA	Pupil size diminished; impaired accommodation
Extraocular movements (EOM) intact	Diminished upward gaze
No ptosis or lid lag	
N. IV: Downward medial movement of eyes intact	
N. V: Sensory perception of pain, light touch, and temperature are intact in ophthalmic, maxillary, and mandibular divisions	Diminished
Motor function strong with clenched teeth	Diminished
Corneal reflexes present	
N. VI: Lateral deviation of eye intact	
No nystagmus	
N. VII: Facial muscles strong and symmetric	
Taste present on anterior tongue	Diminished sense of taste

Physical Findings	Age-Related Changes and Observations
Nervous System (*continued*)	
N. VIII: Auditory acuity normal to ticking watch or whisper AC is greater than BC (Rinne) Lateralizes equally (Weber)	Diminished hearing, especially of high-frequency sounds
N. IX, N. X: Normal gag reflex Soft palate and uvula symmetric with upward movement	
Taste perception on posterior tongue	Diminished taste perception
N. XI: Sternocleidomastoid and trapezius muscles strong, symmetric	Diminished muscle strength
N. XII: Tongue symmetric; no deviation, atrophy, or fasciculation	
Motor nerves	
Normal gait, heel-to-toe, deep-knee bends, walking on heels and toes	Gait wide based, slowed. Omit knee bends and other hazardous procedures. Client may not be able to perform heel-to-shin movement.
Romberg negative	Diminished sense of equilibrium, especially when patient is moving rapidly
Good coordination: Finger-to-nose, patting leg, heel-to-shin	
Grip strong, no tremor or drift of arms	Diminished strength
Muscles: No atrophy, fasciculations, involuntary movements, or abnormal positions	Muscle atrophy
Muscles firm, strong; symmetric strength	Diminished muscle strength and muscle mass
Sensory nerves	
Pain perception intact	Diminished
Perception of light, temperature, and vibration intact	Diminished perception of touch, temperature, and vibration
Normal position sense and point discrimination	Impaired position sense
Normal stereognosis and number identification	Diminished

Physical Findings	Age-Related Changes and Observations
Nervous System *(continued)*	
Mental status and speech	
Orientation to person, place, time	
Recent and remote memory good	Diminished memory of recent events
Serial 7s, 3s normal	Increased time required for responding or reacting to stimuli
Able to think abstractly	
Dress and behavior appropriate	
Mood	
Reflexes (on 0-to-4 scale;	Startle response delayed
normal is 2+)	
Biceps (C5, C6)	Diminished or absent deep tendon reflexes
Triceps (C7, C8)	
Brachioradialis (C5, C6)	
Abdominal (T8, T9, T10↑;	
T10, T11, T12↓)	
Cremasteric (L1, L2)	
Patellar (L2, L3, L4)	
Achilles (S1, S2)	
Plantar (L4, L5, S1, S2)	
MALE GENITALIA	Diminished pubic hair
Penis: Circumcised	If uncircumcised, foreskin retracts without difficulty
No discharge, inflammation, or	
swelling	
No ulcers, scars or nodules	
Urethral meatus: Correct	
location	
Scrotum: No masses, ulceration, or	Pendulous scrotum
lesions	
No inflammation or edema	
of scrotum	
Testes and epididymis:	Small, atrophied testes
Normal size and consistency	
No inguinal or femoral hernia	
Prostate: Soft, nontender, no	Prostatic hypertrophy; median sulcus not palpable
enlargement or nodules,	
edges palpable	

Physical Findings	*Age-Related Changes and Observations*
FEMALE GENITALIA AND PELVIS	
(Use left-lateral position if unable to use lithotomy position)	
Vulva: No inflammation or edema, no tenderness or masses	External genitalia atrophied. Observe for leukoplakia.* Diminished pubic hair
Vagina: Mucosa pink, no lesions, moist, no excessive discharge	Vaginal mucosa pale, thin; scanty amount of vaginal discharge
Vaginal outlet: Good muscle tone, no bulging of mucosa	Weakened muscle tone. Observe for cystcele or rectocele.*
Urethra: No inflammation or discharge	
Cervix: Position normal; no lesions, nodules, or ulcerations; no bleeding or discharge	
Uterus: Anterior and midline, smooth, not enlarged	Uterus small, atrophied. Observe for prolapse of uterus.*
Adnexae: Ovaries normal size and consistency, nontender	Ovaries nonpalpable
Rectovaginal exam: No masses	
Pap smear:	Pap smear should be continued throughout life span.
Rectum and anus	
No inflammation, rash, or excoriation	
No lesions, fissures, or hemorrhoids	
No masses	
Sphincter tone good	Relaxed sphincter tone
No bleeding	
No pilonidal cyst	
Stool	Palpate for fecal impaction.

Source: This physical assessment guide is reprinted with the permission of McGraw-Hill Book Company and is only one part of a more complex learning approach to health assessment. See P. Mayfield, et al., *Health Assessment: A Modular Approach,* New York: McGraw-Hill Book Company, 1980.

Laboratory Tests

Evaluation of laboratory tests is an important part of the comprehensive assessment of the older adult. The nurse must take into consideration the age, history (including medication history), physiologic findings, and the client's health profile. *Normal values*, used for interpreting laboratory tests for younger adults, are inappropriate for the older adult. Instead, *reference interval*, which is closely associated with the particular age group, is used. Table 6-4 gives *reference ranges*, not *normals*, for persons over age 70. The laboratory tests listed in the table include the more common tests in which there are age-related changes.

Table 6–4   Laboratory Values for the Older Adult

Test	Age-Related Changes	Geriatric Values (Over Age 70)
Hematology		
Hemoglobin	Slightly decreased, related to reduced hematopoesis and drop in androgen (male)	M: 10–17g/100ml F: 9–17g/100ml
Hematocrit	Slightly decreased, related to reduced hematopoiesis	M: 38%–54% F:35%–49%
Leukocytes	Decreased, related to decreased T and B lymphocytes, and reduced hematopoiesis	3, 100–9,000 cu mm
Sedimentation rate	Slightly increased	less then 22mm/hr
Blood Chemistry		
ALAT (formerly SGPT)	Decreased	0–22 units
Albumin	Decreased, related to reduced liver size, blood flow, and enzyme production	M: 2.3–4.7g/100ml F: 2.6–5.0g/100m
Alkaline phosphatase	Increased, possibly related to decreased liver function or poor absorption of vitamin D	M: 21.3–80.8 units F: 19.9–83.4 units
Blood urea nitrogen	Increased, related to compromised renal function	M: 8–35mg/100ml F: 6–30mg/100ml
Creatinine	Increased (age and creatinine clearance values must be considered)	0.4–1.9mg/100ml
Calcium	Slightly decreased	M: 8.9–10.9mg/100ml F: 9.1–10.7mg/100ml
Glucose (fasting)	Increased	M: 52–135mg/100ml F: 58–135mg/100ml

Test	Age-Related Changes	*Geriatric Values (Over Age 70)*
Glucose tolerance	Higher peak in two hours with slower decline to baseline	
Potassium	Increased slightly	3.0–5.9mEq/L
Thyroxine (T4)	Decreased 25 percent, related to slowed thyroid function	
Uric acid	Increased	M: 2.6–9.2mg/100ml F: 2.0–8.2mg/100ml
Urine Chemistry Creatinine clearance	Must be calculated to consider decreased glomerular filtration rate:	

$$\frac{(140 - age \times kg\ body\ wt)}{(72 \times serum\ creatinine)} \div\ (men)$$

$$\times\ 85\% \qquad (women)$$

Compiled from Andresen (1989) and Garner (1989)

SUMMARY

A health assessment consists of a health history and a physical assessment that incorporate data about an individual's state of physical and psychosocial health, including the ability to perform activities of daily living while functioning within the family and the community. This information enables the nurse to plan with the client activities that will promote the highest possible state of wellness. A health history is obtained through an interview with the client. If the client is physically or mentally unable to furnish information, then a significant other person may be interviewed.

The physical examination of the older client is similar to the assessment of the younger adult client, with variations in procedure, such as using alternate positions, minimizing position changes to conserve the client's energy, preventing chilling, and allowing ample time. Age-related physical findings must be differentiated from pathologic changes.

The skin of the elderly undergoes many changes. Skin lesions, both benign and malignant, are prevalent. Therefore careful assessment and appropriate referral or follow-up are needed. Hair may become gray and thin and the nails become tough and brittle. Assessment of the eyes and ears may reveal presbycusis, presbyopia, and other visual changes. Cardiac arrhythmias, murmurs, and S4 heart sounds are more common but must be differentiated from cardiac pathology. The musculoskeletal assessment will reveal reduced muscle and bone mass, diminished strength and joint flexibility, and degenerative joint changes.

STUDY QUESTIONS

1. Describe five of the major components of a health history.

2. Explain three ways to alter one's approach when taking a history of an older adult.

3. List the components of a functional assessment of an older adult.

4. Why is it important to assess the personal habits of an older adult?

5. Explain the purpose of including the review of systems in the health history.

6. Discuss five of the elements usually considered in mental status examinations.

7. What are three alterations in the approach that may be necessary during the physical assessment of the older adult?

8. Describe four age-related benign skin lesions.

9. List the major age-related physical changes in each of the following body systems: integumentary, vision, hearing, smell and taste, cardiovascular, respiratory, abdominal, musculoskeletal, neurologic, and genitourinary.

10. Identify the major differences in laboratory values for older adults.

REFERENCES

Andresen, G.P. 1988. A fresh look at assessing the elderly. *RN*. 52(6):28-40.

Campbell, L.A., and B.L. Thompson. 1990. Evaluating elderly patients: A critique of comprehensive functional assessment tools. *Nurse Practitioner* 15(8):11–12, 14–16, 18.

Garner, B.C. 1989. Guide to changing lab values in elders. *Geriatric Nursing* 10(3):144–45.

Hogstel, M.D. 1991. Mental status assessment. *Journal of Gerontological Nursing* 17(5):42–43.

LaGodna, G. 1988. Psychiatric/mental health nursing of older adults. In *Adult Psychiatric Nursing*, edited by J. Lancaster. 3d ed, New York: Elsevier.

Lekan-Rutledge, D. 1988. Functional assessment. In *Gerontological Nursing Concepts and Practice*, edited by M.A. Matteson and E.S. McConnell. Philadelphia, PA: Saunders. 57–91.

Linderborn, K.M. 1988. The need to assess dementia. *Journal of Gerontological Nursing* 14(1):35–39.

Mayfield, P.M., M.L. Bond, M.A. Browning, and J.C. Evans. 1980. *Health Assessment: A Modular Approach*. New York: McGraw Hill. 377–88.

Spencer-Legler, M.A. 1988. The nursing process as a framework for psychiatric nursing. In *Adult Psychiatric Nursing*, 3d ed, edited by J. Lancaster, New York: Elsevier.

7 Psychosocial Assessment

Marta Askew Browning

CHAPTER OUTLINE

FOCUS

The multiple purposes of the psychosocial assessment are discussed in this chapter. There is a strong focus on assessing sociocultural factors that affect the assessment of older adults. Facts to consider in communicating with and interviewing older people also are stressed.

OBJECTIVES

1. Identify the major purposes of psychosocial assessment.
2. Discuss sociocultural factors that affect the assessment of older persons.
3. Relate how poverty, crime, and being a member of a minority group affect the assessment and health care of older adults.
4. Evaluate the effect of folk medicine in the care of older persons.
5. Discuss the role of the family and significant others in the assessment process.
6. Discuss factors that need to be considered when interviewing older clients for the psychosocial assessment.
7. Evaluate how sensory changes affect the ability of older persons to communicate effectively.
8. Identify methods that can be used to increase the effectiveness of communication with older persons.

The effective delivery of nursing care to the older adult requires a broad understanding of the complex psychosocial background from which the individual derives a personal self-concept and identifies the meaning of existence. Understanding this complex pattern of relationships, which includes both people and experiences, is essential to understanding the person who is at its core. Data collected during the psychosocial assessment, added to the data obtained from a review of systems and a physical examination, provide a comprehensive view of the client and form the basis for planning nursing care.

The nursing assessment of the psychosocial status of the client occurs both as a result of simple question-and-answer interviews and as a product of an evolving interpersonal relationship. Thus the nurse not only assesses the complex relationships of the client but also becomes part of one of them. In this position the nurse has an impact on the new patterns that are continuously being formed. If this impact is positive, the client will move toward reaching full potential for physical health and psychologic well-being.

PURPOSES OF PSYCHOSOCIAL ASSESSMENT

In the delivery of nursing care, the psychosocial assessment of the client and family unit as they respond to the internal and external changes in their environment is a major function of the nurse.

Initiation of Relationship

The collection of data for the psychosocial assessment gives the nurse a reason, clearly identified and understood by the client, for initiating nurse-patient interaction. It provides a focus for conversation and reduces some of the initial awkwardness at meeting strangers, thus accelerating the formation of an interpersonal relationship. It further establishes the character of the relationship as therapeutic, with the focus of the interaction on meeting the client's needs.

Conducted properly, the psychosocial assessment provides the nurse with more than answers to questions such as, "Where do you live?" and "How old are you?" It provides the nurse with the meaning these facts have for the client and the relationship of this meaning to his or her identity formation. It is the *feeling* that "My [the client's] home has never been adequate for a family I loved and thus I am a failure," and the *perception* that "66 [years] is the end of the line, life has ended, and no future exists." With this information the nurse can understand better the client's point of view and is more likely to empathize with his or her past, present, and future human struggles, although the nurse may not always agree with the course of action selected. Such an understanding will avoid the application of "standard" plans of care that imply a "routine" solution for every client's problem.

Establishment of Baseline Data

The psychosocial assessment provides baseline data for later comparison. As the client's life evolves and medical problems that require adaptations in lifestyle improve or deteriorate, the progression or regression of the client's disorder can be identified by comparing its present status with the initial baseline data. For example, during an initial home visit a 68-year-old client was quite alert and responded to the interviewer's questions actively, accurately, and with a humorous flair. The client was next seen for nursing evaluation six months later, three months after the death of his wife. His responses to the nurse at this time were slow and halting. The client appeared totally uninterested in his surroundings and his affect remained flat. The nursing assessment of the client during the second visit was radically different from the one conveyed in the initial health assessment. Deterioration was evident in all spheres of activity, and nursing planning and intervention were clearly indicated.

Evaluation of Perception of Health

There is considerable evidence that self-evaluation of health is a significant predictor of mortality in the older adult. Therefore the question "At the present time how would you rate your health?" is an essential query for individuals during the psychosocial interview (Idler and Kasl 1991). The response selected by the older adult from the forced choice set of responses—excellent, good, fair, poor, or bad—has significant implications for the health care provider. Idler and Kasl (1991) noted that older people whose perception that their health status is poor are six times more likely to die than those who perceive their health as excellent.

The power of this question as a predictor of mortality is currently unexplained. The researchers suggested two alternative explanations for this phenomenon. The first explanation is that the individual's perception of health status may prove to be a self-fulfilling prophesy. Over time, perceptions and expectations may impact health status and cause illness. Alternatively, Idler and Kasl (1991) proposed that the question may not really elicit a response regarding present health status as intended. Instead it may yield a subjective, though covert, estimation of life expectancy. The respondent's qualitative response (e.g., excellent, poor) may be a synthesis of many variables such as knowledge of his or her family's chronic disease history, the length of life of parents and/or grandparents, close identification with a relative with whom the respondent shares a physical resemblance, health condition, or lifestyle pattern.

Research suggests that many clients initially appear in the health care setting presenting *signal behavior*—symptoms that are used as an entree to the health care provider's office so that another underlying health care concern may be presented (Stewart, McWhinney, and Buck in Molde 1986). Molde (1986) and Fried, Storer, King, and Ladder (1991) proposed that the medical model, based on eliciting, defining, and speedily diagnosing presenting symptoms, is poorly adapted for discerning the client's real agenda.

Fried's study of models for diagnosing illness presentation in older adults revealed that the "facilitating complaint" (signal behavior) is the one perceived by the client and/or family to represent a legitimate entree into the health care system. Fried et al. (1991) stated that such "facilitating complaints" are presented when clients or families recognize the real health care problem experienced by the older adult but fear that it is not really a medical issue (e.g., functional limitations or caregiving issues) or find the problem to be too threatening to approach directly (e.g., cognitive decline). These researchers also described a variant of the facilitating complaint in which older adults present with a medical chief complaint even when their health and functional status is stable. The underlying cause precipitating such health care visits is usually apprehension about the future, fear of potential frailty and loss of functional independence, and/or significant anxiety or depression.

Chief complaints by older adults need careful analysis. In addition to "facilitating complaints" and their variants Fried (1991) also suggested other models of presenting symptoms that bear exploration. The first of these is the "Synergistic Morbidity Model," in which the client presents with multiple chronic diseases causing cumulative morbidity. In combination these diseases cause a functional decline that the client finds intolerable. This functional decline, not the diseases themselves, becomes the event precipitating entree into the health care system. The client's agenda is relief from the functional impairment, not just diagnosis of the disease.

The second pattern of presentation is called the "Attribution Model." In this situation the older adult senses a decline in well-being and attributes it to deterioration of a previously diagnosed, chronic health condition. However, work-up reveals a new, unrecognized disorder that often has new symptoms the client had not associated with the decline in health status. An evaluation, restricted to the mis-attributed chief complaint alone, would have failed to reveal the new condition.

A third pattern of presenting complaint, identified by Fried and colleagues, is called the "Causal Chain Model." This form of chief complaint becomes the proverbial last straw for the client and/or family members. In this model a chain of events begins with one physical ailment that triggers a domino-like chain of subsequent events. These ultimately culminate in functional decline. Finally Fried and cohorts described what they call the "Unmasking Event Model." In this situation an acute episode or stressor unmasks an underlying, stable or slowly progressive chronic condition that has previously been well compensated and therefore unrecognized. These stressors are usually major life events, such as death of a spouse, retirement, or change in living situations.

The researchers concluded that among their study subjects the application of the classic medical model in response to the presenting or chief complaint would have resulted in a correct diagnosis in less than half of the population. In all other situations the remaining models were more accurate in evaluating and managing the underlying problems of clients and family caregivers.

Molde (1986) stressed the importance of exploring an additional dimension of the client's agenda. After eliciting the presenting or chief complaint, the health care provider should follow with the question "How did you hope that I could help you today?" Her review of the research literature indicated that clients will most often respond, not by asking for diagnosis or relief of symptoms, but with requests for information, support, counseling, advice about diagnosis or treatment, referral, and explanation. Molde suggested that when the interview with clients is limited to testing hypotheses about disease, as in the medical model, nothing is learned about the issues concerning clients or their wishes in relation to diagnosis or treatment.

Identification of Problems

Data collected during the psychosocial assessment aid the nurse in identifying the present overt health and psychosocial problems of the client. In addition the psychosocial assessment focuses attention of the older person on changes associated with aging that may have occurred subtly and imperceptibly. Perhaps the changes have necessitated gradual adjustments in daily habits that the client made without becoming aware of the onset or progression of the adaptation. The following comments of an active 78-year-old gentleman illustrate this phenomenon:

> Until our conversation yesterday, I had never sat down and thought about aging as it applies to me. Of course it had crossed my mind from time to time, but I would usually shrug it off as something I did not like but there was little I could do about it. Now I am wondering how much I have aged—and where do I go from here? There are certain obvious physical signs that I have aged, but I cannot pinpoint the time it began or the rapidity of its progress. . . . How do I know I have aged? For years and years I stood up when putting on my socks, standing first on one foot, then on the other. Since talking to you, I have discovered that I no longer do that (and I doubt that I now could), but I can't recall when I stopped doing it. Now I even find it somewhat of a strain to put on socks while I am sitting on a chair, and it is easier if I stand and put my foot on the chair seat.

Changes such as loss of hearing or decreased visual acuity often foster withdrawal of the older person from activities once pleasurable but now strangely disquieting. The recognition of a physical or psychologic change on the part of the client may lead to the development of strategies that will compensate for the deficit and open the way to a more satisfactory lifestyle.

The evaluation of the data collected in a psychosocial assessment allows the nurse to identify potential health problems and to provide anticipatory guidance for the client that will ameliorate the severity of the problem or prevent its occurrence. For example, during an interview a 74-year-old client told the nurse she was excited about a planned trip to Europe on a chartered tour. The tour was to cover seven countries in ten days. The nurse's awareness of decreased stamina in the older adult led to some anticipatory guidance at this point. Together nurse and client explored alternatives in pacing activities during the trip that allowed the client to maximize her opportunities rather than permit her to overextend her physical limitations and ultimately find the trip exhausting, stressful, and disappointing.

Identification of Teaching Needs

Psychosocial assessment provides a data base for the identification of the teaching needs of the client. These needs may include clarification of misperceptions regarding the client's medical condition and medical regimen, correction of erroneous information regarding bodily changes in aging, and referral to community resources available for assistance. The assessment also provides a basis for consideration of alternative adaptations to physical or psychologic changes brought about by aging or illness. The relevant health information provided by the nurse may range from the importance of taking antihypertensive medication exactly as ordered, through a review of safety checklists for the home environment, to reassurance that sexual desire and relationships are acceptable and normal in advanced age.

Teaching methods and content must be planned by the nurse, recognizing the client's current anxiety level and need to deny illness, effectiveness of prior coping strategies, and intellectual understanding of material to be conveyed. See chapter 16 for a discussion of the nursing role in patient and family teaching.

Utilization of the Family as a Resource

A comprehensive assessment of the client's psychosocial matrix involves the family. Assessment gives the nurse the opportunity to evaluate the state of family relationships and to involve the family with the client in planning care. With an introduction to the nurse via the nurse's relationship with the client, the family receives tacit permission to use the nurse as a source of support, information, and education. The perceptive nurse will understand that patient care is inadequate unless the family is an integral part of the planning of such care.

For example, an older male client suffered a debilitating stroke and required comprehensive skilled nursing care. His older, frail wife felt alienated and separated from her husband of fifty years. Having nursed him through physical and psychologic stresses for half a century, she now perceived herself as a failure when she saw younger, active nurses rapidly and competently meeting all his physical needs. During visits the couple's middle-aged children felt inadequate while "Papa" was hovered over by strangers. In such a situation the sensitive nurse should understand the family's need to demonstrate their love in a tangible way and should develop client approaches that utilize their desire to participate. Procedures like range of motion could be taught to the client's sons, and bathing, hand-holding, and feeding could become the responsibility of the wife. The nurse has then reinforced the operation of the family unit as an integrated system of reciprocal relationships rather than fragmenting and rendering it a superfluous patient appendage.

Because the family is ultimately responsible for the client, the nurse and other members of the health care team should use all available opportunities to keep the family operational as a unit by assisting it in adapting to the physical, environmental, and role changes that accompany declines in health. Such assistance will ultimately serve to ease the transition from institution to home at time of discharge. The nurse is well prepared to mentor the family and friends who are collaborating to form a caregiving network that will support the client at home. (See chapter 19 for a discussion of the nursing role in family caregiving.)

Identification of Other Support Systems

The psychosocial assessment reveals, in addition to familial relationships, any other significant human relationships the client may have. Many years, much love, and much psychic energy probably have been invested in these relationships, and they have become an integral part of the client's self-concept. The nurse must understand the significance of these support figures or significant others, lest serious errors occur that will decrease the client's sense of security and create an environment of acute social deprivation. For example, when incapacitated by short-term illness, an older woman may not fare as well by moving in with her daughter as she would by remaining in an apartment next door to her friend of thirty-five years. Between them may lie a shared history of three decades of living: bearing and raising children, supporting husbands through arduous careers, mourning losses at gravesides, providing mutual support through the new and strange tasks of widowhood, and a rapport based on understanding without the need to exchange words. Out of love the family may be willing and able to supply much more than the daughter out of duty. In addition the nurse must not overlook the value of Sunday School classes, bridge groups, or other organizations in which the client has an emotional investment in providing support during times of client stress.

Identification of Achievement

The process of psychosocial assessment allows the nurse to identify the strengths and achievements of the client and to offer admiration and praise for his or her life successes. Many clients do not realize how successful they have been, nor do they recognize that they have managed difficult life situations with creativity, imagination, determination, and wisdom. A simple "I cannot begin to tell you how I admire your courage—your effort—your warmth—your humor" will provide positive reinforcement and validate the client's self-concept as that of a worthwhile person. It is superfluous to explain how important praise is to the human ego and how much each person longs for and needs to be suffused with the warm glow of appreciation. In addition a review of past successes enables the client to identify coping strategies that have worked well in the past and can be transferred to resolve current problems.

Facilitation of Life Review

The data elicited during the psychosocial assessment encourage life review and provide the client with an active and interested listener. The collection of the data thereby becomes a therapeutic process in itself.

Identification of Sociocultural Factors that Place the Older Person at Special Risk

The psychosocial assessment assists the nurse to identify characteristics of older adults and/or their families that may place them at special risk for health problems. Two significant risk factors are poverty and membership in a minority group.

Poverty. Low income places persons at an increased risk for all of the chronic diseases that head the nation's morbidity and mortality tables. An alarming example is the rate for heart disease that is more than 25 percent higher for low-income people than for the overall population. Correspondingly the incidence of cancer increases as family income decreases; survival rates are lower for low-income clients (United States Department of Health and Human Services 1990). In 1986, 3.5 million elderly persons had incomes below the poverty level. Another 2.3 million, or 8 percent of the elderly, were classified as "near poor." In total, over one-fifth of the older adult population was poor or near poor. Older women had a poverty rate nearly twice that of older men. The nine states with the highest older-adult poverty rates were located in the South: Mississippi (34 percent); Alabama, Arkansas, and Louisiana (28 percent each); Georgia (26 percent); South Carolina and Tennessee (25 percent each); North Carolina (24 percent); and Kentucky (23 percent) (American Association of Retired Persons 1990). While Medicare and Medicaid provide some relief for health-related expenses, many costs are not covered services. The cost of medications and supplies, chore and homemaking services, respite care, dentures, eyeglasses, and transportation to and from clinics may prove to be a substantial barrier to preventive, curative, or maintenance health care.

Women comprise 73 percent of the elderly poor (Davis, Grant, and Rowland 1990). Single women suffer greater poverty than their married counterparts. Three out of five older women are without a spouse. These women are those who never married or are widowed, separated, or divorced. Poverty is exacerbated when individuals are members of a minority group. The highest rates of poverty exist among older African-American women and approach 82 percent when the poor and near poor are added together. Older Hispanic women fare somewhat better but, at poverty rates of 31 percent, are still twice as likely to be poor as women in the general population (Minkler and Stone 1985). Among the 1.6 million older persons who are severely impaired and living in the community, over two-thirds are women; nearly 70 percent of these are poor or near poor. Among widows, poverty often comes after spousal death; one-half of widows were not poor before the death of their husbands (Davis, Grant, and Rowland 1990).

The "feminization of poverty," a term coined in the 1970s (Minkler and Stone 1985, 351) is a result of several factors:

- Lack of employment history outside of the home

- Delayed career entry

- Interrupted career path (often related to caregiving functions such as childrearing or caring for aging relatives)

- Lower pension and Social Security benefits based on lower lifetime earnings than those of men (a result of interrupted careers; lower wage jobs; and jobs without benefits, including pensions)

- Reductions in Social Security or pension benefits to one-half or one-third of the couple's income received prior to spousal death

- Stringent requirements for enrollment in Supplemental Security Income (SSI) and failure of SSI to insure incomes above the poverty threshold

- Lack of entitlement to pension or Social Security benefits if spouse was unwilling to accept reduced annuity payments during his lifetime or if divorce occurred before ten years of marriage were completed

Poverty, or impending poverty, has serious implications for one's ability to procure health care services. Medicare covers less than one-half of all personal care expenses for older adults. While three-fourths of older adults supplement Medicare with Medigap health insurance, the poor or near poor cannot afford such coverage. Therefore among older people nearly 10 percent of women (compared with 5 percent of men) must rely on Medicaid to cover some of the expenses not covered by Medicare (Davis, Grant, and Rowland 1990). For those older adults who have some assets but are near poor (only a few hundred dollars above the poverty threshold), enrollment in entitlement programs may require that they exhaust or deplete their only economic cushion. This is accomplished through a process called spend down (Minkler and Stone 1985). The older adult (or couple) must reduce all assets below thresholds that make them eligible for the desired program, such as Medicaid. This often means that older adults must spend money carefully saved for a rainy day, losing all financial security however minimal. The most profound impact on health care services occurs because, among the poor, health care must compete with other critical priorities such as food and shelter. In such competition, health care must often be placed as a low priority compared to the basic human needs.

Managing on a Low Income. Many older adults shun entitlement programs because they are unaware of their existence, their eligibility for them, or because they do not believe in relying on "taking handouts" or being "on welfare." Proud older adults may go to great lengths to keep children, other relatives, friends, and neighbors from knowing that they are economically strapped. Pensions that in the first years after retirement were adequate may not keep pace in periods of inflation. Interest on savings and investments, essential to economic survival, may decline significantly during cycles of deflation and consolidation in the economy. Often an older adult's net worth is in home equity and few cash savings exist to protect against the negative times of life. Many older adults fear public assistance because in some parts of the country, liens can be placed against the property by the state to recover the amount of the client's welfare grants after the client and surviving spouse die. For older adults who wish to leave property or cash from the sale of the property to their children, public assistance may be soundly resisted. To conserve assets, the client may make choices that baffle health care workers who place a high premium on health. For example, health care may be refused because the client does not have the money to pay the Medicare deductibles or co-pay. Medications may be taken only sporadically because they are so expensive. High-sodium soup may become a steady diet because it is less expensive than meat.

Older persons living on fixed incomes must continuously adapt as the purchasing power of their income declines. At first these adaptations are minor and luxuries are given up. Magazines may be stopped; dinners out are curtailed; women may give up perfume and lipstick purchases; clothing may cease to follow current styles; and gift-giving patterns may change. The small (and particularly the social) pleasures may be gradually eradicated to meet the demanding need for funds for food, shelter, and health care. For those with marginal incomes the occurrence of a life crisis, such as a spousal death, the theft of savings or pension funds in a savings and loan scandal or banking failure, or the cost of a prolonged illness, can prove catastrophic. In a sense older adults who have known poverty throughout their lives are more fortunate than those who face it for the first time in old age. They may have developed survival skills, such as the sharing of resources, communal and extended family living, and maximization of entitlements. Thus for them life in old age may be comparatively more comfortable than in their younger years when a limited income had to be shared with growing children. For the newly poor, coping skills may be inadequate for sound decision making.

The most common cost-cutting measures, after the deletion of luxuries, seem to be related to food and utility costs. Nutritional needs are ignored to make ends meet. Many older adults eat only once a day or skip some days entirely. Some older adults give up their own meals to feed a beloved pet; or noticing that pet food is cheaper than human food, they choose to eat it themselves. Lights and electrical appliances are used as little as possible. Some older adults move about, in peril of falls and other injuries, through darkened houses or apartments to save on the electric bills. Utilities such as heat and water are conserved; it is not unusual to hear of older adults freezing in the winter or dying of heatstroke in the summer. Home repairs are impossible on a limited income; thus safety hazards may proliferate. However, even very poor older adults attempt to maintain phone service. They clearly recognize that the phone may mean the difference between life and death if they suffer from chronic illness. They also know that the phone can maintain a social network when mobility is impaired or one can no longer afford to go out as before.

Treatment by the Health Care System. Nurses must pay attention to the fact that poor clients are treated differently than middle- or upper-class clients. Differential health care treatment is a fact that has long been vigorously denied by many segments of the health care system and the American public. Morbidity and mortality figures for poor and minority populations are making such denials increasingly impossible. The greatest change in public attitude has occurred only recently as the prolonged recession of the early 1990s eroded the health care benefits of the middle class, and rising costs of treating the poor and the old fostered tax increases. Though the public is becoming aware of the tremendous inequities in health care, nothing has yet changed in the health care delivery system. Therefore nurses must recognize the barriers to health care that exist for poor older persons.

Access to health care may be severely limited and the older adult may be shuttled from physician to physician because Medicare or Medicaid clients are not accepted for service or because the client is not able to pay add-on fees above those reimbursed by entitlement programs. Older adults who are poor may have difficulty selecting properly qualified physicians. In inner city neighborhoods many older minority adults select neighborhood physicians or herbalists. These neighborhood practitioners may not qualify for admitting privileges in recognized and accredited hospitals. Therefore when older adults become severely ill and are admitted to a hospital through an emergency room, they must face strange practitioners who may be distrusted.

Because health care is so difficult to obtain, poor older adults seek less of it. Symptoms are ignored, minimized, or denied. Meager financial resources place health care low on the priority scale after shelter and food bills that must be paid first. Thus compliance with health care regimens may be sporadic or absent. If implementation of a health-related regimen (e.g., purchase of medications) involves expenditure

of money, compliance is better if teaching related to the activity is done around the time of the month that pension, Social Security, or entitlement checks arrive. Nurses must be aware that in some instances use of the health care delivery system may carry risks for the older adult who is poor. For example, older adults who live in public housing may have been on a waiting list a number of years before an apartment became available. They may face the loss of that apartment if admitted to a hospital or nursing home for a lengthy stay. Therefore these individuals will go to great lengths to avoid hospitalization.

Even if they are fortunate enough to access health care, the older poor must often wait inordinate amounts of time once they arrive at a clinic or provider's private office. Most often, whole days are consumed by a visit to a health care facility, rather than the two or three hour inconvenience experienced by the younger, more assertive poor, or by the more affluent who would not tolerate such delays. For many older clients, anticipation of the long waits sure to cause physical discomfort from sitting on hard chairs in a crowded waiting room, fear of bladder accidents and the accompanying embarrassment, and the certainty of missed meals are rationale for failing to keep appointments for health care. Furthermore, when seen by young physicians and health care providers, ageism and poverty may combine to create a disastrous combination. The older adult may not receive the same aggressive management of health care problems experienced by more affluent or younger clients. For example, a 72-year-old African-American woman attended a large, inner city hospital medical clinic. During the physical examination she was found to have a lump in her right breast. Even though in the high-risk group for breast cancer, she was given a mammogram appointment for four months from the date of her clinic appointment rather than immediate diagnostic follow-up. This same type of differential treatment occurs often and in subtle ways. For example, the poor may get a manually operated hospital bed for home care rather than an electric bed. They may get tank oxygen rather than an oxygen concentrator if on out-patient oxygen therapy. The old poor may get fewer home visits by home care agencies and be allowed shorter days of stay by hospitals. They may be *dumped* (precipitously closed to service) by unscrupulous health care institutions when their reimbursement benefits expire.

Older adult clients are survivors and most learn to tolerate, with an amazing degree of acceptance, the inconveniences in dealing with the health care delivery system. However, a major barrier to health care seems to be securing transportation to and from health care facilities. Often there is insufficient money to pay for transportation services. At other times, as in the case of the rural older adults, there may be no public or private transportation available. In addition older adults who have canes, walkers, braces, or wheelchairs may find it difficult to negotiate travel in a small car or on a standard city bus. Paratransit services for persons with disabilities are often available in urban areas but seniors may not know how to access or pay for such services. Most of these services charge some fees based on a sliding fee scale. Even if the charge is as low as $1.00 each way, the two dollars for a round trip may prove prohibitive. Emergency transportation by ambulance can also prove disastrous for poor older people. Medicare reimburses some costs of such transportation but the remainder must be paid by the client or by Medicaid. When the clients have Medicaid, the ambulance may refuse to pick them up if the ambulance company has already provided their allotment of reduced-fee service for the month. In many states reimbursement by Medicaid is substantially lower than the actual cost of providing health care services. Therefore providers may try to stringently control the number of Medicaid or no-fee recipients served. Older adults who have Medicaid to supplement Medicare may therefore periodically find that they are refused services even by providers who have served them before.

Impact of Poverty and Crime on Lifestyle. Poverty influences the neighborhood of residence. Many older adults who bought homes in inner cities long ago now find themselves living in deteriorating neighborhoods that are high crime areas. As the neighborhoods declined and the neighbors of decades died, new people moved in and changed the character of the area. Trapped by the declining purchasing power of a fixed income and the declining value of their homes, many of these older adults are now prisoners in their own houses. The neighborhood, once peaceful, may now be occupied by aggressive young drug dealers and/or immigrants whose ways are foreign to the older adult. The older adult may have been or certainly fears becoming a robbery victim. Most know

of an older friend who has been assaulted in the street and has been badly injured or killed.

Intergenerational poverty affects a poor older adult's children and grandchildren. Therefore older adults may have many people living in their household or find themselves responsible for compensating for the results of substance abuse among family members. Impoverished older adults may be raising small children abandoned by other relatives who can no longer care for them. In addition since lack of funding may prevent poor older adults from gaining access to nursing home care, the older adult may also have the responsibility for caring for one or more bedridden or disabled older relatives in the home simultaneously.

Membership in a Minority Group. Statistically a minority is any group (racial, religious, or other) constituting less than a numerical majority of the population. Minority in the sociological sense relates to the lack of power dominance. Minority groups may have unequal access to power or be stigmatized by presumed inferior traits or characteristics (Tripp-Reimer and Laver 1987).

The most common categorization of minority groups is by race. The majority group in the United States is white and will remain that way for the foreseeable future. But national demographics are changing. By the year 2000, Whites will decline from 76 percent to 72 percent of the total population. African-Americans will increase their proportion from 12.4 percent to 13.1 percent and Hispanics, the fastest growing population group, will rise from 8 percent to 11.3 percent. Other racial groups, including American Indians, Alaska natives, Asians, and Pacific Islanders, will increase from 3.5 percent to 4.3 percent of the total (United States Department of Health and Human Services 1990). In 1986 about 90 percent of persons age 65 and older were White, 8 percent were African-American, 3 percent were Hispanic, and 2 percent were other races (American Indian, Eskimo, Aleut, Asian, and Pacific Islanders) (American Association of Retired Persons 1990). Longevity is linked to race and ethnicity; mortality rates are disproportionately higher in minority populations. Much of the difference in health status between Whites and minority groups is the result of poverty (created and reinforced by racism and/or discrimination in employment and education) and social class, rather than race in and of itself.

Burnside (1988) stated that ethnic old adults tend to avoid the mainstream health care delivery system. She identified a number of reasons for diminished use of health care services. These include extreme poverty leading to an inability to pay for services, language barriers, lack of education, inability to access and navigate the bureaucracy, maldistribution of health care services, racism and stigmatization, social isolation, fear, and distrust.

Among minority clients, African-Americans carry special burdens. Though slavery was abolished more than a century ago, racism, bigotry, and discrimination against African-Americans stubbornly persists (Ross and Cobb 1988). Today's older African-Americans have lived through even greater change than their White American contemporaries. That change is hinged on the transition from the injustice of semioutcast status to the right (not yet fully realized or implemented) to finally participate on an equal footing with other groups in American society. Many older African-Americans were active in the Civil Rights Movement of the 1960s. They take great pride in the opportunities that have become available for their children and grandchildren. However, they may not have been able to benefit from these same opportunities themselves. They were already middle-aged when the social changes that opened educational and employment opportunities occurred. The result of the racism that they experienced is most often reflected economically. For example, in 1986 one of every nine Whites was poor but almost one in three (31 percent) older African-Americans suffered poverty. Though African-Americans constitute almost 12 percent of the national population, less than 3 percent of older persons residing in nursing homes are African-Americans (Clavon 1986). African-Americans are often commended for their desire to take care of their own older family members. However, it is possible that they have no choice as poverty and residual racism and segregation may bar them from access to long-term institutional care. Lack of education and poverty make it particularly difficult for older African-Americans to access and use the health care delivery system. It is no accident that the mortality and morbidity rates are higher for African-Americans of all ages.

Ethnic Options and Identity. The minority groups in the United States are generally categorized as follows: African-American; Hispanic American (Mexican Americans, Puerto Ricans, Cuban Americans, and Central and South American immigrants); Asian and Pacific Islander Americans (Laotians, Cambodians, Vietnamese, Hawaiian, Asian Indians, Thai, Samoan, Korean, Filipino, Chinese, Japanese, Guamanian); American Indians and Alaska Natives (Eskimos, Aleuts, Indians). America has one of the most heterogeneous populations in the western world. Health care providers often assume that Caucasians constitute a single cultural group. But White Americans are not homogeneous in terms of ethnic identity and patterns of health behavior. Research has shown that ethnic identity may determine through the fifth generation much of what Americans of European descent believe and do about health. Next to Native Americans, the least studied groups in ethnic gerontology are the older members of European descent in spite of their large numbers in the United States (Tripp-Reimer and Laver 1987).

Ethnic subgroups are important among all racial subgroups. For example, among Whites there are Americans of Italian, Polish, Greek, Norwegian, Swedish, German, Irish, Russian, Ukrainian, and Scottish descent. Within the broad grouping Native Americans, there are over four hundred federally recognized nations, each with its own tradition and cultural heritage (United States Department of Health and Human Services 1990). To further complicate matters of ethnicity, religious affiliations may overlap racial categories; Catholics, Jews, Protestants, and Buddhists may be found in all racial groups.

Older adults belong to a racial group and an ethnic subgroup. They may belong to a religious group as well. They may have been born in this country, been the children of immigrants, or have come to these shores as immigrants themselves. They may have been a part of one of the great migrations within this country, such as the migration of southern Blacks from the rural South to the urban North in search of jobs. If they came to this country in one of the massive waves of immigration that occurred in the early part of this century, they may have worked hard to submerge their cultural differences or ethnicity to assure that their children would be assimilated into the American mainstream. If they are the children or grandchildren of immigrants, they may accentuate and value their ethnic heritage now that they have secured a place in the American hierarchy. If they are more recent immigrants, such as Asian refugees who fled Vietnam as boat people or refugees from Cuba, they may still be struggling to secure a firm foothold on the American dream. Finally, they may be brand new refugees, such as Russian Jews who speak no English and may be bewildered by the bounty of goods on American store shelves and challenged by the value that Americans place on independent effort rather than succor by the State. Older adults may have a clear-cut cultural identity or may have selected an ethnic option from among the many available to them.

Determining the Impact of Culture on Health Beliefs

In this country the pending shift in racial demographics has fostered an obsession with multiculturalism. In an attempt to become culturally literate and culturally sensitive, there has been a proliferation of materials that categorize and compartmentalize the characteristics of racial and ethnic groups. Unfortunately this has led to a fair amount of stereotyping. Examples include: the industrious Asian, the emotional Hispanic, the stoic Indian, and the religious African-American. Such labels and the assumptions that flow from them (and the less positive stereotypical labels) are a dangerous trap for health care providers.

Nurses should approach the issue of cultural identity with an open mind and ask open-ended questions that will encourage the older adult to describe not only his or her own cultural background but that of ancestors and descendants as well. Older adults who arrived as immigrants themselves may still have strong cultural ties to their country of origin. However, their descendants—children and grandchildren—may now be acculturated; cross-cultural conflict may exist in the family system itself. The older adult may thus resist health care practices suggested by both the family and the nurse because they are not compatible with beliefs brought from the original culture. Collecting data free of cultural stereotyping allows the nurse to determine the extent to which the older adult is or wants to be assimilated into American society. Older persons who are more acculturated will require fewer adaptations in health care management.

Certainly nurses should pursue with active inter-

est information regarding biological variations among racial groups. They should enlarge their understanding of health belief systems and folk-medicine practices. However, they must refrain from the temptation to overgeneralize the characteristics studied. The major goal in working with minority clients (or with majority clients if the nurse is a minority) is to gain an accurate idea of their health beliefs and individual perceptions of their health problems. Toward that end the following questions may be more helpful than trying to memorize lists of categorized, cultural characteristics. The responses to these questions by the older adult will be a synthesis of cultural, ethnic, religious, and personal beliefs. They will enable the nurse to conceptualize the client's health belief system and integrate the most closely held values into the plan of care.

- What do you think has caused your problem?

- Why do you think it started when it did?

- What do you think your sickness does to you (how does it work)?

- How bad is your illness?

- Do you think it will get better soon or do you think it will last a long time?

- What kind of treatments have you already used?

- How did they work?

- What kind of treatment do you think you need now?

- What are the most important results you expect from your treatment?

- What problems has your illness caused for you?

- Who is helping you manage your illness? How are they helping?

(Anderson 1990; Redman 1988)

This format allows the practitioner to listen to the clients as they define their own health care beliefs using their personal worldview. It precludes hasty judgments or the impositions of health care regimens that may be totally unacceptable to the older person.

Cross-Cultural Misunderstandings between Provider and Client that Contribute to Noncompliance. The nurse should bear in mind that for racial and minority groups in America a strong determinant in worldviews may be the oppression and subordinate position they have experienced in society (Lash 1991). For those groups who have experienced economic deprivation resulting from unemployment or underemployment, survival may have depended on the development of a complex combination of survival skills and their accompanying attitudes and values. Health counseling, a major role of the nurse, is described by Lash as an "activity of middle-class whites that generates the assignment of many values and characteristics different from those held by racial minorities" (514). She stated that these differences become manifest when the client fails to exhibit the behaviors expected by the health care provider. The provider expects the client to be verbally expressive and open.

- Disclose intimate aspects of their lives.

- Be an equal and active participant in the interpersonal exchange.

- Communicate in standard English.

- Focus on long-range, task-oriented goals.

- Make clear distinctions between physical and mental well-being and cause-and-effect relationships.

Lash (1991) stated that when the majority health care worker confronts minority clients who are reluctant to share intimate aspects of their lives, the practitioner labels the client as resistant, defensive, or uncooperative. They also fail to recognize that individuals who do not use standard English fluently may inaccurately transmit or receive messages. (This can become an acute problem when an interpreter must be used.) She further noted that when the conversation fails to go back and forth between provider and client, the provider may incorrectly interpret the silence as negative. The client may be exhibiting a sign of respect for one viewed to be in a superior or dominant position. For many minority clients health is a manifestation of the harmonious relationship between the body, mind, and spirit. They may become confused when the practitioner tries to separate physical from mental well-being.

Social class can be a significant barrier to the delivery of health care. Most health care providers are members of the middle class, some are members of the upper class. These social classes place great emphasis on goal-directed activity and a high premium on prompt action taken in matters related to health and physical well-being. Many minority clients are disproportionately poor and therefore are members of the lower social class. For them poverty may lead to a preoccupation with tangible, immediate problems and actions related to day-to-day survival. They seek immediate, concrete results from health care providers. Thus the most successful interventions will be those directed toward problems that the client has already identified. Care directed toward anticipatory guidance, reflection of feelings to promote insight, and attempts to discovery underlying intrapsychic problems may be viewed as inappropriate by the client (Lash 1991). Failure to recognize the position of health care in the client's priorities and anger over assumed noncompliance may hurt the relationship entirely. An older minority adult who has survived to advanced age has already proven the ability to make choices that enhance survival. Nurses should recognize and value older adults' skills in selecting among options.

Minority clients often experience powerlessness in their daily lives. Majority-group health care providers who take an authoritarian, demanding approach and take over the decision-making process exacerbate this sense of powerlessness (Freebairn and Gwinup 1979). Care provided in a brusque, hasty manner, considered efficient and professional by health care providers, may be viewed as rude, arrogant, and impersonal by the client. Feeling belittled and shamed, the client withholds information, fails to ask for clarification of instructions, and withdraws figuratively if not literally from the health care delivery system.

Minority clients may come from a cultural value system that does not stress a biophysiological basis for disease. Or they may lack the educational base to understand the application of biophysiological concepts to their health problems. Thus they may not have the necessary background to evaluate the information being given to them.

Most illnesses are self-limiting and heal without medical intervention. Older adults have survived many such illnesses over their lifetime. Furthermore, fiscal constraints prevent many minority adults from seeking health care for any but the most acute symptoms. Even then entry into the health care system may be delayed until functional impairment or severe pain occurs. Lacking a scientific concept of illness, these older adults may find it difficult to seek health care or follow through on health care regimens when no acute or apparent symptoms exist. To such adults relief of symptoms of an illness means that it is healed. Hypertension is an example of an illness for which sustained compliance is difficult to achieve. Many older adults have no apparent symptoms and therefore do not comprehend the devastation that can be wrought by this disorder. The problem is particularly acute among older African-Americans for whom the sequelae—stroke and end-stage renal disease—are particularly destructive. Failure to feel bad particularly impacts medication purchase and compliance. Faced with a choice between food, rent, transportation, or medication, it makes little sense to waste money on drugs when one has no symptoms.

Nurses must recognize that it takes time to build the trust that will glue a relationship together. Many health care providers look like children (even if in their 40s or 50s) to adults of advanced age. Nurses should expect to have to earn acceptance and credibility. Ideas presented will be tested by the older adult and must be found workable or they, along with the practitioner, will be discarded as irrelevant. Patience and forgiveness are the key. Nurses must realize that pressing or conflicting priorities may interfere with prompt compliance with some health care regimens. However, that does not necessarily mean that compliance will not be present at a later date or on another issue. See Appendix A for a sampling of cultural characteristics of the major racial and ethnic groups. This categorization is by no means comprehensive and great caution should be exercised by nurses in the application of these characteristics to minority clients. Generalization of the identified traits to all individuals in a cultural group can blind health care providers to the unique personalities of American clients who may blend many ethnic options to create an individual person.

Integrating Folk Medicine with Traditional High-Tech Care

All cultures, including majority populations, use home remedies and lay practitioners in the management of illness. However, lay healers and the practice of folk medicine may be more important to minority populations. Lay healers are generally well known by the clients and may even be relatives, friends, or neighbors. Thus rapport and interpersonal trust readily exist between healer and client. Lay healers often involve the family of the client in their ministrations and allow management of the illness to remain under the control of family members. Generally lay healers provide advice and give guidance. They do not give orders or make demands (Freebairn and Gwinup 1979).

Lay healers are often thought to have special powers and healing gifts bestowed by God. Since God's power is limitless, all things are possible. Therefore the folk healer's powers may be perceived as potentially stronger than those of traditional Western medical practitioners whose skills may be limited by the confines of human knowledge. Minority populations often use folk healers concurrently with Western medicine or may believe that certain types of disorders may be treated only by the folk healer (Downes 1986).

Major advantages to the use of the folk healer are cost, accessibility, and convenience. Not only are their treatments affordable, they are provided in a culturally acceptable and sensitive manner. Folk medicine is holistic. It most often takes into account all aspects of a person's life, including his or her personal relationships, cultural environment, religion, and personal spiritual beliefs (Freebairn and Gwinup 1979). Folk medicine is familiar. It changes slowly over time and is passed from one trusted individual to another from generation to generation. It has been validated by the experiences of those known and loved.

In contrast, the majority health care provider is a stranger, a representative of a system that is alien and frightening if not frankly hostile to the needs of the minority client. Therefore if majority practitioners wish to attain credibility in the minority community, they must learn about the prevailing folk medicine beliefs and practices. Nurses should seek, whenever possible without active danger to the client, to integrate valued folk medicine practices with those of traditional medicine to create an acceptable approach to the prevention and cure of illness. Many home remedies are equivalent to prescribed medicines and may be safer and cheaper to use. Most folk medicine practices enhance psychological well-being and thus boost the body's immune system in its curative efforts. However, the nurse should remain alert to potential dangers when both folk and traditional medicine are being used together. For example, Hispanics and Asians use many herbal teas. Some of these teas have medicinal properties and may counteract or dangerously potentiate the effect of prescription medications ordered by the physician.

Nurses should recognize that their ethnocentrism—the tendency to consider their own cultural practices as superior to others (Ross and Cobb 1990)—may blind them to the positive aspects of the caregiving systems of others. It can be an adventure to open oneself up to new and different possibilities for health care. It can be a particularly rewarding experience when learning about these options from older minority clients. During their long years they have seen health care go through many trends, often to return and embrace long-forgotten practices. They are the repositories of folk healing practices never known to their younger professional caregivers. They have acquired some valid ideas about what works, though they may not be able to explain why in physiological terms. If nurses give these lay practices a fair evaluation, they may acquire new techniques to adapt to self-care and/or pass along to others.

Goal Setting for Care

Based on an evaluation of the collected data base, the client and nurse set goals for care. Upon reviewing the identified problems and the strengths and limitations in the solutions to these problems, the client is often able to set goals for himself or herself and to suggest and explore alternative methods for reaching these goals. The nurse may not always agree with the client's decision but must understand the significance of the client maintaining the right to make decisions concerning his or her own life. The continued interpersonal association and the nurse's acceptance of the client's decisions increase the client's respect for and trust in the nurse as a caring person. Thus the client may ultimately return to re-evaluate decisions and perhaps even alter them, secure that the nurse will not view this change as a failure on his or her part. In contrast, by insisting on a course of action thought best, the nurse may alienate the client and

fracture the constructive and therapeutic progress of the relationship. The nurse may also become the brunt of the client's anger when an unsatisfactory outcome of an imposed decision occurs.

Collection of Epidemiologic Data

Information collected during psychosocial assessment provides epidemiologic data on the problems and process of aging. Information gained from the assessment of many older adults and analyzed collectively yields information regarding the components of satisfactory and unsatisfactory life adjustments for the older person. Such information can be used to identify the major health problems within this population (Lantz 1976).

Evaluation of Nursing Care

A review of the data collected over a period of time from a variety of clients can reveal the strengths and weaknesses in the nurse's therapeutic approach to clients. An evaluation of these patterns of intervention may indicate a need for a change in the behavior of the nurse or the health care team.

Evaluation of Successful Patterns of Aging

The psychosocial assessment is a learning experience for the nurse. If privileged to work with a large number of older adults (or even one very special one), the nurse can learn about aging and can plan for his or her own arrival at that state by deliberately selecting patterns and approaches to life that have proved effective for others.

Public Policy Planning

Data collected during the psychosocial assessment, together with selected case studies, can be used to influence funding sources, insurance firms, politicians, and lawmakers. The older adult is generally interested in the political process, even if not actively involved. The older adult will often consent to allowing client care information to be shared if the outcome will benefit either individuals or other groups of older adults. Many older adults, both poor and affluent, are willing to personally testify before city councils, insurance review boards, and congressional committees in an effort to improve the health care policies that affect them.

INTERVIEWING THE OLDER ADULT CLIENT

The nature of the data shared with the nurse in the process of psychosocial assessment depends largely on the quality of the nurse-client relationship. Since the commencement and continuation of a satisfactory relationship depend on the effective use of therapeutic communication skills, some additional comments relevant to interaction with older people are in order.

The interview with the client to obtain data for evaluation of psychosocial status is a two-way interaction in which each person has a constant impact on the other. The nurse must maintain continual sensitivity to the client's feelings or responses during the course of the interaction. Attention must be directed toward any verbal and nonverbal cues given by the client that signal that something within the relationship is amiss.

Many older clients approach an interview with some degree of trepidation. Some have resided for a period of time in relative isolation and their skills in verbal exchange may have atrophied from sheer disuse. There may be uncertainty about the purpose of the interaction and a fear of revealing deficits (physical and psychologic) that will cause shame or lead to institutionalization and ultimately the loss of independence. For those who live with a chronically high level of anxiety as they struggle to meet basic human needs on a subsistence level of income or with severely limited social opportunities, the additional anxiety of establishing a new relationship with another person may be almost beyond bearing. Insecurity may exist about the nurse's sincerity in establishing a relationship, and a fear of subsequent abandonment may outweigh the willingness to risk commitment to another.

Preparation for the Interview

Preparation for the interview is essential. The nurse must review the areas to be explored during the interview and put the questions to be asked in a systematic order so that no major area of psychosocial functioning is overlooked. During preparation the nurse should give consideration to the time necessary for complete data collection in relation to the actual amount of time available and to the mental and physical condition of the client.

Care should be taken to plan for the collection of a realistic amount of data in the time allotted. For example with only one hour available it is unrealistic to expect comprehensive data collection. Any attempt to achieve such a data collection in so short a time will create high levels of anxiety for the client, who, feeling pressured, will gloss over significant areas of concern and interest to comply with the nurse's deadline. The client will then view the nurse as disinterested and unfeeling. In the nursing approach to older people it is essential to provide sufficient time to accomplish tasks and achieve goals, because they often require more time to assimilate information and formulate responses. Alterations in thought processes may cause the omission of data, but the older adult has a great desire to respond accurately in regard to the data requested. A sense of pervasive urgency will not result in greater speed but will block both mental and physical performance altogether as the client becomes overwhelmed. Verbal or nonverbal signs of anxiety during the interview should alert the nurse to the possibility that the pace is outstripping the client's ability to keep up competently. Questions fired in quick succession, rapid speech patterns, and body language indicating impatience are negative behaviors producing unsatisfactory results. If the time has been planned properly before the nurse meets the client, situations that engender this behavior by the nurse and elicit a disastrous response from the client may be avoided.

Psychosocial assessment is a lengthy process and continues over the entire span of the nurse-client relationship. The data base is constantly amended and altered to reflect the continuous changes occurring in the client's life situation. When time is limited or the client's condition is marked by confusion, fatigue, or pain, priorities must be determined. Essential data should be acquired initially with branching questions focusing in greater depth on areas of special concern to the client. Additional information may be collected during subsequent meetings.

The nurse's preparation extends to the physical surroundings in which the interview will be conducted. The environment should be prepared as though an honored guest is expected. The interview area should be aesthetically pleasant, well lit, physically comfortable, relatively free from distracting noise, and totally free from disruption. For the period of time allotted the client should be the center of attention. Constant interruptions will impede the ability to recall and convey data, decrease feelings of self-worth, and fracture rapport. If the nurse must enter the client's own environment to conduct an interview, respect for personal space and possessions should be exhibited by such behaviors as knocking before entering and asking permission before moving objects or sitting on chairs. The nurse should try to arrange the interview environment to provide for both intimacy and privacy.

Chairs should be placed at a 45 degree angle to each other and close enough so that touch may be used for positive reinforcement and as a demonstration of concern and understanding, if indicated. Barricading oneself behind a desk or other obstacle will act as both a physical and psychologic deterrent to closeness. If chairs must be near a desk, they should be placed alongside so that no obstruction lies directly between nurse and client. If the interview must be conducted at the client's bedside, the nurse should take great pains to ensure privacy and reduce interruptions. The older adult will find it difficult to participate actively in an interview if treatments and medications are being provided simultaneously by other health team members or if a roommate can eavesdrop on information being exchanged.

The Process of Interviewing

The older adult responds readily to a psychologic environment that projects interest,, encouragement, and support. Therefore unless it is totally impossible to do so because of environmental limitations, the nurse should sit during nurse-client interactions that are designed specifically for the acquisition of data. Sitting communicates important nonverbal messages such as "I have time for you," "I am going to get comfortable so that I can really listen," "I have taken the socially accepted position for meaningful communication." Sitting also places the nurse's face in a position where the client with limited hearing can supplement auditory reception with lip reading. Standing, on the other hand, implies a momentary pause before impending flight. In addition to the nonverbal message sent by the act of sitting, the nurse may be profoundly astonished by the power of the sensitive and discriminate use of touch. Decreased sensory stimulation, altered sensory awareness, reduced social interaction, and at times physical isolation can create in the older adult a strong craving for stroking, caressing, and physical contact that will validate the older person's individuality and convey acceptance.

The nurse should be sensitive to sensory losses that impact communication. The hearing loss that accompanies aging is the second most common condition affecting the health of older adults (Corso 1984), but health care personnel should not assume that all older people are hard of hearing. Clark and Mills (1979) estimated that 30 percent to 50 percent of the population 65 years and older are affected by presbycusis, the most common type of hearing loss in older adults. Too often, however, nurses and other health care personnel automatically raise their voices when talking with older people in the belief that they cannot hear a normal tone of voice. Shouting may be interpreted as hostility or anger by the older person who can hear well.

Signs of hearing loss the nurse should look for are lack of normal response, inattentiveness, difficulty following directions, inappropriate responses, requests to have the speaker repeat words, turning one ear toward the speaker and speech that is very loud or soft (Clark and Mills 1979).

With clients who have minimal hearing losses, nurses can facilitate communication by getting close enough to the client so that the lips can be seen, by assessing which ear has the best hearing and speaking closer to that ear, by using facial expressions and hand gestures, by speaking slightly slower and more clearly, by pronouncing words distinctly, and by using a lower pitch of voice since presbycusis makes it difficult for high-frequency sounds and consonants to be heard and understood. The manner of speaking should be natural and not distorted by vigorous lip movement in an attempt to be understood. The speaker should not eat, smoke, chew gum, obstruct the face with a hand or object such as a pencil, bend the head, or move the face so that the older person cannot see the lips. When it is necessary to repeat a comment because it has not been heard, it is better to rephrase the comment than to repeat the same words.

Background noise should be reduced if possible by turning the television or radio volume down or off, by closing the door, and by asking others in the area to be quiet.

Efforts expended in validating with the client what was actually said usually constitute time well spent. Older people are often not aware of their hearing inadequacies, and their perceptions of what they have heard may not be accurate. Confusion, inaccurate hearing, and other forms of perceptual impairments can occur at a number of points in the communication cycle. The stimulus from the environment may be unclear, ambiguous, or delayed; the receptivity of the sense organs is subsequently affected. Moreover, impaired sense organs have a diminished potential for receiving an accurate message. The processing of information then is affected by the accuracy of the message which was heard.

For those older adults who have certain diagnosed hearing losses, hearing aids may help amplify sounds and thus facilitate the communication process. Hearing aids should be functioning properly before conversation is attempted.

Adequate sight makes communication easier, especially for those who have losses in hearing and comprehension. Eye-to-eye contact can help the nurse evaluate the extent to which the older person has heard and understood what was being said. A perceptive nurse can analyze facial expressions and eye and mouth movements to determine if comments have been heard and understood.

Increased light with no glare, and lighting that comes from behind the client and does not strike the eyes will help the older person see the face and lips of the speaker, thus facilitating communication. Dirty glasses are a common hindrance to clear vision. Older people often do not think to clean their glasses, and if they do, they may use a soiled handkerchief or part of their own clothing, smearing the glasses even more. The nurse should wash the glasses with soap and running water and dry them thoroughly with a substance that will not leave lint on the lenses. It is amazing how much visual acuity can be improved by this simple nursing intervention.

To reduce the confusion caused by a change in environment, the client should be allowed a few moments to adjust before the nurse launches into the interview. This time may be spent in offering a cup of coffee, introducing oneself, and asking the client's name. The nurse should further explain his or her position with the agency or institution and the nature of present and future involvement with the client. The purpose and scope of the interview should be explained, as well as an explanation of how the data will be used. Such an explanation should include the positions of others, if any, who will have access to the information. If the time is restricted, the client should be informed of the limitation.

The most important communication tool for the nurse is the art of listening: listening to what is actually being said and listening for the feeling tone behind it. Listening is far more difficult than talking, because through listening the nurse gives up self and truly places the focus on another. Active listening involves total immersion in the present interaction and requires constant attention to the verbal and nonverbal communication that is being sent and received. Such intense concentration may prove exhausting to the nurse, so schedules should be planned to intersperse client interviews with other activities throughout the day. In this manner the nurse can be "refreshed" and "ready" for the next interpersonal exchange.

The interview should proceed from less personal questions to those that are usually considered personal or intimate. In American culture, questions concerning financial status and sexuality are high on the list of sensitive areas. One cannot always predict, however, the topics that will be sensitive or disconcerting for the client. Some people may be completely unperturbed during the acquisition of their sexual history but may become agitated to the point of tears when they discuss their inability to care properly for a beloved pet. The nurse must therefore be sensitive to the topics that are difficult for the client and refrain from pushing for information beyond that which the client is willing to provide freely. The nurse may also find it difficult to explore certain areas of inquiry because of a personal value orientation that causes certain areas to be labeled as emotionally loaded. Thus the nurse must evaluate whether difficulty in collecting data lies with the client or with the interviewer.

Transition statements should be used when the nurse moves from one type of data to another to signal the client that the focus of the interview is changing and to enable the client to shift mental gears and energy.

Client responses should be acknowledged, and any feelings the client expresses should be accepted without judgmental retaliation. Positive reinforcement should be offered to encourage the client to proceed and to confirm that his or her behavior is indeed appropriate for the situation. A smile added to the simple act of touch is effective positive reinforcement.

During an interview the client may pose questions and should be encouraged to do so. These questions should be answered honestly, thoughtfully, and carefully by the nurse. Problems should not be denied or skimmed over; they should be acknowledged as real concerns calling for consideration and concerted action.

At the conclusion of the nurse-client interview the data should be summarized and the problems and concerns of the client identified. One strategy that often proves effective is to state, "I have been asking you a lot of questions. Before we leave each other today, do you have any questions you would like to ask me?" The client may use this period to expand upon or clarify information that might have been misunderstood or undervalued by the nurse. Together the client and nurse should determine priority problems and evolve appropriate alternatives for action. If possible, time should be scheduled for a follow-up interview to enable the client to provide additional relevant information that may be recalled after reflection. If a face-to-face interview will not be possible, the client should be given instructions for reaching the nurse to correct information or provide an addendum to the information already provided.

Overcoming Language Barriers

There will be times when a significant language barrier exists between the nurse and the client. The client may not speak the nurse's language at all, or more dangerously, may speak it only a little, leading the nurse to assume a fluency that does not exist. Even when the older client appears to be bilingual, the nurse should exercise great caution before concluding that communication is not impaired. During periods of illness and stress, fluency in the acquired or second language may become inconsistent or be lost altogether. Bilingual individuals may also have difficulty communicating thoughts of an emotional or very personal nature in their nondominant language. To surmount the language barrier, there will be times when the use of an interpreter is necessary.

Working with older adult clients through an interpreter is risky business. The three-way interpersonal relationship, in which two participants do not understand one another and must rely on a third party to accurately interpret their intent, is fraught with many more possibilities for misunderstanding than normal communication which is often hazardous. Nurses should assume from the outset that the process will have built-in errors and use every possible means of identifying and correcting them.

Ideally, great care should be taken in the selection of an interpreter. Incongruities between the ages, sexes, and social status of the client and interpreter can create serious difficulties (Tien-Hyatt 1987). When family members are interpreters, the client may limit the range of communication with the professional due to a reluctance to have the relative know about his/her concerns, fears, or business affairs. Conversely, the family interpreter may filter information coming from the client to protect the reputation of the family or to make it more acceptable to the nurse. For example, if a young grandchild must be used as a translator, an older adult male may have great difficulty telling the nurse that he stopped taking his antihypertensive medication because it rendered him impotent. Likewise an older Hispanic woman may have difficulty discussing postmenopausal bleeding through a male intermediary.

It is also critical that the health care provider have some knowledge regarding the relationships between ethnic subgroups. The use of interpreters in public clinics and screening sites can be problematic. For example, in an Hispanic Senior Center English-speaking seniors serve as translators for their peers who speak only Spanish. Hearing difficulties, often shared by both seniors in the interaction, coupled with the assignment of peer translators disliked by some of the clients, create data collection that is not always accurate.

Unfortunately the ideal situation seldom exists, and interpreters are often secured in haste when a crisis is pending. The most readily available individual is seldom well suited for the job they are asked to perform. Whenever possible the nurse should talk to the translator ahead of time and discuss the goal of the planned interaction. The nurse may want to discuss the material to be presented and collaborate with the interpreter on the best way to convey information back and forth. If the translator is not a member of a health care profession, this planning period will also force the nurse to simplify information so that it can be understood by a lay person and remove technical jargon and terminology. If written materials are to be used in the interaction, the nurse and translator may wish to reach a clear agreement on the wording and meaning of what is being conveyed (Freebairn and Gwinup 1979).

During the nurse-client interaction the nurse should direct conversation to the client, not to the translator. It is important that the relationship be established with the client, not the intermediary. Looking at the client while speaking allows the nurse to observe for nonverbal cues that the communication is not clear. Sentence structure should be kept simple and information should be transmitted sentence by sentence, not paragraph by paragraph. Ideas should be simplified and presented briefly. If kept brief, there is less likelihood that the translator will leave out a lot, will project his/her own meaning on what is being said, or will edit by paraphrasing. Great care should be taken to avoid slang, abstractions, or abbreviations.

Some distortion is normal in all communication and more distortion will be present in this type of complex dialogue. Therefore the nurse should request a translation back. The client should be asked to repeat instructions or the main points of the communication in his or her own words back to the nurse through the interpreter (Freebairn and Gwinup 1979). Misunderstandings should then be identified, clarified, and corrected. Since conversation through an interpreter is time-consuming, the nurse will want to ensure that sufficient time is allowed to make the conversation productive. If the client is ill or fatigues easily, conversational sessions may need to be broken into several brief periods. At the time of the initial interaction, priority should be given to the communication priorities identified by the client, and an attempt should be made to establish interim methods of communicating when the interpreter is not available.

OBTAINING DATA FROM THE FAMILY

The family should be an integral part of the psychosocial assessment, although information may be collected from them in a separate session. Contact with the family provides new insights regarding the client. It also enables the nurse to meet the needs of family members who are concerned about the client's well-being and whose lifestyle may have been altered by a change in the psychologic or physical status of the older adult. Data from the family often reinforce the information given by the client. Or discrepancies may come to light that were caused by possible confusion or disorientation on the part of the client.

In some families, conflict exists about the goals of care, the control of the family caregiving network, and/or the ultimate disbursal of an older person's estate and personal possessions. In others, a conflict arises when some family members feel they bear a disproportionate burden of the financial and/or physical care of an older relative. For yet others, unresolved emotional struggles surrounding unmet needs for love, recognition, and achievement exist. It would be wise therefore for the nurse to establish contact with several members of the client's emotional support system, including children, siblings, and friends. Data obtained from several people will enable the nurse to evaluate the quality of family interaction and the accuracy of the perception of the dynamics of the family system by its members. (See "Guide for Family Assessment" in Appendix B and chapter 19 on Family Support and Intergenerational Issues.) If the client is unable to manage his or her own affairs and has no support system or has a family that is acting in a way that endangers the client's psychologic or physical health, the nurse may wish to request an evaluation of the client for the purpose of securing a court-appointed conservator.

PSYCHOSOCIAL ASSESSMENT GUIDES

The guides in Appendices A, B, C, & D are presented as samples of the type and range of data to be used in a psychosocial assessment of the older adult client and his or her family. The reader will note that the client format is lengthy and obvious discretion is required in its use. Different settings, diverse purposes for collection, and individual client needs dictate variation in the components to be used. Questions are presented in a format that the author finds comfortable, but they can easily be adapted to suit the style of another interviewer.

More comprehensive data will be acquired, of course, if the nurse-patient relationship is to be a long one, such as those formed in a skilled nursing home or extended care facility, in the family physician's office, with a nurse practitioner in a community health center, or through long-term contact with a visiting nurse. Abbreviated psychosocial assessment tools with a focus on areas relevant to specific illness are more appropriate for use in acute care settings such as hospitals or emergency care facilities.

All entries should be dated, and additional data should be added during the course of the relationship as indicated. The client should be informed that the nurse may make notes during data-gathering sessions. The nurse should explain that note taking will increase the accuracy of recording and decrease the possibility of error. During the interview, however, the nurse should avoid being so absorbed in recording information that the client becomes distracted. If possible, recording should be kept to the bare minimum. The nurse should remain actively involved in listening and guiding the interpersonal process at hand.

ASSESSMENT OF THE ENVIRONMENT

To focus on the client and family unit alone would be a serious nursing error. Attention must be given to the environment of the older adult, which to a large extent structures and defines his or her life. Most older people wish to remain in the community and within their own homes as long as possible.

An assessment of the home environment is essential for the nurse involved in discharge planning or supervision of the care of an older adult at home. If the nurse possesses an adequate picture of the home environment, adaptations may be made that will aid self-sufficiency and make continued functioning at home possible, thus preventing premature institutionalization. A "Guide for Assessment of Home Environment" (found in Appendix C) will aid the nurse in making decisions concerning the adequacy of the

home environment and the education of the older person who wishes to remain there.

For those clients who must be institutionalized a prior evaluation of the proposed facility by family members is a must. It is no longer a secret that institutions often do great harm while seeking to do good. The growth of the older population has left the nation psychologically and institutionally unable to cope adequately. The problems of too few institutions, shortages of adequately prepared personnel, lack of adequate programming, lack of a cohesive national policy regarding the older population, and the use of institutions as a profit-making investment have all served to create concern over the institution as a therapeutic milieu for long-term care.

The personnel in many institutions that provide care for older adults have for the most part been well-meaning but tragically unaware of the effect their ministrations have on the client. Many are woefully devoid of information concerning therapeutic approaches for older people. In addition, administrative policy, reimbursement guidelines, and profit-making motives may tie the hands of those who wish to implement change.

Gresham (1976) has suggested that nurses infantilize institutionalized older people through a socialization process that creates dependency. Since no clear-cut role exists for older adults, Gresham has suggested that the institution (and often significant others) casts older people in the role of children. Their adult years are negated, together with all the rights, powers, privileges, and responsibilities that accompany them. The client is called by his or her first name, hair is combed in pony tails, and frequent reminders are issued to "be a good girl or boy." Clients, having assessed the prevailing power structure, gradually submit to the socialization process and conform.

Through infantilization, accompanied by sensory, social, and intellectual deprivation, the client is gradually stripped of all identity and purpose. Physical care is perfect, but humanity is lost, and often with it goes the will to live. It is important therefore that the nurse evaluate the "helping" environment critically. The presence of the attributes noted in the "Institutional Assessment Guide" (found in Appendix D) would contribute to the creation of an environment in which the potential of the older adult could be realized and used for continuous growth.

Though intended specifically for extended care facilities such as nursing homes, these criteria are applicable in any environment provided for or created by the older adult. The absence of any of these attributes is a cue to initiate corrective nursing action.

SUMMARY

The major tasks of the nurse who works with the older adult are support in attaining satisfactory life adjustment and recognition of progress on the journey to self-actualization and fulfillment.

Based on the work of Charlotte Buhler (Weiner et al. 1978), self-fulfillment in older adults may be described as involving four factors.

1. The aspect of luck—a sense of meeting the right people, or being in the right place at the right time

2. Realization of potential—a sense of having tapped one's potential and being able to do most of what one wants to do

3. Accomplishment—a sense of having something to show for one's life

4. Moral evaluation—a sense of having "lived right" in terms of moral and religious conviction

Data obtained in the course of psychosocial assessment of the client, family, and environment may be evaluated in light of Buhler's criteria for self-fulfillment. Nursing measures can then be planned to ameliorate the impact of physical or psychosocial aspects of the client's life that prevent self-fulfillment.

Thus the role of the nurse working with the older adult will shift from that of a custodial caregiver to one of a reciprocal human relationship based on mutual respect. Such a relationship will foster the development of self-actualization and fulfillment in the client. Skilled bedside nursing care will still be needed for those older adults beset with radical changes in their physical and psychologic status that confine them to an institutional setting. At present, however, these people comprise only 5 percent of the older population. The remaining 95 percent reside in the community, and for them nursing involvement is no less essential. For community-based older adults, professional nursing care may make the vital difference between a life of self-sufficiency and one of institutionalization. Indeed even within the institution the nurse will make the difference between a life of evolving potential or one devoid of meaning, leading to apathy and despair.

STUDY QUESTIONS

1. Discuss the major purposes of collecting a psychosocial assessment.

2. What are the elements to be considered by the nurse in preparation for conducting a psychosocial interview?

3. Identify eight strategies that can be used by the nurse during the process of interviewing to facilitate the flow of information.

4. What constitutes effective listening and why is it important in collection of a psychosocial assessment?

5. How does the nurse work with the client and family to develop goals and priorities of care?

6. How can friends and significant others be incorporated in the management of the client's care?

7. Explore the nurse's responsibilities to the family.

8. Using the psychosocial assessment guide, identify the items to include on a tool to be used in a thirty-minute interview with a hospitalized, newly admitted, older adult.

9. Using the psychosocial assessment guide in Appendix B, create an interview tool to be used on a 1 1/2-hour home visit to admit an older adult to a health service.

10. Why is an assessment of the environment critical in planning care for an older adult?

11. What major categories of items should be included in an evaluation of a client's home environment?

12. List major categories of items that should be included in an evaluation of an institutional environment.

REFERENCES

American Association of Retired Persons and Administration on Aging. 1990. *A Profile of Older Americans*. Washington, DC: United States Department of Health and Human Services.

Anderson, J.A. 1990. Health care across cultures. *Nursing Outlook* 38(1):12–15.

Burnside, I.M. 1988. *Nursing and the Aged: A Self Care Approach*. New York: McGraw-Hill Book Company.

Clark, C.C., and M.J. Mills. 1979. Communicating with hearing impaired elderly adults. *Journal of Gerontological Nursing* 5(3):40–44.

Clavon, A. 1986. The black elderly. *Journal of Gerontological Nursing* 12(5):6–12.

Corso, J. 1984. Auditory responses and aging: Significant problems for research. *Exp Aging Research* 10(3):171–173.

Davis, K., P. Grant, and D. Rowland. 1990. Alone and poor. *Generations* Summer:43–47.

Downes, N.J. 1986. *Multicultural Health Beliefs and Practices*. HHS Bureau of Health Promotion Grant, # 5031 AH 70058-02.

Freebairn, J. and K. Gwinup. 1979. *Cultural Diversity and Nursing Practice: Instructors Manual*. Irvine, CA: Concept Media.

Fried, L.P., D.J. Storer, D.E. King, and F. Ladder. 1991. Diagnosis of illness presentation in the elderly. *Journal of the American Geriatrics Society* 39(2):117–23.

Gresham, M.L. 1976. The infantilization of the elderly: A developing concept. *Nursing Forum* 15:195–210.

Idler, E.L., and S. Kasl. 1991. Health perceptions and survival: Do global evaluations of health status really predict mortality? *Journal of Gerontology* 46(2):S55–65.

Lantz, J. 1976. Assessment: A beginning to individualized care. *Journal of Gerontological Nursing* 2(6):34–40.

Lash, M.E. 1991. Community health nursing in a minority setting. In *Readings in Community Health Nursing*. 4th ed., edited by B.W. Spradley. Philadelphia: J.B. Lippincott Co.

Minkler, M. and R. Stone. 1985. The feminization of poverty and older women. *The Gerontologist* 24(4):353–57.

Molde, S. 1986. Understanding patients' agendas. *Image* 18(4):145–47.

Redman, B.K. 1988. *The Process of Patient Education*. St. Louis: C.V. Mosby Company.

Ross, B. and K.L. Cobb. 1990. *Family Nursing*. Redwood City, CA: Addison-Wesley Nursing.

Tien-Hyatt, J.L. 1987. Keying in on the unique care needs of Asian clients. *Nursing and Health Care* 8(5):269–61.

Tripp-Reimer, T., and G.M. Laver. 1987. Ethnicity and families with chronic illness. In *Families and Chronic Illness*, edited by L.M. Wright and M. Leahey. Springhouse, PA: Springhouse.

United States Department of Health and Human Services: Public Health Service. 1990. *Health People 2000: National Health Promotion and Disease Prevention Objectives*. [DHHS Publication No. (PHS) 91-50212.] Washington, DC: United States Government Printing Office.

Weiner, M.B., A.J. Brok and A.M. Snadowsky. 1978. *Working with the Aged: Practical Approaches in the Institution and the Community*. Englewood Cliffs, NJ: Prentice-Hall.

8 Dietary Management

Nell B. Robinson

CHAPTER OUTLINE

FOCUS

The focus of this chapter is to provide guidance in meeting the dietary needs of older adults. Adequate nutrition is an essential component of successful aging. This chapter presents factors that hinder the adequate intake of essential nutrients in older adults. The role of the major nutrients in maintaining wellness and preventing disease in the later years is presented. Practical suggestions related to feeding frail older adults also are included.

OBJECTIVES

1. Recognize the role of nutrition in maintaining a healthy body.

2. Evaluate the energy requirements, realizing that the kilocalorie needs may decrease with inactivity and age.

3. Understand the importance of meeting the nutrient requirements for the older adult.

4. Identify standards and food guides available for promotion of healthy eating.

5. Explore the impact of socioeconomic, psychologic, cultural, religious, and physiological factors on food intake.

6. Identify chronic diseases that may occur as a result of inadequate nutrition in older adults.

7. Provide suggestions for feeding patients who cannot feed themselves.

8. Identify resources available that can assist in supplying food and other help to those who need assistance.

9. Provide guidelines for planning healthy meals.

10. Identify ideas for making the food dollar go further while reducing kilocalories.

The nutritional and health status of the older population has become a great concern of health care professionals (Hui 1983). The focus on nutrition for this population has become significant because of the predicted increase in the number and proportion of the older population and the increase in life expectancy (Alfin-Slater 1986). Concern about malnutrition in older people is growing as health care providers and researchers realize how poorly many older Americans eat. It has been estimated that one-third to one-half of the health problems experienced by older individuals are directly or indirectly related to nutritional problems (Community Nutrition Institute 1986). Adequate nutritional care for the older adult deserves considerable emphasis, since the well-nourished older person will not only be more comfortable and energetic but will also be better able to tolerate medical and surgical treatment when it is necessary.

NUTRITIONAL CONSIDERATIONS

Nutrition is important in the aging process. It is not enough merely to survive into the years from 60 to 100; they should be years of health, enjoyment, and mental vigor. The intake of food is one of the greatest variables in life. People have an instinctive appetite for the pleasure of eating, but the desire for food does not necessarily assure availability, adequate intake, or nutritional balance. The food eaten must furnish the building materials from which muscles, organs, teeth, blood, and all other body components are made and repaired. Regardless of a person's age it is necessary for nutrients to be converted into energy, furnish substrates for enzymes and hormones, and regulate and control body functions. Because people do not age physically at the same rate as chronologically, the older population cannot be classified as a homogeneous group. Each older person is an individual, and the health professional must be very careful to avoid stereotyping older people. The information presented in this chapter should serve as a flexible guide for providing nutritional care for older adults.

Energy

It is an important fact of geriatric nutrition that although nutritional requirements remain similar no matter what one's age, the kilocaloric requirements decrease with age. However, disease and ill health in many older adults may actually increase their need for some nutrients while reducing the efficiency of their nutrient digestion, absorption, and metabolism. The unit for measuring energy is the kilocalorie (kcal), the amount of heat or energy required to raise the temperature of one kilogram (kg) of water 1° Celsius. The number of kilocalories needed is determined by *(1)* the number of kilocalories necessary for basal metabolism, *(2)* the number of kilocalories needed for muscular activity, and *(3)* the number of kilocalories required for the digestion and absorption of food.

The kilocaloric requirements gradually decrease with age because of a reduction in the number of metabolically active cells. Moreover, there is an increase in the proportion of body weight that is adipose tissue, along with a reduction in lean body mass, i.e., muscle tissue and bone. The kilocalorie requirements are usually diminished by 10 percent in people aged 51–75 and 20–25% in those older than 75 (Roe 1991a). However, there are large variations in the need for kilocalories according to age, size, occupation, environment, physical activity habits, and the presence or absence of chronic illness. The average recommended dietary allowance for kilocalories beyond age 60 for men of reference size (77 kg) is 2300 kilocalories per day; for women of reference size (65 kg) it is 1900 kilocalories per day. The normal variation of plus or minus 20 percent is accepted (*Recommended Dietary Allowances* 1989).

There is obviously a need for further reduction in kilocalorie intake of a bedridden, immobilized person. The lower intake of kilocalories poses the problem of obtaining sufficient nutrients. The diet of the geriatric patient has less room for so-called empty kilocalories received from high-kilocaloric foods that have few nutrients even though these foods may be inexpensive, easy to eat, and well liked. Sugar, sweets, fats, oils, and alcohol, which are empty kilocalorie foods, should be consumed in limited quantities. It has been determined that for each 3500 kilocalories eaten and not burned, a person gains one pound of body weight. There must be a constant awareness of slight increases in weight, because it is much easier to maintain normal weight than to decrease it after the gain occurs. Obesity, characteristic of adult populations, persists into old age. After the age of 60 about 45 percent of all women and 32 percent of all men are overweight (Weg 1978).

Increased physical activity is important for any person interested in maintaining good health. Not only does exercise help control weight, it also increases blood flow to all body organs, helping to keep them healthy; it helps maintain good muscle tone and slows atrophy associated with chronic disease; it helps avoid constipation problems; it allows for the consumption of more food, which will provide the proper nutrients; it lowers blood sugar levels, often improving glucose tolerance and lowering insulin dosage levels in diabetics; and it is stimulating and may serve to lift an individual's spirits (Kart and Metress 1984).

Proteins

Protein requirements must be met to maintain healthy tissue. Twelve to 14 percent of the kilocalories in the average daily diet should be derived from protein. Foods such as meat, fish, eggs, poultry, milk, and cheese provide high quality protein. Together with whatever other protein foods are in the diet, this high-quality protein should meet the requirements of all older persons. If vegetable and grain proteins are served exclusively, it is necessary to check the amino acid composition of the foods. Good examples of supplementary proteins are cornbread served with pinto beans, cereal with milk, bread with peanut butter, macaroni with cheese, and spaghetti with meat sauce. The daily recommended dietary allowance for protein of 0.8 g per kg of body weight is accepted to be the same for the older adult as for young adults. Because of the difference in body composition, this allowance is higher per unit of lean body mass in an older person and should allow for some decrease in utilization efficiency (*Recommended Dietary Allowance* 1989). Clinical conditions of severe infections,

fever, and surgery lead to increased protein requirements. In older adults, recovery from an illness that causes a protein depletion may increase the protein requirement. The five important syndromes that result in part from protein deficiency in older people are hunger, edema, pellagra, nutritional liver disease, and nutritional macrocytic anemia.

Fats

The Food and Nutrition Board of the National Research Council has been reluctant to make a dietary recommendation for fat. However, some fat must be included in the diet *(1)* to ensure the presence of essential fatty acids; *(2)* to allow an adequate intake and utilization of the fat-soluble vitamins A, D, E, and K; and *(3)* to serve as a lubricating agent. Fats are the most efficient source of energy with twice the energy content per gram as carbohydrates and proteins. Dietary fat is primarily responsible for the feeling of being satiated by food. It also improves the flavor of many foods, making them more appetizing and appealing.

The desirable fat intake for older adults does not differ from that of younger adults. To retard atherogenesis, the American Heart Association recommends that the total fat intake be limited to 30 percent or less of the total energy intake, the saturated fat intake be limited to 10–15 percent of total energy intake with substitution of unsaturated fatty acids for saturated ones, and the cholesterol intake be limited to 300 mg/day or less (American Heart Association 1986).

Carbohydrates

There must be an adequate intake of carbohydrates *(1)* to prevent the breakdown of tissue protein, *(2)* to maintain normal levels of blood glucose for the central nervous system, and *(3)* to make up kilocalorie deficits. Dietary guidelines published for the public by various agencies recommend that carbohydrates contribute 50–58 percent of the total energy intake. Concentrated sweets should account for not more than 10 percent of the total kilocalories. Food intake studies have demonstrated that most older persons do not choose to eat fresh fruits and vegetables. It is not known whether this is related to early dietary habits, expense, or difficulty in storage and preparation. It is important that the diet of these people include more complex carbohydrates such as fruits, vegetables, cereals, and breads and fewer simple sugars such as candy, sugar, jams, jellies, preserves, and syrups (Chernoff 1987).

Older people are susceptible to the development of diabetes, pancreatic malfunction, decreased cellular sensitivity to insulin, and glucose intolerance. Lactose in milk products poses a difficult problem; intolerance to this disaccharide is being recognized more frequently in older people, although the reason is unknown. One should always ascertain if an older person can drink milk and eat dairy products without intestinal discomfort (Hui 1983).

Fiber

Dietary fiber provides bulk in the diet, thus increasing the satiety value of foods. It maintains good intestinal motility, establishes regular bowel movements, and prevents constipation. Because of the large number of highly refined foods on the market today, the population has decreased the daily consumption of dietary roughage. Studies have linked the risk of developing the following diseases and clinical problems with the lack of dietary fiber: obesity, constipation, diarrhea, hemorrhoids, appendicitis, diverticular diseases, colon cancer, blood lipids and cardiovascular disease, and diabetes mellitus (Hamilton, Whitney and Sizer 1991). Foods that are high in fiber content are dried fruits, whole grain cereals, nuts, fresh fruits, and vegetables.

Vitamins

Vitamin deficiencies can be one of the most frequent and serious nutritional problems affecting older adults. Adequate intake of vitamins is essential at all age levels for optimal mental, emotional, and physical health. Older adults with a food energy intake of less than 1500 kilocaries should probably take a vitamin-mineral supplement (Whitney, Hamilton, Rolfes 1990). Taking supplements in quantities that exceed the recommended amount of each vitamin is of no value; excessive dosages may actually be harmful.

Many older people use vitamin and mineral supplements. Studies on vitamin supplementation in this population revealed that the supplements taken were not always the nutrients that were most likely to be deficient in the diets (Garry et al. 1982). Hypervitaminoses in older adults are likely to result from self-medication. Patients should be warned against self-medication with high-potency vitamin preparations. Long-term megadosing with vitamins A and D can result in toxicity and should be discouraged. Ascorbic acid and the B-complex vitamins are frequently consumed at levels ten to one hundred times the RDA on the assumption that excessive ingestion of certain water-soluble vitamins will be excreted. As with fat-soluble vitamins, excessive ingestion of certain water-soluble vitamins carries the potential for toxic effects.

Attention should be directed to the amount of money being spent on vitamin supplements, because older people who have limited incomes may be spending money that would better be spent for nutritious food. They need to keep in mind that food is the best source of nutrients for everyone and that supplements should be used only as supplements to food, not substitutions for it. Administration of specific vitamins should be based on need, defined by clinical and biochemical assessment of nutritional status. Older adults should then be given specific instructions about taking vitamin supplements and not just told to take a multivitamin pill.

Fat-Soluble Vitamins

Vitamin A (retinol). It is not surprising that dietary surveys and biochemical investigations of older subjects have indicated inadequate intakes of vitamin A. Vitamin A, one of the fat-soluble vitamins, is derived either from preformed vitamin A (retinol) or from provitamin A (carotenoids). Vitamin A performs important functions in the body, such as maintaining the skin and mucous membrane (lining of the nose and mouth) and protecting against night blindness. The overt manifestations of vitamin A deficiency occur only after the disease is moderately well advanced. The main external target sites are the eyes and the skin. Loss of visual acuity in dim light (night blindness) and drying of the surface of the conjunctiva (xerophthalmia) usually are the only eye changes associated with vitamin A deficiency in older adults. The dermatologic changes resulting from vitamin A deficiency create a dry, rough skin. There is a growing interest in vitamin A/carotenoid nutrition of individuals and populations because of epidemiologic evidence suggesting a potential anticarcinogenic effect of vitamins A and carotenoids (Diet, Nutrition and Cancer 1982).

Until recently the activity of vitamin A was expressed in International Units (IU), but this value has been changed to retinol equivalents (RE). This unit of measure allows for the variable absorption and conversion of the carotenoids, which were not considered in the previous method. During a period of transition both IU and RE will be used. The daily recommended dietary allowance for vitamin A is 1000 RE (5000 IU) for men and 800 RE (4000 IU) for women (*Recommended Dietary Allowances* 1989). The best food sources of vitamin A are liver, fortified margarine, eggs, butter, and whole milk. Dark green and yellow vegetables, such as broccoli, chard, collards, spinach, turnip greens, carrots, pumpkin, sweet potatoes, winter squash, apricots and cantaloupe, are the best sources of carotene, which the body converts into vitamin A. There is no danger of a toxic level of vitamin A from food sources. But because of the potential of vitamin A toxicity it is advisable to limit intake of the vitamin to approximately the recommended allowance and certainly no more than five times that amount unless there is a medical indication and blood values are closely monitored (Natow and Heslin 1980).

The habitual use of mineral oil as a laxative has been known to decrease the absorption of fat-soluble vitamins, resulting in a vitamin A deficiency. However, excessive vitamin A can be dangerous. Since such excesses are not excreted by the body and are degraded slowly, they are stored and can have a serious toxic effect. Symptoms of too much vitamin A are headache, nausea, and irritability. Other symptoms include enlargement of the liver and spleen, loss of hair, and rheumatic pain. Large doses of vitamin A can lead to the development of intracranial pressure that mimics a brain tumor. Toxic levels are not reached from the intake of food normally consumed.

Vitamin D. Vitamin D is known to aid in the absorption of calcium and phosphorous in bone formation. The deficiency disease is osteomalacia (adult rickets). People exposed to sunlight need no other source of vitamin D, since it can be formed in the skin by ultraviolet rays. Foods fortified with vitamin D are intended mainly for infants and for older adults who may not be exposed to sunlight. Too much vitamin D

causes nausea, weight loss, excessive urination, and calcification of soft tissue.

Vitamin E (tocopherol). Vitamin E belongs to a group of compounds called tocopherols, which are naturally occurring alcohols that have antioxidant and specific biologic properties. The recent interest in vitamin E is not based on science but on misinformation and fantasy. There has been no valid research to back the claims that vitamin E preserves youth; corrects skin disorders; or cures cancer, ulcers, muscular weakness, or heart disease. The daily recommended dietary allowance of vitamin E is 8 mg of @-tocopherol equivalent (TE) for women and 10 mg of TE for men (*Recommended Dietary Allowances* 1989). Since vitamin E is fat soluble, it can be stored in the liver; however, the commonly self-prescribed 800 to 1000 IU daily are generally considered safe but without benefit. The long-term effects of these high doses have not been adequately tested. Vitamin E is present in vegetable oils, whole grains, dark leafy vegetables, nuts, and legumes.

Vitamin K. Vitamin K is essential for the formation of prothrombin and is necessary for proper clotting of blood. There are several forms of vitamin K. Vitamin K1 is found in foods of animal and vegetable origin. Foods rich in vitamin K1 include liver and green leafy vegetables such as spinach, broccoli, and brussels sprouts. Vitamin K2 is synthesized by the intestinal bacteria. Antibiotics interfere with the synthesis of vitamin K2. Prolonged use of mineral oil interferes with the absorption of vitamins K1 and K2. The human requirement for vitamin K is 1g per kg body weight per day (*Recommended Dietary Allowances* 1989). If older adults eat a variety of foods including green vegetables and are not on prolonged use of antibiotics or mineral oil, there is no evidence to indicate a need for vitamin K supplement (Roe 1987).

Water-soluble vitamins

Thiamin. Thiamin has an important role in the process that changes glucose to energy. It functions as a part of a coenzyme that is indispensable in carbohydrate metabolism, providing a supply of energy to the nerves and brain. Thiamin also appears to be essential for fat and protein metabolism. The most common signs of thiamin deficiency are mental confusion, peripheral paralysis, loss of ankle and knee jerk reflexes, weakness, painful calf muscles, edema, and enlarged heart. Poorly balanced or highly refined diets, stress, alcoholism, and impaired intestinal absorption are most often the precipitating factors in thiamin deficiency (Kart and Metress 1984). Based on dietary recall studies, thiamin intakes of most healthy independent older adults in the United States have been judged adequate. However, older adults whose food intake is low have been found to exhibit symptoms of thiamin deficiency (Iber et al. 1982). The daily recommended dietary allowance is 0.5 mg of thiamin per 1000 kcal (*Recommended Dietary Allowances* 1989). Important food sources of thiamin are whole-grain products, enriched flour, organ meats, pork, and legumes.

Because thiamin is a water-soluble vitamin, it is much less stable than those that are fat soluble. Cooking foods at a high temperature in a large amount of water destroys some of the thiamin. If the solution in which the food is cooked is alkaline, more thiamin is lost. For example, if sodium bicarbonate is added to vegetables to retain their bright green color, the thiamin content is diminished. The vitamin remains relatively stable in neutral or acidic solutions. Freezing has little effect on the thiamin content of foods.

Riboflavin. Riboflavin is an essential component of enzymes important in energy metabolism. A deficiency of riboflavin results in dermatitis, lesions around the mouth and nose, hypersensitivity to light, and reddening of the cornea. The best food sources of riboflavin are liver, milk, leafy vegetables, whole grains, and enriched breads. The daily recommended dietary allowance is 0.6 mg of riboflavin per 1,000 kcal (*Recommended Dietary Allowances* 1989). Deficiencies of riboflavin are often associated with high-carbohydrate diets lacking in animal protein, milk, and vegetables. It has been suggested that riboflavin might be the most common subclinical deficiency among the older poor whose diets are high in carbohydrates and notoriously low in milk, meats, and vegetables (Kart and Metress 1984).

Niacin. Niacin is a functional component of coenzymes that are essential for the release of energy from carbohydrates, fats, and proteins. It also plays a significant role in the synthesis of fats and proteins. Niacin is best known for its prevention of pellagra. Pellagra affects the gastrointestinal tract, the skin, and the nervous system. The symptoms of deficiency include fatigue, listlessness, headache, loss of weight, loss of appetite, diarrhea, dermatitis, and mental confusion.

A diet that furnishes the daily recommended allowances for protein also provides enough niacin inasmuch as protein supplies tryptophan for conversion to niacin. Poultry, meats, fish, potatoes, legumes, and green leafy vegetables also contain preformed niacin. The daily recommended dietary allowance for niacin in adults has been set at 6.6 niacin equivalents (NE) per 1,000 kcal and not less than 13 NEs at intakes below 2000 kcal per day (*Recommended Dietary Allowances* 1989). No studies have been done in older subjects that would indicate that niacin requirements should be increased in the older population (Lowenstein 1986).

Vitamin B6 (pyridoxine). Vitamin B6 is actually three closely related chemical compounds—pyridoxine, pyridoxal, and pyridoxamine—that serve as coenzymes for biologic functions involving amino acid metabolism and protein synthesis. It is poorly absorbed by persons with liver disease and is commonly deficient in persons with uremia and gastrointestinal disease. Since these conditions are often present in older adults, these relationships should be monitored.

The drug dihydroxyphenylalanine (L-dopa), a neurotransmitter, is used in treatment of Parkinson's disease. Pyridoxine enhances the conversion of L-dopa to dopamine. Since dopamine cannot cross the blood-brain barrier, such conversion may result in a nullification of the therapeutic effects of the drug. Therefore persons on L-dopa drug therapy should avoid taking vitamin supplements containing vitamin B6 (Kart and Metress 1984). The daily recommended dietary allowance is 1.6 mg for women and 2.0 mg for men (*Recommended Dietary Allowances* 1989).

Vitamin B12 (cyanocobalamin). The most severe form of vitamin B12 deficiency is pernicious anemia. An absence of the intrinsic factor and free hydrochloric acid in the gastric juice of such patients prevents the intestinal absorption of vitamin B12. The deficiency state is characterized by weakness, glossitis, numbness and tingling of the extremities, and macrocytic anemia. If a vitamin B12 deficiency becomes evident because of changes in gastric acidity, a malabsorption syndrome with partial or total removal of the stomach or ileum, or the taking of drugs that interfere with the uptake of vitamin B12, the vitamin should be administered by injection.

The daily recommended dietary allowance is 2 micrograms (*Recommended Dietary Allowances*

1989). The best food sources of the vitamin are beef liver, kidney, whole milk, eggs, oysters, fresh shrimp, pork, and chicken. Since plants are unable to synthesize vitamin B12, it can be found only in food of animal origin.

Folacin (folic acid). Folic acid (or folacin) is important in the metabolism of a number of amino and nucleic acids and especially in hemoglobin synthesis. This vitamin's activities are interrelated with those of vitamin B12. The most notable effect of folic acid deficiency is macrocytic anemia stemming from changes in the bone marrow megaloblasts. A low serum folic acid level is associated with mental disorders. Folic acid intake is frequently reported as low among older people.

Anticonvulsant drugs frequently used by older adults are antagonistic to folic acid. Research indicates that possibly 90 percent of all alcoholics are deficient in folic acid (Kart and Metress 1984). The daily recommended dietary allowance for folic acid is 200 micrograms for men and 180 micrograms for women (*Recommended Dietary Allowances* 1989). Folic acid is available in liver, kidney, yeast, and deep green leafy vegetables.

Vitamin C (ascorbic acid). The requirement for vitamin C for the geriatric patient is still being researched. Since the body cannot synthesize vitamin C, the deficiency state in the older population could be critical. Some people develop an aversion to "acid foods" that bring on heartburn and thus restrict their intakes of vitamin C (Hamilton, Whitney, Sizer 1991). There are frequent reports of extremely low vitamin C intake among older adults (Weg 1987).

The primary function of vitamin C is to promote growth and repair of tissues, including the healing of wounds. It also aids in bone formation and repair. When used as a food additive, vitamin C acts as a preservative. This vitamin deficiency results in scurvy, which is manifested by weakness, irritability, and insidious loss of weight. The signs of deficiency stem from interference with collagen metabolism, capillary leakage, and anemia. The most prominent sign is hemorrhage at points of mild trauma. Gingivitis is a classic consequence of scurvy.

The daily recommended dietary allowance (*Recommended Dietary Allowances* 1989) is 60 mg for men and women. Food sources rich in vitamin C are citrus fruits, tomatoes, strawberries, and green vegetables such as cabbage, broccoli, collards, mustard greens, and turnip greens. This vitamin has received much publicity. Research studies proposing that large amounts of ascorbic acid can cure or prevent the common cold have not been validated.

Minerals

Calcium. Calcium is the most abundant mineral in the human body. Ninety-nine percent of the body's calcium is found in bones and teeth as calcium salts (hydroxyapatite). The remaining 1 percent exists in the blood, other body fluids, and various soft tissues. Calcium is necessary for the proper mineralization of bone. It is important in the growth and maintenance of the skeleton and also plays an important role in blood clotting, cell wall permeability, muscle contractility, micromuscular transmission, and cardiac function. The function of calcium is closely related to that of phosphorus and vitamin D. The ratio of calcium to phosphorus in the diet should be one to one and certainly no greater than one to two. If phosphorous levels are too high, the calcium is withdrawn from the bone to restore equilibrium. Vitamin D must be present for calcium to be absorbed. The daily recommended dietary allowance for calcium for persons 60 years of age and above is 800 mg (*Recommended Dietary Allowances* 1989). However, recent studies of older persons have consistently shown that a calcium intake of 1,000 mg or higher is necessary to achieve calcium balance and decrease the risk of fractures. A number of age-related physiologic and lifestyle changes can increase the need for calcium. Menopause, illness, drug-nutrient interactions, low exposure to sunlight, lactose deficiency, and decrease in physical activity either directly or indirectly decrease the intestinal absorption of calcium and effectively increase the requirement for this mineral (Heaney et al. 1982).

Osteoporosis (loss of bone mass), osteomalacia (demineralization of bone, known as adult rickets), and hypertension may all be related in part to calcium deficiencies. Although the cause of osteoporosis is not understood completely, there is substantial evidence that the disease involves marked changes in calcium and vitamin D metabolism. For example, postmenopausal women do not absorb dietary calcium as efficiently as do younger women. There is also a drop in absorption in men, but this is less marked and occurs at a later age (Allen 1986). The most effective treatment found for osteoporosis is a combination of calcium, fluoride, and estrogen (Riggs et al. 1982). Currently dietary recommendations to the general public to reduce salt (sodium) in the American diet may inadvertently decrease the intake of calcium. This in turn may increase their risk of hypertension and osteoporosis (McCarrion et al. 1982).

The National Institute of Arthritis, Diabetes, and Digestive and Kidney Diseases (1983) recommends 1000–1500 mg of calcium per day for postmenopausal women, particularly those not receiving estrogen supplementation. The American Society for Bone and Mineral Research (1982) supports a calcium intake of 1,400 mg per day to prevent bone loss in postmenopausal women when estrogen therapy is not used.

One of the best ways to prevent or treat diseases related to calcium deficiency is to increase the consumption of calcium-rich foods. Milk and other dairy products are the major dietary sources of calcium. In 1982 the milk group contributed 72 percent of the available calcium in the United States diet (Marston 1984). For individuals who cannot consume milk and other dairy products, calcium supplements may be recommended.

Phosphorus. The daily recommended dietary allowance for phosphorus is 800 mg for men and women (*Recommended Dietary Allowances* 1989). Phosphorus is available from a variety of foods; deficient intakes are unlikely. Older persons taking large amounts of antacids may have increased excretion of phosphorus, which could result in a deficiency.

Magnesium. The daily recommended dietary allowance for magnesium is 350 mg for men and women (*Recommended Dietary Allowances* 1989). No evidence exists for an increased need with aging. A severe loss of body fluid, malabsorption, and liver disease are the conditions that may lead to a deficiency. Dehydration is the most likely factor in older adults. Magnesium is widely available from the food supply, so a deficiency is unlikely to occur.

Sodium. Sodium is the principal electrolyte in extracellular fluid for the maintenance of normal osmotic pressure and water balance. Sodium intake requires particular attention because many older adults have hypertension and are taking antihypertensive medications. Such persons are usually cautioned to reduce their intake of sodium. A safe, adequate intake of sodium is 1100 to 3300 mg, about half the amount of sodium that most adults generally ingest (Robinson, Lawler, Chenoweth, Garwick 1986).

Potassium. Potassium is required for enzymatic reactions within the cell. Potassium deficiencies are not primarily dietary in origin. They may occur in malnutrition, chronic alcoholism, or any illness that seriously interferes with appetite. Any condition that reduces the availability of nutrients for absorption, such as prolonged vomiting, gastric drainage, or diarrhea, may lead to a potassium deficiency. Diuretic drugs sometimes release the sodium in the extracellular fluid, in turn depleting the potassium within the cell. On the other hand, rapid infusions of glucose and insulin used in treating diabetic acidosis bring about such rapid shifts of potassium into the cell that the plasma potassium content may be reduced to levels that could bring about cardiac failure. The safe, adequate intake of potassium by adults is 1875 to 6725 mg per day (Robinson, Lawler, Chenoweth, and Garwick 1986). Meat, poultry, fish, oranges, bananas, and celery are rich sources of potassium.

Iodine. Iodine is an essential nutrient that must be available for the synthesis of the thyroid hormones (thyroxine and tricodothyronine). The public health measure to add iodine to table salt has helped protect people from developing endemic goiter. The daily recommended dietary allowance for iodine in both men and women is set at 150 micrograms (*Recommended Dietary Allowances* 1989).

Iron. Iron deficiency is relatively common in older people because of decreased intake or absorption or both (Alford and Bogle 1982). The most common symptom of iron deficiency in older adults is nutritional anemia, which is characterized by fatigue, weakness, irritability, dizziness, pale skin color, and sore mouth and tongue. The daily recommended dietary allowance for iron is 10 mg for men and women age 60 and older (*Recommended Dietary Allowances* 1989).

There appear to be considerable differences in the absorption of iron from different foods. Iron is more efficiently absorbed from muscle and hemoglobin (for example, red meats and organ meats) than from vegetables and eggs. Iron in whole wheat is better absorbed than iron from enriched bread, in spite of the high phytate content. Conversely, iron in eggs is poorly absorbed, but its absorption can be enhanced by the addition of orange juice. A superimposed iron deficiency anemia can be a serious handicap in an older person with an already impaired, atherosclerotic circulation. The need for iron may be increased in the older person because of mild bleeding from hemorrhoids or other gastrointestinal lesions. Sufficient iron-containing foods, such as green leafy vegetables, meat, and egg yolk, should be incorporated into the daily diet.

Zinc. Zinc is a component of more than eighty metalloenzymes and proteins, where it may have catalytic or structural functions. It is an important factor in the synthesis of deoxyribonucleic acid, ribonucleic acid, and protein. It is thought to stabilize cell membranes. It is essential for growth and cell division, reproduction, taste acuity, wound healing, and normal immune function.

The daily recommended dietary allowance for adult men is 15 mg. The allowance for adult women, because of their lower body weight, is set at 12 mg (*Recommended Dietary Allowances* 1989). Although zinc is available from many foods, decreased absorption occurs with aging (Alford and Bogle 1982). Stresses, such as physical trauma, wounds (including surgery), burns, and muscle-wasting disease, all result in dramatic increases in urinary zinc losses. Many medications (both those sold over the counter and by prescription) used by older people can affect zinc status. Diuretics, chelating agents, antacids, laxatives, and iron supplements may decrease absorption or increase excretion of zinc from the body (Chernoff 1991).

Counseling of older persons should emphasize a varied diet of high nutrient density. Consumption of red meats, poultry, and fish will help ensure adequate zinc intake, because bioavailability of this nutrient is greater from animal foods than from those of plant origin. Among plant foods, legumes and grains are the most significant sources of zinc. For those on a vegetarian diet, consumption of these should be emphasized; vegetables and fruits average less than 0.5 mg zinc per serving (Wagner 1985).

Water

Although water is not often thought of as a food, it has been described as the indispensable nutrient. Without water, survival of a human being is considered limited to four days (Labuza 1977). Insufficient consumption of fluids, for whatever reasons, may precipitate disaster in the organism more quickly than the lack of any other component. Maintenance of fluid balance is essential for the distribution of nutrients to the cellular units, the elimination of water, and the multiple physiochemical processes of life. Total body water decreases with age. In young males 60 percent of total body weight is water compared to 52 percent in the older male. In younger females 52 percent of total body weight is water compared to 45 percent in older females. The normal adult gains and loses approximately 2400 ml of fluids each day (Jaffe 1991).

Although water is available and inexpensive in most parts of the United States, it is a nutrient that older people tend to consume in less than optimum quantities. Many older people do not drink enough fluids because they do not experience thirst as younger persons do or because they are not able to obtain adequate fluids if they are immobile.

Six to eight 8-oz glasses of fluid per day will generally satisfy the water requirement. Older people often find liquids more acceptable in soups, fruit juices, milk products, soft drinks, tea, and coffee. If the patient has difficulty swallowing clear liquids, especially water, foods with the consistency of gelatin, fruit ices, yogurt, custards, or puddings may be more desirable. In prescribing such easily ingested and pleasant liquids, care must be taken to avoid overconsumption of high-kilocalorie beverages and foods. Also, a powdered substance may be obtained to thicken clear liquids so that they can be more easily swallowed.

NUTRIENT STANDARDS AND FOOD GUIDES FOR HEALTH PROMOTION

Recommended Dietary Allowances (RDA)

The Food and Nutrition Board was organized in 1940 as a division of the National Academy of Sciences-National Research Council. One of the projects of this group has been to establish a set of figures for human needs in terms of specific nutrients. *Recommended Dietary Allowances*, which has been referred to throughout the chapter, was first published in 1943. The most recent edition was published in 1989. *Recommended Dietary Allowances* lists the levels of intake of essential nutrients that, on the basis of scientific knowledge, are judged by the Food and Nutrition

Board to be adequate to meet the known nutrient needs of practically all healthy persons (*Recommended Dietary Allowances* 1989).

Adults are divided into two age categories: 25–50 years, and 51 years upward. The researchers agree that the older age groups need to be addressed separately. However, the committee concluded that data are insufficient at this time to establish separate RDAs for people 70 years of age and older (RDA 1989).

This does not mean that the recommended dietary allowances should be rejected in terms of planning diets for older adults, but that their limitations should be recognized and that the older person's specific health problems should be considered. The recommended dietary allowances are expressed in nutrients rather than in specific foods because these recommendations can be fulfilled by a variety of different food patterns.

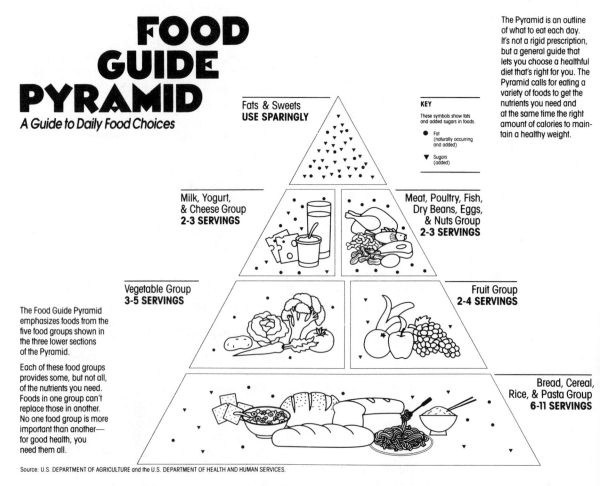

Figure 8–1   The Food Guide Pyramid

United States-Recommended Daily Allowances (US-RDA). The *Recommended Dietary Allowances* should not be confused with the United States-Recommended Daily Allowances (US-RDA). The US-RDA standards were established by the Food and Drug Administration for the purpose of regulating nutrition labeling. Although the US-RDA standards are derived from the National Research Council's dietary allowances, they encompass just a few broad categories. The guidelines for nutrition labeling are currently being revised and there are strong indications that the guidelines will not be labeled as US-RDA to avoid the confusion between RDAs and US-RDAs.

The Food Guide Pyramid. Because most people are not going to take the time to calculate their nutrient intake in terms of kilocalories, proteins, fats, carbohydrates, minerals, and vitamins, *The Food*

How Many Servings Do You Need Each Day?

	Women & some older adults	Children, teen girls, active women, most men	Teen boys & active men
Calorie level*	about 1,600	about 2,200	about 2,800
Bread group	6	9	11
Vegetable group	3	4	5
Fruit group	2	3	4
Milk group	2-3**	2-3**	2-3**
Meat group	2	2	3
	for a total of 5 ounces	for a total of 6 ounces	for a total of 7 ounces

*These are the calorie levels if you choose lowfat, lean foods from the 5 major food groups and use foods from the fats and sweets group sparingly.

**Women who are pregnant or breastfeeding, teenagers, and young adults to age 24 need 3 servings.

Source: U.S. DEPARTMENT OF AGRICULTURE and the U.S. DEPARTMENT OF HEALTH AND HUMAN SERVICES.

Figure 8–2   How many servings do you need each day?

Guide Pyramid (see Figure 8-1) is a convenient plan designed to help a person plan an adequate diet. *The Food Guide Pyramid* allows the menu planner to evaluate the daily intake of milk and milk products, meat, fruits, vegetables, and bread, grains and cereals. Most older adults can name the food groups, but are unable to give quantities of food that should be consumed within each group (see Figure 8-2).

Dietary Guidelines for Americans

There has been increasing concern that overnutrition may be contributing to the illnesses many people suffer from today: heart disease, cancer, diabetes, liver disease, and others. Therefore the *Dietary Guidelines for Americans* (1990) as shown in Table 8-1 places emphasis on prevention of overnutrition and disease.

FACTORS INFLUENCING NUTRITIONAL STATUS OF OLDER ADULTS

Since the health status of a person is influenced by a variety of socioeconomic, psychologic, cultural-religious, and physiologic factors, the nurse should understand these factors and their influence on nutritional needs before adequate health care can be provided.

Table 8–1   Dietary Guidelines for Americans (1990)

1. *Eat a variety of foods daily.* Get the many nutrients your body needs by choosing different foods you enjoy eating from these five groups daily: vegetables, fruits, grain products, milk and milk products, and meats and meat alternatives.

2. *Maintain healthy weight. Check to see if you are at a healthy weight. If not, set reasonable weight goals and try for long-term success through better habits of eating and exercise.*

3. *Choose a diet low in fat, saturated fat, and cholesterol.* Have your blood cholesterol level checked, preferably by a physician. If it is high, follow the physician's advice about diet and, if necessary, medication. If it is at the desirable level, help keep it that way with a diet low in fat, saturated fat, and cholesterol. Eat plenty of vegetables, fruits, and grain products. Choose lean meats, fish, poultry without skin and low-fat dairy products most of the time. Use fats and oils sparingly.

4. *Choose a diet with plenty of vegetables, fruits, and grain products.* Eat more vegetables, including dry beans and peas; fruits; and breads, cereals, pasta, and rice. Increase your fiber intake by eating more of a variety of foods that contain fiber naturally.

5. *Use sugars only in moderation.* Use sugars in moderate amount—sparingly if your kilocalorie needs are low. Avoid excessive snacking. Brush and floss your teeth regularly.

6. *Use salt and sodium only in moderation.* Have your blood pressure checked. If it is high, consult a physician about diet and medication. If it is normal, help keep it that way: maintain a healthy weight, exercise regularly, and try to use less salt and sodium. (Normal blood pressure for adults: systolic—less than 140 mm Hg; diastolic—less than 85 mm Hg.)

7. *If you drink alcoholic beverages, do so in moderation.* If you drink alcoholic beverages do not drive. For individuals who drink, limit all alcoholic beverages (including wine, beer, liquors, and so on) to one or two drinks per day. "One drink" means 12 ounces of beer, 5 ounces of wine, or 1 1/2 ounces of distilled spirits (80 proof).

Source: United States Department of Agriculture, United States Department of Health and Human Services. 1990. *Nutrition and Your Health: Dietary Guidelines for Americans.* 3d ed. Washington, DC: Government Printing Office.

Socioeconomic Factors

Limited income is a major problem among older people. There is a relationship between income and poor nutritional status in the population now institutionalized. (Chernoff 1991).

Income usually decreases sharply with age. The income of persons 55–64 years old is about twice that of the corresponding 65-and-over age group. Not only are older people plagued with decrease in income, they must cope with inflation. As income decreases, people buy less meat and more high-carbohydrate foods, resulting in insufficient nutrients to maintain normal weight (Harman 1979).

Many older people live in substandard housing without adequate food preparation and storage facilities, refrigeration space, and other essentials (Lewis 1978). The nurse will find that a visit to the home may be more useful than an inquiry into diet in evaluating a patient's ability to purchase a balanced diet. Some older people are too proud to admit they are destitute and would rather starve than ask for help. A discussion of food costs, nutritive values, food preparation, and use of leftovers may be helpful in improving the patient's nutrition at the same cost as the original diet or even lower.

Dependence on others for transportation is another problem older persons face. The lack of transportation may force the older person to shop at a neighborhood grocery store where prices are higher and there is a limited selection of food choices.

It is difficult for a person who is taken from familiar surroundings to live with other family members, or for one who is institutionalized in a retirement home, nursing home, or hospital to make adjustments in eating patterns. When an older person is separated from family, friends, or community, such changes often lead to apathy, depression, and loss of appetite.

Alcoholism also can be a problem if an older person is advised to use an alcoholic beverage as an appetite stimulator. Care should be taken to guard against overindulgence, since an excessive intake of alcohol can interfere with the absorption and metabolism of nutrients and may act as a replacement for needed nutrients (Roe 1987).

In seeking relief from chronic aches, an older person is particularly susceptible to the food faddists who claim to have a "miracle cure". Older people often lack nutrition information since they may have received little or no formal nutrition education. In

their youth nutrition was just beginning to emerge as a science.

Psychologic Factors

Authorities believe that malnutrition among older adults is associated with loneliness (Schlenker 1984). The older patient is constantly beset by loneliness, boredom, anxiety, fear, bereavement, or general unhappiness, which leads to isolation and depression. The patient may react to loneliness and depression either by refusing to eat, which leads to malnutrition, or by overeating, which results in obesity, another form of malnutrition. It is important for such older people to avoid isolation. Eating should not become a chore or a dietary experiment. It should remain a genuine pleasure at any age. Mealtime should be one of the highlights of each day.

Socially, food and eating serve as a mode of communication and socialization. Food eaten in solitude lacks these aspects. Socially isolated persons have decreased incentive to prepare and eat food. There is a strong link between isolation and nutrition (isolation can lead to malnutrition). The lonely person who eats little food becomes increasingly apathetic and listless, failing to reach out for social contact (Lewis 1978).

Cultural-Religious Factors

By middle age, eating patterns have become relatively fixed and change is difficult. Familiar food patterns serve as a security blanket (Lewis 1978). Distinctive ethnic, racial, and regional characteristics are still prevalent among older people. Ethnic or racial identity can be reaffirmed by suggesting the use of traditional foods (Kart and Metress 1984).

To determine the cultural-religious influence on the patient's diet, the caregiver should start with an in-depth history of the patient's dietary habits. Question the patient closely on food likes and dislikes, ethnic preferences, and general nutritional knowledge. The patient may eat too much of one type of food and neglect other essential foodstuffs (Luke 1976). It is best to encourage the good food habits of the patient's particular group and to institute improvements gradually rather than impose too many changes at once. A knowledge of the family's food customs plays an important part in establishing good relationships with a patient (Kroog 1976).

The religious customs passed from one generation to another tend to become cultural also. For example, the Jewish dietary laws are observed in varying degrees by Orthodox, Conservative, and Reformed denominations. Orthodox families place great value on the traditional and ceremonial rituals of their religion and observe the dietary laws under all conditions. The dietary laws prohibit using meat and milk at the same meal. (Six hours must elapse after a meat meal before dairy foods may be eaten; half an hour must elapse after eating a dairy food before meat may be eaten.) Orthodox Jews use only the forequarters (rib section forward) of cud-chewing, cloven-hoofed animals such as cattle, sheep, and deer. Animals and poultry must be ritually slaughtered according to specific regulations. Before cooking, meat is koshered by one of two methods: *(1)* the meat is soaked in cold water for half an hour, then salted with coarse salt and drained to let the blood run off; finally it is thoroughly washed under cold running water and drained before cooking; *(2)* the meat is seared quickly (Kroog 1976). The quick-searing method of preparation is preferred for patients on a salt-restricted diet. Separate dishes and utensils must be used for preparing and serving meat and dairy products. It would be wise for the person preparing and serving meat to receive instructions from the patient, since this religious ritual is very important to the patient.

When working with cultural and religious food patterns—whether they be Chinese, Japanese, Mexican-American, Italian, Indian, Jewish, or any other—the health care professional must have a thorough understanding of the patient's cultural and religious preferences.

Physiologic Factors

Body composition changes with age. In later years there is a cell loss as well as reduced cell metabolism. For example, the cell mass may decrease from 47 percent of the total body mass at age 25 to 36 percent at age 70 (Gregerman 1974). The physiologic changes that occur may vary considerably from one person to another, and the aging process may even vary within the same individual. For example, a 70-year-old man may have the cardiac output typical of a 60-year-old and the renal function of an 80-year-

old. It is important to realize that when acute illness occurs, the older person, due to less lean body mass, will suffer depletion of muscle protein to a proportionally greater degree than someone with normal lean body mass. Consequently when a person becomes ill, some attention must be directed to the nutritional status.

Because of the decrease in basal metabolic rate there is a need to decrease the number of kilocalories to avoid weight gain; at the same time, care must be taken to include the necessary nutrients.

Perceptual ability changes with age. Of particular importance to patterns of nutrient intake are changes in hearing, vision, taste, and smell. Loss of hearing may translate into an aversion to talking to grocery clerks, pharmacists, waiters, social workers, or anyone else who might otherwise provide guidance, direction, or helpful information (Roe 1991b).

The visual change that accompanies aging is familiar, as most people require eyeglasses for reading and close work after 40 years of age. Because of visual changes, many older people restrict social activities and in some cases, may become housebound. Reduced peripheral vision may affect nutritional status by restricting driving ability; making it difficult to read labels, prices, recipes, and directions; and making it difficult to operate appliances to cook the food (Roe 1991b).

The ability to taste and smell is also altered with age. Taste and smell are closely related—in lieu of taste, the smell of food is a key factor in acceptability. Although most gerontologists agree that a decline in taste-bud sensitivity is part of the aging process, some hold that it is due to other factors such as smoking and disease. The diminishing senses of taste and smell result in less desire to eat and may lead to malnutrition. Diminishing taste is also accompanied by a decline in salivary flow that accompanies aging. The taste buds are sensitive to sweet, sour, salt, and bitter. Nutrition and age are the two major factors that affect the number of taste cells (Kamage 1982). Although some taste sensations probably decline with age, the sensitivity to sweet is apparently higher, which may account for the older person's preference for sweet-tasting foods. Some loss of sour and bitter taste sensation occurs with new dentures because the palate is covered. However, perception often improves as the patient becomes adjusted to wearing dentures. The patient accepts food better if it is well seasoned. Herbs and spices can be used to season the food, but overuse of table salt should be avoided because of its sodium content. Since flavor perception decreases at very hot or cold temperatures, food served at body temperature (about 95° F) is more acceptable (Lewis 1978).

Abnormalities that increase or decrease sensitivity to one or more of the four basic tastes include nutritional deficiencies such as those of niacin, vitamin A, and trace metals (zinc, copper, and nickel); various disease states such as cancer, renal failure, and diabetes; radiotherapy to the head or neck for cancer; and drug therapy such as tranquilizers, some anesthetic agents, and some amphetamines. Some cancer patients who are undergoing radiotherapy or chemotherapy require as much as five times the usual amounts of sugar for cereal to taste sweet. Cheese and eggs are often more acceptable as a protein source for such patients because meat tastes bitter to them (Carson 1976).

Another obvious change in older people is the loss of teeth. The failure to replace lost teeth with dentures or the use of ill-fitting dentures makes it difficult to bite or chew food. Two opposing incisors for biting and at least two opposing molars for chewing are needed to manage regular food with any degree of success (Lewis 1978). The loss of natural teeth and poorly fitting dentures cause many older people to resort to soft, high-caloric foods such as breads and pastries that lack protein, vitamins, minerals, and fiber. When the loss of teeth and poorly fitting dentures cause older adults to avoid important foodstuffs, it is best to encourage them to return to the dentist for a proper fit. If this suggestion is not successful, give them a list of nutritious soft foods. Cheese, sauces, eggs, beans, yogurt, and ground meat are good sources of protein. Whole-grain cereals, either the cooked or cold varieties softened with milk, provide excellent nourishment, as do cooked mashed vegetables. Some vegetables, such as tomatoes and avocados, are soft enough to be eaten raw. Raw bananas and berries, as well as cooked fruit, make excellent soft desserts (Luke 1976). Aging causes a decrease in the secretion of hydrochloric acid as well as of the digestive enzymes of the stomach, intestine, liver, and pancreas, so that the absorption of many nutrients is diminished, contributing to borderline malnutrition in some older patients.

The majority of older people have one or more chronic diseases. Among the chronic diseases most frequently observed in the older population that are related to nutrition are obesity, cardiovascular diseases, diabetes mellitus, osteomalacia, osteoporosis, hypertension, hiatal hernia, constipation, and dysphagia.

Chronic diseases may alter food intake in different ways. If a modified diet has been prescribed, the nurse should check with the patient to determine if the patient *understands* and *accepts* the diet. If the patient does not understand the importance of the diet or refuses to eat the prescribed foods, in a short time the patient will return to former eating habits. It is important to determine if the prescribed diet includes the required nutrients. If it does not, a dietary supplement should be recommended. Keep in mind that it is best to meet dietary needs by serving a variety of foods. But if variety is not possible, attention must be given to supplementary feedings.

Obesity. Obesity is the most common nutritional problem of public health in the United States. All older people should be encouraged to maintain a normal weight by eating a well-balanced diet with caloric restrictions and by engaging in a planned activity, walking being the most highly recommended exercise. Often weight reduction is necessary to promote successful treatment of a primary condition such as diabetes or arthritis (Natow and Heslin 1980).

Cardiovascular Diseases. Cardiovascular diseases, including heart attack and stroke, are the major causes of death. Factors that have been researched and associated with cardiovascular disease include *(1)* personal factors (heredity, sex, and age); *(2)* lifestyle factors (obesity, smoking, stress, and diet); *(3)* pathologic factors (other diseases); and *(4)* environmental factors (air and water pollutants). Recent research has increased the number of dietary links to cardiovascular diseases, especially lipid metabolism, trace-element imbalances, excess sugar and refined carbohydrates, and dietary fiber (Kart and Metress 1984). The American Heart Association has published easy-to-follow dietary guidelines for the prevention and treatment of cardiovascular diseases.

Diabetes Mellitus. Diabetes mellitus is a chronic metabolic disease characterized by a deficiency in the production and utilization of the pancreatic hormone insulin. The most important aspect of dietary treatment of maturity-onset diabetes is reduction of weight. The American Diabetes

Association and the American Dietetic Association (1986) revised the Diabetic Exchange List in 1986, so anyone giving diet instructions for the diabetic should be familiar with the revised Exchange List for Meal Planning.

Osteomalacia. Osteomalacia is a defective mineralization of bone. The characteristic symptoms are muscle weakness; poorly localized skeletal pain and tenderness; frequent painful rib fracture; and abnormal values for serum calcium, inorganic phosphorus, and serum alkaline phosphatase. Treatment for osteomalacia is usually simple and very effective with vitamin D and calcium supplements. The amount and nature of the supplement depend on the cause and severity of the condition (Kart and Metress 1984).

Osteoporosis. Osteoporosis is a disease due to loss of bone mass. It has been estimated that 15–20 million persons in the United States have osteoporosis. Peak bone mass is achieved at age 30–35 years and declines thereafter. This gradual decrease in bone mass is particularly accelerated in women after menopause (Spencer and Kramer 1987). Osteoporosis can involve most of the bones of the skeleton, but most disability and pain are because of vertebral osteoporosis. About 30 percent of the cases are severe enough to cause fractures. Osteoporosis is treated with a combination of fluoride, calcium, and vitamin D (Kart and Metress 1984). Post menopausal treatment with estrogen for women is perhaps the most effective method of slowing down bone resorption and loss and restoring calcium balance. However, negative effects of estrogen therapy include an increased risk of endometrial cancer (Allen 1986).

Hypertension. Hypertension is identified with high blood pressure. Clinical evidence indicates that moderate sodium restriction can lower blood pressure. Most practitioners who use this approach today prefer reduction of sodium to one gram a day along with the use of a diuretic (Kart and Metress 1984).

Hiatal Hernia. Hiatal hernia appears to be increasing in incidence, and the majority of affected individuals are over 60 years of age. Women appear to be affected more often than men. Surgical correction is rarely recommended and usually has a slim chance of success. Loss of weight, eating smaller meals more frequently, avoiding eating at bedtime, or sleeping with the bed elevated normally provides relief (Kart and Metress 1984).

Constipation. Constipation may be caused by lack of exercise, psychologic stress, or improper diet. After the possibility of disease is ruled out, a modified diet should be planned. Increasing dietary fiber, fluid intake, and physical exercise can prevent constipation. Diets generous in fiber produce larger, soft stools and more frequent bowel movements. High-fiber diets are also used in the treatment of hemorrhoids, diverticulosis, and other colon-related diseases (Kart and Metress 1984).

Dysphagia. Dysphagia is associated with problems in swallowing. This is a result of changes in esophageal motility and decreased secretion of saliva. If the problem is severe, food may be rejected as swallowing becomes difficult. Heartburn from backflow of stomach acid into the esophagus is frequent when the esophageal sphincter has lost control. Dry mouth resulting from reduced secretion of saliva or general dehydration adds to the difficulty in swallowing. Certain drugs such as antidepressants, anticonvulsants, and amphetamines can cause dry mouth, as can dentures, anxiety, or breathing through the mouth. Some older people restrict their fluid intake to limit trips to the bathroom. Increasing intake of fluids or using lozenges can provide some relief (Schlenker 1984).

SUGGESTIONS FOR FEEDING PATIENTS

Older people who are frail, quite dependent, seriously ill, or recovering from illness sometimes are unable to feed themselves. Some suggestions for feeding patients who cannot help themselves are given here.

1. Provide an environment free of odors, clean and orderly, with appropriate temperature and ventilation.

2. Have the patient in a comfortable, upright position. Reclining interferes with chewing and swallowing.

3. Before feeding, assess the patient's ability to swallow. Never attempt to feed a patient who cannot swallow.

4. Sit next to the patient. Have the patient look straight ahead and introduce the food straight

into the mouth. It is difficult for a patient to swallow with head turned at a 45-degree angle.

5. Test the temperature of the food by placing a drop on the back of the wrist. Soups, coffee, and other hot items should not be allowed to burn the patient's mouth.

6. Start by offering liquids or thin soups served in a container with a covered lid.

7. Identify each food as it is given to the patient.

8. Ask the patient to smell the food to encourage chewing and salivating reflexes.

9. Do not mix foods together.

10. Allow time for eating at a slow pace, giving the patient sufficient time to chew and swallow between bites.

11. Blot the mouth. Do not wipe. Wiping stimulates the rooting reflex which opens the mouth, making swallowing more difficult.

12. Have the patient use the upper lip (not upper teeth) to scrape food from utensil. Scraping with the teeth stimulates the bite reflex, which interferes with chewing.

13. Place food well into the patient's mouth to avoid tongue thrust, which pushes food out of the mouth.

14. Keep food moist. Salivation in older people is frequently reduced. Lack of fluid makes chewing and swallowing more difficult. Give sips of fluid frequently during the meal.

15. If the patient is paralyzed on one side of the body, place food in the side of the mouth that is not paralyzed.

16. Observe which textures are easiest for the patient to chew and swallow.

17. Encourage the patient to "think swallow," if swallowing is difficult, by repeating the word "swallow." Pressing up on the chin slightly while the patient swallows may help prevent fluids or thin foods from running out of the mouth.

18. Allow for and accept feelings of frustration, anger, and embarrassment.

19. If the patient is in bed, keep the head of the bed up for at least one hour after meals.

20. Remember that it is not pleasant for an adult to be fed. The attitude of the person feeding the patient often sets the mood. He/she is the single most important factor in the amount of food consumed by the patient who requires feeding. Feed slowly. Be positive and show enthusiasm and encouragement at mealtime.

An individual's attitude toward both food and mealtime is likely to be more positive if self-feeding is possible. Achieving this level of independence supports both physical and mental well-being. Problems in self-feeding may be caused by weakness in the hand or arm making it difficult to lift a cup or spoon. Partial paralysis can limit range of motion or make it difficult to flex the fingers and hand to grasp a cup or fork.

Various devices have been developed to help disabled individuals feed themselves. In many cases, only a slight modification of existing utensils facilitates food handling. A cup with a partial lid or small opening (plastic travel cup) or a straw helps prevent spills. Lightweight plastic cups are easier to handle when filled with liquid than are glass or china cups. Covering a standard utensil (fork or spoon) with foam rubber increases the friction and aids in holding. A suction device on the bottom of the dish or a plate with a broad edge helps those with limited motor skills. Special aids are often available from local hospital supply companies or can be ordered by mail.

Careful selection of food served and a positive approach facilitate progress and encourage effort. A soft diet rather than pureed foods not only is more palatable but requires less skill in eating. Finger foods require less effort and energy for eating. Ideas for making difficult items into finger foods include putting ground meat in a roll, folding a pancake in half so it can be picked up, or serving hard-cooked eggs or small fruit slices (Schlenker 1984).

NUTRITION PROGRAMS FOR OLDER ADULTS

There has been an increased social concern for the plight of older Americans. In 1965 Congress passed the Older Americans Act, which provides for various programs designed to improve the quality of life for older people. One of the programs provided under this legislation is the Nutrition Program for the Elderly. This program has been referred to in the past as the Title VII Meal Program because it came under Title VII of the Older Americans Act. As a result of amendments to the Act in 1978 the program is now referred to as the Title III Meal Program. The congregate program is designed to provide inexpensive, nutritionally balanced meals for older persons. Low-cost meals are served in group settings to people who are 60 years or older and to their spouses. Meals are designed to provide at least one third of the recommended dietary allowances. Older people are not required to pay, but they may contribute voluntarily toward the meals. In addition to food various supportive services are also provided as part of the program. Transportation to and from the meal, information and help for other services, health counseling, nutrition education, and recreation activities are some of the other services. Information about the program and how to participate in it are also provided to eligible older people (Chernoff 1987).

The Title III Meal Program helps meet the nutritional needs of many older people through the Meals-on-Wheels program. This program provides hot meals that are delivered to homebound older adults. This service is provided at the community level. The extent of the service varies from one to three meals daily (one hot and one or two cold) for a varying number of days per week (three to seven). Cost is based on the ability to pay.

Many older people qualify for the Food Stamp program. This program allows the person on a very limited budget to purchase more food.

Program aides, who are trained through the Expanded Food and Nutrition Program of the United States Department of Agriculture, are providing basic nutrition to low-income families. While the program aides' focus is families with young children, they also work with other families as their priorities permit. Aides provide information on wise shopping, basic food needs, and food preparation techniques. Teaching is done on a one-to-one basis, with the aide going to the home.

Neighborhood food-buying cooperatives are available in some communities. While the structure and goals of cooperatives vary, food is generally available at a lower cost than at the supermarket. In return, members contribute time to running the cooperative. Advantages of membership for older people are *(1)* reduced food costs (often as much as 20 percent) and *(2)* the social aspects of working with a neighborhood group (Lewis 1978).

RECOMMENDED GUIDE FOR MENU PLANNING

Here are some nutritional guides to menu planning for older people.

1. Plan to serve meals on a regular schedule.
2. Include a variety of foods.
3. Plan to serve smaller amounts of food more frequently.
4. Keep abreast of new trends in nutrition education.
5. Make older people aware that money spent on nutritional food is money well spent.
6. Recognize food and drug interactions.
7. Prepare and serve food attractively.
8. Increase fluid intake.
9. Include fibrous foods for proper elimination.
10. Recognize social, economic, cultural, and religious factors.
11. Season foods to stimulate taste buds.
12. Use polyunsaturated oils and margarines.
13. Select complex carbohydrates.
14. Learn to identify intolerances.
15. Use meat substitutes such as cheese, dried beans, and peanut butter.
16. Use various forms of milk—skim milk, nonfat dry milk, or buttermilk.
17. Serve fresh fruits and vegetables.
18. Serve whole-grain or enriched breads and cereals.
19. Follow instructions for therapeutic diets.
20. Check the menu against the daily food guide. A sample menu using the *Food Guide Pyramid* is illustrated in Table 8-2.

Table 8–2   Sample Menu Plan

Breakfast	Morning Snack	Noon Lunch	Afternoon Snack	Supper	Evening Snack
Orange juice	Graham crackers	Baked chicken	Banana	Tuna noodle casserole	Ready-to-eat cereal
Oatmeal	Peanut butter	Buttered rice	Milk	Chopped broccoli	Sugar
Milk	Tea, coffee or	Cooked carrots		Lemon, butter or	Milk
Tea or Coffee	other beverage	Green beans		margarine	
		Fresh fruit salad		Cherry gelatin	
		Roll		Sugar cookies	
		Tea or coffee		Tea or coffee	

Sample menu is one example of how foods that supply the needed nutrients can be selected from the Food Guide Pyramid

	Bread, Cereal, Rice, & Pasta Group	Vegetable Group	Fruit Group	Milk, Yogurt, & Cheese Group	Meat, Poultry, Fish, Dry Beans, Eggs & Nuts Group	Fats & Sweets and Other Foods
Breakfast	Oatmeal (1/2 cup cooked) = 1 serving		Orange juice (3/4 cup) = 1 serving	Milk (1/2 cup) = 1/2 serving		Tea or coffee (black) Sugar for cereal (optional)
Morning Snack	Graham crackers (3) = 1 serving				Peanut butter (2T) = 1 serving	Tea, coffee, water
Noon lunch	Rice (1/2 cup, cooked) = 1 serving Roll (1) = 1 serving	Carrots (1/2 cup cooked) = 1 serving Green beans (1/2 cup) = 1 serving	Fresh fruit salad (1/2 cup) = 1 serving		Baked chicken (3 oz.) = 1 serving	Tea or coffee (black) Butter on rice

(Table continued)

	Bread, Cereal, Rice, & Pasta Group	Vegetable Group	Fruit Group	Milk, Yogurt, & Cheese Group	Meat, Poultry, Fish, Dry Beans, Eggs & Nuts Group	Fats & Sweets and Other Foods
Afternoon Snack			Banana (small) = 1 serving	Milk (1 cup) = 1 serving		
Supper	Noodles for tuna noodle casserole (1/2 c) = 1 serving	Chopped broccoli (1/2 cup cooked) = 1 serving		Milk for casserole (1/2 cup) = 1 serving	Tuna for tuna noodle casserole (2 oz) = 2/3 serving	Butter or margarine Cherry gelatin Sugar cookies Tea and coffee (black)
Evening Snack	Ready-to-eat cereal (1 oz) = 1 serving			Milk (1 cup) = 1 serving		Sugar for cereal (optional)
Actual total from menu	6	3	3	3	2-2/3	—
Minimum total recommended following the Food Guide Pyramid	6	3	2	2–3	2	—

MONEY-STRETCHING IDEAS TO MAKE THE FOOD DOLLAR GO FARTHER AND REDUCE KILOCALORIES

1. Plan menus and shop from a prepared list. Be careful to avoid foods containing large amounts of fat and sugar.

2. Avoid costly, instant, or convenience items.

3. Take advantage of vegetables and fruits in three forms: fresh, canned, and frozen. Select fruits and vegetables that are in season and locally grown.

4. Select juices for vitamin C content. Rule out fruit-flavored choices supplying only sugar.

5. Meat generally requires the larger part of the food dollar. Lower-cost cuts can be as nutritious but must be cooked and stored properly to prevent shrinkage. Serve more fish and chicken. Avoid frying.

6. Avoid prepackaged, sliced, or processed meats. They are usually more expensive and higher in kilocalories than bulk meats.

7. Check the price of canned meats such as tuna, chicken, and fish, noting that the boneless meat could be the most economical buy. Avoid canned meats packed in oil.

8. Read labels. Avoid high-kilocalorie foods.

9. Buy cereals that require cooking rather than ready-to-serve cereals. Avoid presweetened cereals.

10. Use nonfat dry milk solids in cooking. These may be used dry in recipes for bread and cake but should be in liquid form or recipes such as gravies, sauces, and puddings. Use larger amounts of nonfat dry milk than recommended on the package to increase nutrient density.

SUMMARY

The increasing number of older Americans presents health care professionals with a unique challenge. Adequate nutritional care for the older patient deserves considerable emphasis because the well-nourished patient not only is more comfortable and energetic but is better able to tolerate medical and surgical treatment.

The daily *Recommended Dietary Allowances*, the *Food Guide Pyramid*, and the *Dietary Guidelines for Americans* are designed to be beneficial in planning a diet that will furnish the needed nutrients. Factors contributing to nutritional deficiencies in older adults include poor food habits, reduced income, racial and cultural patterns, poor dental health, and chronic diseases.

Nutrition education during the entire life span, as well as during later life, is needed. Good food habits can best be achieved by people who have accurate knowledge of nutrition and are motivated to use it.

The nurse must emphasize to the older patient the importance of good nutrition. Although the nurse cannot reverse the effect of poor nutritional habits developed early in life, nutrition education can positively influence the quality of life for the older person.

STUDY QUESTIONS

1. In what ways can physical activity contribute to nutritional balance in older adults?

2. What are the major problems associated with carbohydrates, fats, and protein among older people?

3. Discuss the pros and cons of vitamin supplements for older people.

4. Identify the role and some of the major problems among older people with regard to fat-soluble vitamins, B complex vitamins, and vitamin C.

5. Why is the absorption of minerals inefficient?

6. Identify the role and some of the major problems among older people with regard to calcium, phosphorus, magnesium, sodium, potassium, iodine, iron, and zinc.

7. Discuss the role of water and major problems associated with water imbalance among the aged.

8. Explain the purpose of having RDAs, US-RDAs, the *Food Guide Pyramid*, and *Dietary Guidelines for Americans*.

9. Discuss the socioeconomic, psychologic, cultural-religious, and physiologic factors influencing the nutritional status of older adults.

10. List suggestions for feeding a patient who must have assistance in eating.

REFERENCES

Alfin-Slater, R.B. 1986. Special report: Nutrition and the elderly. *Nutrition and the M.D.* Van Nuys, CA: P.M. Inc.

Alford, B.B. and M.L. Bogel. 1982. *Nutrition During the Life Cycle.* Englewood Cliffs, NJ: Prentice-Hall.

Allen, L.H. 1986. Calcium and osteoporosis. *Nutrition Today* 21(3):6–10.

The American Diabetes Association, The American Dietetic Association. 1986. *Exchange Lists for Meal Planning.* Chicago, IL.

American Heart Association. 1986. *Dietary Guidelines for Healthy American Adults: A Statement for Physicians and Health Professionals by the Nutrition Committee.* Dallas, TX: American Heart Association.

The American Society of Bone and Mineral Research. 1982. *Osteoporosis.* Kelseyville, CA: The American Society of Bone and Mineral Research.

Carson, J.A. and A. Gormican. 1976. Disease-medication relationships in altered taste sensitivity. *J Am Diet Assoc* 68:550–53.

Chernoff, R. 1987. Aging and nutrition. *Nutrition Today* 22(2):4–11.

Chernoff, R. 1991. *Geriatric Nutrition.* Gaithersburg, MD: Aspen Publishers Inc.

Community Nutrition Institute. 1986. *Nutrition Week* 16:4.

Diet, Nutrition and Cancer. 1982. Washington, DC: National Academy of Sciences Press.

Garry, P.J., J.S. Goodwin, W.C. Hunt, E.M. Hooper, and A. Leornard. 1982. Nutritional status in a healthy elderly population: Dietary and supplemental intakes. *Am J Clin Nutr* 36(2):319–31.

Gregerman, R.I. and E.I. Bierman. 1974. In *Textbook of Endocrinology*, edited by R.H. Williams. Philadelphia: W.B. Saunders.

Hamilton, E., E. Whitney and F. Sizer. 1991. *Nutrition Concepts and Controversies.* 5th ed. St. Paul, MN: West Publishing Co.

Harman, D. 1979. Geriatric nutrition. In *Quick Reference to Clinical Nutrition*, edited by L.H. Seymour. Philadelphia: J.B. Lippincott.

Heaney, R.P., J.C. Gallagher, C.C. Johnston, R. Neer,

A.M. Parfitt, M.B. Chir, and G.D. Whedon. 1982. Calcium nutrition and bone health in the elderly. *American Journal of Clinical Nutrition* 36(5): 986–1013.

Hui, Y.H. 1983. *Human Nutrition and Diet Therapy.* Belmont, CA: Wadsworth.

Iber, F.L., J.P. Blass, M. Brin, and C.M. Leevy. 1982. Thiamin in the elderly—relation to alcoholism and to neurological degenerative disease. *American Journal of Clinical Nutrition* 36(5):1067–82.

Jaffe, M. 1991. *Geriatric Nutrition and Diet Therapy.* El Paso, TX: Skidmore-Roth Publishing.

Kamath, S. 1982. Taste acuity and aging. *American Journal of Clinical Nutrition* 36(4):766–75.

Kart, C.S., and S.P. Metress. 1984. *Nutrition, the Aged and Society.* Englewood Cliffs, NJ: Prentice-Hall.

Kroog, E.J., H.T. Corzine, R.T. Frankle, M.E. Johnson, T. Ogata, and R.V. Robbins. 1976. *Cultural Food Patterns in the U.S.A.* Chicago: The American Dietetic Association.

Labuza, T. 1977. *Food and Your Well-Being.* Los Angeles: West Publishing Co..

Lewis, C. 1978. *Nutrition: Nutritional Considerations for the Elderly.* Philadelphia: F.A. Davis.

Lowenstein, F.W. 1986. Nutritional requirements of the elderly. In *Nutrition, Aging and Health*, edited by E.A. Young. New York: Alan R. Liss.

Luke, B. 1976. Good geriatric nutrition is a lifelong nursing matter. *RN* 39(7):24–26.

Marston, R.M. and S.O. Welsh. 1984. Nutrient content of the U.S. food supply in 1982. *National Food Reviews* 25:7–13.

McCarron, D.A., C.D. Morris, and C. Cole. 1982. Dietary calcium in human hypertension. *Science* 217:267–69.

National Institute of Arthritis, Diabetes, and Digestive and Kidney Diseases. 1983. *Osteoporosis: Cause, Treatment, Prevention.* NIH Publication No. 83-2226. Washington, DC: Government Printing Office.

Natow, A.B., and J.A. Heslin. *Geriatric Nutrition.* Boston: C.B.I. Publishing Co.

Recommended Dietary Allowances. 1989. 10th ed. Washington, DC: National Academy Press.

Riggs, B.L., E. Seeman, S.F. Hodgson, D.R. Taves, and W.M. O'Fallon. 1982. Effect of the fluoride/calcium regimen on vertebral fracture occurrence in post-menopausal osteoporosis. *N Engl J Med* 306:446–50.

Robinson, C., M. Lawler, W. Chenoweth, and A. Garwick. 1986. *Normal and Therapeutic Nutrition.* 17th ed. New York: Macmillan.

Roe, D.A. 1987. *Geriatric Nutrition.* 2d ed. Englewood Cliffs, NJ: Prentice-Hall.

Rose, S.N., ed. 1991a. *Geriatric Patient Education Resource Manual.* Gaithersburg, MD: An Aspen Publication, Aspen Publishers, Inc. Vol 1.

Roe, S.N., ed. 1991b. *Dietician's Patient Education Manual.* Gaithersburg, MD: An Aspen Publication, Aspen Publishers, Inc. Vol. 1.

Schlenker, E.D. 1984. *Nutrition in Aging.* St. Louis: Times Mirror/C.V. Mosby.

Spencer, H. and L. Kramer. 1987. Osteoporosis, calcium requirement, and factors causing calcium loss. *Clinics in Geriatric Medicine* 3(2).

United States Department of Agriculture, United States Department of Health and Human Services. 1990. *Nutrition and Your Health. Dietary Guidelines for Americans.* 3d ed. Washington, DC: Government Printing Office.

United States Department of Agriculture, United States Department of Health and Human Services. 1992. *The Food Guide Pyramid.* Home and Garden Bulletin Number 252.

Wagner, P.A. 1985. Zinc nutriture in the elderly. *Geriatrics* 40(3).

Weg, R. *Nutrition and the Later Years.* 1987. The Ethel Percy Andrus Gerontology Center, Los Angeles, CA: University of Southern California Press.

Whitney, E.N., E.M.N. Hamilton, and S.R. Rolfes. 1990. *Understanding Nutrition.* 5th ed. St. Paul, MN: West Publishing Co.

9 Management of Medications

Janice Knebl
Howard Graitzer

CHAPTER OUTLINE

FOCUS

This chapter provides an overview of the pharmacologic differences in prescribing medications for an older population. Knowledge of the physiologic, psychologic, sociologic, and functional changes that occur with aging are necessary for health care providers to prevent potential adverse medication reactions that could affect the older person's health.

OBJECTIVES

1. Analyze the reasons for polypharmacy.

2. Define pharmacodynamic and pharmacokinetic changes in the older patient.

3. Describe common medication interactions.

4. Explain the special differences when administering medications to older adults.

5. Discuss the value and problems associated with generic medications.

6. Analyze the effects of medications commonly used by older adults.

The ability to cure and prevent certain diseases with medication is one of the major achievements of modern medicine. However, the challenge of appropriately utilizing our ever-expanding medication array has become more and more complex, particularly in older adults. Recent studies have shown that older patients may respond differently than younger patients to medications because of the effects of normal aging (Montamat, Cusack, and Vestal 1989a). Our data base is limited, however, as much clinical pharmacology in older patients is extrapolated from data on younger people.

POLYPHARMACY

Little data are available regarding medication use in patients over the age of 70. The Food and Drug Administration does not require any manufacturer to evaluate the impact of aging on drug toxicity (Spencer, Nichols, Waterhouse, West, and Bankert 1986). Multiple diseases, environmental factors, and genetic variation combine with the normal physiologic changes of advancing age to affect drug metabolism, efficacy, and toxicity (Montamat et al. 1989a). Older patients are two to three times more likely to experience an adverse drug reaction than are younger patients (Nolan and O'Malley 1988a). Older patients underreport their symptoms, and signs of disease may be subtle. This, combined with atypical presentations and chronic illness, results in an underestimation of adverse drug reactions (Klein, German, Levine, Feroli, and Ardery 1984). These issues also lead to increased difficulty in detecting drug-induced disease.

One-third of all medications in the United States are prescribed for individuals age 65 and older; yet these people comprise approximately 12 percent of the United States population (American Association of Retired Persons and Administration on Aging. 1990. *Profile of Older Americans*). With multiple diseases and resultant polypharmacy there is the increased likelihood of drug-drug, drug-disease, and drug-nutrient interactions. Despite a belief that such patients have an increased incidence of adverse medication reactions, there is controversy whether this is a result of normal aging or a manifestation of multiple disease states (Nolan and O'Malley 1988a). Polypharmacy correlates strongly with the incidence of adverse medication reactions, and older hospitalized patients receive more prescription medications than do younger patients. Additional factors include more severe illnesses, multiple pathology, smaller body size, female sex, diminished hepatic and/or renal function, and prior drug reactions (Vestal, Jue, and Cusack 1985a). Drugs most frequently associated with adverse drug reactions are listed in Table 9-1.

Medication therapy may influence or precipitate many major clinical problems in older patients, e.g., incontinence, impaired mental status, falls, iatrogenesis, and impaired homeostasis.

PHARMACODYNAMICS

Pharmacodynamics is the study of drug effects at the receptor level. It has also been referred to as what a drug does to the body. Pharmacodynamic changes appear to be due to the effects of normal aging, but the mechanisms are not well understood. As aging occurs, some drugs demonstrate enhanced efficacy, while others show diminished activity. Potential explanations for these differences include alterations in

Table 9–1   Medications Associated with Adverse Reactions in Older Patients

Digoxin
Beta blockers
Calcium channel blockers
Diuretics
Sympathomimetics/antihistamines
Nonsteroidal anti-inflammatory
    drugs
Corticosteroids
Theophylline
Benzodiazepines
Neuroleptics
Antidepressants

the blood/brain barrier or possible target organ dysfunction. Whether this is a consequence of normal aging or due to underlying disease is not known. An example of altered pharmacodynamics in aging is the enhanced central nervous system (CNS) depressive effect of diazepam in older patients (Reidenberg, Lavy, and Warnter, et al., 1978).

A controversy exists regarding the use of warfarin in older patients (based on its pharmacodynamic properties) (Coon and Willis 1974; Gurwitz et al., 1988; O'Malley et al., 1977; Reidenberg 1987; Shepherd 1977). Therefore, particular attention should be given to the prothrombin time when adjusting warfarin. Many drugs interfere with metabolism. For example, cimetidine inhibits the cytochrome P-450 system that retards the metabolism of warfarin and increases the risk of bleeding. Warfarin is highly protein-bound and may be displaced by other drugs that are highly protein-bound, such as the oral sulfonylureas and salicylates. Although normal aging is not a contraindication to oral anticoagulant therapy, factors such as gait instability, a history of falling or syncope, peptic ulcer disease, concomitant drug therapy,

or poor compliance increase potential adverse effects.

Older persons seem less sensitive to drugs that affect beta-adrenergic receptors (e.g., isoproterenol, propranolol). This differential effect in the older patient may be due to a decreased number of high affinity receptors and a decreased sensitivity to those receptors (Vestal, Wood, and Shand 1979; Scarpace 1986; Montamat and Davies, 1989; Pan 1986). Even though the effects of beta-adrenergic agonists and antagonists appear to diminish with aging, the clinical significance of these findings is not known. Available studies on alpha-adrenergic receptors have not revealed any significant change or decrease in the number and affinity of receptors with normal aging (Buckley, Curtin, Walsh, and O'Malley 1986).

PHARMACOKINETICS

Pharmacokinetics is the study of drug absorption, distribution, protein binding, hepatic metabolism (biotransformation), and renal excretion. Changes in pharmacokinetics with aging may cause higher drug

Table 9–2   Factors Affecting Pharmacokinetics in Older Patients

	Normal Aging	Disease States
Absorption	No change affecting drug	Malabsorption
		Pancreatitis
	↑ gastric pH	Gastric surgery
	↓ gastrointestinal motility	
	↓ gastrointestinal blood flow	
Distribution	↓ total body water	Congestive heart failure
	↓ lean body mass	
	↓ serum albumin	Hepatic or renal insufficiency
	↑ body fat	
Hepatic metabolism	↓ liver size	Congestive heart failure
	↓ liver blood flow	
	↓ enzyme activity	Thyroid disease
		Cancer
Renal clearance	↓ renal blood flow	Volume depletion
	↓ glomerular filtration	Chronic renal insufficiency
	↓ tubular secretion	

Table 9–3   Examples of Medications with
High Protein Binding

Phenytoin
Warfarin
Many nonsteroidal agents
Diazepam
Furosemide

concentrations at the site of action. Knowledge of the normal age-related changes in disposition should lead to more rational drug dosing. Table 9-2 lists the altered pharmacokinetics in aging.

Drug Absorption

There is currently no evidence that normal aging affects drug absorption to any significant degree. There is an increase in gastric pH, decrease in gastric emptying, diminished intestinal blood flow, and impaired intestinal motility (Cusack and Vestal 1986). However, some drugs have high first-pass extraction as they go through the liver following oral administration. Their bioavailability may actually be increased because of the decreased liver size seen in normal aging. In young, healthy adults the gastrointestinal tract receives 28 percent of the cardiac output, while older patients have a 40–50 percent reduction in blood flow to the liver and GI tract (Wilkinson and Shand 1975). This reduction is further accentuated in the presence of congestive heart failure. However, disease states can affect drug levels in young or old persons, such as the impaired absorption of quinidine and procainamide in congestive heart failure.

Drug Distribution

Drug distribution depends on body composition, plasma protein binding, and blood flow. Age-related changes affecting drug distribution include reduced lean body mass, relative decrease in total body water, reduced serum albumin, and increase in the percentage of body fat (Vestal and Dawson 1985). Lean body mass accounts for 82 percent of ideal body weight in a younger individual, compared to 64 percent in an older person. The proportion of adipose tissue increases with age from 18 percent to 36 percent in men and from 36 percent to 48 percent in

women (Bruce, Andersson, Arvidsson, and Isaksson 1980; Novak 1972; Forbes and Reina 1970). For example, digoxin is not very fat-soluble and does not distribute in adipose tissue. Therefore a reduction in lean body mass and a decrease in total body water results in elevated serum digoxin levels as long as dose and creatinine clearance remain constant in normal older persons. Examples of fat-soluble drugs are barbiturates, phenothiazines, benzodiazepines, and phenytoin. As a result of the higher percent body fat in older patients, these drugs can be stored in this depot, resulting in prolonged half-life. Drugs such as lithium, aminoglycosides, and cimetidine are water-soluble and because of reduced total body water have higher serum concentrations in older patients.

Plasma protein binding can affect drug distribution, especially for drugs that are highly protein-bound. Albumin concentrations are minimally decreased in normal aging and therefore not clinically significant (Campion, deLabry, and Glynn 1988). However, older individuals with multiple chronic diseases often have significant reductions in serum albumin (Woodford-Williams, Alvarez, Webster, Landless, and Dixon 1964). When serum albumin is reduced, the number of available binding sites is reduced, resulting in increased amounts of free drug that is biologically active. Most drug levels measure total drug (bound and unbound) and therefore serum levels may not be accurate in the face of hypoalbuminemia. However, it is only the free (unbound) drug that is capable of binding to its receptor site of activity or of undergoing biotransformation or elimination. Additional examples of drugs that are highly protein-bound are listed in Table 9-3.

Diminished blood flow as a result of normal aging can affect the amount of drug delivered to the various organ sites. Cardiac output decreases by about 1 percent per year after the age of 30, while renal and hepatic blood flow decrease slightly more. Therefore the amount of blood flow delivered throughout the body can change according to the cardiac output and distribution of blood flow.

Hepatic Metabolism

The transformation of drugs that enter the body depends on the activity of hepatic enzymes, the hepatic blood flow, and the number of functioning liver cells. Despite normal liver function testing in older patients, all of the determinants of hepatic metabolism can be significantly altered. As mentioned earlier, hepatic blood flow declines with aging and is further reduced in the face of congestive heart failure.

There are two phases of hepatic metabolism that account for the biotransformation of drugs. Some phase I enzyme reactions involve oxidation, reduction, or hydrolytic reactions. Phase I reactions involving the cytochrome P-450 enzyme system are also known as the mixed function oxidase system. The hepatic enzymes most affected by normal aging are phase I.

Phase II enzyme reactions involve conjugation glucuronidation, or acetylation reactions. The metabolites of phase II are generally inactive and not affected by normal aging. Some drugs undergo both phases of hepatic metabolism. Table 9-4 shows examples of phase I and phase II biotransformation. Hepatic metabolism is highly variable from individual to individual and therefore unpredictable.

Both enzyme induction and enzyme inhibition of drug metabolism can occur in older people. While in animal models enzyme induction usually declines with aging, some studies have shown that cigarette smoking induces hepatic microsomal enzyme activity (Vestal, Norris, Tobin, Cohen, Shock, and Andres 1975; Campbell and Hayes 1974).

Therefore older smokers would metabolize theophylline to a greater extent, potentially producing inadequate levels of the drug. Serum levels should be used for dosing adjustments, particularly in older patients with a drug like theophylline, with its narrow therapeutic range. Cimetidine, on the other hand, inhibits microsomal enzymes (cytochrome P-450) (Drug Interaction Facts 1985). Simultaneous use of theophylline and cimetidine decreases theophylline clearance. However, this occurs to the same extent in young and older patients. Table 9-5 lists examples of drugs inducing or inhibiting cytochrome P-450. In older adults it is generally advisable to reduce the dosage of drugs undergoing extensive first-pass metabolism and use serum levels when available to monitor therapy.

There are drugs with high rates of first-pass metabolism, which may be affected by the normal changes occurring in the liver with aging (e.g., liver blood flow and size). When the magnitude of this initial hepatic metabolism is extensive, there may be a large difference in achieved serum levels after oral and intravenous doses of some drugs (e.g., proprano-

Table 9–4   Medications Undergoing Biotransformation

Phase I	Phase II
Diazepam (Valium)	Temazepam (Restoril)
Chlordiazepoxide (Librium)	Oxazepam (Serax)
Flurazepam (Dalmane)	Lorazepam (Ativan)
Alprazolam (Xanax)	
Quinidine (Quinidex)	
Theophylline (Theo-dur)	
Nortriptyline (Pamelor)	
Propranolol (Inderal)	
Ethanol (alcohol)	

Table 9–5 Medication Interactions Affecting the Mixed-Function Oxidase (Cytochrome P-450) System

P-450 Inducers	P-450 Inhibitors
Phenobarbital	Cimetidine
Rifampin	Influenza vaccine
Phenytoin	Erythromycin
Carbamazepine	Allopurinol
	Metronidazole

lol and verapamil). There is a more extensive list of drugs undergoing first-pass hepatic metabolism in Table 9-6.

Renal Elimination

The most predictable age-related pharmacokinetic change is the reduced rate of elimination of drugs by the kidneys. Glomerular filtration rate and renal tubular secretion diminish with aging (Rowe, Andres, Tobin, Norris, and Shock 1976). Normal renal function testing (e.g., BUN and creatinine) does not reflect actual renal function in older patients. BUN is a reflection of protein intake, hepatic metabolism and detoxification of ammonia, and renal clearance. Decreased protein intake may cause a low BUN unrelated to renal function. Creatinine is dependent on the amount of muscle mass, which decreases with normal aging, especially in a frail, older person with muscle wasting. As a result, serum creatinine may be falsely low in the face of actual declining renal function. To obtain an accurate measure of renal function, the Cockcroft-Gault formula is used to calculate creatinine clearance (Cockcroft and Gault 1976).

For a male:

$$\text{creatinine clearance} = \frac{140 - \text{age} \times \text{weight (kg)}}{72 \times \text{serum creatinine}}$$

For a female:

$$\text{creatinine clearance} = \frac{140 - \text{age} \times \text{weight (kg)}}{72 \times \text{serum creatinine}} \times .85$$

The formula is accurate in ambulatory and hospitalized patients but may be less useful in nursing home patients, for unknown reasons (Drusano, Munice, Hoopes, Damron, and Warren 1988). Creatinine clearance predictably declines linearly with

Table 9–6 Medications With Large First-Pass Metabolism

Tricyclic antidepressants
Beta blockers
Narcotics
Nitrates
Hydralazine
Verapamil
Labetalol
Most major tranquilizers
Most antiarrhythmic agents

aging in cross-sectional studies. This decline in renal function is less predictable in longitudinal studies (Rowe et al. 1976). Table 9-7 lists drugs that are predominantly renally eliminated. Drugs that undergo renal elimination with a narrow therapeutic range should be monitored with serum levels when available (e.g., aminoglycosides, digoxin, lithium, procainamide).

DRUG INTERACTIONS

Drug-Drug Interactions

As the number of drugs administered to an older person increases, an increased incidence of reactions between drugs occurs. Some of the drug-drug interactions are predictable, based on the altered pharmacodynamics and pharmacokinetics (Lamy 1986). For example, the amount of digoxin available for action is increased with the concurrent administration of quinidine, due to a reduction in the renal excretion of the digoxin (Lanoxin) (Sloan 1986). Therefore digitalis toxicity is more likely to occur when these two drugs are administered together. Other examples of drug-drug interactions have already been described in the sections of pharmacodynamics and pharmacokinetics.

Drug-Disease Interactions

Currently there are no scientific data to highlight this type of interaction. Common sense dictates that drugs used to treat an intercurrent disease may well worsen another disease or negate its treatment or possibly trigger another medical problem (Lamy 1986). For example the use of timolol (Timoptic)

ophthalmic solution for glaucoma has been reported to cause symptomatic bradycardia, heart block, and decompensated congestive heart failure in older patients. These drug-disease interaction effects may necessitate the discontinuation of the medication. Antihistamines and anticholinergics are widely available in "cocktail" multi-ingredient cold, allergy, and sleep aids. These could cause urinary retention in an older male patient with benign prostatic hypertrophy or delirium in someone with an underlying dementing disorder (Koford 1985).

Drug-Nutrient Interactions

Drugs have been shown to interfere with the nutritional status of older persons in four basic ways: the suppression or stimulation of appetite, an alteration in nutrient digestion and absorption, an alteration in metabolism or utilization of a nutrient, and alteration in the excretion of that nutrient (Roe 1986).

Antipsychotic agents (including lithium carbonate), antianxiety agents, and antihistamines can stimulate appetite. Malabsorption of calcium can occur with ingestion of broad-spectrum antibiotics, such as tetracycline. There is an enhanced excretion of certain ions, i.e., potassium, magnesium, and zinc during the administration of thiazide diuretics. Laxatives such as bisacodyl (Dulcolax), phenolphthalein, and mineral oil decrease glucose and thiamine uptake (Oppeneer and Vervoren 1983), with mineral oil containing laxatives also impairing the absorption of fat-soluble vitamins.

Food can alter the bioavailability of some medications, reducing their efficacy. Older nursing home residents, for example, may be receiving enteral formulas that could affect absorption of the medication.

Table 9–7 Medications with Decreased Renal
Elimination in Old Age

Digoxin
Cimetidine
Aminoglycosides
Lithium
Procainamide
Chlorpropamide
Most antimicrobials

Another hazard includes closing of an enteral feeding tube when medication is instilled during the course of formula infusion. In a study conducted by Cutie, Altman, and Lendel (1983) several cough and cold medicines, formulated as elixirs, formed gelatinous masses capable of clogging a tube. Concurrent administration of phenytoin with continuous enteral tube feedings may lower the serum concentration and therefore its therapeutic effectiveness (Bauer 1982).

Malnutrition can alter the pharmacokinetics of many drugs. Subclinical malnutrition may contribute to the increased incidence of drug toxicity seen in older people (Rikans 1986). In fact, nutritional hazards in older patients are greatest in those with pre-existing subclinical nutritional deficiencies and in those being treated for chronic illness (Rikans 1986).

GENERIC MEDICATIONS

All medications have three names: chemical—e.g., acetylsalicylic acid; generic—e.g., aspirin; and trade name—e.g., Bayer, St. Joseph's. The generic name is determined by a national council and the trade name (brand name) is invented by the pharmaceutical company.

Drug manufacturers who develop and market new drugs have a patent on the drug for seventeen years. By the time the Food and Drug Administration has approved the drug for market, several of those years have passed. The current law gives the manufacturer up to fourteen years patent regardless of the length of time the FDA takes to approve a drug (Radios 1983). The law states that generic drugs must meet the standards for effectiveness, safety, purity, and strength that the original drug met. Consumer groups have advocated greater use of generic drugs because of the cost advantage. The generic manufacturers have not spent money developing, testing, and marketing the product, so their cost is less. All fifty states now have laws allowing for the substitution of generic drugs. However, some state laws allow the physician to restrict dispensing of a brand name drug only.

According to consumer groups the savings realized by substituting generic drugs for brand name drugs is between 30 percent and 40 percent (Rados 1983). In 1984 the Hatch-Waxman amendments passed by Congress were signed by the president. These amendments seek to increase the number of generic drugs available while protecting the patent of the originator of the drug. To obtain FDA approval of a generic drug, the manufacturer would need to show only that the drug is safe and effective. The FDA determines whether the generic drug is therapeutically equivalent to the brand name drug (Rados 1983). Each manufacturer is subject to inspection by the FDA for building maintenance and quality control. The FDA publishes a list of "Approved Prescription Drug Products with Therapeutic Equivalence Evaluations," which is available from the Superintendent of Documents in Washington, DC. Consumer groups are stressing the savings from the use of generic drugs.

The question concerning efficacy of generic medications is considered by physicians and consumers. If proper attention is not given to the vehicle in which the *active* drug is packaged, the drug may be generically equivalent, that is, the same amount of active ingredient as the trade name drug, but therapeutically nonequivalent. If this occurs, the generic medication will not act in an identical fashion to the brand name product (Lieberman 1986). In addition, generic drugs are granted approval after checking for equivalence in as few as twelve persons (Lamy 1986). It is often difficult to assess when a drug is not bioequivalent. A physician or nurse failing to see a clinical response to a drug may wrongly assume that the drug is inappropriate, not suspecting a bioequivalency problem. Use of generic medications in older patients is further complicated by the normal physiologic changes of aging and coexistent disease states. Therefore bioequivalency of generic drugs is complicated by increased variability in the older patient.

Lamy (1986) has suggested that there are critical patients, diseases, and drugs for which generic substitution should not be allowed. He further stated that persons over the age of 75 or aged women living alone should not have substitutions made. Therefore nurses need to be aware if an older patient's prescriptions have been filled with a generic drug and observe for any side effects or lack of efficacy of the drug.

MEDICATION ADMINISTRATION

Pills can be either tablets or capsules containing the drug, *active ingredients*, and *inactive ingredients* such as fillers, lubricants, dyes, or gelatin. Tablets come in many forms, such as chewable, coated, effervescent, lozenges, and sublingual; whereas capsules only come in two forms, either hard or soft gelatin.

Pills may also be controlled release to deliver the medication in a constant amount over a long time period. Therefore pills should not be crushed and tablets or capsules should not be broken without consulting a physician, pharmacist, or drug reference manual. The long action of the medication could be destroyed because all the drug could be released at once and be dangerous to the patient. In addition the protective coating on the tablet could be destroyed and cause irritation to the stomach. Examples of some common medications that should not be crushed include Cardizem (diltiazem), Dulcolax (bisacodyl), Feldene (piroxicam), Feosol (ferrous sulfate), Theo-dur (theophylline), and Symmetrel (amantadine).

Problems of Self-Medication

Most older people continue to live at home and are responsible for taking their own medications. There are many reasons why problems develop when medications are self-administered. One reason cited by Myers, Meier, and Walsh (1984) is the failure of health care personnel to give clear instructions on how and when to take each medication ordered. Myers et al. (1984) gave a number of reasons she found for failure to take medications correctly, including the failure of the physician or pharmacist to inform the client of the exact time to take a drug or the expected side effects of the drug. Other reasons found were forgetfulness by the client and the lack of funds to purchase the medication. Pepper and Robbins (1987) found that multiple prescriptions and complex regimens—for example, medications at many different times of the day—contribute to noncompliance. Over 25 percent of older patients incorrectly take prescription medicines as instructed on the medication bottle labels. In addition an estimated 10 percent of older patients swap prescription medications with friends and relatives (Collet 1988).

People often take over-the-counter drugs along with prescription drugs without consulting their physicians about the effects of adding the extra drug and without even realizing that over-the-counter medicines are drugs. Failing vision contributes to the in-

ability of many older people to read instructions on drug labels. Pharmacists often neglect to determine the patient's ability to understand or remember how and when to take the drug.

Studies of ambulatory patients in a family practice clinic found some of the reasons for problems in self-administering medications by older clients included errors of omission, failure to take the entire prescription, obtaining drugs from more than one physician (thus taking drugs that interact adversely), and failure to understand how to take the drug (Myers et al. 1984). Other problems of self-medication arise when people take large doses of laxatives daily, various medications for colds frequently, and antacids regularly. These people never consider that this information should be reported to the prescribing physician. In fact, if not directly asked about the purchase or use of over-the-counter medication, older patients will not readily provide this information.

Older people who take multiple drugs or drugs that decrease mental alertness, such as tranquilizers, sedatives, or hypnotics, are prone to making errors in taking drugs due to confusion. They usually take too much rather than too little, since they often forget they have already taken the drug and will repeat the dose. In an interesting study of noncompliance with prescribed drug regimens, Myers et al. (1984) found that the ability to name the drug and state why it was being prescribed did not increase the patient's compliance with taking medication as ordered. One reason a patient will give for discontinuing a prescribed drug is that the patient has experienced no particular symptom to alert him or her to the need for continued therapy. This problem is particularly true when a medication is needed to control a condition such as hypertension. There are few, if any, symptoms until late in the course of the disease, so that clients of all ages are prone to discontinue their medication in the belief that they no longer need it. Another reason some clients discontinue medication for hypertension is the occurrence of side effects that may be unacceptable to the client. Teaching the need for medical care and prescribed therapy at the time hypertension is discovered is essential. Depending on the regimen of drugs, clients should know what to expect from the drug and why therapy must be continued (Myers et al. 1984).

Facts a person should know about the prescribed medicines are

- the name of the drug

- why the medicine is ordered

- when to take the medicine, i.e., before meals, after meals, or at bedtime

- whether to take the medicine with food and which food should not be eaten at the time the medicine is taken

- the major side effects of the drug

- what to do if the side effects occur

- whether the medicine is to be swallowed, chewed, or placed under the tongue

If the older person has poor vision, the pharmacist should be requested to use large print on the medication label. Also, containers that are easily opened are usually preferred by older people. Older patients should be reminded to tell each of their physicians about *all* of the drugs they are taking. Before purchasing over-the-counter drugs, the pharmacist should be consulted about possible drug interactions with prescribed medications.

NURSING INTERVENTIONS IN PATIENT EDUCATION

Wade and Finlayson (1983) have divided nursing interventions to reduce the occurrence of adverse drug reactions into three domains: vigilance, accountability, and responsibility.

Vigilance is the constant assessment by the nurse of the patient's response to drugs or an adverse or toxic effect. This is done in the hospital, nursing home, and community environments. The nurse must always maintain a high index of suspicion in older patients receiving multiple drug regimens. This requires knowledge of pharmacogeriatrics, careful observation, judgment, and appropriate documentation.

The nurse is accountable for all aspects of medication administration. The consideration of accountability may take on medicolegal aspects in today's health care practices.

Lastly, nurses are responsible for teaching patients about their medications, including self-administration techniques and behaviors to remove any barriers to compliance (Schwertz and Buschmann 1989). Schwertz and coworkers outlined several nursing actions to reduce adverse drug reactions, Table 9-8.

Knowledge as to the differences between young and older learners is imperative to the effectiveness of nursing interventions in reducing adverse drug reactions and improving compliance. Adult learners tend to be self-directed and learn more readily if the knowledge can be applied in solving an immediate problem. Also, previous life experiences can be very important in teaching older patients, allowing them to integrate new information on a familiar foundation

Table 9–8   Nursing Actions to Reduce Adverse Medication Reactions

- Establish a baseline health and drug history

- Monitor physiologic status prior to administering new drugs

- Consider pharmacokinetics and pharmacodynamics

- Monitor for polypharmacy

- Consider nonpharmacologic treatment modalities

- Initiate medication education and teaching

- Assess mental and physical abilities

(Collett 1988). (See chapter 16 for more details on the teaching and learning needs of older patients.)

EFFECTS OF MEDICATIONS COMMONLY USED BY OLDER ADULTS

Medication therapy in an aging population needs to take into account the interrelated changes in various organ systems and the variability of physiologic changes found among people as they age. Some of the differences in the effects of drugs in older persons have been outlined in the pharmacokinetic and pharmacodynamic sections. Prescribing practices should include the principles of pharmacokinetics, pharmacodynamics, disease states, aging factors, drug interactions, and patient related factors such as compliance.

Cardiotonic Drugs

Digoxin is the most frequently prescribed digitalis glycoside because it has a short half-life. However, it has a narrow margin of safety. Toxicity is frequent in the older patient because of a marked reduction in the rate of its renal clearance. The maintenance dosage needs to be adjusted in accordance with the glomerular filtration rate (Montamat and Davies 1989).

Digoxin was the only medication in the top five of four studies evaluating the most common drugs leading to hospitalization (Caranaso, Stewart, and Cluff 1974; Miller 1974; Black and Somers, 1989; Crymonpre, Mitenko, and Sitar, et al. 1988). The most serious side effects are disturbances in cardiac rhythm. Noncardiac symptoms of digoxin toxicity include fatigue, listlessness, anorexia, and nausea (Rikans 1986). Therefore digoxin toxicity should be suspected in an older digitalized patient with substantial weight loss and nonspecific symptoms.

Any digitalis drug causes a higher incidence of toxicity in the presence of the low serum potassium levels that accompany treatment with thiazide diuretics such as hydrochlorothiazide (HydroDiuril) or the more potent drug furosemide (Lasix), or when there is a low intake of potassium with normal renal output. When propranolol hydrochloride (Inderal) is given to a patient who is also receiving digitalis, the effect of digitalis is decreased and arrhythmias may occur.

Antiarrhythmic agents have a low therapeutic index. Alterations in their kinetics place older persons at a higher risk than younger patients. In the case of quinidine, clearance is reduced along with prolongation of the elimination half-life (Montamat and Davies 1989). Therefore monitoring of plasma levels becomes essential in the older adult.

Antihypertensive Agents

Hypertension is the second most prevalent chronic-disease process reported in older persons; arthritis is the most common (American Association of Retired Persons and Administration on Aging. 1990. *Profile of Older Americans*). High blood pressure in an older patient should be confirmed by several supine and standing blood pressure readings before treatment with medication is begun. Overzealous treatment of hypertension in older patients may cause orthostatic hypotension, which could result in falls, altered mental states, or renal and cardiac physiologic alterations.

An initial approach to treatment of hypertension in an older patient should include a review of all medications being taken to rule out drug-induced hypertension. Salt-intake reduction, weight reduction, restriction of alcohol to less than 1.5 ounces/day, and exercise are other nonpharmacologic recommendations to make.

Because of the heterogeneity of the older population when initiating pharmacologic antihypertensive therapy, the coexistence of other disease states and conditions needs to be considered. Compliance, cost, and potential side effects merit additional considerations.

Diuretics are effective in lowering blood pressure in older patients, but consideration should be given to use of the lowest effective dose. As a group, diuretics are the least costly and have a long duration of action, making once-a-day dosing possible. However, several special concerns associated with diuretic use include hypernatremia, hypokalemia, hyperuricemia, and glucose intolerance.

Centrally-acting adrenergic inhibitors include methyldopa hydrochloride (Aldomet) and clonidine hydrochloride (Catapres). Caution should be exercised when utilizing these agents in an older patient because of the troublesome side effects of orthostatic hypotension, dry mouth, impotence, and sedation.

Beta-adrenergic blocking agents may be suited to

the older hypertensive with angina, choosing cardioselective agents such as metoprolol (Lopressor) or atenolol (Tenormin). However, primary among the disadvantages are central nervous system disturbances such as depression and confusion, symptomatic bradycardia, and possible development of heart failure.

Angiotensin converting enzyme (ACE) inhibitors have shown efficacy in controlling hypertension and reducing left ventricular hypertrophy in older patients (Tuck et al. 1988). Utility has also been shown in decreasing pre- and afterload in hypertensives with congestive heart failure.

Calcium channel blockers are very effective in the treatment of hypertension and angina. However, all calcium channel blockers do not exert the same primary and secondary effects on the cardiovascular system. For example, diltiazem (Cardizem) has more effect on conduction through the sinoatrial (SA) node and can lead to bradydysrhythmias in the older patient. Verapamil (Clan, Isoptin) has more effect on atrioventricular (AV) conduction than on the SA node and can therefore lead to heart block. Nifedipine has no clinically significant effect on the SA or AV nodal conduction system. But it can affect heart rate via stimulation of the sympathetic nervous system in response to its vasodilatory effect and cause a reflex tachycardia.

Analgesics

Drugs such as the narcotic analgesics, which act on the central nervous system, should be used in low doses in older people because they may depress respirations and cloud consciousness. For example, both morphine sulfate and meperidine have increased peak serum levels and lower plasma clearance rates in older persons. When equivalent doses of morphine sulfate or pentazocine were given for pain, both the total amount of pain relief and the duration of relief were greater in older than in younger patients (Montamat, Cusack, and Vestal 1989).

Analgesics such as the salicylates, which are available over the counter and by prescription, are used to relieve not only the discomfort of arthritic-related pains but also nonspecific pain such as headaches and oral pain. If taken in large amounts, tinnitus and hearing loss can occur (Mongan et al. 1973). If renal function is impaired, an increased serum level of salicylate results and the risk for salicylism.

Nonsteroidal anti-inflammatory drugs (NSAIDs) are frequently used in the management of osteoarthritis, rheumatoid arthritis, and other chronic inflammatory diseases. These drugs, such as ibuprofen (Motrin, Advil), inhibit prostaglandin synthesis, which can affect other organ system functioning such as renal blood flow and gastrointestinal mucosal protection. Older NSAID users are 2.5 times more likely to develop a major complication than are younger patients (Jones and Schubert 1991). Gastrointestinal complications have ranged from mucosal erosions to peptic ulcers (acute and chronic) with bleeding and perforation (Freston and Freston 1990). Unfortunately the majority of older patients who develop NSAID-induced gastropathy remain asymptomatic prior to the complication (Jones and Schubert 1991). For those older patients in whom NSAID therapy is required, it has been suggested to use lower dosages initially, shorter half-life agents, enteric coated products, and (when appropriate) coadministration of antacids or food. It has also been suggested to reassess the need during each patient encounter for the continued use of the NSAID (Jones and Schubert 1991). NSAID use in older patients with compromised circulation and mild azotemia requires monitoring of renal function. The risk of NSAID-induced renal failure is related to daily NSAID usage, those with age- and/or disease-related vascular compromise, underlying renal insufficiency, coexistent diuretic use, and ethanol use (Sandler et al. 1991).

Geriatric Psychopharmacology

Psychotropic medications are generally categorized as antipsychotics, antidepressants, and sedative/hypnotic agents. These include the most misused and overused class of drugs in the geriatric population (Kane, Ouslander and Abrass 1989).

Psychotropics. In the past, indications for the use of psychotropic medications, particularly in institutionalized older adults, have been vague. In a study by Buck and coworkers in 1988, over half of the nursing home residents studied were prescribed at least one psychotropic drug (Buck 1988). The Omnibus Budget Reconciliation Act of 1987 developed prescribing parameters for psychotropic use in long-term care institutions. Each nursing home must ensure that each resident's drug regimen is free from unnecessary drugs and dosages, undue adverse consequences, and significant medication errors or significant medication error rates (Lamy and Michocki 1988). When psychotropic medication is considered in older patients, a comprehensive assessment will ensure that antipsychotic drug therapy is necessary to treat a specific condition. Patients taking antipsychotic agents should receive gradual dose reductions, drug holidays, and behavioral programming in an effort to discontinue these drugs (Lamy and Michocki 1988). The antipsychotic agents or major tranquilizers can be beneficial in the treatment of psychosis, paranoid illness, and agitation associated with dementia. The choice depends on the syndrome being treated and the patient's other clinical problems. Prior to initiating therapy, a thorough evaluation should exclude any underlying medical illness. In general, psychotropic medications should be prescribed at doses 30–50 percent as large as those for younger patients (Thompson 1983a). The dosage is then titrated gradually until the therapeutic goal is reached or until adverse side effects develop (Thompson 1983). The older patient is particularly vulnerable to the side effects of these agents such as delirium or extrapyramidal symptoms including tardive dyskinesia, arrhythmias, and postural hypotension (Montamat, Cusack, and Vestal 1989a).

The antipsychotic agents have side-effect profiles that vary with potency. A listing of selected antipsychotics in order from most to least potent includes chlorpromazine, thioridazine, thiothixene, haloperidol, and fluphenazine. The higher potency neuroleptics have more sedating and anticholinergic side effects; the lower potency agents exhibit predominantly extrapyramidal side effects (Thompson 1983b). For example, haloperidol (Haldol) is utilized in older patients because of its low sedative effects, minimal anticholinergic effects, and virtually no cardiac side effects; but an increase in extrapyramidal side effects occurs.

Antidepressants. Antidepressants are utilized to treat major clinical depression, which has been reported to occur at any given time in at least 10 percent of the older population (Thompson 1983). Diagnosis of clinically significant depression should follow the criteria established in the Diagnostic and Statistical Manual III (DSM III-R).

When tricyclic antidepressants are used, the drug is chosen on the basis of a person's response to side effects. Tricyclic antidepressants can produce a variety of cardiac side effects, such as an increase in heart rate, prolonged P-R interval, QRS duration, QT time, and flattening of the T wave. Desipramine and doxepin are reported to have a low incidence of cardiovascular effects (Thompson 1983a). Orthostatic hypotension is another common side effect; however, it is not seen to the same degree with all tricyclic antidepressants. For example, nortriptyline and desipramine tend to cause fewer hypotensive episodes than other tricylics (Thompson 1983).

Anticholinergic side effects secondary to tricyclic antidepressant therapy include change in mentation (including delirium), impaired visual accommodation, delayed gastric emptying, urinary retention and decreased sweating, hyperthermic reactions, and sexual dysfunction (Thompson 1983). For example amitriptyline is the most anticholinergic drug in its class along with a prolonged half-life in an older person; desipramine is the least anticholinergic. Amitriptyline and doxepin are the most sedating of the tricyclic antidepressants.

Antianxiety Agents, Sedatives, and Hypnotics. Benzodiazepines have both anxiolytic and hypnotic effects and are the most frequently prescribed drugs for antianxiety and anti-insomnia properties (Thompson 1983). The effects of aging on the distribution and elimination kinetics cause a prolonged half-life in the older patient. Diazepam (Valium) has a half-life of approximately twenty hours in a 20-year-old to ninety hours in an 80-year-old (Thompson 1983b). Chlordiazepoxide's (Librium) half-life increases from seven hours in the young adult to forty hours in those over 80. However, because of little alterations in the pharmacokinetics of lorazepam (Ativan) and oxazepam (Serax), there are no major changes in half-life with aging. When antianxiety drugs are needed in the older person, they should be started at the lowest effective dose for a short period of time (Cohen and Eisendorfer 1985).

Buspirone (Buspar) is a newer medication marketed as an anxiolytic that improves symptoms of anxiety, though no more effectively than benzodiazepines. However, it is less sedating than diazepam (Valium) and does not cause withdrawal symptoms when discontinued. Current experience with this drug in treating anxiety in the older patient is limited (Ballinger 1990).

Prior to prescribing an hypnotic agent, the particular cause of insomnia should be sought. Benzodiazepines that are prescribed as hypnotics are divided into those with shorter or longer durations of action. The shorter-acting benzodiazepines, such as triazolam (Halcion) and temazepam (Restoril), are suitable for older people because they have less residual daytime effect. The longer-acting benzodiazepines in general should be avoided in older patients. The aim of treatment with hypnotics is for a short period of time—approximately four weeks maximum—or intermittent use if possible (Ballinger 1990).

SUMMARY

Over the past decade our knowledge of the physiologic changes that occur in the older adult has broadened. Better prescribing parameters have been developed, based upon the pharmacodynamic and pharmacokinetic alterations that occur. This improved knowledge base in the pharmacology of older individuals will assist practitioners in geriatric medicine. However, further research is much needed regarding medication effects in the frail older population.

Nurses assist older patients in many different settings: hospitals, nursing homes, clinics, adult daycare centers, senior centers, and through home health care programs. Nurses need to obtain an accurate medication history and should question the need for all of the drugs being taken. This is particularly true when the nurse discovers changes in the older patient's mental or physical status. Also, many times the nurse is the lone health care provider evaluating the patient in the home environment, where medication bottles can be reviewed with attention to prescribing physician, expiration dates, number of pills, and ability of the patient to access the medication. Nurses can and should play a major role in the reduction of polypharmacy in the older patient.

STUDY QUESTIONS

1. State one reason why the older adult is more likely to experience an adverse drug reaction.

2. Define pharmacodynamics and pharmacokinetics.

3. Discuss three important pharmacodynamic properties of warfarin when prescribed for an older patient.

4. Why is drug distribution altered with age?

5. Which phase of hepatic metabolism is affected with aging?

6. Identify three drugs with a large first-pass metabolism in the liver.

7. How can decline in renal function with aging be assessed?

8. Name two reasons older persons might not follow the prescribed medication regimen.

9. State at least six facts older people should know about their prescribed medications.

10. Describe the differences between *generically equivalent* and *therapeutically equivalent*.

11. Discuss examples of clinical signs and symptoms of digoxin toxicity.

12. Identify two potential side effects of NSAID use in an older patient.

13. When an older person receives a tricyclic antidepressant, what are three potential side effects?

REFERENCES

American Association of Retired Persons and Administration on Aging. 1990. *A Profile of Older Americans*. PF 3049 (1288, D996). Washington, DC: United States Department of Health and Human Services.

Ballinger, B.R. 1990. Hypnotics and anxiolytics. *British Med J* 300(17):456–58.

Bauer, L.A. 1982. Interference of oral phenytoin absorption by continuous nasogastric feedings. *Neurology* 32:570.

Black, A.J. and K. Somers. 1989. Drug-related illness resulting in hospital admission. *J Royal Coll Phy* 18:40–41.

Bruce, A., M. Anderson, B. Arvidsson, and B. Isaksson.

1980. Body composition. Prediction of normal body potassium, body water and body fat in adults on the basis of body height, body weight and age. *Scand J Clin Lab Invest* 40:461–73.

Buck, J.A. 1988. Psychotropic drug practice in nursing homes. *JAGS* 36:409.

Buckley, C., D. Curtin, T. Walsh, and K. O'Malley. 1986. Aging and platelet a2-adrenoreceptors. *Br J Clin Pharmacol* 21:721–22.

Campbell, T.C. and J.R. Hayes. 1974. Role of nutrition in the drug-metabolizing enzyme system. *Pharmacol Rev* 26:171–97.

Campion, E.W., L.O. deLabry, and R.J. Glynn. 1988. The effect of age on serum albumin in healthy males: Report from the Normative Aging Study. *J Gerontol* 43:M18–M20.

Caranaso, G.J., R.B. Stewart, and L.E. Cluff. 1974. Drug-induced illness leading to hospitalization. *JAMA* 228(6):713–17.

Cockcroft, D.W. and M.H. Gault. 1976. Prediction of creatinine clearance from serum creatinine. *Nephron* 16:31–41.

Cohen, D. and C. Eisdorfer. 1985. Major psychiatric and behavioral disorders in the elderly. In *Principles of Geriatric Medicine*, edited by R. Anders, E. Bierman, and W.R. Hazzard. New York: McGraw-Hill.

Collett, C. 1988. Assessing the patient education needs of the elderly. *Medical Time*s November:95–99.

Coon, W.W. and P.W. Willis. 1974. Hemorrhagic complications of anticoagulant therapy. *Arch Intern Med* 133:386–92.

Cusack, B.J. and R.E. Vestal. 1986. Clinical pharmacology: Special considerations in the elderly. In *The Practice of Geriatrics*, edited by E. Calkins, P. Davis, and A. Ford. Philadelphia: W.B. Saunders.

Cuties, A.J., E. Altman, and L. Lendel. 1983. Compatibility of enteral products with commonly employed drug additives. *JPEN* 7:186.

Drug Interaction Facts. 1985. *Facts and Comparisons*. St. Louis, MO: Drug Interaction Facts.

Drusano, G.L., H.L. Munice, J.M. Hoopes, D.J. Damron, and J.W. Warren. 1988. Commonly used methods of estimating creatinine clearance are inadequate for elderly debilitated nursing home patients. *J Am Geriatr Soc* 36:437–41.

Forbes, G.B. and J.C. Reina. 1970. Adult lean body mass declines with age: Some longitudinal observations. *Metabolism* 19:653–63.

Freston, M.S. and J.W. Freston. 1990. Peptic ulcers in the elderly: Unique features and management. *Geriatrics* Jan 45(1):39–45.

Grymonpre, R.E., P.A. Mitenko, D.S. Sitar, et al. 1988. Drug-associated hospital admissions in older medical patients. *JAGS* 36:1092–98.

Gurwitz, J.H., R.J. Goldberg, A. Holder, N. Knapic, and J. Ansell. 1988. Age-related risks of long-term oral anticoagulant therapy. *Arch Intern Med* 148:1733–36.

Jones, M.P. and M.L. Schubert. 1991. What do you recommend for prophylaxis in an elderly woman with arthritis requiring NSAIDs for control? *Amer J of Gastroenterology* 86(3):264–68.

Kane, R.L., J.G. Ouslander, and I.B. Abrass. 1989. *Essentials of Geriatrics*. 2d ed. New York: McGraw-Hill.

Klein, L.E., P.S. German, D.M. Levine, E.R. Feroli, Jr., and J. Ardery. 1984. Medication problems among outpatients: A study with emphasis on the elderly. *Arch Intern Med* 144:1185–88.

Koford, L.L. 1985. OTC drug overuse in the elderly: What to watch for. *Geriatrics* 40(10):55–60.

Lamy, P.P. 1986. Drug interactions in the elderly. *Journal of Gerontological Nursing* 12(2):36–37.

Lamy, P.P. and F.J. Michocki. 1988. Medication management. *Clinics in Geriatric Medicine* 4(3):623–39.

Lieberman, M.L. 1986. *The Essential Guide to Generic Drugs*. New York: Harper and Row.

Miller, R.R. 1974. Hospital admissions due to adverse drug reactions. *Arch Intern Med* 134:219–23.

Mongan, E., P. Kelly, K. Wies, W.W. Porter, and H.E. Paulus. 1973. Tinnitus as an indication of therapeutic serum salicylate levels. *JAMA* 226:142–45.

Montamat, S.C., B.J. Cusack, R.E. Vestal. 1989. Management of drug therapy in the elderly. *N Engl J Med* 321:303–9.

Montamat, S.C. and A.O. Davies. 1989. Physiological response to isoproterenol and coupling of beta-adrenergic receptors in young and elderly human subjects. *J Gerontol* 44:M100–M105.

Myers, M., D. Meier, and J. Walsh. 1984. Pharmacology: General Principles. In *Geriatric Medicine*, edited by C. Cassel and J. Walsh. New York: Springer-Verlag.

Nolan, L. and K. O'Malley. 1988a. Prescribing for the elderly. Part I. Sensitivity of the elderly to adverse drug reactions. *J Am Geriatr* 36:142–49.

Novak, L.P. 1972. Aging, total body potassium, fat-free mass, and cell mass in males and females between ages 18 and 35 years. *J Gerontol* 27:438–43.

O'Malley, K., I.H. Stevenson, C.A. Ward, A.J.J. Wood, and J. Crooks. 1977. Determinants of anticoagulant control in patients receiving warfarin. *Br J Clin Pharmacol* 4:309–14.

Oppeneer, J.E. and T.M. Vervoren. 1983. *Gerontological Pharmacology*. St. Louis: C.V. Mosby.

Pan, H.Y.M., B.B. Hoffman, R.A. Pershe, and T.F. Blaschke. 1986. Decline in beta-adrenergic receptor-mediated vascular relaxation with aging in man. *J Pharmacol Exp Ther* 239:802–7.

Pepper, G.A. and L.J. Robbins. 1987. Improving geriatric drug therapy. *Generations* 12(1):57–61.

Rados, B. 1983. *Generic Drugs: Cutting Costs, Not Corners* (Publication #[FDA] 86-3156). Reprint from FDA Consumer, Department of Health and Human Services. Rockville, MD: Public Health Service-FDA.

Reidenberg, M.M. 1987. Drug therapy in the elderly: The problem from the point of view of a clinical pharmacologist. *Clin Pharmacol Ther* 42:677–80.

Reidenberg, M.M., M. Lavy, H. Warner, et al. 1978. Relationship between diazepam dose, plasma level, age, and central nervous system depression. *Clin Pharmacol Ther* 23:371–74.

Rikans, L.E. 1986. Minireview: Drugs and nutrition in old age. *Life Sciences* 39(12):1027–36.

Roe, D.A. 1986. Drug-nutrient interactions in the elderly. *Geriatrics* 41(3):57–74.

Rowe, J.W., R. Andres, J.D. Tobin, A.H. Norris, and N.W. Shock. 1976. The effect of age on creatinine clearance in men: A cross-sectional and longitudinal study. *J Gerontol* 31:155–63.

Sandler, D.P., R. Burr, and C.R. Weinberg. 1991. Nonsteroidal anti-inflammatory drugs and the risk for chronic renal disease. *Ann Intern Med* 115(3):165–72.

Scarpace, P.J. 1986. Decreased B-adrenergic responsiveness during senescence. *Fed Proc* 45:51–54.

Schwertz, D.W. and M.T. Buschmann. 1989. Pharmacogeriatrics. *Crit Care Nurs Q* 12(1):26–37.

Shepherd, A.M., D.S. Hewick, T.A. Moreland, and I.H. Stevenson. 1977. Age as a determinant of sensitivity to warfarin. *Br J Clin Pharmacol* 4:315–20.

Sloan, R. 1986. *Practical Geriatric Therapeutics*. Oradell, NJ: Medical Economics Books.

Spencer, R.T., L. Nichols, H. Waterhouse, F. West, and E. Bankert. 1986. *Clinical Pharmacology and Nursing Management*. Philadelphia: J.B. Lippincott.

Thompson, T.L., II, M.G. Moran, and A.S. Nies. 1983a. Drug therapy: Psychotropic drug use in the elderly. (First of the papers.) *NEJM* 308(3):134–38.

Thompson, T.L., II; M.G. Moran, A.S. Nies. 1983b. Drug therapy: Psychotropic drug use in the elderly. (Second of two parts; review article.) *NEJM* 308(4):194–99.

Tuck, M., et al. 1988. Hypertension in the elderly. *JAGS* 36:630–43.

Vestal, R.E. and G.W. Dawson. 1985. Pharmacology and aging. In *Handbook of the Biology of Aging*. 2d ed., edited by C.E. Finch and E.L. Schneider. New York: Van Nostrand Reinhold.

Vestal, R.E., S.G. Jue, and B.J. Cusack. 1985. Increased risk of adverse drug reactions in the elderly: Fact or myth? In *Therapeutics in the Elderly: Scientific Foundations and Clinical Practice*, edited by K. O'Malley and J.L. Waddington. Amsterdam: Excerpta Medica.

Vestal, R.E., A.H. Norris, J.D. Tobin, B.H. Cohen, N.W. Shock, and R. Andres. 1975. Antipyrine metabolism in man: Influence of age, alcohol, caffeine, and smoking. *Clin Pharmacol Ther* 18:L425–32.

Vestal, R.E., A.J.J. Wood, and D.G. Shand. 1979. Reduced beta-adrenoceptor sensitivity in the elderly. *Clin Pharmacol Ther* 26:181–86.

Wade, B. and J. Finlayson. 1983. Drugs in the elderly. *Nurs Mirror* 156:586–92.

Wilkinson, G.R. and D.G. Shand. 1975. A physiological approach to hepatic drug clearance. *Clin Pharmacol Ther* 18:377–90.

Woodford-Williams, E., A.S. Alvarez, D. Webster, B. Landless, and M.P. Dixon. 1964. Serum protein patterns in "normal" and pathological aging. *Gerontologia* 10:86–99.

10 Mental Disorders

Brenda Botts Riley

CHAPTER OUTLINE

FOCUS

The focus of this chapter is mental disorders that are commonly found in the older population. The major disorders are depression, organic mental disorders, schizophrenic disorders, and substance abuse disorders. Older individuals often manifest symptoms in ways that do not necessarily fit into established categories because they may possess symptoms of more than one disease simultaneously. For these reasons it is sometimes difficult to diagnose mental disorders in this age group.

OBJECTIVES

1. Discuss factors related to aging that may cause depression.

2. Analyze symptoms of depression in older people that nurses must be aware of when assessing the physical and mental status of patients.

3. Describe specific nursing interventions for the depressed older patient.

4. Give examples of para or benign suicide.

5. Categorize nursing assessment for the suicidal older person.

6. Discuss nursing interventions for the suicidal older patient.

7. Compare nursing interventions for dementia and delirium.

8. Identify nursing diagnoses that are commonly found in the patient with Alzheimer's disease.

9. Describe nursing interventions for older persons with a diagnosis of schizophrenia.

10. Discuss nursing interventions for the older person who is a substance abuser.

When the mental problems of older adults are studied, it is apparent that they cannot be separated from the social, physical, economic, and political dynamics of modern society. As many people reach older-age status, they are relegated to positions in society in which they are relatively powerless to control their destinies. Having feelings such as powerlessness, helplessness, and hopelessness, older adults react in ways that are often mistakenly regarded as signs of mental illness. Through sensitivity to the special problems of older people, nurses can intervene in ways that help older persons overcome problems or at least make difficult situations more tolerable.

DEPRESSION

When studying the physiologic problems associated with old age, the strong correlation between aging and depression becomes apparent. As age increases, so does the incidence of depression. This problem is found to be most acute for that segment of the population between the ages of 55 and 70. Indeed, depression is the most common functional mental disorder of older adults. It is estimated that 15–20 percent of persons over 65 years of age suffer from clinical depression (Fry 1986) and that 20–30 percent have less severe symptoms (Gurland 1982). Weisman (1979) and Rosenfeld (1978) state that 20–50 percent of older persons have milder symptoms of depression. It is obvious that depression is a significant problem among older adults.

Individual Variations in Depression

As might be expected, the degree of depression varies considerably from one person to another or within the same person from one time to another. This variation in emotional state may range, for example, from feeling "blue" to thoughts of suicide. Furthermore this emotional state may be complicated by the differences in each person's varying tendency or ability to let others know about his or her thoughts and feelings. It is important to identify the thoughts and feelings of older adults for effective interpersonal relationships and treatment.

Causes of Depression

It is helpful to understand not only the emotional state of the older person but also the general experiences of older people within specific social milieus. In some situations the causes of depression may be apparent, for example, when there is an obvious loss of self-esteem, possessions, or loved ones. In other situations the cause may not be clear at all. There may be no obvious cause, even to the depressed person. He or she may experience a sense of overall letdown. The causes may be vague or too numerous to list. Laboratory tests for identifying biological markers of depression are being explored. They hold promise but are not conclusive at this time (Blazer 1989a).

Culture and Depression. One basic social factor to consider in relation to the problems of aging is culture. For example, minority groups in the United States (e.g., African-Americans, Oriental-Americans, Mexican-Americans, and American Indians) differ somewhat from the dominant culture in their attitudes and practices toward their older members. These attitudes and practices, along with certain economic circumstances, contribute to a unique consciousness about older adults in these groups.

Cultural differences help to explain the fact that the incidence of depression varies among social groups. For example, older African-Americans seem to experience less depression than the older population as a whole. This difference may be attributed to economic, religious, and familial factors. First, many African-Americans cannot afford to retire; therefore they tend not to suffer from the crises of loneliness, feelings of uselessness, and loss of status that frequently accompany retirement. Second, the African-American church is typically a strong source of emotional support for older adults, as well as an arena for greater social involvement. Finally, contrary to popular belief, African-American families offer a cohesiveness and support for older adults that is not readily evident in the general population (Butler and Lewis 1982; Leslie 1976).

Other minority groups share similar economic, religious, and familial characteristics regarding their attitudes and care of older adults. These similarities among minority groups and their differences from the general population should not be overgeneralized or oversimplified, however. Indeed the dominant American culture, with its early retirement age, small nuclear families, high rates of mobility, and the casual–to–negative attitudes toward older people, who are no longer felt to be "productive" (Butler and Lewis 1982), is being incorporated gradually into the living patterns of all American subcultures.

In general, American society is youth oriented. Older adults are seen as a burden and are unpleasant reminders of the inevitabilities of human life. Hence the aging process is denied. This denial makes it difficult for older adults to be accepted in society as useful members with a healthy sense of self-worth. Thus the stage is set for many older adults to become depressed.

Depression of Older Adults as a Crisis. Another way to understand the "problem" of aging as related to depression is to view it as a crisis. Aging is accompanied by many crises. More losses occur during this stage of psychosocial development than during any other period of life. Friends and loved ones are dying, there is a sudden loss of status through retirement, and many older people eventually are asked (or forced) to move from their own homes to the homes of a son or daughter or to an institution. Meaningful treasures that represent fond memories and security have to be left behind. The experience of closing a household and selling or giving away possessions accumulated over a period of fifty years or more, for example, must be very sad. Frequently accompanying these moves is the loss of independence. Many decisions are made for older people by those around them. Again, self-esteem and feelings of self-worth are diminished. As loss is heaped upon loss, each successive deprivation may become more difficult to tolerate. The stages of recovery and resolution in the grief process become more difficult to achieve. There are fewer people available to take the place of those who are gone. Normal grief turns into depression because of increased feelings of worthlessness and lack of meaning in life.

Aging women in American society, especially among whites, bear special burdens. Many older women live alone (Butler and Lewis 1982). Most no longer feel useful as mothers. Many are husbandless. The roles they had thought most important in the past exist no longer. They feel useless, as though there

were no place for them. Also, the physical signs of aging affect women more than their male counterparts. Many older women spend much time and money trying to preserve a youthful look only to appear old in spite of their efforts. Since women have been led by American culture to believe that youthful beauty is one of the major assets of the female, they also believe that to lose youthful appearance is to lose status and self-esteem. A woman may feel that as a woman she has been discriminated against all her life, and as she grows older the problem of aging is added to the problem of being a woman, exacerbating the discrimination problem.

Loneliness. Among the many problems older people face, loneliness is one of the most painful. Although loneliness is experienced by some people in all age groups, older adults, as a group, are most chronically affected. A large number of older people in the United States experience loneliness daily. For many it is a constant fact of life. Approximately two of every ten older people in the United States live alone (Butler 1982). Although not all who live alone are lonely, many are. The consequences of loneliness can be devastatingly cruel for those older people who are socially neglected.

Generally loneliness is a state of being in which the person feels helpless to meet the basic needs of belonging, intimacy, and relatedness to others. This state results in decreased self-esteem and self-worth. A person may be in a crowd or may live with many people, as in a nursing home, but if the person experiences no intimacy, no bonds of belonging with those close by, that person will be socially isolated and lonely.

Causes of Loneliness. There are many causes of loneliness among older adults. Often with retirement comes an end to feelings of usefulness and a separation from work and friends. As a person grows older, friends and loved ones are lost through death and geographic mobility. As the body grows older, health often deteriorates, limiting physical mobility and the ability to maintain emotional ties with others. Older people are commonly viewed as less desirable partners for intimate or meaningful relationships. As spouses die, they leave feelings of emptiness and desolation. Hopes of finding someone else to share life may seem slim. Helplessness and dependency frequently increase with aging and illness. For these reasons families may decide that it is best to place the aged mother or father in an institution. Thus familiar surroundings and people are left behind, bringing feelings of loneliness.

Results of Loneliness. In some institutions and even in the private homes of some older people the environment may not stimulate thought or feeling. With limited movement and ability older adults must depend upon others to make contact with them. When those closest to them fail, they suffer from a form of sensory deprivation. Sensory deprivation is a type of loneliness, since there is no perceived opportunity for relatedness.

Loneliness is thought to cause not only emotional problems in older adults but physical problems as well. The attention of older adults is focused on body functions and pains; ailments may be magnified. Older people in desperation may develop physical complaints as a result of loneliness and they will visit their family physician in search of help. They often are sent away with a prescription for medication, leaving the basic problem of loneliness undetected and untreated. Older adults are left with feelings of hopelessness, since there seems to be no chance that life will get better. They do not know where else to turn for help.

Loneliness may result in emotional problems ranging from isolation to depression and psychoses. With depression the person feels undesirable and worthless, with no sense of identity. No one seems to value her or him as an intimate friend or lover, and no one seeks the person out for companionship regularly or frequently. With psychosis the older person may want so much to have intimate contact with another that the mind invents someone to talk to. Or else the person may choose to live in the past, thinking about more pleasant days. Those with whom such a person happens to come into contact are confused with people from past times. A young nurse may be mistaken for the older person's son or daughter. Such confusion may be temporary, as if the person were interrupted in the middle of a daydream; or the confusion may last for some time, particularly if it is not treated.

Prevention of Loneliness. There is no sure way to prevent loneliness, since relationships end for a variety of reasons. When the loss is of sufficient magnitude, loneliness will result. Certain factors seem to lessen the impact, however, and perhaps decrease the chance of loneliness. Maintaining a sense of identity through one's occupation may be helpful. A retired

lawyer, for example, may still have a strong identity with his or her profession. A social network that includes close relationships among various age groups will help decrease the impact of losing significant others.

Many older people claim that television programs and personalities have helped decrease their boredom and loneliness. For some the radio or television set is never turned off, since the companionship of the voices helps these people sleep. Pets may be used in the place of human relationships. They help the person feel needed and loved. Pets respond affectionately. The death of a pet may also be very traumatic, however. Even plants provide a reprieve from loneliness. A strong religious belief can provide a hedge against loneliness, since many believe that help and companionship are constantly available from God. Religious faith can give strength to endure physical isolation. Membership in a church group offers companionship with others who have common goals and beliefs.

Finally, creativity and curiosity help fill the mind with thoughts other than the self and direct energies outward. Materials that can be used to express creativity may be made available through such community resources as senior centers. Accomplishments help build self-esteem. Efforts should be made to prevent or treat loneliness, since it may lead to more severe problems such as depression, physical illness, psychosis, or suicide.

Widowhood. For a man or a woman the death of a spouse is particularly traumatic, especially if the couple has been very dependent upon each other. Holmes, when studying life crises, found that the death of a spouse was considered the most traumatic event in a person's life (Holmes and Rahe 1967). Roles and responsibilities change. If the husband is left, he may have to learn to cook for the first time in his life. The wife may have to manage finances, something she may never have done. Goals and plans must be adjusted or relinquished.

Some older people are dependent on their spouses in special ways. For example, people who are chronically ill depend on the spouse to provide care and security. The death of the caregiver husband or wife in such cases is doubly difficult, since it seems almost impossible to adjust to living without this help. With children and other relatives living far away, the survivor is left with little choice. Options may include leaving home, friends, and familiar surroundings to live with a son or daughter, who usually has a busy schedule and problems of his or her own, or going to an institution such as a nursing home. So the death of a spouse often brings grief from several causes: plans, goals, and dreams must be abandoned; physical possessions and familiar surroundings are lost when the widowed person is forced to move.

Many feelings besides sadness may be experienced by the bereaved after the loss of a spouse. There may be feelings of loneliness, emptiness, abandonment, and anger. The spouse may wander through empty rooms, not sure of what to do next. Physical and emotional illness increases (Butler and Lewis 1982; Lynch 1977). The spouse may take on the characteristics of the deceased, including the physical symptoms of the illness before death. Statistics have shown that there is greater mortality among survivors within the first six months after the loss of a spouse than in the general population of the same age group. Also, 22.5 percent of deaths of husbands that occurred within the first six months after the deaths of their wives were attributed to the same general causes as the deceased wife's (Butler and Lewis 1982; Lynch 1977). The incidence of suicide is also higher among widowed people (Lynch 1977).

Working through the grief process may take a year or more. Anniversaries, holidays, and special times and places bring on renewed grief as the person reminisces about experiences shared with the loved one. Emotional problems such as depression are often the end result. The problems of the widow or widower may continue to increase unless help is received from friends, loved ones, or professionals.

If the death is expected, there may be time to make such plans as different living arrangements or the use of resources such as Meals-on-Wheels to fill in gaps. The nurse should try to get the bereaved involved with others to fill some of the lonely hours.

If the death is unexpected, the person who is left may be emotionally devastated, since there has been no time for anticipatory grief or to formulate plans for adjustment. This is a crisis situation. The nurse must be direct and specific in an attempt to clarify the survivor's plans and options. Most often, the nurse involved will be on the staff of the hospital where the death has occurred or where the person was pronounced dead. The nurse may refer the survivor to a crisis unit, a visiting nurse, or other resources such as the Widowed Persons Service. Many times the widow or widower is left with no help and no follow-up and becomes sick, depressed, or suicidal.

The same nursing intervention applies to the spouse whose husband or wife is dying at home. Nurses making home visits should assess the coping abilities and resources of the survivor before the death occurs. Proper referrals should be made and resources should be contacted so that follow-up care and support will be available when it is needed. Thus stress may be reduced with the help of the nurse.

The bereaved should be given the opportunity to express feelings about the dead spouse, even such negative emotions as guilt and anger. After such a free expression of feelings, the bereaved will be better able to put thoughts and events into perspective. Feelings that are released through discussion are more manageable and less overwhelming than those experienced in emptiness and loneliness.

After the bereaved has had some time to grieve, some of this energy should be turned to planning for the future. What living arrangements are possible and acceptable? What about meal planning, grocery shopping, and cooking? What must be done to help this person maintain the activities of daily living in an acceptable fashion? What can be done to resocialize this person? The widowed person's social life will be different now; even old acquaintances will react differently to the newly single man or woman.

As these questions are discussed, resources such as relatives, friends, and community services should be contacted and specific plans made. Ongoing evaluation of the program by the client is essential in meeting identified needs. If such programs were devised and implemented to the client's satisfaction early in a crisis such as the death of a spouse, the incidence of depression and suicides of the older age group would surely be reduced.

Physical Changes. Physical changes may decrease a person's self-concept and thus lead to depression. Not only does physical appearance change as the body ages, but physiologic functioning changes. Decreased hearing and sight lead to isolation and loneliness, increased dependence, and decreased mobility, all of which decrease self-esteem.

Physical Illness. Depression is common after a diagnosis of chronic illness. Problems resulting from conditions such as strokes, parkinsonism, and cancer may cause dramatic changes in body image, resulting in decreased feelings of self-worth.

As the ability to take care of oneself decreases, the quality and amount of nutrition, exercise, and general self-health care also tend to decrease. Poor nutrition and lack of exercise frequently aggravate existing problems. Intellectual and physical functioning declines, adding to depression (Cadoret and Widmer 1988).

Financial Problems. Physical and emotional illness is often accompanied by financial problems. Older adults worry about using all their resources to pay medical bills. For example, Mr. B. suffered from a chronic illness. The first time he went to the hospital, Medicare and his hospital insurance policy paid most of his bills. Subsequent hospitalizations, however, took his life's savings and he had to sell his home to pay medical bills. When he died, his wife was left without a home and none of the $15,000 that they had saved for the two of them to enjoy in their later years. Such situations are frustrating, humiliating, devastating, and depressing. Income and perceived health are closely associated with self-esteem (Lee 1976). As income and health deteriorate, self-esteem decreases. And as self-esteem decreases, depression increases.

Medications. Some medications prescribed for physical illness may cause depression. For example, reserpine, frequently used to treat hypertension in older adults, is known to cause depression in a significant number of patients (Blazer 1989a). Tranquilizers, especially the phenothiazines, may also cause depression (Butler and Lewis 1982). Many other drugs cause symptoms similar to those seen in a person who is depressed. Examples of these drugs are lithium carbonate, thiazide diuretics, digitalis, methyldopa, propranolol hydrochloride, levodopa, corticosteroids, anticancer agents (cytostatic and immunosuppressive drugs), barbiturates, and propanediols (Salzman and Shader 1979; Buckwalter 1990).

Types and Symptoms of Depression

Diagnostic, or clinical, depression is a type of affective mood disorder. Two diagnoses that include symptoms of depression only are major depression and dysthymic disorder. The diagnosis of major depression may be used for a single episode or a recurring problem. As individuals age, recurring episodes occur more frequently and may last longer (Blazer 1989a). The symptoms of dysthymic disorder and major depression are similar. However, dysthymic patients have symptoms that are less severe and of shorter duration than those of patients diagnosed as having a major depression. Other affective disorders that may have depressive elements include bipolar, cyclothymic, and atypical disorders (American Psychiatric Association 1987).

Bipolar disorder may include manic episodes as well as mood shifts to depression. Symptoms of mania and depression are often severe. However, manic episodes are not often seen in late life (Blazer 1989a). Patients with symptoms similar to those having bipolar disorders but who are less severely ill are diagnosed as having a cyclothymic disorder. These persons experience periods of depression and hypomania. The patient with an atypical depression has a brief illness and does not have all the symptoms that are usually seen with a major depression or one of the other diagnostic categories mentioned previously.

It is important to note that uncomplicated bereavement is not considered a mental illness and should not be confused with depression. However, prolonged or unusually severe bereavement may develop into a major depressive episode.

A person who experiences a maladaptive reaction to an identifiable precipitating stressor is diagnosed as having an adjustment disorder. Social and occupational functioning is disturbed. When the stressor is removed, the person is able to function satisfactorily. If the stressor cannot be removed, then the person learns to adapt at a new level. Although the person may experience depression, it is not of major proportions as seen in major depression. Older adults may experience an adjustment disorder when changing places of residence, for example. The individual who has a major depression loses interest and pleasure in living. The facial expression is often one of sadness and the person speaks of being worthless and hopeless. Eating and sleeping problems occur frequently. Slowed thought processes and speech may be evident. Suicidal ideation is not uncommon. In addition the person may experience psychotic features such as delusions or hallucinations (American Psychiatric Association 1987).

The symptoms of depression are many and varied

Table 10–1   Common Symptoms of Depression in Older Adults

Thoughts	Behaviors—Actions	Feelings	Other
Self-deprecation resulting from guilt	Withdrawal	Irritable	Appetite disturbance
	Loss of sexual interest	Fearful	Anorexia
Worthlessness	Agitation	Sad	Weight change
Suicidal	Slowed movements	Angry	Constipation
Obsessive	Crying	Hopeless	Fatigue
	Tearful	Helpless	Somatic complaints
	Compulsive	Indecisive	Sleep disturbance
	Dependent	Dissatisfied	Difficulty concentrating or thinking
		Bored	
		Anxious	
		Depersonalized	
		Apathetic	

(see Table 10-1). Each patient's experience may be somewhat different, and depression may mask other problems. On the other hand the patient diagnosed as having other problems can also experience depression. General somatic complaints and decreasing physical health sometimes indicate depression (Cohen 1977). Nurses often overlook signs of depression when concentrating on the more obvious physical problems, since depression is accepted by some as a normal part of the aging process, although it is not.

Nursing Assessment

A thorough assessment is necessary so that the many problems associated with aging may be identified. A history aimed at eliciting information about the client's life changes, losses, and signs and symptoms of depression is necessary. The length of the current illness, a history of past episodes, and the patient's response to treatment should be explored (Blazer 1989a). Depression screening instruments, such as the Beck Depression Inventory or the Zung Self-rating Depression Scale may be helpful tools to be used as a part of the nursing assessment (Keane and Sells 1990). A thorough health assessment may iden-

tify problems of which the patient is only vaguely aware. The nurse should plan to spend ample time with the older person who has symptoms of depression. Responses are often slow and the patient may want to tell the nurse in greater detail about his or her problems.

When possible, nurses should talk with the patient and family about the history, nursing problems, making plans for action, and setting realistic goals. These plans should be written clearly and kept so that they are available to any staff member working with the patient and family. It is important that the patient and the family, if the patient depends on them for care and assistance, be a part of the problem-identification and -solving process. Patients should be encouraged to make decisions about their care to the extent they are capable.

Nursing Interventions

Nurses' Feelings and Attitudes. When providing care for the older depressed patient, nurses should first consider their personal attitudes toward their own aging. If aging is not seen as a normal part of the developmental sequence but as something to be avoided and denied, the nurse will probably have a difficult time caring for the older person. Negative attitudes, such as avoidance or disdain, are quickly perceived by older adults, who are usually sensitive to derogatory feelings and attitudes about themselves.

Nurses may also have the feeling that since older adults frequently have chronic illnesses, there is little hope for recovery or improvement; they find working with the older age group discouraging. However, remarkable improvement or recovery may be seen when working with depressed older adults, even though they may also have chronic physical conditions (Cohen 1977; Burnside 1988).

When working with depressed patients, nurses often find themselves feeling depressed. They should analyze the situation objectively and realize that they may be assuming the patient's problem as their own. So, although the nurse should accept the patient and the patient's problem, the nurse must remain a separate individual with thoughts and feelings apart from the patient's.

Encouraging Self-expression of Older Adults. Depressed people need to express feelings that are bothering them. Many patients welcome this opportunity for catharsis. They often have guilt feelings that need to be discussed. They can talk for hours about their "bad" feelings, "bad" thoughts, "bad" actions, or the "bad" things that have happened to them. Others find talking about their inner thoughts and feelings difficult. These people will need encouragement and patience. The nurse must demonstrate a willingness to sit in silence. The nurse will often need to meet with the patient many times before beginning to understand what is happening emotionally to the patient. Through empathy the nurse provides the patient with a beneficial experience. It is therapeutic for a patient to share his or her feelings of despair with someone who is willing to listen. In fact an empathetic listener may be the only help the patient needs.

Increasing Self-esteem. Depressed patients function better if they are given a routine schedule that they are expected to follow. Each day should be filled with activities and tasks to accomplish. Such a structured plan serves two functions. First, it gives the patient something to focus on other than the patient's own life and problems. Second, as tasks are accomplished, self-esteem is improved.

As self-esteem decreases, so does interest in one's physical appearance. A once neat, clean, and tidy person may have dirty hair, show no interest in bathing or changing to clean clothes, and be satisfied to live in an environment of dirt and foul smells. Comments such as "You have on a nice dress today" will reinforce cleanliness. Helping the older woman with makeup may be especially gratifying. As appearance improves, self-esteem will increase and depression will decrease. The reverse is also true. As depression decreases, appearance improves. By stating simply "It's time for your bath now," the nurse will let the patient know what is expected and will discourage the patient from choosing not to bathe.

While providing nursing care, the nurse should be careful to treat the patient with respect; otherwise an attitude of worthlessness and hopelessness may be reinforced. The nurse should be aware of the patient's personal space and respond to the patient as if visiting in a neighbor's home. The nurse should knock before entering the room. The purpose of being there should be explained in sufficient detail. When the nurse leaves, the nurse should avoid appearing rushed or too busy to care for the patient. Since the patient frequently feels exploited by others, he or she may hesitate to trust the nurse. By keeping appointments and treating the patient with respect, the nurse can reduce the patient's suspicion and lack of trust. Patients should be taught to block negative thoughts about themselves by thinking instead of pleasant times and experiences or people and places they like. If the patient is anxious, teaching relaxation techniques may be helpful.

Caring for Physical Problems. The nurse should pay scrupulous attention to the patient's physical condition. Fluid intake and output should be noted as well as what and how much the patient is eating. Steps should be taken to encourage the patient to eat. The nurse will have to observe and talk with the patient to see what works best. Sometimes eating with another patient will help. Sometimes the nurse's presence and verbal encouragement will induce the patient to eat. If the patient consistently refuses to eat, nasogastric intubation with tube feedings should be considered, but all other methods of encouragement should first be attempted.

Depressed patients are frequently constipated, since their whole body, including the gastrointestinal tract, slows down. Balanced diets are not eaten and exercise is avoided. Proper measures should be instituted to deal with this problem. High-bulk foods, sufficient fluids, warm drinks before breakfast, and laxatives as ordered by the physician should be used to avoid this problem. The most successful plan may be to follow the patient's usual routine as practiced at home.

Hypochondriasis. As noted in the discussion of the symptoms of the older person suffering from depression, many have physical complaints. These patients find it difficult to talk about anything but their physical problems. Nurses may think this annoying, especially when it seems as though the physical complaints are being used manipulatively to avoid tasks or uncomfortable situations. Nurses must look at their own feelings, which often include frustration, anger, and hostility. The nurse should determine what the patient's behavior means to him or her. Complaints of physical symptoms are sometimes accompanied by suicidal ideation (Blazer 1989a). By emphasizing—putting oneself in the patient's position as much as possible while maintaining objectivity—the nurse can begin to understand the patient's plight and work with the patient toward resolution of the problems. The nurse must encourage or reassure some patients; they have so little confidence in their own ability to care for themselves, they have learned to manipulate others to do so instead. By learning how they can meet their own needs, such patients may increase their self-satisfaction and decrease their need to manipulate. Some patients may respond best if their manipulative behavior is ignored, although all physical complaints must be investigated and treated appropriately.

Dependency. Depressed patients are often very dependent. By using the emotional tools of sadness or crying, they frequently arouse pity or a motherly desire to make everything all right. The patient may be able to manipulate the nurse who has accepted the mothering role into taking care of needs and problems the patient alone is capable of resolving. However, such successful manipulation can only lower the patient's self-esteem because it causes the patient to feel an increasing dependency. The nurse must look objectively at the care provided for the depressed older adult. In order to make the care most therapeutic for the patient, independence must be encouraged. At the same time, the patient must be allowed to be dependent as needed to reach a state of emotional health that is as good as or better than before the depression occurred.

Regression. As is true of any depressed person, older persons show signs of emotional regression. It is especially important for the nurse not to succumb to the temptation to treat older adults like children. With the already low self-esteem from which the depressed suffer, such treatment confirms their self-diagnosis of worthlessness and helplessness. Unless otherwise requested by the patient, the nurse should address the patient in a manner of respect, using the last name.

Anger and Guilt. Anger is a feeling common to depressed patients. They may be angry at what they perceive as mistreatment by the world or by specific people or groups. They feel powerless to deal with the situation or to gain control over their lives. They may feel let down by significant others who have died, leaving them lonely and with other burdens to bear. The depressed person feels powerless to regain a sense of well-being. Angry feelings may be dissipated by being expressed.

As stated earlier, depressed patients often experience feelings of guilt and remorse. Things done or left undone may haunt older people as they review their lives. The nurse should listen and encourage them to talk about their lives and what bothers them. Providing older people with individual attention will help them have hope that their situations can be improved and that there will again be meaning in their lives.

Suicidal Precautions. Deep feelings of regret and remorse may turn to feelings of despair and then to suicidal thoughts. Since suicide is a major problem in the older age group, the nurse should be aware of the possibility of suicidal behavior by a patient who has been diagnosed as having a terminal or chronic illness or who has suffered any significant loss. A patient may become suicidal around the time of anniversaries and special occasions. Proper precautions must be taken to protect the patient from harming herself or himself. The nurse should acknowledge the patient's feelings of desperation and help him or her work through them in order to preserve the patient's life.

Group Therapy. Groups of various types have been formed to aid the depressed older person. Patients suffering from losses (or adjustment disorders) are treated in short-term, open groups. They learn from observing each other and the therapist how to communicate effectively, share feelings, and cope with crises and stress situations.

Depressed patients in nursing homes or extended care facilities may be grouped together, depending on the patient's ability to respond verbally. Open discussions help alleviate guilt and anger (Butler and Lewis 1982). Reminiscing may be encouraged as a way to help patients discuss their lives and problems (Hamner 1984). The technique of remotivation is often used for the more severely withdrawn. Nurses have more freedom in choosing treatment techniques in these facilities than in most other types of institutions. Nurses are most often the therapists in these groups.

Activity groups are also used. In these groups the interaction is centered around accomplishing a task or playing a group game. Regressed and nonverbal patients may find it easier to participate in these groups than in others.

Medications. Depressed patients frequently receive antidepressant medication therapy. The tricyclic antidepressants are the medications most often used for treating depression in older adults. Smaller than average doses are generally recommended. The physician may order a small dose at first and then increase the dose in accordance with the patient's response. The nurse should be aware that it may take several weeks for the tricyclics to reach a therapeutic blood level. It is particularly important to know if the patient has suicidal thoughts, so that special precautions can be taken to prevent self-harm. The patient who receives amitriptyline (Elavil) may actually feel worse for two to five weeks (Butler and Lewis 1982). This possibility should be explained to the patient; it should be stressed that the period of feeling bad will be temporary. Amitriptyline is a potent cardiotoxic agent, and its use for older adults has been strongly discouraged (Nickens, Crook, and Cohen 1986). Desipramine (Norpramin) and nortriptyline (Pamelor) produce fewer side effects in older adults than do most of the tricyclics. The side effects of tricyclic antidepressants that older adults find particularly irritating are twitching, tremor, ataxia, hypotension, dry mouth and problems with dentures, constipation, and urinary retention. Patient anxiety may be alleviated by the knowledge that the symptoms are drug side effects that should subside. The patient should be cautioned to rise from sitting and lying positions slowly. Hard candy or chewing gum will help allevi-

ate the discomfort of dry mouth. The nurse should question patients about constipation and urinary retention and take measures to prevent both (Gotz and Gotz 1978). The monoamine oxidase inhibitors are generally not recommended for treatment of older adults because of the frequency of side effects (Butler and Lewis 1982). Newer nontricyclic drugs such as amoxapine (Asedin), maprotiline (Ludiomil), and trazodone (Desyrel) are available, but they have side effects that mandate that they be used with caution for older adults (Nickens, Crook, and Cohen 1986).

Lithium carbonate is often the drug used in the treatment of bipolar depression. This drug, if taken as prescribed, is believed to reduce recurring episodes (Mendlewicz 1976). Its side effects include gastrointestinal symptoms such as nausea, vomiting, and abdominal pain; other side effects are thirst, fatigue, tremor, and muscle weakness. The serum lithium level should not exceed 1.5 milliequivalents (mEq) per liter and levels should be checked regularly. Lithium intoxication may lead to death (Spencer et al. 1986).

Electroconvulsive Therapy. Electroconvulsive therapy is used to decrease depression in older adults. The number of treatments should be kept at a minimum (Butler 1982), since older people are more prone to confusion and recover more slowly as the number of treatments is increased. Treatments may be spaced farther apart than the usual three per week. Older patients may receive one per week based on their response and amount of confusion (Kral 1976). The nursing responsibilities for the older person receiving electroconvulsive therapy are the same as for a person of any age. The physician's explanation of the procedure should be reinforced and the value of the treatment explained. The nurse will be responsible for seeing that the patient receives no food or drink from midnight the night before the treatment until after the procedure is completed. It may be the nurse's responsibility to administer pretreatment medication such as a sedative. The nurse or a familiar person should accompany the patient to the treatment room. After the convulsive therapy is completed, the nurse must remain with the patient until the patient has recovered and is fully conscious. The patient must be observed closely for possible respiratory problems (Butler 1982). The nurse will need to take vital signs frequently until they are stable. When the patient has responded fully, the nurse's goal should be reorientation. The nurse should call the patient by name and say that he or she has just received electroconvulsive therapy and that although there may be a feeling of confusion, the patient will regain memory soon. The nurse should inform the patient of the date, the time, and the name of the hospital. Then the nurse should accompany the patient to breakfast and remain to answer questions and provide support.

Nursing Care Plan. A nursing care plan for a depressed patient is shown in Table 10-2. The nursing staff will need to evaluate the care plan and change nursing orders and expected outcomes as new data are obtained through continued assessment. New problems may be identified and old problems may be resolved. The nursing staff should indicate, when charting, the progress made toward resolving problems and the patient's reaction to the care given, new problems identified, and the results of nursing interventions based upon nursing orders as stated in the nursing care plan.

Family Therapy. The patient and family often find discussions among the nurse, patient, and family helpful. To mend relationships between family and patient, an exchange of feelings may be necessary. Unless the nurse has special training in group work or psychiatric nursing, however, a more qualified assistant will be needed, since a group situation may be harmful unless proper support is given and emotions are dealt with constructively. Families often feel overwhelmed when dealing with their older relatives. They feel guilty about taking the older member to a nursing home against the relative's will. On the other hand they realize that it may be dangerous to leave the older people in their homes alone if they are confused and forgetful. Most are not aware of the community resources available to help deal with problems of older adults. So in desperation and with feelings of guilt, they turn to the nursing home for assistance. This plan may be the best choice. If the patient can be maintained at home, however, this solution may be much more satisfying to patient and family than institutionalization.

Once in a nursing home, the patient should be given as much independence and be allowed to make as many decisions as his or her condition allows. Depressed patients have difficulty both in being independent and in making decisions. As they improve, however, these qualities should be encouraged, since both will add to the patient's self-esteem.

Outpatient Care. Many depressed patients can be treated on an outpatient basis. Such patients come to institutions for group or individual therapy, evaluation, and medication. Home visits are used to assess the environment as well as to provide support for the family and patient. A patient may be maintained indefinitely in the home with regular visits from a nurse. Many older people neglect their physical health until a problem becomes significant enough to warrant medical attention. As nurses make home visits, the physical well-being of the patient should be assessed regularly by the nurse. Home health aides are employed to assist the patient in meal planning and preparation, to provide companionship to relieve loneliness and boredom, and to ensure a safer environment for the forgetful.

Referrals. The nurse should recognize personal limits in providing care to the older depressed patient. If it becomes apparent that the patient in any setting is getting increasingly worse, the nurse should ask for assistance from appropriate sources and encourage the patient who is at home to seek help from others.

Prevention of Depression

Since many of the causes of depression in older adults are known, nurses should be able to prevent some problems. Well before such nursing action becomes necessary, as people reach middle age, they should begin to plan for retirement if they have not already done so. Interests other than work should be developed. Employment agencies, mental health centers, and educational systems should provide retirement planning and counseling assistance. Those older adults who want to work should be allowed to do so. More jobs for older citizens are being advertised, and this practice should be encouraged.

Table 10–2 Nursing Care Plan for a Depressed Patient

Data	Nursing Diagnosis	Expected Outcomes	Nursing Orders
Subjective: 9/21 "I hate you! Let me out of here! What does my son know? He knows I shouldn't be here. They just want my home. I don't want anything to eat. I'm not hungry." Objective: 9/21 8:30 A.M.—Began crying as she talked about family leaving her here. 9:45 A.M.—Shouted to nurse to leave her alone. Angry look on face. Subjective: 9/22 "Leave me alone. I don't want to make cookies this morning. I don't feel like it. I just want to stay in my room. I don't feel like getting up." Objective: 9/22 Curled up in bed with covers around shoulders. Not as talkative as in past. Refused breakfast, ate 1/2 serving turnips and 1/2 serving cornbread for dinner. Drank 1/2 carton of milk.	Coping: ineffective, individual anger related to feelings of rejection.	1. Patient will discuss how she came to the nursing home. She will also discuss her thoughts and feelings about her situation in a one-to-one relationship with the nurse and in group discussion by 9/28. 2. She will follow the schedule developed for her by 9/24.	1a. Encourage her to discuss in detail how she came to the nursing home. 1b. Encourage her to state how she feels about being left here. 2. Using an attitude of kind firmness, encourage her to follow this schedule: 7:00 A.M.—Arise, bathe, dress, wash face and hands for breakfast 8:00 A.M.—Eat breakfast in dining room seated with other patients 8:30 A.M.—Back to room to brush teeth, wash face and hands 9:00 A.M.—Exercises in day room (calisthenics) 9:30 A.M.—Free time 10:00 A.M.—Adjunctive therapy—sewing, cooking 11:30 A.M.—Free time, get ready for lunch 12:00 noon—Lunch 12:30 P.M.—Outside activity, walking or gardening *(continued)*

Data	Nursing Diagnosis	Expected Outcomes	Nursing Orders
			2:30 P.M.—Free time
			3:00 P.M.—Group discussion of personal problems led by psychiatric nurse and social worker
			4:00 P.M.—Free time, get ready for supper
			5:00 P.M.—Supper
			5:30 P.M.—Patient government
			6:30 P.M.—Visiting with family and friends or attending programs provided by volunteers (group singing, birthday parties, bingo, movies)
			9:00 P.M.—Preparation for bed
			9:30 P.M.—In bed
		3. She will maintain her weight and will eat a balanced diet by 9/24.	3a. Intake and output
			3b. Encourage fluids—she likes buttermilk and lemonade. Offer these (240ml) or water every two hours.
			3c. Observe what she eats; if she isn't eating, sit with her and encourage her to eat.
			3d. Seat her with other patients for each meal—do not allow her to eat alone.
			3e. Weigh the patient every third day.

By planning with the family for the care of the disabled older adult, much heartache and sorrow may be prevented. Community educational programs provided by health and educational institutions can alert the populace to the need for advanced planning in caring for the older adult. Families and communities should realize how important it is for older people to maintain their independence and be surrounded by a familiar environment. Such a realization will encourage these groups to make decisions that are more palatable for older adults, thus decreasing the incidence of depression. An older person's involvement in voluntary associations, clubs, and senior citizens groups lessens feelings of isolation and loneliness, increases the meaning in life, and gives older persons something to look forward to. These activities also help the older person to maintain positive feelings about self. The older population should be made aware of the availability of crisis intervention services. Most people believe these services are only for the young with specific problems. As stated earlier, however, the older adult has a higher rate of crises than any other age group. A special effort, therefore, should be exerted to reach them.

Helping the older person remain physically well will decrease depression. A thorough health assessment will aid in identifying problems early and preventing further deterioration. Screening programs that are readily accessible to older people can be of great benefit. Patients should know about their medications: what to expect of them and when to seek help.

In summary there are many things the nurse can do as a professional and as a citizen to improve conditions for older adults and thus decrease older people's feelings of depression. The nurse can begin by being aware of the resources and limitations of the community. Gaps in services need to be identified and solutions found. As the number of older adults in America increases, the problem of depression will also increase.

SUICIDE

Suicide is a leading cause of death in older adults. Twenty-five percent of the suicides that occur in the United States yearly are in the 65-and-older group (Richardson, Lowenstein, and Weissberg 1989; Brant and Osgood 1990). The suicide rate for older men is even more dramatic; it reaches a peak among white men who are in their 80s. This group is most vulnerable to suicidal behavior because men of other cultures and women in general experience the loss of power and prestige to a far lesser degree than the aging white man whose employment and financial status are more likely to change rapidly (Butler and Lewis 1982; Gurland 1976). As in the younger population, suicide is lowest among married men and highest among divorced men.

Causes

The reasons for suicide are varied. Some older people see no meaning in life. Many older adults feel there is no longer any reason to live. They may rationalize that since everyone they love has gone, they would rather destroy themselves and, if the concept is part of their religious beliefs, join their loved ones in heaven than live in isolation and loneliness on earth. Others, knowing that they have chronic, incapacitating, or terminal illnesses, prefer to end their lives of suffering. Similarly there are those who, finding that they have a chronic illness, prefer to destroy themselves rather than leave their families penniless. Patients with many physical complaints have a high suicide rate. The physical complaints may conceal severe depression, which may be difficult to identify unless the observer is particularly attuned to suicide problems among older adults (Gurland 1976). Confused, psychotic patients may commit suicide. Some of these patients also suffer from depression. Others seem to kill themselves almost accidentally. For example, they may believe that they have special powers and step in front of oncoming traffic thinking that they can cause it to stop. Another tragic situation can occur when, during lucid moments, confused patients may realize what is happening to them and, feeling useless, worthless, hopeless, and helpless, they decide to terminate their lives.

Common Methods of Committing Suicide

In contrast with younger people who may make several attempts at suicide, perhaps hoping to be discovered each time, most suicides by older people are planned so that the results will be fatal. In the United States, firearms are used most often. Other commonly used methods are drug overdose, hanging, and jumping from high places. Of all the people who attempt suicide, those over 50 are more likely to succeed than younger people, and it is rare that anyone above 65 years of age fails. Conversely, suicide threats by people over 65 are rare; they simply kill themselves (Butler 1982).

Benign or Para Suicide. Not included in the suicide statistics are those who just decide to stop living. They stop eating, withdraw, and give up. Such behavior probably occurs frequently, but accurate statistics are difficult to obtain. Research in this area is urgently needed. Such patients refuse to take medication, to get needed treatment, or to cooperate with prescribed treatment. Slowly but surely they die. Many benign suicides are thought to occur in nursing homes. The life expectancy of patients after they have been admitted to the average nursing home is 1.1 years, with one-third of them dying within the first year and another one-third dying between the first and third years (Butler and Lewis 1982). Some enter the nursing home in fairly good physical condition; but because they perceive their lives as useless, meaningless, and filled with hopelessness, they feel that they have nothing to look forward to and many choose to stop living by refusing to maintain their bodies.

Medical Care for the Suicidal Patient

Medical care for the suicidal patient usually includes antidepressant medications. Also, electroconvulsive therapy has been an effective life-saving device for patients who are determined to destroy themselves. After a few treatments, dramatic improvement may be seen in the patient's will to live. The patient's energy level increases, and facial expressions are less sad and more responsive to others. The nursing responsibility for medication administration as well as for electroconvulsive therapy is the same as that discussed under depression.

Nursing Assessment

The nursing assessment of the suicidal patient consists of a thorough history. The nurse may need to obtain information from relatives. Recent physical or material losses sustained by the client, anniversaries of such losses, and disappointments and changes, such as moving from one's home to the home of a

relative or an institution, should be noted particularly. Also, the nurse should note changes in the client's physical or emotional status. If the possibility of suicide is suspected, the nurse should ask the patient specifically if he or she is contemplating suicide. If so, the nurse should determine if the patient has made specific plans of how and when suicide will be attempted. Significant others associated with the patient should be asked about significant changes that they may have noticed in the patient recently. Evidence of depression, as listed in Table 10-1, should be ascertained.

Nursing Interventions

Patients who live in the community and who threaten suicide should be referred immediately to a facility that provides psychiatric care. Suicidal thoughts, threats, or attempts are emergencies and provisions for proper treatment should be made with expediency and efficiency. A life is in danger, just as in medical emergencies.

Safety Precautions. In an institution, suicidal patients should be afforded every opportunity to express their feelings to an individual therapist as well as in group therapy. Safety precautions should be taken. These precautions include close observation of the patient and perhaps removal of objects that may be used as suicidal implements. Officials in some facilities hesitate to remove personal objects such as razors, thinking that such an action demonstrates to the patient that he or she is considered untrustworthy, thus further decreasing the patient's self-esteem. Others argue that in a suicidal crisis, the patient is not to be trusted and that it is the staff's responsibility to help the patient maintain self-control by removing objects that may be used in self-destruction. Since the older adult commonly uses the surest method, it seems wise to pay close attention to objects that might be used to commit suicide and to keep the patient under close observation as well. However, these measures cannot ensure the safety of the patient. People who are determined to destroy themselves will find a way, such as the woman who dug into her veins with a hair pin and bled to death. Working on the patient's desire to live will have more lasting effects but generally takes time. During that time the patient's safety must be a priority nursing concern.

Since institutionalized older patients are frequently depressed, it is beneficial for them to follow a routine daily schedule of activities. When the patient's mind and hands are kept busy, there will be less time to plan and carry out suicide. This axiom is also true for the patient who has decided to "stop living." The patient who is involved, along with other people, in projects and activities in which tasks are accomplished experiences a greater sense of self-esteem; the person feels needed and useful and may begin to feel that there is a purpose in life.

Special precautions should be taken for patients who have been practically immobilized by depression and who suddenly show improvement; they may have finally formalized a suicide plan and have decided to carry it out. The energy that was being sapped by the inner conflict between living and dying has suddenly been liberated. Now that the conflict is resolved, the energy is available to be used in carrying out the act of suicide.

Providing for Basic Needs. The nursing interventions for patients who are involved in benign suicide will be different than for patients who are more actively intent on destroying themselves. Safety and protection are not the overriding considerations in dealing with benign suicide. The focus must be on the physiologic method the patient has chosen in order to die. If the patient has chosen to stop eating, measures to encourage eating and drinking must be instituted. If these fail, the possibility of feeding by nasogastric intubation must be considered. The patient who has chosen to stop taking medicine must be encouraged to take the medicine. Rewards might be offered, if the nursing staff can discover what kinds of things the patient desires. Close observation, helping the patient follow a schedule, and one-to-one group therapy are all important measures in the care of potential benign-suicide patients as well as those who are more actively suicidal.

Nurses' Attitudes toward Caring for Suicidal Patients. Nurses should investigate their own attitudes when taking care of suicidal patients. Many nurses seem to find it difficult to tolerate patients who are trying to destroy themselves while they (the nurses) are trying so hard to save lives and so many who want to live must die. However, psychologists say that most people have considered suicide at one time or another, and, therefore, if nurses look into themselves deeply enough they may find some common strands upon which empathy can be built. Certainly

patients who are this desperate need much care and understanding.

The nurse should also realize that personal efforts will not always be successful despite the best nursing care. Some patients are determined to die. It is painful for nurses to deal with their own feelings of guilt and anger that are aroused after they have worked intensely with a patient only to see the patient die despite all their efforts. However, nurses must remember their limitations. Certainly, most of the time and emotional energy spent working with suicidal patients brings positive results. Other patients in an institutional setting will ask about patients in their group who have committed suicide. It is generally thought best to discuss the loss in group meetings rather than to try to hide or deny the facts, since such denials lead the patients to mistrust the staff. Because nurses are in a close working relationship with many older people, they should think of ways that will make patients' lives more fulfilling, thus improving the quality of life and decreasing the number of suicides.

Some older people advance this argument: If they are dying of an incurable disease, or if they are mentally incapacitated, why should they not be allowed to end their misery and die with dignity? Why should they be forced into a living death? This thought-provoking question has inspired a great deal of debate, with few, if any, generally acceptable answers.

ORGANIC MENTAL DISORDERS

Dementia

Dementia is a generalized impairment in intellectual functioning that interferes with social and occupational functioning. Deterioration is seen in memory, judgment, and abstract thought. Appointments are missed and the older person gets lost in a new environment. These changes affect the personality so that the person has different characteristics as the condition progresses. Selected premorbid traits become predominant. For example, a person who was suspicious and quick to anger in the past may become hostile and paranoid. Other alterations in the personality may occur. The person who had previously been active and sociable may become withdrawn and apathetic. This condition in advanced stages results in dependence on others for total care and the person becomes oblivious to environmental surroundings (American Psychiatric Association 1987; Butler and Lewis 1982; Linderborn 1988).

Linderborn (1988) stated that between 10 percent and 20 percent of the older adults living in the community have a significant cognitive impairment, compared with an estimated 50–75 percent of institutionalized older people. The likelihood of an individual developing dementia after 80 years of age is 20 percent (Raskind 1989).

A number of causative factors have been identified for dementia. The most common in older adults is primary degenerative dementia, such as Alzheimer's disease (American Psychiatric Association 1987). The second most prevalent cause of dementia in older adults is multi-infarct dementia, a vascular disease that involves multiple occlusions of small cerebral arteries. These two diseases account for 80 percent of the dementias experienced by older adults (Butler and Lewis 1982). Other categories of causes include central nervous system infections, brain trauma, toxic metabolic disturbances, normal pressure hydrocephalus, neurologic diseases, and postanoxic or posthypoglycemic states (American Psychiatric Association 1987; Rabins 1983). Dementia may occur suddenly, as in brain trauma, or it may develop insidiously. Many causes of dementia may be treated, resulting in complete recovery; other types may be kept from progressive deterioration by early, appropriate treatment.

The American Psychiatric Association (1987), in the *Diagnostic and Statistical Manual of Mental Disorders*, third edition revised (*DSM-III-R*), took the position that reversibility of dementia is based on the underlying pathology. Therefore it may be progressive, static, or remitting; it may be reversible or irreversible.

Irreversible forms of dementia include Alzheimer's, Parkinson's, Pick's, and Huntington's diseases. In other dementias the more widespread the structural damage to the brain, the less likely it is that clinical improvement will occur (American Psychiatric Association 1987; Linderborn 1988).

Rabins (1983) stated that up to 33 percent of older adults experiencing cognitive decline may be successfully treated so that symptoms are reversed. Examples of conditions that may be reversed are those caused by toxic substances such as medications, those caused by infections such as meningitis, and those caused by brain trauma such as hematomas. Butler and Lewis (1982) noted that treatment is the only reliable way to determine whether a condition is reversible.

The individual who experiences a demented condition will react based on the specific causes, the basic personality traits, and the environmental support available. Memory loss begins insidiously and may be embarrassing and cause anxiety. The person may confabulate by fabricating forgotten details of events or situations. Other persons may attempt to cope with memory loss by planning and arranging the environment to help them remember. Lists are made and neighbors and relatives assume responsibility for reminding demented older people of important events and times, such as when to take medications and what the dose should be. Feelings of helplessness, hopelessness, and worthlessness are not uncommon. As faculties continue to deteriorate, the person may become depressed and suicidal. Institutionalization often becomes the best choice for providing safety, security, adequate nutrition, and other essentials for life (Butler and Lewis 1982).

Treatment and Nursing Care. Medical treatment for the two major types of dementia found in older adults, primarily degenerative dementia and multi-infarct dementia, is symptomatic since there is presently no known cure for these conditions (National Institute on Aging 1980). However, nursing care cannot be overemphasized. Much can be done by the nursing staff to help prevent further deterioration and to reverse dementias that are treatable.

The primary nursing diagnosis listed by the North American Nursing Diagnosis Association (McLane 1987) that most applies to patients experiencing cognitive impairment is "altered thought processes." Based on individual symptoms and problems, patients may also have diagnoses such as

- Body Image Disturbance
- Self-Esteem Disturbance
- Personal Identity Disturbance
- Sensory-Perceptual Alterations
- Hopelessness
- Powerlessness
- Nutrition, altered

- Constipation

- Diarrhea

- Urinary elimination, altered patterns

- Injury, high risk for

Each nursing diagnosis will be individualized by stating specifically what the diagnosis is related to and what specific evidence supports the diagnosis for a particular patient. For example, a nursing diagnosis for a patient experiencing dementia could be "Thought processes, altered" related to brain injury.

Assessment of the individual with cognitive impairment, including dementia, involves a thorough physical examination, psychosocial assessment, and a mental status test. This assessment is necessary whether the nurse is meeting the patient for the first time in the home or on admission to an institution. Continued assessment is desirable through observation, and updated tests and examinations are indicated to provide optimal care.

Mental status examinations help identify the patient who is at risk of acute confusional states. These tests help determine the degree of cognitive impairment, thus assisting the nurse in developing an individualized plan of care for the patient with dementia (Linderborn 1988; Yazdanfar 1990). Many tools exist, each with its own advantages and disadvantages. Some take a long time to complete and are not suitable for the patient with a limited attention span. The mental status examination is just one part of assessment. See chapters 6 and 7 for a more detailed overview of assessment.

A thorough social, medical, and psychiatric history from the family and significant others can provide valuable information that may help determine the cause of the dementia and may help differentiate it from depression. A depressed older person might appear demented. It is particularly helpful to have the family list the prescribed as well as the over-the-counter drugs that the patient is taking. Medications can cause or exacerbate cognitive impairment (Rabins 1983). Also, the amount of cognitive decline may be estimated through description of the patient's past functioning, including the work and social histories. The person who has made contributions to the family and community through work and social involvement and who is now unable to carry on a conversation most likely has significant cognitive

impairment. A thorough assessment is necessary to help determine the care that is needed.

The plan of care is based on the degree of cognitive impairment as indicated by the mental status exam, the history, and the observed symptoms or problems (Burnside 1979; Johnson and Keller 1989). The American Psychiatric Association (1987) lists three levels of severity for dementia and describes the characteristics of each.

The first level is mild severity. The person in this stage is able to live independently even though work and social activities are significantly impaired. The person is forgetful and anxiety may be increased due to the recognition that the mind does not function as it once did. The family needs to be aware of the potential for deterioration; frequent checks on the functioning and well-being of the person are necessary.

The second level is moderate severity. The person in this stage can no longer live independently without supervision. Although the patient can be managed in the home with adequate support, institutionalization may be necessary. Major concerns of the nurse for patients at this level include safety, nutrition, fluid intake, exercise, orientation, and maintaining self-esteem. Patients in this stage may function adequately in an open unit with other patients.

The third and last level is severe. Total patient care may be necessary as the disease progresses. The person is unable to take care of personal needs for hygiene, elimination, nutrition, fluids, or exercise. Communication becomes progressively more difficult and the person eventually becomes incoherent and mute (American Psychiatric Association 1987). These patients are often better served on a closed unit that is designed especially for demented or Alzheimer's patients (McCracken and Fitzwater 1989).

A major focus for nursing care of the patient with dementia is providing a safe environment. Memory impairment, a criterion of the diagnosis of dementia, causes disorientation. The disorientation that occurs may be progressive so that the person experiences confusion related to time. As the disease continues, orientation related to place and person becomes problematic. It may be difficult to get the patient to go to bed at bedtime or there may be a problem with the person getting up in the middle of the night thinking that it is time to go to work. The person often lives in the past and tries to maintain the schedule of years past when there was a family to support. The demented person may wander from the present place of residence looking for the home or workplace of years ago. Close friends and relatives may be mistaken for others or strangers. For example, an older man with dementia told his wife she had better leave their house because it was almost dark and he did not know what the neighbors would think if she, a stranger, stayed late. A stable staff and a routine schedule are helpful when caring for disoriented patients.

As dementia increases, the ability of the patient to communicate decreases. The patient and the nurse may become frustrated as a result. The nurse should avoid open-ended questions, speak slowly, avoid giving a lot of new information in a short period of time, and use words and sentences that may be more easily understood (Lee 1991).

Since the demented person is often psychologically living in a different world, in a different time and place, there is a periodic or constant search by the person for the reality that exists in the mind. Therefore wandering, pacing, agitation, and increased anxiety may occur. It is imperative that buildings be secured so that patients cannot wander outside without being noticed. Halls and rooms should have sufficient light at all times so that the person getting up at night can see to walk without falling over items. Unnecessary furniture and equipment should be removed from the living area; equipment should be locked in a secure place. In some instances it may be better for the patient to eat alone or with one or two other persons. Stimulation, without a purpose, should be minimal to prevent increased agitation. At the same time, sensory deprivation must be avoided since this can be causally related to dementia. Thus activities should be individually planned to meet the patient's needs. Walking, touching, listening to quiet music, and eating favorite foods can reduce agitation (Struble and Sivertsen 1987). In addition, distraction, praise, eye contact, and a light-hearted approach are effective when providing care for an upset patient (Burgener and Barton 1991). Mayers and Griffin (1990) described a stimulus play project in which agitated Alzheimer's patients were given toys for designated periods of time. The patients demonstrated interest in the toys and seemed to particularly like the mechanical toys with knobs and dials that could be manipulated. Soft toys were stroked and cuddled. Care must be given so that the patient is not demeaned or belittled in any way when using toys to decrease agitation and increase stimulation.

Pets also have been found to decrease agitation and increase stimulation in some demented patients. In some nursing homes, pets are permanent residents with the patients providing care. In others, pets are brought in by volunteers to visit those residents for whom it has been predetermined that pets will offer benefit (Gammonley and Yates 1991).

Confronting the patient with symptoms or deficits increases anxiety, decreases self-esteem, and may initiate development of other maladaptive behaviors. Increasing the patient's insight into disease etiology, symptoms, or prognosis is not desirable with irreversible dementia.

It is important to maintain or increase self-esteem of the older person with dementia. Self-confidence is often diminished, and the person experiences feelings of failure, shame, and humiliation. Independence, decision-making, and self-care should be encouraged if the person can safely manage these behaviors. Verbal suggestions and encouraging remarks increase self-care. Discussing the past, looking at old family pictures, and group therapy with various foci, such as reminiscing or remotivation, may help the person concentrate on a time when life was good and productive and the patient was important and useful. Therapy may also need to focus on finding meaning in the present if the person is intellectually capable.

Reality orientation may be a helpful tool when assisting the disoriented person maintain orientation to time, place, and person. Reminders of the date, the time, and the place may be posted in conspicuous places. Name tags should be worn by personnel. Personnel should state their names and the patient's name often to help the disoriented person remember their own names and the names of others.

Reality-orientation group meetings may be held for thirty minutes several days a week at the same time and place. The instructor assists the group members in discussing simple, concrete objects or ideas that will help patients concentrate on reality. Examples of topics for discussion include flowers, food, pets, trees, and pictures. Each session begins with members stating their names.

Other types of therapeutic groups may be beneficial for the patient who has dementia. Abramson and Mendis (1990) stated that patients should be evaluated and placed in groups with similar abilities. The goals of the sessions should be commensurate with the patients' abilities. The group experience should be positive for the members.

Remotivation groups follow a schedule so that the patient and staff anticipate the meeting. Small groups meet with a leader for about thirty minutes to one hour several times a week. The members are encouraged to become acquainted with each other, to share past experiences and interests, and to participate fully in the group discussions. Topics for discussion vary considerably, and occasionally visual aids are used. The daily newspaper is a good source of reality in the environment; or travel films may be borrowed from a local library or university. The use of all the senses is encouraged. For example, objects such as unusual sea shells and rose petals may be brought in for the group members to touch, or they may be given wild flowers to smell. The leader should focus the sessions on interesting and pleasant discussions rather than on the physical and/or psychological problems of the patients.

After using reality orientation for several years with "severely disoriented old-old people," Feil (1982) found that it was unrealistic to help these people return to reality. Instead, she developed *validation therapy*, with the primary goal of accepting the disoriented old where they are and helping them reach *their* goals instead of the goals of others. Validation therapy "means accepting the disoriented old-old adult who lives in the past" (Feil 1982). Warm, supportive, understanding, accepting, and empathic communication is an important part of validation therapy. Allowing the disoriented old-old to live in the past, to be comfortable in their fantasy, and to escape from the realities of the often painful and stressful present helps them survive.

Nurses may want to modify patient behavior when it is problematic or maladaptive. The specific maladaptive behavior must be identified. Rather than identifying combative behavior, which does not describe a specific activity, it is better to state "hits caregiver when not allowed to leave the building." After the behavior has been identified, the caregivers should observe the patient for a designated amount of time to determine when and how often the behavior

occurs. In addition the consequences of the behavior are noted. The observers attempt to determine what rewards the patient is receiving from the maladaptive or problematic behavior. Plans are made to withdraw rewards for the problem behaviors and to reward adaptive behaviors. The caregivers must identify appropriate rewards that will be effective for the identified present. All caregivers should participate in planning and implementing the behavior modification program and relate to the patient in a consistent manner.

Some types of dementia may result in the patient becoming incontinent. Many products and techniques are available to deal with incontinence. The caregiver assisting the patient with this problem should make every effort to maintain the dignity of the patient. Privacy and frequent care are necessities (Butler and Lewis 1982).

It is usually the family of the patient with dementia who brings the person to the health care facility for diagnosis and treatment. The patient often is not capable of initiating entrance into the health care delivery system. The family should be made a part of the planning and caring team from the beginning, based on their ability and interest (Riefler and Larson 1985). They should be informed of the cause and prognosis of the patient's condition as they are able to tolerate such information. The nurse should be careful not to overwhelm the family with too much negative information all at once. Group sessions in which topics related to dementia are discussed over a period of time and with the support of other members can be advantageous.

Families sometimes feel guilty because they are unable to maintain the older person at home, but they can find support in groups where other families have had to make similar decisions and have worked through their feelings. The nurse should praise the family members for the care that they have provided for the patient. Encouraging their participation in continued care of the patient also reduces the guilt feelings. Many self-help groups have been organized in communities across the nation to assist families in dealing with family members who have dementia, especially those who have Alzheimer's disease.

Since depressed older people may exhibit symptoms such as disorientation and memory loss and may complain of difficulty in thinking and concentrating, it is not uncommon for the caregiver to assume that the problem is dementia (deterioration

Table 10–3　Factors that Help Distinguish Depression from Dementia

Major Depression	*Dementia*
Disturbance of mood.	Disturbance of intellect.
Patient complains of memory impairment, difficulty thinking, difficulty concentrating, reduction of intellectual abilities.	Patient may complain of cognitive impairment or ignore symptoms of decreased ability to function intellectually. The patient may attempt to cover up symptoms, especially as the condition progresses.
Poor performance on mental status examinations due to affective disturbance. If motivated to perform, can do so with a degree of success.	Poor performance on mental status examinations due to intellectual deficit. No amount of motivation can significantly improve performance.
Past performance on mental status examinations may be variable.	Past performance on mental status examinations demonstrates increasingly poor performance.
Clinical history indicates approximate date of onset of problem with symptoms progressing comparatively rapidly.	Clinical history indicates an insidious onset with symptoms becoming gradually worse.
May have history of previous mood disturbance.	

of intellectual capacity) rather than depression. When depression masks as dementia, it is known as pseudodementia (American Psychiatric Association 1987). Table 10-3 lists factors that help distinguish major depression from dementia. A thorough history from relatives, friends, and the older person can be invaluable in making the final diagnosis. It is not unusual for the person experiencing depression to have a history of depressive episodes.

If in doubt about whether an older person should be considered depressed or demented because of symptoms of poor intellectual functioning, the person should be treated for depression since the person, the family, and the caregiver will respond differently based on the prognosis of the two. The older person with depression can recover completely, especially if treated by a professional person. The person accurately diagnosed as having dementia may continue to deteriorate. With depression, the intellectual functioning will improve as the depression lifts.

Delirium

Delirium is an organic mental disorder that is most often defined as a clouded state of consciousness or an acute confusional or stuporous state. In contrast, the person suffering from dementia has a clear con-

sciousness. The American Psychiatric Association (1987) indicates that other characteristics of delirium may include incoherent speech; perceptual disturbances, such as illusions or hallucinations; increased or decreased psychomotor activity, disorientation; and disturbance in the sleep cycle. A patient history often reveals a specific organic cause for the delirium. Causes for delirium include alcoholic intoxication, systemic infections, withdrawal from drugs, side effects of medication, electrolyte imbalance, and postoperative states (American Psychiatric Association 1987; Butler and Lewis 1982; National Institute on Aging 1980).

The onset of delirium is rapid and duration is short as compared with dementia. However, delirium that results from a metabolic imbalance may develop over a period of time. The older person is more susceptible to delirium than the young adult or the middle-aged individual. This is especially true for the aged person who has experienced delirium earlier in life (American Psychiatric Association 1987; Rabins 1983; Butler and Lewis 1982).

Other differences between delirium and dementia exist. Symptoms observed in the patient with delirium fluctuate in a twenty-four-hour period. They may become more acute or they may subside. For example, the person with delirium may hallucinate more actively, perspire more, become more agitated, and appear more frightened at 10:00 p.m. than at 7:00 p.m. Whereas the person with dementia will remain approximately the same in a twenty-four-hour period. Delirium is usually reversible, while dementia is usually not. Dementia is chronic and usually irreversible (Gomez and Gomez 1989).

Treatment and Nursing Care. As with dementia it is very important for the nurse to obtain an accurate history from significant others. The delirious patient is usually unable to provide a history. A detailed history will help determine cause, time of onset, and appropriate treatment. Early diagnosis and treatment are especially important. In one study 50 percent of the patients who had untreated delirium died (Butler and Lewis 1982). Delirium should be treated as an emergency, and more accurate treatment can be initiated when the cause is known. When there is doubt about whether the person is experiencing delirium or dementia, the treatment should be for delirium (American Psychiatric Association 1987). Table 10-4 lists factors that help distinguish delirium from dementia.

Fluid and nutritional requirements when caring for the delirious patient must be met. Tranquilizers may be ordered to reduce agitation or restlessness. A behavioral medication assessment, as illustrated in Figure 10-1, is necessary since medications may cause paradoxical or other ill effects in the older adult. Noting the effect of medications administered cannot be overemphasized in the care of the delirious patient.

Table 10–4 Factors that Help Distinguish Delirium from Dementia

Dementia	*Delirium*
Hallucinations are associated with memory impairment.	Hallucinations are associated with inability to maintain or shift attention to external stimuli.
Person is alert.	Reduced level of consciousness.
Clinical picture usually develops over a long period of time, except in the case of an accident.	Symptoms develop over a short period of time.
Etiology often not known.	Specific causative factors can often be identified.
Irreversible except in cases such as hypothyroidism, subdural hematoma, normal-pressure hydrocephalus, and tertiary neurosyphilis.	Reversible except when it progresses to dementia.
Symptoms are usually stable.	Symptoms fluctuate, usually clearing in hours or days.

Adapted from the American Psychiatric Association. 1987. *Diagnostic and Statistical Manual of Mental Disorders*. 3d ed. revised. Washington DC: American Psychiatric Association.

Date	Behavior Observed	Medication Administered	Dosage & Route Administered	Time Administered	Effect Observed	Time of Observation	Nurse Initials
Example 2/15	Agitation—pacing	Lorazepam	1 mg orally	9:15 A.M.	2, 4	10:45 A.M.	B.R.

Directions:

Describe the problem behavior in a word or a phrase. List the medication given, the dosage, the route, and time of administration. Using the descriptors below, write the corresponding number of the descriptor in the column titled "Effect Observed." The nurse giving the medication should initial the record.

Effect Observed:

1. Incidence of observed behavior within a given time (one hour) decreased.

2. Incidence of observed behavior within a given time (one hour) increased.

3. Patient oversedated (drowsy, sleeping, reaction time slowed, etc.).

4. Patient more agitated.

5. Side effects detract from the effectiveness of the drug.

6. No noticeable effect.

7. Other—describe briefly.

Figure 10–1 Behavior medication assessment

The environment should be safe with adequate lighting to avoid the possibility of misinterpretation (illusions). Shadows can be frightening. Only the bare essentials should be kept in the patient's room to reduce the risk of injury to self or others. The delirious patient who mistakes the nurse for someone who may cause harm may attempt self-defense by throwing loose objects, such as soap dishes; therefore it is best to remove those items from the room. The room should be quiet with little stimulation since noises, strange lights, and people cause fear and agitation.

Familiar surroundings and caregivers help to decrease stimulation and increase comfort and trust. The person with delirium should be maintained in the same room with the same people providing the care whenever possible.

Verbal communication should be concise and simply stated. Long statements and complicated directions are confusing to the patient who cannot think correctly.

SCHIZOPHRENIC DISORDERS

Other psychiatric disorders besides depression and dementia are a problem for older adults. According to a study done by Pfeiffer and Busse (1973), 18–25 percent of the older age group have major psychiatric syndromes. Four to 8 percent of this group have psychoses; 5 percent have senile, arteriosclerotic, or other organic syndromes; and 2.4 percent have major functional psychoses. Neuroses afflict 8.9 percent of older adults, while 3.6 percent have character disorders (Pfeiffer and Busse 1973). Blazer (1989a) stated that the prevalence of schizophrenia decreases in the older population.

Symptoms of mental disorders may be overlooked since many people assume that they are a part of growing old. The symptoms of mental illness in older adults are the same as for younger individuals. Society at times blames the symptoms on eccentricity and "senility," so that the ill older person may be ignored. Problems that could be helped are pushed aside and older adults are left to suffer alone.

Paranoid Schizophrenia

Emotional problems that were controlled in earlier years become exaggerated as crises increase in frequency and methods of coping decrease. People who,

when they were younger, had a tendency toward suspicion and lack of trust often become paranoid. There may be rational basis for their suspicion, since many factors in society do work against the older person. Older people experience delusions of persecution, delusions to cover feelings of inadequacy, and hallucinations. However, many older people who were once diagnosed as paranoid schizophrenic are no longer as adamant about the reality of their delusions as they were; their hallucinations may become less frequent (Verwoerdt 1976); some become calmer even though they are being maintained on the same amount and kind of medications as earlier in their lives. *Paraphrenia* is a term that is sometimes used in geriatric psychiatry, especially in Europe. It is used to describe the patient who experiences late-life onset of schizophrenic symptoms, usually with paranoid characteristics (Butler and Lewis 1982; Nickens, Crook, and Cohen 1986).

Since symptoms and anxiety become more acute when an emotionally ill person is threatened, the nurse should intervene to reduce the anxiety and keep it at a minimum. Changes in living arrangements, such as a new roommate or a move to a different part of a building, tend to increase anxiety in such a person. It is important to establish trust in any relationship, but it is vital with a paranoid person who has trusted few, if any, people throughout life. The nurse must keep promises, be completely honest, and show respect. The nurse should be on time and avoid violating confidences.

The daily schedules of an emotionally disturbed person should reflect routine and sameness. The patient should be allowed to choose whether to have new experiences. These patients usually choose to remain somewhat distant in their relationships with others. The nurse should respect this preference and allow the patient to make the overtures in their relationship and avoid pressuring the client to interact. The nurse might say, "Let me know if you need anything or if you want to talk. I'll be at the nurses' station for awhile. Come and get me if you like." That way, the choice of interaction is left to the patient, creating less threat.

The aging person has fewer and fewer significant others because people die or move away. Therefore, the number of people available for help and comfort decreases. Paranoid patients in the community need special help, since they are hesitant to make new friends and, in fact, generally discourage overtures made by others. The visiting nurse should maintain frequent contact without threatening the patient by trying to get too close.

Many older patients with paranoid characteristics are maintained as outpatients with medication. They must return to clinics periodically for re-evaluation. The follow-up procedures give the nurse an opportunity to assess the patient's coping abilities and to note any changes. If coping seems adequate, the nurse should refer the patient to appropriate resources.

Catatonic Schizophrenia

An older woman came to an acute psychiatric center. She would lie very still in her bed, and nothing about her body seemed to move except her angry eyes. She would slowly get out of bed only after strong encouragement and assistance and then sit almost motionless in the day room in the midst of constant activity. She was diagnosed as suffering from catatonic schizophrenia. The nursing care that helped this woman included sitting near but not too close to her, calling her by name, speaking to her as if the nurse expected her to respond, and maintaining her on a nondemanding schedule in which she was not allowed to withdraw to her bed. Each morning she was awakened, assisted with bath and dressing, and then taken to breakfast. She was placed in groups that required little interaction for her, similar to remotivation groups. She was allowed to spend time sitting in the day room but not in her room alone. At first she responded only with angry one-word answers or requests. She received medication and, as time passed, she became less angry and responded more spontaneously. Later she was discharged, much improved. Patients as acutely ill as this woman are difficult to manage in the community, since their families have difficulty taking care of them. Once discharged, however, this woman could be maintained indefinitely on medication in her home with periodic visits to clinics for re-evaluation.

Many schizophrenic patients face problems when they are discharged; they stop taking their medication, and do not keep clinic appointments. A visiting nurse who begins follow-up soon after the patient's discharge can often identify such problems and encourage the family and patient to continue the plan of care in the home. Visiting nurses can be an important link in maintaining the person with schizophrenia in the home with less cost and usually more satisfaction to the patient than hospitalization.

Undifferentiated Schizophrenia

Many older schizophrenics do not have clearly defined specific symptoms. Rather, they exhibit a flat affect, they relate poorly with others, get little joy or reward from living, and have a rigid, guarded appearance. Most have been functioning in what society considers a less-than-acceptable manner for years. These patients are often diagnosed as chronic undifferentiated schizophrenics. In an institution, nursing care for these people includes establishing rapport, giving the patient as much responsibility as possible for his or her own care, and involving the patient in a routine schedule of activities. Jobs involving routine tasks with some type of reward may be undertaken successfully by many patients with this diagnosis. In the community such schizophrenics may be maintained in semiprotected settings such as halfway houses, day-care centers, or apartment houses in which there is some supervision.

Treatment and Nursing Care

Medical treatment for psychoses often includes an antipsychotic medication such as a phenothiazine or haloperidol (Haldol). Haloperidol has been found to be relatively safe for use in older adults (Nickens, Crook, and Cohen 1986). As with other drugs antipsychotics must be used cautiously with older adults. Side effects occur more often and tend to be more dramatic among older people. Hypotension can be a threat to the patient's safety. The patient should be warned and encouraged to rise slowly from sitting and lying positions. After receiving parenteral doses, the patient should be instructed to lie down for an hour. Constipation may be a problem. Other observed side effects are extrapyramidal effects such as muscle rigidity, shuffling gait, tremors, and dyskinesias. When first receiving the drug, the patient may also complain of dry mouth. The older person should receive a smaller dose of phenothiazines than the average adult. Nursing responsibilities include observing for side effects, reporting the side effects to the physician, taking such safety precautions as staying with the patient when he or she rises from a sitting or lying position, and providing chewing gum, drinks, or hard candy to help deal with dry mouth (Gotz and Gotz 1978). Older patients should also be warned against taking central nervous system depressants (including alcohol) along with the major tranquilizers. Roughage in the diet, adequate fluid intake, and a regular daily routine will help with problems of constipation.

Older patients receiving neuroleptics are at risk for developing tardive dyskinesia. Symptoms of tardive dyskinesia include primary involuntary facial movements but may also include movements of the extremities and the trunk. The patient may exhibit buccal, masticatory, sucking, smacking, lateral jaw movements, and tongue thrusting. Tardive dyskinesia may be first manifested upon withdrawal of a neuroleptic. The symptoms may subside after several months; however, in some cases they are irreversible.

No effective treatment has been found for tardive dyskinesia. It is best not to administer neuroleptics unless they are necessary and no better alternative can be found to deal with the presenting problem. If the patient must take neuroleptics, they should be discontinued as soon as possible. Tardive dyskinesia is less likely to occur with short-term use (Gierl, Dysken, Davis, and Lesser 1987; Christison, Christison, and Blazer 1989).

SUBSTANCE ABUSE DISORDERS

Substance abuse is most commonly associated with young and perhaps middle-aged people. However, older adults too frequently have problems with drugs. Many substances such as alcohol, caffeine-containing drinks, and nicotine products are used for relaxation and to satisfy physiologic dependence. Some drugs are prescribed and have been for years; others are over-the-counter drugs that may be more "psychologically" addicting than the prescribed drugs. Many over-the-counter drugs contain substances such as alcohol that may be habit forming. Often the older adult is addicted to several substances. Older people should be educated about drugs through such agencies as churches, senior centers, or the media.

Alcoholism

There is disagreement about alcoholism being a common problem among the older population. Krach (1990) stated that it is and yet only 15 percent of older alcoholics are receiving treatment. Lasker (1986) stated that alcohol consumption increases after the age of 50. Older drinkers are more likely to drink daily and to remain socially isolated (Krach 1990). Nurses should be aware that their older clients could be using alcohol to cope with depression, loneliness, and other problems. Nurses working in general hospitals often see patients who are admitted for a medical or surgical problem and soon show signs of delirium tremens. An example of this situation is a 74-year-old woman who was admitted to a medical unit of a general hospital because of an edematous abdomen. After several days of tests, her nurses observed that she could hardly hold her coffee cup because her hands shook so badly. They also noted that she became confused more often as time went on. Her nurses discovered in talks with her that the patient normally drank alcohol in one form or another with meals, between meals, and often before going to bed at night to help her sleep. When this information was conveyed to her physician, the patient was given chlordiazepoxide hydrochloride (Librium) to help calm her.

A 78-year-old man was admitted to an orthopedic unit because of a broken hip. After returning from surgery, he became restless and attempted to remove himself from his traction. During a lucid moment he told his nurse that if she would get him a "shot of whiskey," he would be all right. The nurse shared this information with the physician, who ordered that the older patient be given a certain amount of whiskey routinely. The patient became much easier to care for after the whiskey routine began.

These are examples of a common problem—alcoholism—in the older age group. Older adults drink for many reasons: grief, loneliness, hopelessness, and depression. Being inebriated helps one forget, if only temporarily, problems and conditions that seem overwhelming (Butler and Lewis 1982).

An important complication in older alcoholics is cirrhosis of the liver, which is one of the leading causes of death in the United States (Blazer 1989b). A relationship also seems to exist between alcoholism and esophageal carcinoma in older adults (Kart et al. 1978).

Delirium Tremens

The treatment for older alcoholics should be both psychologic and physical. Physically, the nurse must be aware of the signs and symptoms of delirium tremens. Within two to four days after withdrawal from a routine intake of alcohol, symptoms such as tremors, confusion, fearfulness, increased temperature with diaphoresis, illusions, and hallucinations may occur. These symptoms last from two to three days but may be reduced with medication such as chlordiazepoxide. Delirium tremens should not be ignored, since there is a 5 percent mortality rate among treated cases and a 15 percent mortality rate among untreated cases (Zamoa 1978; Burkhalter 1975). The physician frequently orders an increase in fluid intake to replace lost electrolytes or to correct dehydration. Many patients with delirium tremens are malnourished. Vitamins and minerals, as well as a diet high in protein, high in carbohydrates, and low in fat, are usually ordered. Since some patients are prone to seizures, precautions to protect the patient are necessary. The environment should be safe; there should be no objects close at hand with which the patient may harm himself or herself should a seizure occur. If the patient is ambulatory, close observation should be maintained. A padded tongue blade should be kept within easy reach. Anticonvulsant medication may be ordered. Patients who are not given antianxiety medications may be extremely fearful. In fact they may appear terrified. A quiet environment with few external stimuli should be provided.

Nursing Care

An evaluation of alcohol consumption can help detect potential and current problems. Having the older person describe the amount and type of beverage consumed daily will give clues about possible alcoholism (Lasker 1986). Also, a thorough history and physical are important. Self-neglect, confusion, and repeated falls are clues that substance abuse may be a problem.

Treatment for the older alcoholic is the same as for a younger person. Before treatment can be satisfactory, the alcoholic must want help and be prepared to change life patterns. At first the alcoholic may try to hide the problem of alcohol addiction, but with help from significant others, the client may be motivated to seek assistance in breaking the habit.

The nurse should inquire about employment, social, and health histories in order to assess the possibility of substance abuse. Habitual absence from work, frequent job changes, several marriages, and a history of physical problems may indicate that alcoholism must be considered when planning care. Once it has been established that the older person has a problem with substance abuse, questions should be asked about amounts or dosage, names and types of substances, time of day usually consumed, and perceptions of the effects on daily life. The nurse should discuss negative effects of drug interactions between the abused substance and prescribed or over-the-counter drugs.

In working with the alcoholic, the nurse must have a nonjudgmental attitude and a respect for the person and must make an attempt to understand the person's problems. A consistent approach by the staff, using a matter-of-fact attitude and limit setting, will discourage the manipulative behavior that is often a characteristic of the alcoholic. This program should increase the alcoholic's trust of the staff and may avoid much of the disappointment and frustration staff members often feel when dealing with the manipulative alcoholic.

The patient should be encouraged to participate in a program of planned activities. As improvement becomes apparent, the patient should be given increased responsibility for managing personal affairs and belongings.

The alcoholic who returns to the community should be encouraged to join such groups as Alcoholics Anonymous for support. Other resources such as halfway houses and day hospitals may also be available. The family may need special assistance. The nurse can offer support by listening and by appropriate referrals for family therapy or for financial help.

SUMMARY

Mental disorders that older adults may experience include depression, organic mental disorders, schizophrenia, and substance abuse disorders. As spouses, friends, and relatives die, chances for intimacy and significant interaction are limited. Lack of human contact may lead to loneliness, depression, and other problems. Nurses can make a difference by establishing a meaningful relationship and by assisting in the use of community resources.

Depression occurs frequently as a separate specific condition but also occurs in conjunction with other problems. It is difficult to differentiate depression from some other diagnoses, such as those occurring with organic mental disorders. Neither depression nor organic mental disorders necessarily accompany old age. Both can be treated with positive outcomes. Attitudes of caregivers, persistence, and patience of those working with older adults are required for lasting improvements to be seen. The determined nurse can develop interventions and special programs that will benefit older clients who have depression and organic mental disorders.

Schizophrenia may be seen in more concentrated numbers in institutions, such as state mental hospitals, than in the general public. Patients with schizophrenia present behaviors such as paranoias, withdrawal, manipulation, and hostility. Individualized nursing care plans must be developed for each patient so that interventions are consistent, evaluated, and revised as needed.

Suicide, although frequently a result of depression, may occur with other types of diagnoses or with persons who have not been labeled as being ill. Self-destruction is a significant problem for persons over 65 years of age, especially men. Nurses caring for patients in the community or in institutions should be constantly alert to clues for suicidal ideation and behaviors. Patients who are suspected of being suicidal should be assessed for the possibility of suicide and should be asked specifically if suicide is being contemplated. Appropriate interventions and referrals are crucial.

As the number of older people in society increases, it becomes imperative to find and implement ways of making this developmental stage more satisfying so that emotional problems may be avoided or prompt and efficient treatment provided. The older adult represents a vast untapped resource. Putting this resource to use would benefit society as well as older adults. By letting them be useful, society can give meaning to their lives and decrease their chances of experiencing depression or other emotional and mental problems. Nurses can work in society to change attitudes through teaching and example. By providing the best care possible for older adults, nurses can help return them to a productive and meaningful life or allow them a dignified death.

STUDY QUESTIONS

1. Evaluate the effect that loneliness has on the physical and mental well-being of an older person.

2. Discuss nursing interventions to help the older person deal with loneliness in a health care facility or in his or her own home.

3. How are culture and depression related?

4. How are crises and depression related for older adults?

5. Discuss examples of problems of the depressed older patient and identify specific nursing interventions for those problems.

6. What percentage of the suicides that occur in the United States yearly are in the 65-and-older age group?

7. Differentiate between the symptoms of delirium and dementia.

8. Explore nursing interventions for the wandering person who has dementia.

9. Describe nursing care for the older person with paranoid behavior.

10. Describe extrapyramidal effects the nurse should anticipate when the patient is receiving antipsychotic medications.

REFERENCES

Abramson, T. and K. Mendis. 1990. The organizational logistics of running a dementia group in a skilled nursing facility. In *Mental Health in the Nursing Home*, edited by T.L. Brink. New York: The Haworth Press.

American Psychiatric Association. 1987. *Diagnostic and Statistical Manual of Mental Disorders*. 3d ed., revised. Washington, DC: American Psychiatric Association.

Blazer, D. 1989a. Affective disorders in late life. In *Geriatric Psychiatry*, edited by E.W. Busse and D.G. Blazer. Washington, DC: American Psychiatric Press, Inc.

Balzer, D. 1989b. Alcohol and drug problems in the

elderly. In *Geriatric Psychiatry*, edited by E.W. Busse and D.G. Blazer. Washington, DC: American Psychiatric Press, Inc.

Brant, B. and N. Osgood. 1990. The suicidal patient in long-term care institutions. *Journal of Gerontological Nursing* 16(2):15–18.

Buckwalter, K. 1990. How to unmask depression. *Geriatric Nursing* 11(4):179–81.

Burgener, S.C. and D. Barton. 1991. Nursing care of cognitively impaired, institutionalized elderly. *Journal of Gerontological Nursing* 17(4):37–43.

Burkhalter, P.K. 1975. *Nursing Care of the Alcoholic and Drug Abuser*. New York: McGraw-Hill.

Burnside, I.M. 1979. Alzheimer's disease: An overview. *Journal of Gerontological Nursing* 5(4):14–20.

Burnside, I.M. 1988. *Nursing and the Aged*. 3d ed. New York: McGraw-Hill.

Butler, R. and M. Lewis. 1982. *Aging and Mental Health: Positive Psychosocial and Biomedical Approaches*. 3d ed. St. Louis: C.V. Mosby.

Cadoret, R.J. and R.B. Widmer. 1988. The development of depressive symptoms in elderly following onset of severe physical illness. *Journal of Family Practice* 27(1):71–6.

Christison, C., G. Christison, and D. Blazer. 1989. Late-life schizophrenia and paranoid disorders. In *Geriatric Psychiatry*, edited by E.W. Busse and D.G. Blazer. Washington, DC: American Psychiatric Press, Inc.

Cohen, G.D. 1977. Approach to the geriatric patient. *Med Clin Nort Am* 61(4):855–66.

Feil, N. 1982. *Validation*. Cleveland, OH: Edward Feil Productions.

Fry, P.S. 1986. *Depression, Stress, and Adaptations in the Elderly: Psychological Assessment and Intervention*. Rockville, MD: Aspen Publishers.

Gammonly, J. and J. Yates. 1991. Pet projects: Animal assisted therapy in nursing homes. *Journal of Gerontological Nursing* 17(1):12–15.

Gierl, B., M. Dysken, J. Davis, and J. Lesser. 1987. Neuroleptic use in the elderly. In *Schizophrenia and Aging*, edited by N.E. Miller and G.D. Cohen. New York: the Guilford Press.

Gomez, G. and E. Gomez. 1989. Dementia? Or delirium? *Geriatric Nursing* (May/June):141–42.

Gotz, B., and V. Gotz. 1978. Drugs and the elderly. *Am J Nurs* 78(8):1347–51.

Gurland, B.J. 1976. The comparative frequency of depression in various adult age groups. *J Gerontol* 31(3):283–92.

Gurland, B.J. 1982. Depression in the elderly: A review of recently published studies. In *Annual Review of Gerontology and Geriatrics*, edited by C. Eisdorfer. New York: Springer.

Hamner, M.L. 1984. Insight, reminiscence, denial, projection: Coping mechanisms of the aged. *Journal of Gerontological Nursing* 10(2):66–68, 81.

Holmes, T.H. and R.H. Rahe. 1967. Social readjustment rating scale. *J Psychosom Res* 11(3):213.

Johnson, L. and K. Keller. 1989. Staging Alzheimer's disease. *Geriatric Nursing* 10(4):196–97.

Kart, C., E. Metress, and J. Metress. 1978. *Aging and Health—Biologic and Social Perspectives*. Menlo Park, CA: Addison-Wesley.

Keane, S. and S. Sells. 1990. Recognizing depression in the elderly. *Journal of Gerontological Nursing* 16(1):21–25.

Krach, P. 1990. Discovering the secret: Nursing assessment of elderly alcoholics in the home. *Journal of Gerontological Nursing* 16(11):32–38.

Kral, V. 1976. Somatic therapies in older patients. *J Gerontol* 31(3):311–13.

Lasker, M.N. 1986. Aging alcoholics need nursing help. *Journal of Gerontological Nursing* 12(1):16–19.

Lee, R.J. 1976. Self-images of the elderly. *Nurs Clin North Am* 11(1):119–24.

Lee, V. 1991. Language changes and Alzheimer's disease: A literature review. *Journal of Gerontological Nursing* 17(1):16–20.

Leslie, G.R. 1976. *The Family in Social Context*. New York: Oxford University Press.

Linderborn, K.M. 1988. The need to assess dementia. *Journal of Gerontological Nursing* 14(1):35–39.

Lynch, J.J. 1977. *The Broken Heart: The Medical Consequences of Loneliness*. New York: Basic Books.

Mayers, K. and M. Griffin. 1990. The play project: Use of stimulus objects with demented patients. *Journal of Gerontological Nursing* 16(1):32–37.

McLane, A.M., ed. 1987. *Classification of Nursing Diagnoses*. St. Louis: C.V. Mosby.

Mendlewicz, J. 1976. The age factor in depressive illness: Some genetic considerations. *J Gerontol* 3(3):300–3.

McCracker, A. and E. Fitzwater. 1989. The right environment for Alzheimer's. *Geriatric Nursing* 10(6):293–94.

National Institute on Aging. 1980. Senility reconsidered: Treatment possibilities for mental impairment in the elderly. *JAMA* 244(3):259–63.

Nickens, H.W., T. Crook, and G.D. Cohen. 1986. Psychotropic drugs. *Generations* 10(3):33–37.

Pfeiffer, E. and E.W. Busse. 1973. Mental disorders in later life—affective disorders, paranoid, neurotic, and situational reactions. In *Mental Illness in Later Life*, edited by E. Busse and E. Pfeiffer. Washington, DC: American Psychiatric Association.

Rabins, P.V. 1983. Reversible dementia and the misdiagnosis of dementia: A review. *Hosp Community Psychiatry* 34(9):830–35.

Raskind, M.A. 1989. Organic mental disorders. In *Geriatric Psychiatry*, edited by E.W. Busse and D.G. Blazer. Washington, DC: American Psychiatric Press, Inc.

Refilfer, B.V. and E.B. Larson. 1985. Alzheimer's disease and long-term care: The assessment of the patient. *J Geriatr Psychiatry* 18(1):9–26.

Richardson, P., S. Lowenstein, and M. Weissberg. 1989. Coping with the suicidal elderly: A physician's guide. *Geriatrics* 44(9):43–47.

Rosenfeld, H. 1978. *New Views on Older Lives.* Washington, DC: United States Department of Health, Education, and Welfare, Publication No. 76-687.

Salzman, C. and R. Shader. 1979. Clinical evaluation of depression in the elderly. In *Psychiatric Symptoms and Cognitive Loss in the Elderly*, edited by A. Raskin and L.F. Jarvic. New York: John Wiley and Sons.

Spencer, R., L. Nichols, G. Lipkin, H. Waterhouse, F. West, and E. Bankert. 1986. *Clinical Pharmacology and Nursing Management*. 2d ed. Philadelphia: J.B. Lippincott.

Struble, L.M. and L. Sivertsen. 1987. Agitation behaviors in confused elderly patients. *Journal of Gerontological Nursing* 13(11):40–44.

Verwoerdt, A. 1976. *Clinical Geropsychiatry*. Baltimore, MD: Williams and Wilkins.

Weisman, M.M. 1979. The psychological treatment of depression. *Arch Gen Psychiatry* 36(10):1261–69.

Yazdanfar, D. 1990. Assessing the mental status of the cognitively impaired elderly. *Journal of Gerontological Nursing* 16(9):32–36.

11 Death: The End of the Aging Process

Patricia Bohannan

CHAPTER OUTLINE

FOCUS

In this chapter dying and death are viewed as important parts of life that need to be discussed openly and frankly among patients, families, and health care providers. Nurses have an important role in caring for patients who are dying and families who are grieving.

OBJECTIVES

1. Describe the death trajectory.

2. Evaluate the attitudes of older persons about death and dying.

3. List the major fears of the dying person.

4. Explain health care providers' attitudes about caring for dying older adults.

5. Discuss the advantages and disadvantages of the various locations where older people die.

6. Evaluate the concept of the hospice movement.

7. Discuss the meaning of death with dignity.

8. Explore your own feelings about caring for older persons who are dying.

9. Describe the role of the nurse in providing care to an older person who is dying.

10. Describe support services for nurses who routinely care for dying persons.

Dying is a normal process that occurs in all living beings. It is as much a part of life as birth. For every individual person it is a unique experience. It represents the culmination of the entire aging process. For some people the dying process occurs rapidly, in just a few hours or days. For others the dying process is a slow, deteriorating process that extends over months and possibly years.

DEATH TRAJECTORY

Humans are physical and psychosocial beings. Therefore discussion of a death trajectory, or the course that one follows to death, must include not only a description of the death of the physical body but also the death of the person. Aristotle described death in old age as exhaustion: "Finally, when motion is no longer possible, the breath is given out and death ensues" (Hutchins 1952). Science has added so much to our knowledge of the process of death that there are no longer sharply defined criteria by which to define it. When is a person really dead?

Human beings are made of many cells. Some of these cells can rejuvenate themselves and some cannot. Some organs can continue to function long after others have ceased. Some systems must function to maintain life while others are not essential. A perplexing question has arisen that is yet unanswered: Do people age because their systems wear out or do systems wear out because people age?

Since the early nineteenth century the traditional signs of death have included the absence of a heartbeat (which may also include the absence of a pulse); the absence of breathing, demonstrated by the extremities, mouth, and lips turning blue; and a lack of reflexes in the pupils of the eyes. With advances in medical technology these signs have become difficult to ascertain. Respirators, cardiac resuscitation units, and dialysis machines can maintain these vital functions with little or no brain activity. Using brain death as the criterion for determining death is highly controversial. The electroencephalograph records the electrical activity of the brain. Although the cerebrum contains the center of consciousness, it can be destroyed and the heart and lungs may still function. Therefore accepting brain death as the criterion for death is a judgment based on the value of a human being's ability to think, reason, feel, and interact with others. The conflict occurs when the brain of a dying person shows little or no electrical activity but the heart and lungs continue to function, especially with the aid of machines.

Many older people in our society begin their psychosocial death long before their body develops physical disabilities. According to the theory of aging proposed by Cummings and Henry (1961) older people progressively disengage from their environment and live in an increasingly detached state. Chronic illnesses cause disruption in social relationships because they impair mobility, speech, and hearing, among other problems. In the final stages of life older people may take steps to isolate themselves. They often limit their visitors to one or two close family members or friends. Older people are particularly apt to behave this way if a long illness has caused drastic changes in their appearance. Nurses should not assume that everyone values having many family members and friends present when they are dying. Many older people have detached themselves from family and friends and do not wish to re-establish these relationships. Scanlon (1989) suggested that disengagement from the environment and relationships are natural characteristics of the dying person's adaptation, not a reflection of lack of love.

A patient who was dying of melanoma had a daughter whom he had not seen or communicated with in a number of years. When she came to see him, he was rude and angry with her and she left, never to return. Several days later, when talking with a nurse, the patient tried to explain his behavior. He said, "No, I don't want to see or talk to her again. That pain has passed. Why revive it now?" He died a week later—alone, as he chose.

The social segregation that occurs in a nursing home should also be considered. Usually, the more disabled a person becomes, the more he or she is segregated from residents with normal physical and mental functions. Watson and Maxwell (1977) stated that socially structured dying or progressive social withdrawal may be as deadly to the mind and emotions of a patient as irreversible biologic deterioration is to the body. The will to live is more powerful than any medication. The degree of social interaction that will be therapeutic for the dying person, therefore, is highly individual.

Some patients seem to rely heavily on their spiritual beliefs during the death experience. Sometimes a strong religious faith provides peace and reassurance for the person who is facing death. Other times this faith enhances feelings of guilt about past experiences and creates anxiety and fear. Carey (1975) conducted a study in which he measured emotional adjustment in eighty-eight terminally ill patients. Fifty-six of these patients were over 50 years of age.

He found that intrinsically religious people (those who tried to integrate their spiritual beliefs into their lifestyle) had the greatest ability to cope with their limited life expectancy.

Many older people in our society are associated in some way with a religious group. It is important to determine the religious faith of the dying patient. Usually the patient will share his or her belief with the nurse, but sometimes it is necessary to ask for this information. Often a visit from a minister, priest, rabbi, or religious friend can be helpful. These visitors may pray with dying patients or read scripture to them. These patients usually find it easier to express their spiritual concerns to someone of their own faith.

Although the minister, priest, or rabbi is best qualified to provide spiritual support, the nurse may furnish it. Reading scripture and praying with the dying older adult at night may provide tranquility and comfort when medications will not. Nurses should not assume that everyone welcomes spiritual support. Some people even resent being asked about their religious preference. To some patients, calling the minister is an admission that death is imminent and this acknowledgement may create hostility and anxiety.

From this short review it is clear that every death trajectory is individual. There seems to be no pattern, and little can be predicted. It is hard to die, because dying means giving up life. Death is the inevitable end of life, however, and something all must do. Most of all it is a fundamental right of all human beings to die in such a way that their death complies with their individual values.

WHAT IT MIGHT FEEL LIKE TO BE DYING

Moody (1975) has done extensive research among people who have been brought back to life through resuscitation. From an analysis of these patients' descriptions of death, several things can be predicted about the experience of death. Hearing seems to be present after breathing and heartbeat have stopped. The voices may be "far off," but the patient probably hears and understands them. Several people reported hearing the doctor pronounce them dead.

Most of the patients in Moody's research reported very pleasant feelings. They seemed to feel peace and quiet. There was a variety of references to dark and light and visual experiences. Some people were able to view their own bodies and what was being done to them. Some people seemed to return to different times in their lives or have rapid flashbacks of past experiences. They did not want to leave their bodies at first, but after they experienced the pleasant feelings they did not want to return to their bodies. One of this author's patients, dying of renal failure, asked his family not to pray for him to live because he had been close enough to death to know that it was better than living.

ATTITUDES OF OLDER PEOPLE TOWARD DEATH

The older person is prepared for death only because of the prediction that life is nearing its end. However, an emotional adjustment to a terminal diagnosis may be as difficult to accept as it would be for a 20-year-old. Many older people who live in nursing homes feel that death is their only future. Only the actual time is unknown. Older people tend to set short-term goals or adopt a policy of living only one day at a time. Younger dying patients tend to continue to make long-term plans and deny their prognosis.

Many older people are concerned about the burden their care places on the family, especially on an older spouse. Some older adults choose to go to a nursing home to live because they feel that living with their children is destructive to their families. Younger patients with chronic illnesses seldom express concern about the effect that their illness has on the family.

Esberger (1980) provided a good review of the literature concerning the attitudes of older people toward death. This review stated that older people are more familiar with death, funerals, and cemeteries than are younger people. They are also more likely to have made preparations for their own death. They may even welcome death if their life is lacking in love and personal interaction. Older people adhere more closely to religious traditions and are more likely to believe in life after death than are younger persons. Oberst, Thomas, Goss, and Ward (1989) found older caregivers more accepting of death and more prepared to deal positively with the demands it placed upon them.

Anyone who is facing death has fears. Williams-

Ziegler (1984) identified three major fears: the fear of pain, the fear of loneliness, and the fear of meaninglessness. Some aspects of these fears are unique to the older patient.

Fear of Pain

The fear of pain is universal. Pain in the older adult is somewhat different. According to Woodrow et al. (1975) pain tolerance, measured by pressure on the Achilles' tendon, decreases with increasing age. However, others have found that as people age, their tolerance of pain in response to peripheral or skin stimuli actually increases. Pain is subjective and frightening, whether it is real or imagined. The relief of pain is a primary objective in the care of the dying patient. Nurses should not assume that older patients always require less pain medication. Herr and Mobily (1991) warn that older clients may deny pain, either because they do not want to admit that their condition is getting worse or they do not want to appear weak.

As the patient nears death, the need for narcotics may decrease and the patient may sleep for long periods of time. The nurse should not assume that such patients have no pain because they do not complain. They may be hurting severely and are too weak to ask for medication. Cardiorespiratory failure may cause slow, irregular breathing. Narcotics may be administered to prevent suffering even in the presence of low respiratory rates if death is imminent. Carey (1975) found that the level of discomfort that the terminally ill patient experiences is negatively related to the patient's ability to cope with a limited life expectancy. In another study, Dobratz et al. (1991) demonstrated that 66 percent (N=30) of the subjects had escalating pain up to death. This pain required increasing opioid requirements and alterations in the routes of administration. Therefore, providing comfort for older patients may involve the use of many innovative nursing skills.

Fear of Loneliness

The fear of loneliness is magnified for the institutionalized older people who are dying. They may demonstrate this fear in many ways. Some patients make many requests of the nursing staff. Patients who could do many of these things for themselves just want the reassurance of knowing that someone is there. Some patients express their loneliness by becoming hostile toward the nursing staff or their family. The nurse can help the family members by explaining this fact. Nurses and family need to be understanding and accepting of this type of hostile behavior.

Dying a lonely experience. Each of us must do it alone. Interacting with other humans, those who are alive and well, may help take our minds off the fears we have about dying. Yet it also reminds us of all that we will be leaving behind. Some people desire social interaction to forget their fears, while others avoid it to depress their grief. Again, each person has a unique attitude toward death.

Fear of Meaninglessness

The fear that life has been meaningless is most apparent in older adults. If older people experience few achievements and view their current life as unproductive, they may continually recall previous situations that illustrate their independence and productive capacity. Older dying adults may spend many of their last hours or days reminiscing. Butler (1974) said that the function of life review is to reconcile the past with the present so that life can continue to evolve and change to the end. He suggested that this mental process enables the older person to adapt to the changing circumstances at the end stage of life. For the dying, life review helps reconcile past conflicts and failures and establishes a meaning of life. Recalling the past can also be simply pleasurable. A pleasant memory can act as a tranquilizer and relieve stress and grief.

ATTITUDES OF HEALTH CARE PROVIDER TOWARD DYING OLDER ADULTS

Physicians are taught the art and science of diagnosis and treatment of illness with the goal of alleviating the illness. Physicians often make decisions concerning treatment based on their knowledge of the disease and its treatability. Many physicians do not believe they have the right to place a value on the patient's age or quality of life.

The effects of treatment, both surgical and medical, are also considered. The aging process causes a decrease in the ability of the body to tolerate trauma. Therefore the older patient with multiple problems may be given milder or more conservative treatment. Kastenbaum (1981) described how health care providers may decide to withhold treatment that could extend life and improve quality because of assumptions that the older person is ready to die. Decisions concerning treatment should be made on factors other than age alone.

Frequently, the older patient has a number of complex chronic illnesses that challenge the physician's skill. The treatment of one disease may compound another disease. Some physicians find this possibility discouraging. Decisions not to treat a disease are often based on the knowledge that ultimately the patient will die of another complicating illness. As an example, a physician may elect not to treat sepsis in a patient dying of metastatic cancer.

Nurses are also taught to assist the ill patient to become well. When the patient is old and has multiple problems, the nurse may be less aggressive in initiating nursing interventions. This is especially true if these interventions are painful. A nurse may hesitate, for example, to help an old, arthritic patient walk. If the patient's prognosis is poor, the nurse may have difficulty initiating such basic hygienic activities as the bed and bath and oral hygiene. Some nurses are reluctant to give care to the dying because they are afraid the activity may cause the patient to die.

The physician's attitude toward caring for the dying is often reflected by the other health care providers. Once the physician makes the choice not to treat the patient's disease actively, the nurse will redirect his or her goals to providing a peaceful and painless death. This choice may be made with age as a consideration, but usually it is motivated by the patient's ability to tolerate the treatment. Conflict can arise between the physician and other care providers when these decisions are not made jointly. The nurse may believe that the older patient should be allowed to die in peace, whereas the physician may actively seek a specific diagnosis, cure, or remission or the reverse may be true.

Sometimes older patients believe that their lives are useless and they would be better off dead. If the goal of the physician is to provide a remission or cure, the conflicts that arise are enormous. Nurses become discouraged because they get little cooperation from the patient, and physicians become frustrated because regardless of what they do, the patient does not progress. An example of this kind of situation is seen in the case of a 72-year-old man with nonresectable cancer of the esophagus who was provided with a gastrostomy for feeding purposes. For weeks this man cried, "I want to die. Please let me die." In spite of routine tube feedings and other care he became progressively worse. During the final three weeks of his life he passively allowed the nurses to care for him. He remained in a fetal position and refused to speak a word. Finally, the gastric tube became dislodged and he was allowed to die.

Even though health providers know that the natural end to life is death and that death is more likely to occur in old age, they often experience grief when the patient dies. Chaplain Herman Cook, director of Chaplaincy Service at Parkland Hospital in Dallas, Texas, has referred to the grief of the health care provider as the "third grief."

Physicians who have invested much time and energy in the diagnosing and treatment process will experience professional failure after the death of a patient. Nurses also experience a sense of professional failure when they have had a heavy investment in lifesaving activities and comfort-oriented care.

There are three other factors that may arouse grief in the health care provider. One is the *openness* that exists between the dying patient and the health care provider. This sharing seems to create a mutual feeling of positive regard that has great value for the patient, the nurse, and the physician. The loss or termination of this relationship results in grief.

The second factor that may affect the amount of grief experienced by health care providers is the degree to which they *identify* with dying patients. Patients who are the same age, race, and socioeconomic status as the health care provider remind the professional of his or her own vulnerability to death. The loss of patients who remind the health professional of significant people in their own lives also increase the grief experienced.

The third factor that affects the amount of grief experienced is the *social value* the health care provider places on the contribution the patient may be making to the lives of others. Because the status of the older adult in our society is considered to be nonproductive by many people, the death of an older patient may not generate a great deal of grief for the health care provider. If, however, the physician or the nurse identifies and has an open, caring relationship with the patient, they will encourage a sense of loss and the grief that accompanies this loss.

LOCATION OF DEATH

If we choose the place we are to die, most of us would probably choose our own homes. In an unpublished survey in 1975, of 150 nurses, 60 percent said they would like to die at home. However, many patients have no choice. They may be comatose and require care that cannot be given at home. Stein et al. (1982), in a study of older people in Miami, found that 35 percent of the sample lived alone and had no one nearby to help. As in most decisions, there are advantages and disadvantages to dying either at home or in a hospital or nursing home.

Death at Home

Most people want to die at home because they feel they will be able to control their death trajectory. Probably one of the most important considerations in choosing to die at home is financial. With the rising cost of hospital care, dying at home has become more popular. There is the advantage of being in familiar surroundings with one's own belongings. Another important advantage to dying at home is the opportunity to interact with family. This is especially true of the older patient who wishes to be with grandchildren and great-grandchildren.

The disadvantages of dying at home are equally great. The burden that is placed on the family is often a problem. Older patients may not wish to interfere with the family life of their children. Some older people do not feel that their aged spouse can assume the responsibility for the intense nursing care that is necessary. Older caregivers may not be physically able to care for a dying spouse because of chronic illness or physical limitations. Fengler and Goodrich (1979) described this caregiver as the "hidden patient." Thompson, Breckenridge, and Gallagher (1984) found an increase in health problems in older bereaved widows or widowers. A person who decides to die at home is asking loved ones to assume the responsibility of allowing death to occur. This obli-

gation is often more than the family can accept emotionally, a situation that is demonstrated when the family rushes the person to the hospital during the final stages of dying. It is a tremendous request to ask someone you love to assume the responsibility of allowing you to die.

Death in the Hospital

The advantages of dying in the hospital are many. The convenience and availability of care is an important factor. Also, it is reassuring to many dying people to know that equipment and skill are available to control many of the fearful symptoms they may experience. For the family, the release from the complete responsibility of care is sometimes viewed as an asset. The principal advantage of dying in the hospital is that the health caregiver shares the responsibility of the death with the family. The family can be assured that they have done everything that could be done to make dying as easy as possible for their loved one.

However, there are many disadvantages to dying in a hospital. In most hospitals patients cannot eat, sleep, or move about as they choose. Their privacy is invaded and they are put into a strange bed in strange clothes. They are subjected to needles, tubes, tests, and drugs without their consent. If they refuse, they are considered uncooperative and punished verbally and nonverbally as if they were children. If the death trajectory lasts a long time, dying in the hospital becomes a tremendous financial sacrifice for the family. This situation is particularly true of the older patient who is living on a retirement income and has a long-term illness that requires several hospitalizations. Not only is the spouse left without resources, but he or she is often left with medical bills and no way to pay them.

Death in the Nursing Home

In society today, many older people are placed in nursing homes for the final days of their lives. Most family units are small and many times both adults in the family have to work to support the family financially. Therefore there is really no one to assume that constant responsibility for the care of an ill older adult at home.

Nursing homes may provide an alternative during a long death trajectory that is less disruptive to the family unit. Today many nursing homes encourage their residents to bring their own belongings and some have homelike furnishings. Patients are not subjected to multiple invasive procedures, and skilled personnel are available to assist with activities of daily living. Many nursing homes now provide hospice care, with hospice staff managing part of the dying patient's care.

Nursing homes also have disadvantages. Dying patients are required to adhere to a time schedule similar to the hospital. Older patients often have negative attitudes about living in a nursing home. The increased demand for physical care that occurs at the end of a death trajectory places additional burdens on an often overburdened nursing staff. In an attempt to protect the residents from the realities of death, the dying patient is often separated from the other residents. Therefore he or she feels alone.

Nursing home care, like hospitalization, is expensive. Many older people have limited insurance coverage for nursing home care. Often the older spouse or the children must assume additional financial burdens to provide this care.

The Hospice Concept

Lay people and health care providers have been aware of the need to have better ways to manage death. In as few as fifteen years, the hospice movement has achieved widespread publicity and growth. In 1974 there was one hospice in the United States. Today there are thousands, ranging from small volunteer groups to larger institutions that care for hundreds of dying patients and their families (Amenta 1984).

According to the National Hospice Organization, incorporated in March of 1978, *hospice* is defined as a palliative and supportive service that provides physical, psychologic, social, and spiritual care for dying people and their families. The purpose of hospice is to provide support and care for people who are in the last phase of incurable disease so that they may live as fully and comfortably as possible (National Hospice Association 1979).

The hospice movement in America is patterned after the popular British model, St. Christopher's Hospice of London. Several variations of St. Christopher's exist, including inpatient hospital-based programs, home care programs, and freestanding inpatient hospice facilities. Basically, all hospice programs provide the palliative and supportive services of physicians, nurses, social workers, counselors, clergy, and volunteers. The goal of these programs is to reduce the physical, emotional, spiritual, social, and economic stresses experienced during the final stages of the illness period, the dying process, and bereavement (McCabe 1982).

The National Hospice Reimbursement Statute passed by Congress in 1983 provided, for the first time, for Medicare reimbursement benefits for hospice services provided by certified hospice programs. To be certified, hospice programs must have a medical director and must provide *(1)* twenty-four hour nursing care, *(2)* social services, *(3)* physicians' care, *(4)* counseling, *(5)* homemaker services, *(6)* outpatient medication and medical supplies, and *(7)* bereavement counseling. All certified hospice programs must be able to provide both inpatient and outpatient services. Currently there are more than 1700 hospice programs that assist families in providing home care for their dying relatives (National Hospice Organization 1989).

Older patients who are eligible for Medicare Part A may elect hospice care if they are certified by their physician to be terminally ill with a life expectancy of six months or less. Effective January 1989 there was no cap on the number of covered days for hospice care. Previously, Medicare reimbursement for hospice was a maximum of $6,500 (Hamilton and Neubauer 1989).

The passage of this landmark legislation established the hospice program as a viable component of the United States health care system. It clearly establishes standards that assure more uniform quality of care. Finally, it provides a source of income for hospice programs that before were dependent upon local fundraising efforts and direct charges to the patients.

Hospice nursing requires intensive care in the home. Most of this care is provided by family members. The hospice nurse's role is to educate, supervise, and support the family caregivers. A review of previous studies reveals that family caregivers need honest information concerning the condition of their relative, assurance that comfort will be provided, and knowledge of how to perform nursing skills (Hull 1989). Family caregivers identified important caring nursing behaviors to be twenty-four-hour accessibility, practitioner skills, communication skills, and nonjudgmental attitude (Hull 1991). The hospice nurse must be an expert practitioner, teacher, and counselor and must be able to collaborate closely with other members of the hospice team.

Many issues surrounding hospice care still confront older patients and their families. The hospice physician must assume medical responsibility. Many physicians and patients do not want to make this transition. The patient must sign an informed consent form that clearly states the patient is revoking curative treatment. This decision is often frightening. Critically ill older people who have no primary caregiver might require inpatient services. Therefore hospice organizations may hesitate to accept these individuals.

Eighty percent of hospice patient days must be in the home. Virtually all Medicare beneficiaries who elect to receive hospice benefits must have a home, a competent primary caregiver, and enough money so that the caregiver can be unemployed for an extended period (Lynn 1986).

A national survey of 400 terminally ill patients in hospital-based, home-based hospices and conventional care sites demonstrates that hospice patients and families were highly satisfied. Economic analysis indicated that cost per patient was $1,100 less for home-based care than for hospital-based hospice care (Greer 1983).

Carney and Burns (1986) found that the majority of patient services provided by hospice programs were performed by registered nurses. They cited the underserved patients as the very old, the poor, racial minorities, and persons living alone or with relatives who were unable to provide full-time care.

Hays (1986) found that inpatient hospice patients experienced more pain, nausea/vomiting, and respiratory distress. Their families had more anxiety and fatigue than home-care hospice patients and families. However, Grobe et al. (1981) identified that families of home-care patients had to learn ambulation skills, bowel management, comfort care, dietary control, pain management, and wound/skin care in order to facilitate home care. More than one half of the primary caregivers in Holling's (1986) study experienced significant physical difficulty that resulted in severe fatigue and exhaustion. However, they also described a closeness during the terminal events that was perceived as joyful. Cantor (1983) reported on a study of 178 frail, older primary caregivers in New York City who experienced high levels of stress from both the physical and financial demands that were a result of the home care required by the dying patient.

These studies indicate that hospice care, like hospital care and nursing home care, has certain assets as well as liabilities. Therefore the nurse who is counseling the terminally ill patient and family must consider many social and financial variables in order to direct the patient to the resource that will be most effective for each individual situation.

DEATH WITH DIGNITY

Television and motion pictures have depicted death simply as the act of closing the eyes and ceasing to breathe. Unfortunately, this is the only type of death many Americans have viewed. In reality, death rarely occurs this way. Seldom is a person healthy looking and active one minute and dead the next. Most Americans equate "death with dignity" with "death without machines" (respirators, monitors, and intravenous fluids). The decision not to employ these advances in medical technology, however, does not in any way ensure a death that is of the quality seen on the television screen.

The American social structure places great emphasis on the human being's ability to master nature. Our heritage supports this value, demonstrated by the people who endured the hardships of the passage West. Also, our society places a great value on productivity, which is so highly valued that we fail to learn to enjoy doing nothing. Finally, American society considers social isolation second only to death in severity of punishment. With these values ingrained from birth, it is no wonder that Americans fear the process of dying more than death itself.

In 1980, 40 percent of all direct care in hospitals was given to people 65 years of age and older. By 2050, nearly 80 percent of all hospital care will be required by older citizens (Oakley 1986). These figures show that nurses can expect to be giving care to older clients. More patients will require compassionate, supportive care as they experience their death trajectory.

Nursing Implications

Nursing literature abounds with specific skills that should be performed for the dying patient. The concept of "death with dignity" is used freely with few specific criteria that are largely undefined.

On December 15, 1973, *Science News* (p. 375) reported that the American Medical Association had passed a "Death with Dignity" resolution that included the removal of machines and the use of large doses of pain-killing drugs with patient or family permission. Simns (1975) said that death with dignity includes stable and comfortable surroundings and an opportunity for physical, psychologic, and spiritual comfort. Fayback (1975) stated that death with dignity calls for comfort, minimization of pain, calmness, and the absence of heroic measures to sustain life. Cooper (1973) stated that death with dignity should depend on cultural preference.

In her classic work Dr. Elizabeth Kubler-Ross et al. (1972) identified five emotional responses seen in dying patients: *(1)* shock and denial, *(2)* anger, *(3)* bargaining, *(4)* depression, and *(5)* acceptance. Denial may be a protective emotional response because the dying person is not able psychologically to handle the idea of his or her own death. Therefore nurses should be willing to allow the patient to deny without supporting the denial. Acceptance is the response seen in patients who have come to grips with the idea that they have a disease that will ultimately end in their death, but such acceptance does not include giving up hope. In fact Kubler-Ross (1972) says that hope is an essential component of quality death. But can the patient reach the stage of acceptance and still have hope?

Nurses often expect older people to fear death less than younger persons. Older patients who express anger or resentment may be classified as "problem patients." Nurses should not expect older people to have a passive acceptance of death.

A minister who has done work on death and dying visited a 92-year-old woman who was severely crippled with arthritis and was bedridden in a nursing home. He assumed that because she was 92 years old and in poor physical condition she would probably want to talk about death, a topic he came prepared to discuss with her as a concerned, knowledgeable, and interested person. At his first mention of the topic, however, she sat straight up in bed and said to him in a firm voice, "Listen here, Tom. I'll take life to death, any way I can get it." That incident taught him a lesson about the meaning of death to an older person.

Interfering Factors and Their Control

Although dying is a unique experience and every person may have individual preferences, sometimes unavoidable factors interfere with a dignified death.

Pain. A dignified death implies an absence of physical pain. Since pain is a subjective symptom, nurses must rely on the patient's assessment of its severity. Many older people feel that the need to ask for pain medication is a sign of weakness and dependence or that there is dignity in being able to endure pain. Some older people who are aware of the loss of their mental acuity do not wish to take drugs, which they believe will increase this problem. For many people, the fear that drugs might damage their body is worse than the pain itself. Austin et al. (1986) reported that 50 percent (N = 40) of the patients in their study were noncompliant with prescribed analgesics even though they were experiencing severe pain. When asked why, the most common answers were *(1)* fear of addiction and *(2)* loss of personal control. Ferrell and Schneider (1988) found that 83 percent (N=75) of the cancer patients in their study took less pain medication than was ordered. They identified fear of addiction, fear of tolerance, misunderstanding of dosage, and feeling that the pain could not be treated as reasons for not taking the drugs.

Billings (1985) recommended that pain medication be prescribed regularly by the clock to maintain a drug blood level that would provide pain relief for the dying patient. He also recommended use of heat, cold, hypnosis, relaxation, guided imagery, and biofeedback to help control pain.

Nursing care during the dying process must be directed toward providing comfort. Although at this stage dependence on drugs is not important, the patient's tolerance to the drugs must be considered. The longer a person takes a drug, the greater the dose that person will require to relieve pain. Many older people have a decreased ability to metabolize and excrete narcotics. Therefore drugs given close together may produce a cumulative effect. Interestingly, Austin et al. (1986) also found that half of the subjects in the 71–85 age group (N=12) reported pain that was not easily controlled. Dobratz, Wade, Herbst, and Ryndes (1991) found that only 23.3 percent (N=30) of their subjects required continuous subcutaneous morphine before death. The remainder, 76.7 percent, were managed with oral and rectal routes of administration. Pain management for the older dying patient clearly needs further investigation.

Because of these considerations, the nurse must make an accurate assessment of the older patient in pain. Herr and Mobily (1991) provided several guides for assessing pain in an older patient. Special attention must be given to assessing the cognitive and functional status of the older patient. It is most important for the patient to know that pain medication is available when needed and that the nurses will continue to do everything possible to relieve pain until death. Oral narcotics are the drugs of choice for pain relief in terminally ill patients. Morphine liquid is now available in the United States. Oral morphine 55–60 mg is usually considered equivalent to 10 mg of morphine given intramuscularly. However, after prolonged use this may be reduced to under 30 mg. Constant monitoring is necessary to balance pain relief, mental status, and respiratory status (Blues and Zerwekh 1984).

In the final stage of dying, people frequently become semicomatose or completely unconscious and the assessment of pain becomes difficult. The possibility that the semiconscious state is a result of excessive use of narcotics is real; such overuse should be avoided. Often, nurses medicate dying patients because of family demands; the family can cope with the loved one dying if he or she is sleeping peacefully. This attitude reflects our concept of death as a process in which we simply go to sleep and never wake up.

Loss of Control. The amount of control the patient is able to retain also contributes to the quality of death. The power to make decisions concerning one's future is highly valued. At a time when so many uncontrollable things are happening, dying patients often aggressively try to make decisions about their care—even if the decisions are contraindicated—so as to reassure themselves that they still have some control.

Because institutions are such structured environments, many people may choose to die at home. There they can decide when they will sleep, when and what they will eat, and what and how much medication they will take.

Nurses should actively allow dying patients to direct their own trajectories. Many old people seem to think they are too old to make decisions. They leave the decisions to their family, physicians, and nurses. Scanlon (1989) stated that the most valuable questions a nurse can ask a dying patient are "What are your greatest concerns?" and "How can I be of help?" Nursing intervention must respond to these answers. Mutually establishing realistic goals with the dying patient helps to support the hope that is essential for a quality death.

The inability to control body functions is a constant reminder to the patient that he or she is losing control. For example, as a control measure, catheters can be placed in the bladder, but the loss of bowel control can be devitalizing to the older patient. Every effort should be made to keep patients clean and dry in such a way that their feelings are protected and their privacy is maintained.

Respiratory Distress. The inability to breathe easily during the final stage of life causes anxiety and fear in everyone. A dying patient may become restless and anxious, increasing the respiratory rate and air hunger. The family becomes disturbed when they perceive the discomfort of the patient. The physician may order drugs to depress the respiratory center of the brain and thus decrease the patient's air hunger. Morphine is usually the drug selected. If the patient has developed a tolerance to this drug, large doses may be necessary to provide relief from air hunger.

Several nursing measures can be used to break the air-hunger cycle. The atmosphere must remain calm. Just talking quietly while encouraging the patient to take deep breaths and relax is often effective. The patient should be positioned to achieve maximum ventilation. Every effort should be made to provide rest for the patient. Sometimes it becomes necessary to sedate the patient with continuous intravenous medication. Nurses may be hesitant about giving sedation in large doses to dying patients. The respiratory center may be depressed so much that the patient's respiratory rate may not be high enough to provide adequate ventilation. Nurses must be able to assess this situation accurately. In the final hours before death, the patient may develop noisy or gurgling respiration. This may cause the family great concern. The nurse should try positioning the patient on his or her side. If this does not allow the removal of the pooled secretions in the pharyngeal areas, a suction may be needed. The physician may order small doses of atropine to reduce the secretions. If comfort is the goal, then care that includes medications that will provide comfort is usually the appropriate intervention.

Body Image. The concern that people have for their personal appearance is not limited by age. Older patients with chronic diseases have usually sustained progressive changes in their appearance. The fear of a deteriorating appearance in the final stage of life is often a contributing factor to depression among such patients.

Nurses can help decrease depression by taking the time to assist patients with the daily tasks that contribute to their personal appearance. A case in point is that of a lovely lady who had breast cancer. Every morning, at the patient's request, the nursing staff went through the ritual of cleaning her face and applying makeup. She died one afternoon in her beautiful pink gown with her face completely made up, including eye shadow. Even her nails were manicured. Her death was an important event in her life and she was dressed for the occasion.

In summary, dying is never easy but much can be done to make it more dignified. The nurse is often the primary person to aid the dying patient. By relieving pain and assisting people to control their own deaths, the nurse helps to provide dignity with death, which is the right of every human being.

DEVELOPING POSITIVE ATTITUDES ABOUT NURSING THE DYING

How can health professionals work with and closely relate to dying patients and their families and still enjoy their practice and their lives? Paraphrasing Kubler-Ross (1975), sharing in the death of those who understood its meaning can use this experience to grow.

A Philosophy of Dying for Nursing

The nurse must establish what service is to be offered and to whom this service is directed. A service that is offered to a dying client must be care oriented, not cure oriented. Many nurses labor under the misconception that their service has no value unless it helps the client to move from an ill state to a well state. The ill client may need the nurse's services regardless of his or her progression toward wellness. In fact the closer a person is to death, the greater is the need for nursing care.

The services the nurse may render are varied, but the goal is to help the individual die as peacefully and comfortably as possible. As far as possible, the client should be able to direct this care according to his or her own particular values. Therefore it is important to establish what those values are. This information should be readily available to the entire health care team.

Grief

Part of the response to the loss of a relationship is a feeling of grief, and nurses may experience this emotion when a patient dies. Each person grieves in his or her own way. Nurses should express this grief and not feel that professionalism is lost. Sometimes a sharing time with other members of the health team offers an opportunity to express this grief. If the nurse realizes that grief is a measure of his or her involvement with the patient, the grief will be seen as something positive. Frequently, nurses must be reminded that without grief there is no caring.

Evaluation

A specific task that is often overlooked after the death of a client is evaluation. Each value the client had expressed and how the death met that criterion should be reviewed. Also, the ways in which different people affected the dying process should be reviewed. Although this analysis may reveal weaknesses in the dying patient's care, it also emphasizes the positive activities that improved the quality of the patient's death. This may be an effective means of changing the nursing staff's attitudes toward themselves and their professional abilities in a positive way. Table 11-1 illustrates a tool that can be used by the staff of an oncology unit to evaluate a death trajectory. This tool can be helpful to an individual nurse or to a group in a patient care conference. During these conferences, staff support each other because they also go through a grieving process at the loss of a patient.

Table 11-1   Death with Dignity: Evaluation Tool

- Did the death occur where the client wanted to die?
- Was the client kept clean?
- Was the client kept comfortable?
- Was the client afraid?
- Did the client control his or her death?
- Were loved ones present during the dying process?
- Was support given to the remaining family?

SUMMARY

The process of dying is unpredictable. As much as possible, this process should conform with the values of the dying person. The older person may or may not be more accepting of a terminal diagnosis than a younger person. Most older people experience fear of pain, fear of loneliness, and fear of meaningless as part of the death trajectory.

Although health care providers may accept death as the natural end to life, they still experience grief. Three factors that affect how much grief is experienced are: *(1)* openness with the patient, *(2)* identification with the patient, and *(3)* the social value of the contributions made by the patient.

Because of the problems associated with dying in the current health care delivery system, the hospice concept has become a reality. Although the idea of a home hospice environment is promising, the demands placed on the primary caregiver are often physically and financially demanding. Many older people live alone or with a spouse who is also old and physically handicapped, making home care hospice programs incapable of providing the necessary support. Therefore older people will continue to need inpatient hospice programs, hospitals, and nursing homes for care during the death trajectory.

With an increasing older population and an increase in chronic disease, nurses will be caring for more dying older patients in the future. Nurses have the opportunity to assist older people in dying with dignity. Their contributions in the area of pain control and the relief of respiratory distress require expert clinical management. By actively seeking to maintain the patient's body image and allowing the dying patient to direct his or her own death trajectory, the nurse can help the patient attain a quality death. Finally, nurses caring for dying patients must actively evaluate their methods of care to develop positive attitudes.

STUDY QUESTIONS

1. Define death trajectory.

2. What does the term *brain dead* mean?

3. Identify three major fears associated with dying.

4. Describe common conflicts that surround decisions to treat or not treat older patients.

5. Identify three factors that may influence grief experienced by the health care provider when the patient dies.

6. Evaluate the assets and liabilities of dying
   a. At home
   b. At a hospital
   c. At a nursing home
   d. In a hospice

7. Describe how age influences one's attitude toward death.

8. Identify three factors that may influence a dignified death.

9. Describe appropriate nursing interventions to control factors that contribute to a dignified death.

10. Identify an evaluation method that will assist the staff with the development of positive attitudes about caring for the dying patient.

REFERENCES

Amenta, M. 1984. Hospice USA 1984—Steady and Holding. *Oncology Nursing Forum* 11(5):68–74.

Austin, C., P. Eyres, E. Hefferin, and R. Krasnow. 1986. Hospice home care pain management: Four critical variables. *Cancer Nursing* 9(20):58–65.

Billings, J.A. 1985. *Outpatient Management of Advanced Cancer*. Philadelphia, PA: J.B. Lippincott.

Blues, A. and J. Zerwekh. 1984. *Hospice and Palliative Nursing Care*. Orlando, FL: Grune and Stratton.

Butler, R. 1974. Successful aging and the role of life review. *J Am Geriatr Soc* 12:529–35.

Cantor, M. 1983. Strain among caregivers: A study of experiences in the U.S. *The Gerontologist* 23(6):597–604.

Carey, R.C. 1975. Living until death: A program of service and research for the terminally ill. In *Death, the Final Stage of Growth*, edited by E. Kubler-Ross. Englewood Cliffs, NJ: Prentice-Hall.

Carney, K. and M. Burns. 1986. Hospice care: Some insights on nature, demand and cost. In *Hospice Handbook: A Guide of Managers and Planners*, edited by L.F. Paradis. Rockville, MD: Aspen.

Cooper, R.M. 1973. Euthanasia and the notion of death with dignity. *The Christian Century*, February:226.

Cummings, E. and W.E. Henry. 1961. *Growing Old*. New York: Basic Books.

Dobratz, M.C., R. Wade, L. Herbst, and T. Ryndes. 1991. Pain efficacy in home hospice patients: A longitudinal study. *Cancer Nursing* 14(1):20–26.

Esberger, K.K. 1980. Dying and the aged. *Journal of Gerontological Nursing* 6(1):11–15.

Fayback, M. 1975. Death with dignity. *Journal of Gerontological Nursing* 1(3):42–44.

Fengler, A. and N. Goodrich. 1979. Wives of elderly disabled men: The hidden patients. *The Gerontologist* 19(3):175–83.

Ferrell, B.R. and C. Schneider. 1988. Experience and management of cancer pain at home. *Cancer Nursing* 11(2):84–90.

Greer, D. 1983. National hospice study analysis plan. *J Chronic Dis* 36(11):737–80.

Grobe, M., D. Ilstrup, and D. Ahmann. 1981. Skills needed by family members to maintain the care of an advanced cancer patient. *Cancer Nursing* 4(5):371–75.

Hamilton, C.L. and B.J. Neubauer. 1989. Hospice nursing: Serving ambivalent clients. *Nursing and Health Care* 10(6):321–22.

Hays, J. 1986. Patient symptoms and family coping: Predictors of hospice utilization patterns. *Nursing* 9(6):317–25.

Herr, K.A. and P.R. Mobily. 1991. Pain assessment in the elderly. *Journal of Gerontological Nursing* 17(4):12–19.

Holing, E. 1986. The primary caregiver's perception of the dying trajectory: An exploratory study. *Cancer Nursing* 9(1):29–37.

Hull, M.M. 1989. Family needs and supportive nursing behaviors during terminal cancer: A review. *Oncology Nursing Forum* 16(6):787–92.

Hull, M.M. 1991. Hospice nurses caring support for caregiving families. *Cancer Nursing* 14(2):63–70.

Hutchins, R.M., ed. 1952. *Great Books of the Western World*. Vol. 8. Chicago: Encyclopaedia Britannica.

Kastenbaum, R.J. 1981. *Death, Society and Human Experience*. 2d ed. St. Louis: C.V. Mosby.

Kubler-Ross, E., S. Wessler, and L. Avioli. 1972. On death and dying. *JAMA* 22(2):174–79.

Kubler-Ross, E., ed. 1975. *Death, the Final Stage of Growth*. Englewood Cliffs, NJ: Prentice-Hall.

Lynn, J. 1986. Ethics in hospice care. In *Hospice Handbook: A Guide for Managers and Planners*, edited by L.F. Paradis. Rockville, MD: Aspen.

McCabe, S. 1982. An overview of hospice care. *Cancer Nursing* 5(2):103–8.

Moody, R.A. 1975. *Life after Life*. Covington, GA: Mockingbird Books.

National Hospice Organization. 1979. *Standards of a Hospice Program of Care*. Branford, CT: National Hospice Organization.

National Hospice Organization. 1989. *A Guide to the Nation's Hospices.* Arlington, VA: National Hospice Organization.

Oakley, D. 1986. Projecting the number of professional nurses required for in-hospital direct care of older people: 1970–2050. *Western Journal of Nursing Research* 8(3):343–49.

Oberst, M.T., S.E. Thomas, K.A. Goss, and S.E. Ward. 1989. Caregiving demands and appraisals of stress among family caregivers. *Cancer Nursing* 12(4):209–15.

Scanlon, C. 1989. Creating a vision of hope: The challenge of palliative care. *Oncology Nursing Forum* 16(4):491–96.

Simns, L. 1975. Dignified death: A right, not a privilege. *Journal of Gerontological Nursing* 1(5):21–25.

Stein, S., M. Linn, and E. Stein. 1982. The relationship of self-help networks to physical and psychological functioning. *J Am Geriatr Soc* 30(8):764–68.

Thompson, I., J. Breckenridge, and D. Gallagher. 1984. Effects of bereavement on self-perception of physical health in elderly widows and widowers. *J Gerontol* 39(4):309–14.

Watson, W. and R. Maxwell. 1977. *Human Aging and Dying.* New York: St. Martin's Press.

Williams-Ziegler, J. 1984. Allaying common fears. In *Dealing with Death and Dying.* 2d ed. (Nursing Skillbook series), edited by P.S. Chaney. Springhouse, PA: Nursing 84 Books.

Woodrow, K., G. Freidman, A. Siegelaub, and M. Collen. 1975. Pain tolerance difference according to age, sex, and race. In *Pain, Clinical and Experimental Perspective,* edited by M. Weisenberg. St. Louis: C.V. Mosby.

Part 4

SPECIALIZED NURSING CARE

12 Hospitalized Older Adults

Rhonda Keen-Payne

FOCUS

This chapter explores why hospitalization is often a new and frightening experience for older persons. Nurses need to focus on adapting the nursing process to meet their needs and preventing major iatrogenic conditions.

OBJECTIVES

1. Discuss the concerns and needs of older persons who become hospitalized.

2. Identify the roles of hospital staff in meeting the specialized needs of older patients.

3. Explain possible effects of prospective payment systems (PPS) on an older patient with multiple chronic illnesses.

4. Give examples of functional health assessment in the hospital setting.

5. Evaluate the need for balance between autonomy and safety in the hospitalized older patient.

6. Discuss major causes of iatrogenesis in the older hospitalized patient.

7. Identify two preventive interventions for each of the major causes of iatrogenic conditions discussed.

8. Explain possible causes for family stress in the care of hospitalized older patients.

As the largest consumers of the major components of health care, including ambulatory services, acute care hospitalization, and long-term institutional care, the per capita cost of health care for older adults in 1985 was over $4,200, compared with about $1,700 for the population as a whole (Kane, Ouslander, and Abrass 1989). Close to half of those expenditures are for hospital care (Schrier 1990). A study of Medicare recipients conducted by the Health Care Financing Administration (HCFA) in May 1991 verified the extensive utilization of medical facilities and identified the leading medical causes for hospitalization and rehospitalization. The study revealed 9.1 million hospitalizations among older persons in 1988. Stated another way, approximately 21 percent of all Medicare beneficiaries were hospitalized at least once in 1988. The data indicate that those in the oldest age group (85 and over) had twice as many admissions as the youngest (65–74). The top eight admission diagnoses were

- Acute ischemic heart disease
- Cerebrovascular disease
- Congestive heart failure
- Pneumonia
- Chronic ischemic heart disease
- Cardiac dysrhythmias
- Hip fracture
- Fluid/electrolyte problems

Certain illnesses had higher rates of readmission. There was approximately one readmission per four initial admissions for bladder and cervical cancers, affective psychoses, and congestive heart failure (May, Kelly, Mendlein, and Garbe 1991). About 44 percent of all inpatient days are accounted for by other individuals; the average length of hospital stay is 8.9 days.

SIGNIFICANCE OF GERONTOLOGICAL NURSING TO HOSPITAL PRACTICE

Comprehensive services are needed to promote wellness, care for those with illness, and provide rehabilitation. The acute care setting may be an appropriate site for these activities because of the frequency with which the older person uses hospitalization (Golightly, Bossenmaier, McChesney, Williams, and Wyble 1984). Acute care facilities are changing to meet the needs of consumers as well as to expand their own markets. Services that are offered by hospitals include such diversities as senior day-care centers, rehabilitation centers, outpatient clinics especially focused on the older person, transportation services, home care and homemaker services, and respite care for families caring for the dependent older person in the home (Dean 1987). Health care is usually a priority for the older individual, and the

hospital may find partial resolutions to economic problems in this population's needs.

Distinguishing between normal aging and pathology is a constant challenge, even in the well older person. A highly complex level of care is required for an acutely ill older patient. Ideally nurses, dietitians, physicians, social workers, and pharmacists in hospitals should have special education in gerontology. For example, a pharmacist with gerontological preparation would be familiar with patient responses to certain medications that are common in older persons. A multidisciplinary specialized team is a goal to work toward in most hospitals.

The use of a specially prepared nurse or staffing system is helpful in the acute-care setting where a mix of patients is usually present that includes a high proportion of older patients. For example, nursing care of the older patient can be improved by the use of a gerontological clinical nurse specialist or a gerontological nurse practitioner in the hospital setting. The vulnerability of older people means that the nurse must be prepared to discuss such issues as the right to life and death, autonomy, and sanctity of life with clients, families, and peers (Heine 1988).

Additionally, older patients often present the most complex illnesses because adaptation is slowed and reserves are rapidly depleted. A nurse specialist would provide ongoing education to nursing staff about older persons, serve as a community resource, and coordinate care for patients as a whole. Such a nurse could also serve as a consultant to the nursing and medical staff with specific patients especially in functional assessment of older patients (Reilly 1989).

The gerontological resource nurse is another alternative. This nurse is usually a staff member who volunteers to work closely with the clinical nurse specialist in order to become more knowledgeable in the common problems associated with older patients. After about six months this nurse is able to serve as a resource for a unit, giving care to a group of patients but also being available to help other nurses. This system not only promotes sensitivity to older patients but it also improves the overall care (Fulmer 1991).

Case management is a third approach to improving the care of older patients during hospitalization. Case management is a method of delivering care that is characterized by a nurse coordinating all of the care for a patient and family within a service network or organization (Putney, Hauner, Hall, and Kobb

1990). Similar to the primary nurse, the case manager is able to focus on holistic care because all services are provided through one system. In these systems, patient outcomes are defined and payment is linked to the projected length of stay. Rather than simply discharging the patient, however, the case manager continues to coordinate care. Case management is especially important in the care of older people because gerontological patients require a variety of services. It is also a cost-effective way of providing care for older persons in their communities (Wood 1991).

Nurses must be prepared to meet the needs of such a large group of patients. From the time of the patient's admission to the hospital until discharge plans have been carried out, nurses have closer contact with the patient than does any other member of the health care team. Nurses must understand not only the normal aging process but also the common deviations from this normal process, the individual differences among older adults, and the many problems that confront these people and their families.

Few persons are admitted to a hospital without anxiety and some illness or loss of function. The older patient, though, is more vulnerable than younger adults are. In addition to this vulnerability the older patient is likely to be stereotyped as incompetent and frail (Cohen 1990). Older people may not be treated as adults because they are perceived as dependent, helpless, and unable to make decisions. Additionally, older persons are much more likely to receive negative generalized labels as a result of one behavior or incident. For example, forgetting the day of the week is of no consequence if the patient is younger, but may result in an erroneous label of dementia in an older person.

Some of these problems can be prevented through education and consciousness-raising or sensitivity training. Harmful stereotypes and prejudices may be exposed and countered through classes in growth and development of older persons. Media, such as films or board games, are available that help in confronting prejudices and false information (Dempsey-Lyle and Hoffman 1991). Gerontological nurses have an excellent opportunity to challenge stereotypes and assist other health team members in examining their values about aging.

ADMISSION

Common Reasons for Hospital Admission

Many older persons enter the hospital on an elective rather than emergency basis and are hospitalized because of a complication associated with a chronic illness. Older persons are hospitalized more frequently than younger adults because they have a diminished reserve and deteriorate quickly with an acute illness. The older individual most at risk is one with a chronic condition that is aggravated by a superimposed acute condition.

The most commonly occurring conditions are arthritis, hypertension, heart disease, orthopedic limitations, and diabetes. Visual and hearing impairments also are common.

Fears of Patients

Admission to a hospital is a crisis for many older adults. Some of them reach old age without ever having been hospitalized before. They enter the hospital not knowing what to expect. Some think of the hospital only as a place to die. Others fear that they may never be able to go back to their own homes again, especially if they recognize that they will need help in caring for themselves. Often, being in the hospital separates them from loved ones. Perhaps they are separated from a spouse for the first time in their marriage, or perhaps the spouse is also ill and arrangements have had to be made for his or her care. The older person may enter the hospital suffering from an uncontrolled chronic condition after the recent death of a spouse and he or she fears what may happen. Hospitalization of the widowed person often occurs within the first year after the death of the spouse.

Older adults may be anxious about their diagnoses, the tests to be performed, the consequences of the tests, and their ability to understand what the physicians and nurses tell them. Patients often request that a son or daughter be present when the physician speaks with them. When they enter a hospital, older people who have been independent in all their activities and decision making at home are suddenly faced with the need for help in understanding the implications of their illness.

Concerns About Hospital Costs

Although Medicare and private health insurance help meet health care costs, there are still financial problems for many older adults. For the many older people who live on fixed incomes, the share of costs is rapidly increasing. Medical bills may already be high for older people who have several chronic health problems. Admission to a hospital places an additional financial burden on them and on their families. Older adults often enter the hospital wondering whether they will be able to pay the bill. Each time a different physician or other health care person sees the patient, he or she may wonder or ask how much it will cost. Older patients often tell nurses that they are "just on Medicare," hoping that the nurse and others will understand that they cannot afford more services than Medicare benefits provide.

Most older patients and their families are familiar enough with the payment system for health care to dread its complexities. Implemented in 1983, the Medicare Prospective Payment System (PPS) reimburses agencies and caregivers on a flat-fee basis. This fee is determined by the patient's classification into one of 473 diagnosis-related groups (DRGs). The agency will be paid the set fee, regardless of the patient's length of stay or accumulation of costs. Therefore losses must be absorbed if patient costs exceed the fixed rate. On the other hand the agency receives the revenue if a patient's care is delivered at a cost less than the DRG fixed rate. In many states all third party payors, in addition to the government, pay on the basis of DRGs.

After the introduction of DRGs, observers and participants in the system began to worry that older patients would be discharged too soon. The financial incentive for a rapid resolution to the patient's problems is certainly realistic. Many studies have illustrated an increase in the acuity of hospitalized patients. For older patients the risk of inadequate care may be greatest for those with more than one diagnosis. When multiple diagnoses are present in the older patient, the possibility of being discharged too soon should be considered (Grau and Kouner 1991).

Room Accommodations

The type of room accommodation may cause problems. Although semiprivate rooms are often those most easily available in the hospital, many older adults, because of their physical or mental condition, can best be cared for in a private room. A study by Williams et al. (1979) showed that confused patients do better in private rooms because there are fewer distractions.

The older ill person who has a choice may not want to share a room with a total stranger or be where family members cannot visit freely. Privacy is important when the patient is giving personal information to the physician or nurse. The giving or collecting of information continues throughout the hospital stay, and often the patient in a semiprivate room has no control over what or how much other patients hear.

Some older patients request a semiprivate room, however, because they want company. Others request a semiprivate room because their insurance normally covers this type of accommodation, whereas a private room is allowed only if it is medically necessary.

There are special problems for patients and their families if the older adult must spend some time in an intensive care unit. The activity, the strange noises, the critical condition of the patient, and the limited visiting time all contribute to the fears and anxiety of both the patient and family. Refer to chapter 15 for an expanded discussion of this problem.

Room assignments, except for the intensive care unit, are usually made by admitting personnel who are aware only of a symptom or perhaps of an admission diagnosis. Assignments are made according to the diagnosis or the medical service of the patient's physician, with little knowledge or concern about specific patient needs. This problem can result in the need to transfer a very ill or uncomfortable patient at an inconvenient time.

Nursing Interventions During Admission

Nurses must be sensitive to the problems older adults face at the time of admission to a hospital. As people age, their ability to cope with problems and new situations may not be as good as when they were younger; this ability may be weakened further with illness or anxiety. Ryan and Robinson-Smith (1990) suggested that older patients who are able to cope with stressful life events such as hospitalizations may further develop their understanding of life and their experience in living. Nurses should be able to actively assist these patients by decreasing disorientation and fear. Actions that promote the patient's control of life events, such as active participation in care planning, should be implemented.

Some understanding of Medicare and other insurance coverage helps the nurse appreciate the dilemma many older patients face. The nurse should make appropriate referrals to the hospital social service staff to help the patient with problems and needs that are beyond the nurse's knowledge and ability.

When the patient is called by name, is introduced to "his" or "her" nurse, and knows that the nurse has been expecting him or her, the patient feels that there is someone on whom to depend. The nurse should determine how the illness and hospitalization affect the patient. One way is to sit down and talk with the patient. Often, patients will tell a nurse about their personal problems, their concerns about their health, and their anxieties about the future. The older patient thinks of the nurse as an experienced and knowledgeable person who understands problems, even though the nurse may be young.

The nurse can be helpful to those who make room assignments by requesting that the older patient be placed in the room best suited for him or her. If the patient must be in the same room with other patients, as much privacy as possible should be provided, even if all that can be done is to limit visitors. Wherever the room assignment may be, the nurse who admits the patient has the responsibility for extending warmth and sincerity to the patient and family and for making the admission to the hospital a smooth process.

Like any other set of patients, older persons' reactions to illness and crisis are widely varied. People become more different the older they become. Some are gracious and cooperative, even in dire circumstances. Others are cantankerous and impossible to please. One cannot group all older patients together; to do so increases the risk of making mistakes in identifying and managing the patient's problems. By avoiding stereotypical labelling of the patient, the nurse will be better able to deliver compassionate, individualized care.

Special Precautions

Before implementing uniform safety precautions, the threat to personal control and autonomy should be reviewed. Older persons are sometimes perceived as so fragile that their needs for safety outweigh the right to autonomy (Lidz and Arnold 1990). The conflict between autonomy and safety is inherent in our society's stereotypical image of the dependent older person. Promoting autonomy is extremely difficult for the nurse when faced with regulations and policies, written to enhance safety, that may violate the older person's right to make decisions as an adult. In general, autonomy is best promoted in a setting where patients' rights are valued, patient education is systematically provided so that patients can participate in their care, and individual adaptations are encouraged rather than simply tolerated. For example, nurses should question the importance of patients being required to wear a hospital gown to prevent their own clothing from being soiled. Should patients be encouraged to leave the unit and visit the hospital gift shop or restricted uniformly for their safety? Because of the desire to protect the older person from injury, many policies and procedures may unnecessarily violate the person's autonomy.

Older patients require special attention because of their heightened vulnerabilities, decreased reserve, and possible complex disease and drug interactions. Additionally, older patients may take longer to adjust to hospital admission. These factors require informed, committed nurses to plan and administer care. Hospitals may wish to investigate the development and use of a unit devoted to those senior clients with multiple communication, ambulation, orientation, or elimination impairments (Golightly et al. 1984). If the older population is integrated throughout the hospital, the geriatric component of in-service education topics should always be addressed. Topics specifically on aging and the older individual should also be included.

In general the nursing care of the older patient requires a holistic approach. One of the major risks that the older person faces is the deterioration of one body system while experiencing a problem in another system (Tobis 1982). Another major risk is that the older patient frequently exhibits subdued signs and symptoms of problems. Infections may not cause temperature elevations until the patient is very ill; pain is often not experienced by older patients having myocardial infarctions. Increasing confusion may be the only sign of complications or problems.

Confusion and communication problems are

sometimes misinterpreted by nurses. The older patient may have sensory losses that inhibit communication. These losses are too often falsely interpreted as cognitive deterioration. Confusion may be caused by relocation, electrolyte imbalances, medications, or infection. These explanations should be explored before cognitive assessments are completed.

Orientation to New Surroundings

The older client may exhibit acute confusion when faced with relocation. Usually short-term, this disorientation may be quite marked, and may include the inability to accurately identify time, place, or persons in the setting. The nurse should be aware that this is not an unusual response to change in some older patients; it might be worse in those admitted from long-term care settings. Patience and support of the person are essential. The nurse should seek additional history to determine if the patient was previously well-oriented, as well as identify additional changes or stressors that might contribute to the confusion. Sometimes confusion is due to medications or an electrolyte imbalance related to changes in nutritional status. The nurse should postpone as many interventions as possible, including taking a history from the patient, until the patient begins to be more aware of the surroundings. Most importantly, caution should be used in labelling the confusion as dementia.

The older individual has relocation considerations that may not be a problem for a younger person. Hospitalization may mean drastic changes in the older person's support system, especially if the family is unable to travel back and forth to the hospital. Physical environment alterations are also threatening to the older person who has some sensory losses. These patients have a decreased ability to adapt rapidly to changes in environment and nurses should be sensitive to this extended adaptation period (Pergrin 1987). Patients also exhibit fears about hospitalization because it may represent the end of independence (Golightly et al. 1984). Orientation to the environment is critical to the well-being of the older person. Falls are most likely to occur early in the hospitalization and may be partially due to a disorientation to surroundings. Cognition may be temporarily disrupted in a new environment, and confusion is also a factor in client safety (Palmateer and McCartney 1985).

Orienting patients to their new surroundings helps them feel at ease. They must learn how to summon the nurse. If there is an intercom system, patients must be shown how to use it. Patients may be intimidated by electronic controls or may be unable to read or understand identifying labels. The operation of the electric bed and the television must be explained and demonstrated to the patient. Visiting hours, meal times, and other similar hospital routines should be explained. Printed brochures explaining hospital policies may be given to patients, but there is no assurance that they can or will read them. To put patients at ease, the nurse should give them simple, clear instructions and allow the patients to demonstrate that they can use the nurse call switch, for instance.

ADAPTING THE NURSING PROCESS FOR THE OLDER PATIENT

Some adaptations must be made in the nursing process in the care of the older adult in the hospital setting.

Assessment

A thorough assessment is important and can be completed in several short time segments, if needed. The patient is usually overwhelmed by all the activity and questions during the admission process and needs some time to adapt to the new environment. The patient's physical and mental conditions should be the primary considerations in determining when and how the assessment can be done. The nurse's judgment is essential at this point.

There is considerable difficulty in assessing patients with either physical or cognitive impairments. Several different tools are available to guide these assessments, but they usually require that the nurse or physician be trained to use the guide (Kane and Kane 1981; Andersen 1989). Ideally the gerontological clinical nurse specialist or nurse practitioner will be available to assist in the assessment of older patients with multiple impairments. In general the nurse should be aware of the importance of focusing assessment on the patient's ability to perform the activities of daily living and the degree of assistance needed on a regular basis.

Assessment of older persons must be functionally based rather than disease based for a variety of reasons. Many older individuals have lived with a chronic illness for a long time and have successfully adapted to activities of daily living. The most important assessment focuses on the patient's capacity to perform activities associated with independent existence (Panicucci 1983). In this way the patient's strengths, weaknesses, goals, and limitations are identified rather than simply listing diagnoses. Additionally, assessment should not be limited to the admission period. Frequently, patients are temporarily confused because of relocation, infection, or effects of medications. Difficulty in communication also inhibits assessment. Difficulties such as hearing or speaking impairments often are identified after the initial assessment period. Assessment data should be evaluated daily until the patient seems settled and the data do not change significantly.

In the acute-care setting it would be helpful to use some kind of formal assessment tool, especially for cognition assessment. Cognition is the ability to process, store, and recall information. It is essential to independent functioning. Accurate assessment is vital, not only for planning hospital care, but also for discharge planning. Some studies show that cognition is frequently omitted from assessment or inaccurately assessed (Palmateer and McCartney 1985).

The nurse should evaluate patients' functional abilities, because all nursing activities are centered around helping them in self-care. Can they feed themselves? Can they get in and out of bed and to the bathroom safely? How long can they stay out of bed? Other considerations may include how they managed at home. Do they use a cane or walker? How much assistance did they need at home? How much assistance will they need in the hospital? Patients often describe how they managed at home in familiar surroundings before they became ill. The nurse should ask questions in such a way that clear answers will be given and must listen carefully and communicate effectively.

The nurse should determine what patients know or understand about their medical diagnoses, but the older adult may have difficulty giving accurate or adequate information. If they have multiple chronic problems, they often do not remember important facts about each condition. As one patient said, "Too many things have happened." Also, they frequently have made adaptations to their disabilities to the point that they do not consider them problems and only mention what is bothering them at the moment. Asking the patient about all drugs being taken at home will provide information about medical problems that might not otherwise have been mentioned.

The nurse should try to learn as much as possible about the patient's usual day at home. The habits of daily living provide information that is useful in planning hospital care and future home care. Many older people sleep late in the morning, eat only two meals daily, and stay up late at night. Patients' patterns of living make a difference in how some medications will be taken. Do they take naps? Do they sleep well at night? How many times do they get up to go to the bathroom? Are they active at home? Older people who usually work or stay active may become bored when they must remain in bed in the hospital room. The restrictions that may be imposed upon them, of course, will depend upon the reason for hospitalization.

Older patients frequently bring numerous medications with them to the hospital. The nurse should learn about all medications the patient is taking, including prescription and over-the-counter drugs. It is important to determine how and why specific medications are being taken as well as the patient's understanding of the action and side effects of these drugs. Do the patients have a regular medication schedule? Do they take their medicines according to directions? Have they worked out a method to remember to take them? Do the patients know the names of their drugs and why each drug is being taken? The nurse should be alert for clues to errors and to symptoms that might be drug related.

The nurse should learn the patient's eating patterns, food likes and dislikes, and cultural eating habits. Does the patient snack? Does he or she eat something before going to bed? Although the dietitian usually takes diet histories and sees that the patient gets the prescribed diets, it is important that nurses know enough about the patient's preferences and prescribed diets to make requests or provide the necessary nourishment in special circumstances. Planned snacks may be necessary when the patient is not eating well at mealtime or when he or she needs extra food because of the danger of hypoglycemia. The nurse may determine other needs for snacks or the patient may need food with medications, but the foods that are given must be within certain prescribed limits. When the patient is on a prescribed diet, the nurse must know how well the patient is tolerating the diet.

A thorough physical assessment is necessary to determine the patient's current physical condition. During the physical assessment, the nurse will determine special problems and learn from the patient how he or she has been managing these problems at home. It may be necessary for the same type of care to be continued in the hospital. The nurse may be able to suggest a more comfortable or easier way to take care of the situation and, with an adequate explanation, the patient may readily accept the change.

Some special precautions are necessary in gathering data for the physical examination. Perhaps most importantly, the patient should be allowed time to adjust to the hospital setting before major procedures are performed. Unless time is urgent, the physical examination can be completed in small sections over several days. In general the patient should be protected from cold and chilling. Additionally, the older patient may have difficulty with balance and sudden movements and should be protected from falling. The older patient's diminished sight and hearing may necessitate special instructions or adaptations. Finally, the older patient will probably tire easily. The examination should minimize position changes and be conducted in short intervals.

Laboratory work is an important component of physical assessment and may be even more important for the older person. Some laboratory values are slightly different than those for the general adult population, and the persons who care for older patients must be aware of these variations. Unfortunately, many of the laboratory variations for older people are unknown or poorly documented. (See chapter 6 for further information on laboratory values.)

Special procedures such as roentgenography and other diagnostic studies cause problems for the older adult. Some special diagnostic procedures can be traumatic for the older patient. Nurses should explain to the patient what to expect. If a test requires special preparation, the nurse may need to give repeated instructions. Everyone who is involved in the patient's care should be alert for such special problems as difficulty in hearing, blindness, or an inability to stand, walk, or move from stretcher to table without assistance. The patient with knee flexion contractures will need to sit for a chest X-ray film.

Older patients who receive large amounts of laxatives to completely cleanse the bowel before a barium enema or colonoscopy should be observed closely during the evening and night shifts before the diagnostic test. The action of the laxatives may be delayed because of normal decreased peristalsis in older people. Therefore these patients have repeated bowel movements during the night. If they are slightly confused because of the late hour and a new environment, they may fall trying to go to the bathroom. Also, these patients are usually very tired and weak after having been awake part of the night and having had numerous bowel movements. Therefore they should be carefully assisted to wheelchairs or stretchers when going to the endoscopy or radiology departments. Also, patients who are unable to retain enema solutions will be embarrassed if they cannot wait for a bedpan. They may fear that the health care personnel will think they are uncooperative.

Nurses should be sure that other personnel are aware of the patient's special problems that could affect the patient during a special procedure. Nurses should accompany patients to provide continuity and support during lengthy or stressful procedures. For example, a patient must often remain on a hard table for a long period of time for some of the procedures, a particularly uncomfortable experience for the emaciated or thin older patient. Patients are also expected to move into different positions that are difficult for them to assume.

The older ill person often returns to bed completely exhausted after many diagnostic studies and is sometimes understandably unhappy. Nurses should listen to the problems the patient describes and try to work with personnel from other disciplines in solving them.

When blood is drawn for laboratory tests, the nurse, if present, should apply pressure to the venipuncture site immediately to prevent blood from leaking into the subcutaneous tissue. If adhesive bandages are applied, they should be removed after several hours to prevent further trauma to the skin.

During an assessment, a variety of adaptations that people use to cope with their health problems may be identified. For example, an older woman may manage urinary incontinence by wearing a disposable brief to keep dry. An 80-year-old man may wear a condom catheter connected to a leg drainage bag during the day when he is up and about, while during the night the catheter is connected to a bedside drainage bag. Such a patient may have to stand, each time he has a bladder spasm, to void through the catheter. Another special problem is seen in the older adult who has had a colostomy for years and has never been properly fitted with an appliance. Also, there are patients who have worn trusses for years for the reduction of a hernia. Many of these adaptations may be left alone. If a better solution to the problem is available, the alternative should be explained to the patient.

Family, friends, and physicians can supply additional information. Assessment will continue throughout the hospitalization period. Often, patients can recall events more easily and correctly when they are not rushed to respond. They remember more and answer more completely when the nurse talks and works in a calm manner.

Planning

As with any other patient, the care of the older adult should be individualized. Because the older person may have multiple problems, the nurse must make plans to give immediate attention to the acute problems and the prevention of additional ones. Skin breakdown, respiratory complications, and loss of muscle strength are potential problems for the older adult who must be placed on bed rest in the hospital.

Specific ideas for working with present problems and preventing future problems should be incorporated into the overall planning. The professional nurse is responsible for writing the plan of care. The plan must reflect changes in patient condition, appropriate nursing diagnoses, and how nursing care is to be revised. Care plans will vary, depending on the institution, but a brief form is helpful if it is individualized and kept up to date.

Intervention

Nursing intervention includes all the action the nurse takes in giving, supervising, and coordinating care. Even though professional nurses do not give all the direct care personally, they are responsible for supervising that care. Good communication is essential among the nursing team members. Nursing assistants and others have a contribution to make in recognizing changes in patients' conditions that must be reported and in suggesting action. They may be in closer contact with the patient than the nurse for longer periods of time.

During all the time care is given, there should be good communication with the patient. The patient should know the name of the person who gives the care. If one person gives care over a period of days, the patient begins to develop trust in that person. It is unfortunate for the older patient that assignments must be changed so often, because some people have difficulty adjusting to different personnel. A primary-nurse system has merit in that the patient often has the same nurse for an extended period of time. This plan seems to be beneficial for the older patient. Some nurses have found that older patients who are uncooperative or confused often respond better to one nurse whom they recognize than to new staff. Patients who are confused when admitted or who become confused during the hospital stay must be kept oriented to their surroundings, to the time of day, and to the events of the day. A clock, a calendar, a television, and the use of reality-orientation techniques by personnel will help.

Nursing interventions in the hospital may be used as examples for the patient to follow at home. An example is the medication schedule. If medications are scheduled at times that patients find convenient to continue at home, drug compliance—a major problem with older people at home—may be improved. A hospital self-medication program can be an excellent learning experience for selected older patients, during which they are supervised and evaluated in taking their own medications.

The nurse's use of medical terminology is often a source of confusion for older patients. Nurses should use clear language that the patient can understand. The nurse should use terms that patients commonly use to be able to communicate with them.

A delay in answering a patient's call light may cause a problem. Although an answer through the intercom system may seem adequate to a patient who is waiting for someone to come into the room, the time always seems longer than it really is. Time perception is a particular problem with older patients. Patients who must have assistance to get up may not wait for help if they need to go to the bathroom.

Prevention of Iatrogenesis

Perhaps the most critical nursing interventions for hospitalized older people are those that prevent iatrogenesis. For the older patient, iatrogenesis is usually related to falls, immobility, infection, and drug misuse.

Falls are a leading cause of iatrogenesis in older persons. Recognizing the patient's need for mobility and right to autonomy, the nurse must protect the patient from environmental and personal factors that contribute to falls.

The risk of patient falls is correlated with age. Falls frequently mark the end of independent living for the older individual. In a large, retrospective chart and incident report review, Lund and Sheafor (1985) investigated characteristics and circumstances of older persons who fell and who did not fall in a community hospital. Most patients fell at the bedside and were most likely to fall on the night shift. Contributing factors identified were the use of restraints, getting up alone, loss of balance, and sedation. Patients who were transferred three or more times were at as high risk for falling as were those admitted in the autumn. Other high-risk factors identified were the use of ambulatory assists, the use of certain medications including diuretics and hypotensives, and cognitive impairment (Lund and Sheafor 1985).

Riffle (1982) surveyed several studies and identified a variety of physiologic factors related to falls: *(1)* bone fragility, *(2)* postural hypotension, *(3)* decreased reaction time, *(4)* visual changes, and *(5)* changes in balance and mobility. Riffle also noted pertinent nursing interventions useful in preventing falls. These interventions ranged from the prevention of osteoporosis to the avoidance of sudden position changes. Encouraging regular physical exercise, gradual lighting changes, and heightened chair seats were also suggested safety measures. Ross (1991) suggested the use of a risk assessment tool that predicts persons likely to fall, administering the tool on admission and again if the person's condition changes significantly. Several studies have been conducted regarding risks associated with falls. Risk factors identified include poor health status, confusion, geographic location, sleeplessness, and decreased mobility (Janken, Reynolds, and Swiech 1986). In a study of falls in nursing homes, older age was a significant factor. Other factors identified were time of day—with midmorning being the most frequent time—and physical and mental impairments (Gross, Shimamoto, Rose, and Frank 1990).

Confusion is also a major factor in falls. Factors that contribute to confusion were identified by Campbell, Williams, and Mlynarczyk (1986). These factors included a new and different environment, alterations in sensory input, a decrease in control of the environment, pain, immobility, altered elimination patterns, and changes in life patterns.

In terms of ambulation, the patient's environment should be designed around functional status. For example, if the patient uses a walker or a cane, the bed should be placed toward a wall so that maximum space is available for the device. The first week of hospitalization is the most common time that patients fall, and most falls occur as the patient moves from a wheelchair or bed. Staff should be well trained on inpatient transfer techniques and should be expert in assessing the need for assistance. If possible, the area should be decorated with bright, contrasting colors toward the red and yellow end of the color spectrum. Clear demarcations should be visible between wall and floor; linens and bed; and buttons, knobs, and handles. This color scheme assists the older person with diminished sight to note differences in contours and levels in the room. Chairs should be padded; firm; with nonskid legs, arms to grip while rising, and a fairly high seat. The patient should be oriented to the physical setting at least every shift for the first two or three days and more frequently if possible. A night light or a light turned on in the bathroom provides some safety for the patient who has to get up at night. Some patients who have neuritis with burning in the feet may be accustomed to getting up and walking at night for relief. Nurses should provide the best safety measures possible.

The hospital bed should be kept in the low position for the ambulatory patient. Raised top side rails are helpful to the patient in turning and getting out of bed. They also serve as a reminder of the width of the bed. Full side rails may be a hazard unless the patient is inactive and moves very little. It is safer for the patient to have only top rails if he or she gets into and out of bed without help. Some older patients who are persistent may climb over the rails or over the foot of the bed if the rails restrict them from getting up. The nurse, patient, and family must determine the best safety precaution.

Immobility is a constant threat to the older patient, with environmental and human features, such as policies that restrict activity for everyone rather than evaluating each individual for risk (Mobily and Kelley 1991). A philosophy or perspective that actually promotes activity, rather than a more passive approach of attempting to relieve immobility, helps patients maintain mobility. The mandates of the Omnibus Budget Reconciliation Act of 1987 (OBRA 1987) are useful in the promotion of activity in long-term care settings, for example, because they require that restraints can be used only after other interventions have been tried and have failed. Policies of this sort can assist the nurse in negotiating for adequate staffing so that mobility can be provided for compromised patients (Kelley and Mobily 1991). The use of restraints is frequently associated with negative responses from both patients and nurses. In a study by Strumpf and Evans (1989), patients reported such feelings as demoralization and humiliation after being restrained. Nurses also described feeling guilty and frustrated for having restrained patients. These same patients offered several alternatives to restraints, most of which centered around increased availability of staff.

Alternatives to restraints require plans for ongoing assessments and rapid interventions for the patient who experiences a cognitive change and begins to wander or for the patient whose physical condition deteriorates to the point that safety seems threatened (Brower 1991).

Physical restraints should be used only as a last resort. There must be a physician's order to impose them, and nurses must know hospital policies regarding their use. If a restraint must be used, care should be taken not to restrict or impair circulation or cause undue pressure on nerves or cause skin and tissue damage. The best restraint may be a familiar person who can talk with the older patient and keep him or her oriented to time, place, and person.

In a related iatrogenic condition, pressure ulcers and other losses of skin integrity occur frequently and are expensive and dangerous to the older patient (Kelley and Mobily 1991). In addition to promoting mobility, nurses should recognize the additional risks of poor nutrition, incontinence, and increasing age.

Nosocomial infections are a significant factor in iatrogenesis. The most common body systems involved are the respiratory, gastrointestinal, genitourinary, and integumentary (Stolley and Buckwalter 1991). Infection control procedures should be followed carefully to protect the older person. The nurse should be especially alert to early signs of infection in this population because the usual symptoms are frequently depressed, late, or absent (Stolley and Buckwalter 1991).

The susceptibility of older people to drug misuse is well accepted. Factors contributing to this misuse are the use of multiple prescription and nonprescription drugs, the variety of physicians prescribing and treating the patient, and the physiological reactions of older people to drugs. The first step in intervention is to determine exactly what medications the patient has been taking as well as when and how they have been taken. The nurse will need to evaluate possible interactions and side effects of the various drugs that the patient has been taking. The pharmacist is a valuable resource for this information, and most pharmacists are willing to assist in patient education. Once the drugs are identified and characterized, the physicians involved in the care of the patient will determine appropriate medications to be given. The nurse should carefully evaluate patient response to medications and begin teaching about medications early in the hospital experience, even though the majority of teaching will occur as discharge planning.

Older patients often need someone to be with them when they smoke, if smoking is permitted. They might doze off or if vision is a problem, these patients may not see the edge of the ash tray; they might drop ashes or the lit cigarette itself, causing a fire.

Nurses must make sure that patients are able to chew and swallow food easily. Patients who have had strokes may choke on their food. Food should be cut into small pieces, and the patient should be encouraged to chew well and swallow each bite. These patients should be observed while they are eating.

The nurse should be certain to document safety precautions taken in the older patient's environment. For example, the patient's record should consistently reflect that appropriate bed rails are raised and that the call light is within reach of the patient. Any specific teaching or orienting measures should also be documented.

Evaluation

Evaluation is an ongoing process throughout the patient's hospital stay. Peer review and quality assurance of nursing records and patient care may be used while the patient is still in the hospital. Discharge nursing audits may also be made to evaluate care and to determine what should be done to improve nursing care. Specific criteria should be developed to measure effective nursing care for the older adult.

Many hospital nursing services are changing the focus of their evaluation from one of process to outcome. An example of a positive evaluation would be that the person was discharged with the ability to meet daily needs—such as eating, dressing, and moving about the room—without assistance. Outcome criteria are tailored to meet the individual patient and are both measurable and realistic. Another example would be that a person was discharged with the ability to meet the daily needs of dressing and preparing meals with the assistance of a home care aide.

The nurse should write these criteria with the help of the patient and family. The criteria should reflect functional status, so that the patient's ability to manage daily activities is described.

REHABILITATION

The value of rehabilitation for the older adult cannot be underestimated. Independence in the functions of daily living is extremely important for older people and for those assisting in their care. The rehabilitation process is usually longer and involves more effort than for younger people, but it can help the older person maintain independence and feelings of self-worth. The early initiation of a program of physical therapy often improves the patient's range of motion and relieves pain.

Rehabilitation does not always restore normal function completely, but it can lead to such a degree of improvement that the patient can perform many of the activities of daily living. Nurses should recognize the benefits of the rehabilitative process and encourage and participate in the process.

Nurses should encourage patients to help them master doing things for themselves. Not only should nurses help older patients to be capable of functioning independently, they also should help them to develop a desire for independence.

The cost of rehabilitation measures are not covered by some insurance policies, and payments are limited under Medicare. This kind of insurance coverage must be improved. Older adults often live more happily and independently in their own homes with reasonable rehabilitative goals and care through a multidisciplinary health care group. Nurses can help make this goal a reality by becoming involved in the continuing care of the patient.

THE FAMILY OF THE OLDER ADULT

During illness older adults often turn to their families for help. Most older adults have families to which they are closely tied. The family suffers when the family members suffers. The older person's illness often places a burden on the family. Family members become concerned and are quite disturbed at times. Some families are supportive, whereas others appear unconcerned. Many families harbor fears and guilt feelings toward the older member. They blame themselves for not being more attentive to the older person and suddenly become interested and overprotective. Their reactions and behavior can be disturbing to nurses.

In the past few years, research has been conducted on the caregivers of older persons. Families of chronically ill older persons struggle with financial burdens, lack of qualified and available assistance, and anxiety about the older person and other family members. Several studies have documented the stress and strain on families as they have attempted to keep the older individual out of an institution (Wilson 1989; Schirm and Fenell 1991; Baillie, Norbeck, and Barnes 1988).

The nurses should include the family as much as possible in the plan of care for the hospitalized older patient. Families should be kept informed and encouraged to be involved in the older patient's care. It is essential to include the family in plans for the patient's home care, so that they can help the older family member remain as independent as possible.

At this time the nurse should recognize that some families may use the hospitalization as a time to rest or to catch up on other obligations. Family members may have many outside responsibilities and cannot be as attentive to the patient in the hospital as many nurses and hospital personnel would like. The nurse should express an understanding of their problems.

The nurse should be able to refer families to resources to help them cope. These resources may include such things as written material, support groups, senior day-care centers, or home health agencies. Families are an important resource for the older patient and the nurse's ability to help them will also help the patient. See chapter 19 for more details on family caregiving.

SUMMARY

Because the older population is steadily growing larger, there are more older people who require hospitalization. They deserve specialized care, and nurses should be prepared to give that care. Nurses must understand the normal aging process and recognize deviations from the normal. Also, nurses should be aware of the numerous problems related to hospitalization that can occur as a result of the aging process. The nurse should prevent iatrogenic conditions from developing while the older person is hospitalized.

The patient in the hospital must deal not only with the medical diagnosis but also with the psychologic, social, and economic problems associated with aging. Solutions to all these problems should be sought throughout the patient's hospital stay.

Nurses should assess the problems and needs of every hospitalized older adult in their care. The nurse should enlist the help of people in all health care disciplines to enhance the total care the patient receives. Nurses should use every opportunity, in or out of the hospital, for improving the nursing care of the older adult. The patient often learns how to prevent problems or illness and how to manage care at home as a result of the care and instruction gained from the nurse in the hospital. Sometimes this type of comprehensive care will make it possible for patients to stay in the familiar surroundings of their own homes and postpone their admission to another health care facility.

The nurse must recognize that the older person's responses may be slower and should therefore give nursing care in an unhurried manner. Nurses should have patience, understanding, and genuine concern for the older person in the hospital. Gerontological nursing also includes care and support of the family of the older adult.

STUDY QUESTIONS

1. Apply demographic characteristics of older persons in the United States to statistics on health problems and hospitalization.

2. State common reasons for hospitalization of older persons.

3. Identify potential relocation considerations for older patients.

4. Describe the differences between disease assessment and functional assessment.

5. Explain the role of the nurse in admitting an older person to the hospital.

6. Describe special considerations before and during diagnostic studies when the patient is old.

7. Discuss the major causes of iatrogenesis in the hospital and how to prevent them.

8. Describe the role of the nurse in assessing medication use by the older hospitalized patient.

9. Identify common interventions used to deal with confusion in hospitalized older adults.

10. Discuss family concerns when an older person is hospitalized.

REFERENCES

American Association of Retired Persons (AARP) and Administration on Aging. 1991. *A Profile of Older Americans.* Washington, DC: United States Department of Health and Human Services.

Andersen, G.P. 1989. A fresh look at assessing the elderly. *RN* 31(6):28–39.

Baillie, V., J.S. Norbeck, and L.E. Barnes. 1988. Stress, social support, and psychological distress of family caregivers of the elderly. *Nurs Res* 37(4):217–22.

Brower, H.T. 1991. The alternatives to restraints. *Journal of Gerontological Nursing* 17(2):18–22.

Campbell, E., M. Williams, and S. Mlynarczyk. 1986. After the fall—confusion. *Am J Nurs* 86(2):151–54.

Cohen, E.S. 1990. The elderly mystique: Impediment to advocacy and empowerment. *Generations* (supplement). 14:13–16.

Dean, A. 1987. The aging surgical patient: Historical overview, implications, and nursing care. *Perioperative Nursing Quarterly* 3(1):1–7.

Dempsey-Lyle, S. and T.L. Hoffman. 1991. *Into Aging*. Thorofare, NJ: Slack, Inc.

Fulmer, T.T. 1991. Grow your own experts in hospital elder care: The gerontological resource nurse. *Geriatric Nursing* 12(2):64–66.

Golightly, C., M. Bossenmaier, J. McChesney, B. Williams, and S. Wyble. 1984. Planning to meet the needs of the hospitalized elderly. *J Nurs Adm* 14(5):29–30.

Gross, Y.T., Y. Shimamoto, C.L. Rose, and B. Frank. 1990. Why do they fall? Monitoring risk factors in nursing homes. *Journal of Gerontological Nursing* 16(6):20–25.

Grau, L. and C. Kovner. 1991. Comorbidity, age, and hospital use among elderly Medicare patients. *Journal of Aging and Health* 3(3):352–67.

Heine, C.A. 1988. The gerontological nurse specialist: Examination of the role. *Clinical Nurse Specialist* 2(1):6–11.

Janken, J.K., B.A. Reynolds, and K. Sweich. 1986. Patient falls in the acute care setting: Identifying risk factors. *Nurs Res* 35(4):215–19.

Kane, R.A. and R.L. Kane. 1981. *Assessing the Elderly: A Practical Guide to Measurement*. Lexington, MD: Lexington Books.

Kane, R.L., J.G. Ouslander, and I.B. Abrass. 1989. *Essentials of Clinical Geriatrics*. 2d ed. New York: McGraw-Hill.

Kelley, L.S. and P.R. Mobily. 1991. Iatrogenesis in the elderly: Impaired skin integrity. *Journal of Gerontological Nursing* 17(9):24–29.

Lidz, C.W. and R.M. Arnold. 1990. Institutional constraints on autonomy. *Generations* (supplement) 14:65–68.

Lund, C. and M. Sheafor. 1985. Is your patient about to fall? *Journal of Gerontological Nursing* 11(4):37–41.

May, D.S., J.J. Kelley, J.M. Mendlein, and P.L. Garbe. 1991. Surveillance of major causes of hospitalization among the elderly, United States, 1988. *Morbidity and Mortality Weekly Report* (April) 40 (SS-1):7–17.

Mobily, P.R. and L.S. Kelley. 1991. Iatrogenesis in the elderly: Factors of immobility. *Journal of Gerontological Nursing* 17(9):5–10.

Palmateer, L. and J. McCartney. 1985. Do nurses know when patients have cognitive deficits? *Journal of Gerontological Nursing* 11(2):6–16.

Panicucci, C. Functional assessment of the older adult in the acute care setting. 1982. *Nurs Clin North Am* 18(2):355–63.

Pergrin, J. 1987. Are we sensitive enough? *Journal of Gerontological Nursing* 13(4):11.

Putney, K.A., J. Hauner, T. Hall and R. Kobb. 1990. Case management in long-term care: New directions for professional nursing. *Journal of Gerontological Nursing* 16(12):33.

Riffle, K. 1982. Falls: Kinds, causes, and prevention. *Geriatric Nursing* 3(3):165–69.

Reilly, C.H. 1989. The consultive role of the gerontological nurse specialist in hospitals. *Nurs Clin North Am* 24(3):733–40.

Ross, J.E.R. 1991. Iatrogenesis in the elderly: Contributors to falls. *Journal of Gerontological Nursing* 17(9):19–23.

Ryan, M.C. and G. Roginson-Smith. 1990. What does it mean? Making sense of the hospital experience. *Journal of Gerontological Nursing* 16(8):17–20.

Schirm, V. and S. Fennell. 1991. Nurse empathy to caregivers of chronically ill elders. *Journal of Gerontological Nursing* 17(10):26–28.

Schreier, R.W. 1990. *Geriatric Medicine*. Philadelphia: W.B. Saunders.

Stolley, J.M. and K.C. Buckwalter. 1991. Iatrogenesis in the elderly: Nosocomial infections. *Journal of Gerontological Nursing* 17(9):30–34.

Strumpf, N.E. and L.K. Evans. 1989. Physical restraint of the hospitalized elderly: Perceptions of patients and nurses. *Nurs Res* 37(3):132–37.

Tobis, J. 1982. The hospitalized elderly. *JAMA* 248(7):874.

Williams, M.A., J.R. Holloway, and M.C. Winn. 1979. Nursing activities and acute confusional states in elderly hip fracture patients. *Nurs Res* 28(1):25–35.

Wilson, H.S. 1989. Family caregiving for a relative with Alzheimer's dementia: Coping with negative choices. *Nurs Res* 38(2):94–98.

Wood, L.A. 1991. Geriatric case management: The time is now. *Journal of Gerontological Nursing* 17(4):3.

13 Emergency Care

Carol A. Reynolds

CHAPTER OUTLINE

FOCUS

The focus of this chapter is to examine why and when older people utilize emergency medical services and the nurse's role in making the experience safe and less threatening.

OBJECTIVES

1. Identify the reasons why older people often utilize emergency services as their primary health care.

2. Discuss a few selected medical conditions that present some unique problems to the older emergency patient.

3. Explore ways to decrease the prevalence of accidents in older adults.

4. Discuss the physiologic problems that can complicate the assessment of the older patient and provide suggestions for facilitating the process.

5. Discuss the special needs of older patients in the emergency room and ways a nurse can meet those needs in the emergency setting.

Little attention has been paid to the use of emergency services by older adults despite the fact that utilization continues to increase. In fact many older adults list hospital clinics, emergency departments, or outpatient departments as their regular source of medical care (Lowenstein, Crescenzi, Kern, and Steel 1986). Utilizing these types of services is not necessarily an arrangement of convenience. But it is one of necessity because many older adults may have problems with self-care, lack of family support, have difficulty finding a physician who accepts Medicare assignment, or lack insurance coverage for outpa-

tient care. Getting to the emergency department is difficult for many older adults because they often do not have their own transportation and must rely on others or take public transportation. Upon admission to the emergency department, their evaluation is more time-consuming because their condition is usually more complex. They often have multiple chronic problems. They also have a greater chance of having a serious medical problem. Doubtless, the older patient population presents a multifaceted challenge for the emergency setting. Much progress is yet to be made in learning of the specific health characteristics and emergent needs of this age group (Dunne and Strauss 1986; Strauch 1986).

REASONS FOR EMERGENCY DEPARTMENT VISITS

The emergency department services older adults in three ways: *(1)* as a primary care provider, *(2)* as a place for receiving emergent and urgent care, and *(3)* as an entry into the acute or long-term health care system (Lowenstein et al. 1986). Older patients who use the emergency department as their primary care resource often do so because of limited economic resources. They have insufficient funds to access and pay for health care, so they go to the emergency department because those services are reimbursed in part through Medicare. Older patients are frequently unaware of available supportive community services. They do know, however, that the emergency department can provide immediate and comprehensive care as well as entry into the health care system if appropriate (McDonald and Abrahams 1990).

Many older people have self-care problems that they are unable to resolve. If they have little or no personal or family support, they are forced to look elsewhere in times of need. This is the group that utilizes the emergency department seven to thirty times more frequently than those older people with a supportive extended family who live in the area (McDonald and Abrahams 1990).

Emergent and urgent care for older adults accounts for a very significant percentage of visits to the emergency department. Lowenstein's study found that only 31 percent of the visits to the emergency department by those under 65 years of age were urgent or emergent compared with 37 percent of those 65–74 years of age and 45 percent of the visits of those 85 years and over (Lowenstein et al. 1986). The outcome of emergency care resulted in a higher percentage of older people being admitted to the hospital: 18 percent of those under 65 years, 33 percent of those between the ages of 65 and 74, and 47 percent of those over 75 years of age. It was also noted that of those released from the emergency department, a significant percentage of those over 75 years of age returned within fourteen days for additional treatment for the same medical problems. This may occur because many of the patients who are over

75 years of age have problems with self-care (Lowenstein 1986).

Because of its role in giving primary care as well as emergent care to patients who have little knowledge of available services, the emergency department becomes the natural agency for the referral of older patients to appropriate agencies in the community. Vitally important, then, is the access of up-to-date information regarding supportive community services (Wilson et al. 1983).

COMMON CONDITIONS REQUIRING EMERGENCY CARE

It is beyond the scope of this chapter to discuss all the major conditions requiring emergency care. Rather, a few major emergency conditions have been selected because of the consequences that occur in older adults.

Constipation

Constipation does not seem to compare in gravity to such critical emergencies as heart attack, congestive heart failure, stroke, or hip fracture. It is, however, a common malady that can cause a great deal of anxiety and discomfort and in some cases impair cognitive functioning. Incapacitation can occur when the condition progresses to a state of fecal impaction (Kane et al. 1989). Fecal impaction often occurs because it was recognized too late or because self-care measures were not successful. At this point the patient often presents to the emergency department. Relieving the condition is often difficult and can be very exhausting. Occasionally the procedure is not immediately successful. In those cases inpatient hospitalization may be necessary so that evacuation methods can be continued after the patient has had time to rest.

In the older adult several factors frequently contribute to constipation: faulty diet (too little fiber and too little fluid intake), loss of rectal sensation, and prolonged or excessive use of laxatives (Pemberton 1989). These factors should be investigated by the nurse. Appropriate predischarge counseling on how to prevent recurrence should be discussed with the patient and/or family. They need to be informed of the ill effects of chronic laxative use, the need for establishment of a daily routine for bowel evacuation, and the need to increase fluid intake to a minimum of two liters per day (more during hot weather). Taking adequate fluids may require specific planning with older people because they often see it as too large an amount to take. Plans for increasing fiber should also be discussed. Fiber can easily be added to the diet with high-fiber items such as bran cereal, fruits, vegetables, beans, and dried fruits. Phyllis Summers, M.S., R.N. (1991), a Gerontology Clinical Nurse Specialist, offers a high-fiber fruit ball recipe that she has found to be effective as one element in a program to prevent constipation, Table 13-1.

The essence of a successful preventive plan is to keep it simple and gain the patient's cooperation by discussing and planning rather than merely providing instructional statements. Preventive measures will enhance the patient's sense of well-being and independence through the development of better self-care skills (Kenny 1990).

Environmental Emergencies

Body temperature is maintained by an internal thermostat that triggers physiologic mechanisms for heating or cooling the body. This maintains a constant core temperature despite the extremes in the surrounding environment. Older people are less able to adjust to extremes in environmental temperatures. Therefore both hypothermia and hyperthermia are

conditions found primarily in this age group. Although these disorders tend to be underreported, there is information that indicates that morbidity and mortality increase during very hot and very cold periods. There are numerous factors that contribute to the risk of hyperthermia and hypothermia, including alterations in thermoregulatory, cardiovascular, respiratory, and central nervous system functions. Older persons are often on medications that can affect perception of a physiologic adjustment to changes in surrounding temperatures. They may also have abnormalities in fluid balance as well as changes in lean body mass and in the proportion of fatty tissue. Socioeconomic status often plays a significant role when older people cannot afford adequate housing or adequate heating and cooling to protect themselves from the elements.

Heat Illness. Heat illness includes several entities: heat edema, heat syncope, heat exhaustion, and heat stroke. The first three are not lethal in themselves but could compromise the older adult to a greater degree than a younger person. These four conditions will be addressed separately even though they may very well be related and progressive.

Heat Edema. Symptoms of a heat edema condition are swollen feet and ankles. The swelling can be relieved by elevation of extremities. Though this is a relatively benign condition, in the older adult with a

---

Table 13–1   Fruit Ball Recipe

1 cup dried raisins

1 cup dried prunes, chopped

1 cup dried figs, chopped

1 cup dried apricots, chopped

1 cup chopped peanuts (may omit if hard for patient to chew)

1 ounce psyllium (as found in products such as Metamucil)

1 cup mashed bananas

May add coconut for taste if desired

Mix all together and form into one-inch balls

Freeze entire fruit ball and take one out in the evening an hour before bedtime.

Eat one fruit ball every night before bedtime.

Anonymous

cardiovascular condition the patient may need to be evaluated for electrolyte balance and possible need for diuretics (Judd and Dinep 1986).

Heat Syncope. Heat syncope can occur as a result of vasodilation and pooling of blood in the lower extremities. It is more likely to occur if there has been excessive perspiration. Patients may require some fluid replacement either orally or intravenously, depending on the condition of the patient (Judd and Dinep 1986).

Heat Exhaustion. Heat exhaustion is the result of sweat dehydration following exposure to heat, humidity, and overexercise. Patients may present with vasomotor collapse manifested by low blood pressure; thready, rapid pulse; fatigue or weakness; profuse perspiration; pale, cool, and clammy skin; and perhaps some confusion. Body fluids need to be replaced and electrolyte status evaluated (Judd and Dinep 1986).

Hyperthermia (Hyperpyrexia/Heat Stroke). Heat stroke is the loss of body temperature regulation. Patients present with hot, dry skin; no perspiration; and a core temperature of greater than 104° F (40° C). The pathophysiology of hyperthermia is that the thermostat has been reset to an abnormally high level. This in turn decreases warmth perception, and blocks the cooling mechanisms of sweating and peripheral vasodilation. Retained heat eventually has a negative effect on all the major organs of the body. This effect is most likely ischemia, because the metabolic demand for oxygen exceeds the supply. Hyperthermia has a 50 percent mortality rate for a person of any age, but especially for the older adult (Judd and Dinep 1986).

Environmental hyperthermia in the young person is almost always brought on by exertion. Exertion-induced heat stroke is rapid in onset, so the need for emergency treatment becomes quickly and dramatically obvious; in an older person it progresses more slowly and insidiously. Predisposing factors are environmental and socioeconomic as well as physiologic. Prolonged heat wave is the primary environmental factor; cardiovascular disease is the most important physiologic factor. A typical situation of affected older adults is that of being subjected to temperatures higher than 90° F (32° C) and a relative humidity above 50 percent for over forty-eight hours. Other complicating factors may be underlying debilitating

disease, infection, or obesity. Patients experience gradual dehydration, confusion, lethargy, and delirium over a period of days and then may go into coma. Cardiovascular disease may precipitate a hypodynamic state preventing heat dissipation. Medications are frequently prescribed which can further compromise their ability to handle hyperthermia. Examples of commonly used medications are phenothiazines and antihistamines, which inhibit sweating, and haloperidol and propranolol, which inhibit the thirst mechanism. Many receive diuretics, which decrease circulatory volume and further limit the vasodilation and perspiration needed for heat elimination. Because of gradual development, the condition goes unrecognized and treatment is often delayed (Judd and Dinep 1986; Kane et al. 1989).

There are also some contributing socioeconomic factors. Older people, particularly those on a fixed income, often live in older homes that are not adequately cooled. Many older people live in lower socioeconomic urban areas where fear causes them to keep their windows bolted shut depriving them of any natural cooling that could be gained from air movement through open windows (Judd and Dinep 1986).

Hyperthermia carries a high mortality rate. Treatment must be geared to the rapid reduction of body temperature before irreversible brain damage can result. One of the simplest methods for fast heat reduction is sponging the patient with cool water or placing the patient, wrapped in wet towels, in front of a fan. Immersion in a bath of cold water is a rapid but extremely awkward method. It must be accompanied by rubbing of the skin to produce vasodilation. Inserting a nasogastric tube and irrigating with iced fluids may be used. Irrigating the peritoneal cavity with cold, isotonic saline (peritoneal lavage) may be helpful, but this takes specially skilled personnel and would therefore not be the first treatment of choice (Judd and Dinep 1986; Reed and Anderson 1984). Shivering may have to be inhibited by the administration of chlorpromazine hydrochloride (thorazine). Grand mal seizures are not uncommon and can be controlled with diazepam (Valium). Mannitol may be given to control cerebral edema. Cooling is to be continued until the patient's temperature falls to 102°F (38°C). Oxygen is given to meet the hypermetabolic needs of the tissues. If the patient is found to be in shock, acidosis, or cardiac failure, treatment modalities must be instituted to reverse these conditions. The mortality for hyperpyrexia increases with duration and degree of condition (Judd and Dinep 1986; Reed and Anderson 1984).

Hypothermia. Hypothermia is characterized by a body core temperature of 95°F (35°C) or lower. See Table 13-2.

Several reasons are offered to explain why older adults are at particularly high risk for hypothermia. In general they are in a poorer state of health with reduced resistance to and ability to recover from stresses. They also have a diminished sensation to cold and impaired sensation to changes in temperature. They do not always perceive a need to add clothing or seek a warmer environment. They are

Table 13–2 Degrees of Hypothermia

Classification	Core Temperature	Symptoms
Mild	90°–94°F/> 32.2°C	• Shivering (may be absent in older persons because of illness or drugs) • Conscious • May be confused • Normal blood pressure • Fatigue • Weakness • Apathy • Slurred speech • Cool skin • Sensation of cold (+/-)
Moderate	80°–89°F/ 26.6°–32.2°C	• Semiconscious • Combative • No shivering • Muscle rigidity • Dilated pupils/poorly reactive • Ventricular fibrillation with agitation • Decreased respirations • Blood pressure difficult to obtain • Bradycardia • Slowed reflexes • Cyanosis • Cold skin
Severe	80°F/< 26.6° C	• Comatose • Muscles flaccid • Apnea • Spontaneous ventricular fibrillation • Very cold skin • Areflexia

Adapted from Britt, Dascombe, and Rodriquez 1991; Kane et al. 1989.

often on medications that reduce the body's ability to protect itself against the cold. Their ability to generate heat is attenuated by decreases in metabolic rate, immobility, and defects in the thermoregulatory mechanism of the brain that inhibits shivering. Additionally, shivering is less effective due to decreased muscle mass. Heat is lost more readily because there is less-efficient peripheral vasoconstriction to shunt blood to the body core and there may be less body fat to provide insulation. Socioeconomic factors again play a part. Many older people do not have enough money to adequately heat their homes.

Little information is available from research data in the United States, but one study did show how age affects the death rate in cases of hypothermia. The average death rate from hypothermia for people ages 65–74 is nearly three times the national average. The death rate for people ages 75–84 jumps to nearly five times the national average. Those 85 and older are at greatest risk, with death rates nearly eight times the national average.

The chance for recovery is fairly good if the body core temperature does not drop below 90°F (32°C). If it drops to 80°–90°F (26°–32°C), the patient may recover but will sustain damage to kidneys, liver, heart, or pancreas. A person who experiences a core body temperature below 80°F (26°C) will probably die (Kane et al. 1989; O'Seipel 1986).

Recovery rates are related to duration, severity of the situation, presence of any underlying disease, and age. Recognition of hypothermia may be difficult because of a stereotypical association of hypothermia with obvious intense exposure to the cold. Older people, however, may experience hypothermia from prolonged exposure to house temperatures as mild as 60°–65°F. Because of this, if an older patient is brought in for apparently psychological problems, the problem may in fact be hypothermia. Belligerence, mental confusion, problems with coordination, lack of cooperation, and even apparent intoxication may be symptoms of hypothermia (Boswick, Martin, and Schultz 1986; Britt et al. 1991).

Rewarming techniques for the hypothermic older patient depend on the degree of hypothermia, the accessibility of resources, and the contraindications for each rewarming modality. Types of rewarming are listed in Table 13-3.

Slow passive external rewarming is generally preferred for hemodynamically stable older patients with mild or moderate chronic hypothermia, but who may have some intravascular volume contraction. Active external rewarming may also be used, but it should always be monitored because it has been associated with increased morbidity and mortality. The dangers with this method are further dropping core temperature by shunting peripheral blood back too quickly thereby resulting in peripheral vasodilation that can precipitate hypovolemic shock by decreasing circulatory volume. Core rewarming is necessary for those who are hemodynamically unstable or severely hypothermic. Selection of the core warming method will depend on equipment and personnel availability. Those methods that could most realistically be carried out in the emergency department include inhalation rewarming, heated intravenous solutions, and peritoneal lavage. In this latter method, dialysate is heated through a warming coil and exchanged until the internal temperature attains an acceptable level (Britt et al. 1991; Judd and Dinep 1986; Kane et al. 1989).

Confusion

Confusion is not a diagnosis in itself, but it is frequently the reason for the admission of older persons to the emergency department. In assessing an older client who is confused, the nurse must determine the circumstances surrounding and the progression of the confused state. Confusion can be caused by anxiety, hypoxia, pain, pulmonary edema, stroke, pneumonia, drugs, or other physiologic processes or emotional states. Confusion should never be automatically labeled dementia. In some instances confusion may be a chronic problem, but a thorough investigation is always warranted.

The geriatric population has a two to three times larger incidence of medication reactions than those in younger age groups. That incidence rate exceeds 20 percent in patients over the age of 80 (Schrier 1990). Confusion is a common adverse medication reaction that can be manifest by acute symptoms as well as longer-term cognitive impairment (Kane et al. 1989). A case example was 87-year-old Mrs. Tucker. She had been dismissed from the hospital after workup for severe headaches. The neurologist had ordered nortriptyline and chlorpromazine for her headaches. Mrs. Tucker received her first doses in the hospital. For home use, the nortriptyline dosage was to be increased at bedtime. Mrs. Tucker was somewhat confused on discharge from the hospital, but by the next morning she was extremely confused. She had difficulty walking and was talking to her husband, her mother, and her sister, who had all died many years before. Her daughter brought her to the emergency department because she suspected a stroke. According to her daughter, Mrs. Tucker was a very bright and very independent individual. She drove her own car, worked part-time as a receptionist, and completed the daily *New York Times* crossword puzzle "without looking up words or cheating." She had never had any

prior episodes of confusion. Examination revealed no stroke, no organic cause for Mrs. Tucker's symptoms. Her confusion was the result of an adverse reaction to nortriptyline and/or chlorpromazine. Because of the long half-life of the nortriptyline and Mrs. Tucker's sensitivity, the physician said it could be three weeks before she was back to normal, but hospital care was not deemed necessary. Her daughter made arrangements with relatives and friends to help care for Mrs. Tucker at home because the severity of her symptoms required twenty-four-hour care. During this time a long-term effect was manifest—the erosion of Mrs.

Table 13–3 Types of Rewarming

Type	Technique
Passive	Warm environment
	Heat generation via shivering
	Blanket insulation
Active	
External	Heating pads
	Immersion in warm water
	Hot water bottles
	Environmental heaters such as room heaters and hot air blankets, warm water circulating blankets or pads
	Electric blankets
Core	Heat IV solution
	Hemodialysis
	Gastric/colonic lavage
	Mediastinal lavage
	Inhalation rewarming
	Diathermy
	Peritoneal lavage
	Extracorporeal blood warming
	Cardiopulmonary bypass

Sources: Britt et al. 1991; Kane et al. 1989.

Tucker's confidence in her thinking and judgment. As the confusion began to clear, she had difficulty at times deciding if some of her thoughts were a part of her real-world thinking or a part of her confusion. Mrs. Tucker did regain her ability to complete those crosswords. But because it was such a devastating experience, some insecurity or lack of confidence persisted for a long time and affected her independence. Her daughter says she still has not recovered 100 percent of her self-confidence.

In another instance, a 90-year-old man was brought to the emergency department by his grandson. The gentleman lived alone but was seen daily by his grandson. This relative related that his grandfather had not been feeling well and that he had had the flu. He had become confused since his illness and was unable to care for himself. The grandson wanted his grandfather examined to determine if he would have to place him in a nursing home because of his "senility." Further history and a physical examination indicated severe dehydration. The old man's fluids and electrolyte balance were restored and he was released from the hospital some days later fully recovered and quite rational.

Care must be exercised in history taking lest the patient's confusion go unnoticed. Many patients appear to give accurate data, but they may use methods to cover up a loss of memory such as not answering, talking around a question, or responding without answering. An example of the latter method is:

Question: "Do you know where you are?"

Answer: "Yes."

Question: "Do you know who X is?" (referring to someone well known to the patient)

Answer: "Of course I do."

Questions should be phrased to elicit specific information and not merely a response. In cases of doubt, it is best if the information can be confirmed by a family member or other reliable source.

An additional problem closely related to confusion is that words have different meanings to people of different ages and cultures. A client who says, "I think I got bad blood," could mean any number of things. The nurse must determine what the patient means. A client 40, 50, or 60 years older than the nurse is probably viewing the world from an entirely different perspective. A 90-year-old man who remembers when medicine was primitive and a doctor was called only as a last resort when someone was dying may view the efforts of modern scientific medicine with suspicion and may not follow the needed medical regimen. The patient may appear confused but in actuality is only acting on his earlier belief that medicine and doctors are really unable to help. He may not be able to accept the opinions of a young doctor who has long hair or a beard or who is of a different race. Some older men react negatively to a nurse who is a man, because they have always perceived of nursing as a profession for women. A similar situation may occur with a woman physician.

On occasion a fear or worry is so overwhelming that the person appears confused. A 72-year-old woman who had been in a motor vehicle accident kept crying that there was no one to care for "Phyllis." She repeated again and again, "What will happen to Phyllis?" She pleaded with the nurse to go see about "Phyllis." All efforts to calm her failed and she would not answer any questions regarding her injury. After several minutes a nurse asked if she could contact Phyllis for her. The older woman finally explained that Phyllis was her dog and that if she were hospitalized, there would be no one to care for her pet. As soon as she was assured that someone would take the dog to a boarding kennel, the woman became calm and no longer appeared disoriented. She was then ready and able to relate the details of her accident. Many older people have inadequate family or friend support systems. They often turn to pets or even plants as companions, and the threat of their loss may cause temporary panic or confusion.

Accidents

Accidents are probably equated more closely with emergency department care than some other types of illnesses, even though they fall far below the incidence of heart disease, neoplasms, and cerebrovascular accidents. Accidents are ominous for older adults. An older person may die from what might otherwise be considered a minor injury because of the inability to cope physiologically. When it is considered that trauma is imposed upon a cardiopulmonary system that is weakened by age, a high mortality is understandable. When the older person does survive, the period of convalescence is longer and frequently the recovery is incomplete. Psychologically, injuries that occur as a result of accidents and fractures are frequently devastating and can result in the loss of independence.

Burns. Burns account for 8 percent of accidental deaths in older people (Bobb 1988). They are at greater risk of burn injury because of decreased sensory perception, visual and hearing losses, and decreased mobility and agility that contribute to slower response to environmental problems (Copeland 1986). There are numerous examples of what circumstances can evolve: burning a hand on an electric burner because the ON light was not seen; tripping over a space heater and catching a nightgown on fire; catching a sleeve on a pot handle, causing hot liquid to spill; stepping into a bathtub of scalding water and not being able to get out quickly enough.

Burns stress every major organ. Because of normal aging as well as the presence of underlying disease, the older patient does not have sufficient reserves to deal with the increased metabolic, cardiac, renal, pulmonary, and immunologic requirements. This increases the risk of dying among older burn patients compared to younger adults with the same extent of burn injury. This concept is depicted in a two-factor scoring system called the BAUX rule. It is used in the emergency department to predict survival from a burn injury. The method adds the patient's age to the percentage of body surface area that is being burned. A score of 75 or greater indicates a poor prognosis and high mortality probability. For example, a 25-year-old and a 75-year-old with 30 percent burns have BAUX scores of 55 and 105 respectively, giving the older person a much poorer prognosis.

The case of an older woman with a scald burn is a good example. Scald burns are not uncommon because tap water of 130 degrees can produce a third-degree burn in thirty seconds (Bobb 1988). Mrs. Patterson, 76 years old, was brought to the emergency department by ambulance following a bathtub scalding. She had drawn her bath water but did not realize how hot the water was. She stepped into the tub before sensing it was too hot. Being frail, she was unable to stop herself from lowering her body all the way into the water. By the time she was able to get out of the tub, she had sustained burns on her buttocks, perineum, feet and lower legs, and one hand.

Her total body burn was approximately 30 percent second degree. The BAUX rule gave her a poor prognostic score of 106.

Mrs. Patterson also had significant underlying cardiovascular disease, which manifested itself during the initial resuscitation. She did not tolerate the initial fluid load, her blood pressure elevated significantly, and she became tachycardic. This intolerance to initial fluid load is not uncommon in older persons (Kravitz 1988). The patient was transferred quickly to a regional burn center, where the staff concurred that her prognosis was extremely poor. She died a day or two later. The staff found this to be a very difficult situation to accept because they "had done everything by the book" and the burn "didn't look that bad."

There are a number of other predictive formulas of mortality using other predictive factors, but the BAUX rule is a quick, simple, and reliable tool for use in the emergency department (Copeland 1988).

Scalds (hot baths, showers, hot liquids on the stove) and flame burns (ignition of clothing, flammable liquids, house fires) are the most common thermal injuries. Contributing factors include use of alcohol and smoking. Older people often have proportionately larger burns compared to younger patients. This may be due, in part, to older persons' decreased ability to escape from flames in house fires. They also have a much higher number of complications and therefore much longer hospitalizations. A greater effort needs to be directed toward prevention because of the poor prognosis associated with burns in this age group.

Motor Vehicle Accidents. Motor vehicle accidents account for approximately 25 percent of accidental deaths in persons over 65 years of age. This is expected to increase as the number of drivers over age 65 increases (Bobb 1988). Patterns of injury in motor vehicle accidents are the same for older people as for younger populations. These injuries often involve multiple systems. The priorities of early diagnosis and treatment are the same regardless of age group. The problems inherent in caring for older adults involve their physiologic responses and the presence of any underlying disease(s). Shock is a common problem in the multiple trauma victim. In the older adult it can be catastrophic if there is significant underlying cardiovascular disease. The patient may progress rapidly from a state of impending shock to frank shock (Strauch 1986). Shock becomes an ominous sign as shown in a study of geriatric injury where all victims who died had suffered shock, while only six percent of survivors had experienced shock (Oreskovich, Howard, Copass, and Carrico 1984).

Falls. Falling is reflective of the fragility that comes with aging. Therefore there is a high incidence of falls among older adults. Complications of falls progress beginning with injury, then hospitalization and its intrinsic hazards of immobilization and iatrogenic illnesses, disability, possible institutionalization, and lastly death. Death from falls accounts for two-thirds of the accidental deaths among older people. Such statistics suggest that falls may be "predictors of death as well as causes" (Kane et al. 1989).

Fracture of the proximal femur is the most common fracture in older people and carries with it a very high mortality rate. Approximately 25 percent of these patients die within six months of fracture, which is twenty times the expected death rate for a similar older population. Morbidity is also high and often related to loss of the ability to walk (Heckman and Williams 1986).

Falls can be classified according to cause:

1. *Accidental.* These falls are often due to a combination of environmental factors (e.g., poorly lighted stairs, loose rugs, low tables, pets, ice, grease) and physiologic factors (e.g., changes in postural control and gait, incidence of pathologic conditions such as impaired vision and hearing, and decreased muscle strength and coordination). The single most frequent cause of falling is tripping (Exton-Smith 1977).

2. *Drop attacks.* These falls happen without any apparent cause and are thought to result from temporary muscle paralysis. One suggested explanation for this phenomenon is the movement of the head and neck in the presence of cervical arthritis. The cervical arthritis causes spondylosis, which in turn compromises the blood supply to the reticular formation in the medulla (Kane 1989).

3. *Dizziness and/or vertigo.* Lightheadedness, a common nonspecific complaint among older people who fall, can be related to a number of disorders including postural hypotension and volume depletion. Postural hypotension is a drop of more than 20 mm Hg in systolic blood pressure which can occur when the person rises too fast from a lying or sitting position. Vertigo is technically different from lightheadedness. It is a sensation of rotational movement most commonly associated with inner ear disorders. It is probably not a common cause of falls (Kane et al. 1989).

4. *Medications.* Many medications contribute to falls because of their side effects. Examples include: diuretics (hypovolemia), antihypertensives (hypotension), hypoglycemics (acute hypoglycemia), psychotropic drugs (postural hypotension), excessive sedation (postural hypotension, muscle rigidity), and alcohol (loss of coordination) (Kane et al. 1989).

5. *Dysfunctions of the central nervous system and the cardiovascular system.* These can include acute episodes (such as strokes or cardiac dysrhythmias) or disease processes that produce disability (such as Parkinson's disease).

Keeping in mind the changes in bone structure that are inevitable in the aging process, the deduction is simple that the most common injuries resulting from falls are fractures. For older adults, fracture often means immediate immobilization. Local newspapers often have news stories of older people who have spent days on the floor because the immobility and pain resulting from a fracture prevented them from reaching the telephone.

Emergency care of a person who has fallen includes

1. Thorough assessment of acute injuries.

2. Treatment of any life-threatening emergencies, such as hemorrhage or subdural hematoma.

3. Investigation of the underlying cause of the fall.

4. Allaying anxiety.

Anxiety may result from the incident and resultant injuries, the treatment, the unfamiliar surroundings, and concern about loss of independence (Grigsby 1986).

Prevention of Accidental Injuries. Some areas of prevention merely require instruction. Others require modifications of the physical environment or of certain activities. Some preventive measures may be executed by older people themselves, whereas others require assistance from other people. Some of these prevention measures may, however, be resisted, resented, or rejected by the older person, while other measures are denied them for financial reasons.

Older people should avoid abrupt motion. Rising too quickly from a sitting or lying position or turning one's head too fast may lead to hypotensive vertigo. In colder weather, older adults should be instructed to dress warmly outdoors and indoors if the temperature is 70°F (21°C) or below. If appliances such as gas space heaters are used for warmth, older people should be advised of the need for adequate ventilation to prevent asphyxiation by carbon monoxide. Space heaters should be positioned carefully so that the older person does not fall over them and start a fire. The heaters should be kept at a safe distance so that clothing will not be caught in the coils or catch fire—a common occurrence in the South, where open gas heaters are widely used. Setting the water heater thermostat below 120°F is a very good measure to prevent accidental bath scalding. Because there are many causes for house fires, smoke alarms should be installed and checked regularly. The members of the household should have escape routes planned in advance to ensure orderly and timely escape in the event of a house fire. The Burn Prevention Committee of the American Burn Association has a variety of educational materials regarding fire and burn protection. Because of the older adult's decreased pain sensitivity and agility, it is important to test the water temperature before an older person gets into the tub or shower. Smoking in bed may not be common among older people, but when it is practiced, it is hazardous and should be avoided.

Some simple and relatively noncostly measures that will help prevent accidents are nonskid treads on stairs, painting the top and bottom stair steps a highly visible color (for example, orange or red), and nonskid wax on floors. If rugs are used, they should be rubber backed or tacked down well so that they do not skid and so the older person will not catch a toe under the edge, trip, and fall. The stove should be clearly marked so that the person can tell if the burners or oven are off or on.

Other preventive measures, such as avoiding the use of high beds, throw rugs, rickety furniture, and casters on furniture, may be difficult to implement. Why might these and other changes be resisted or re-

jected? Older people usually consider their personal belongings dear, and their "way of doing things" may have become set. For example, for years an older man had his rocker in a corner of his living room with a rug in front of it. The rug "kept his feet warm." The chair looked nice against the shining hardwood floors, and just because he "had a little hard time getting around was no reason for taking his rug away." It had been there for so long without causing a problem that he did not feel he would begin to slip and fall over it now. The answer in this situation was to glue nonskid strips onto the back of the rug. Not all hazards, however, are remedied that easily.

Some preventive measures require outside intervention that may not be appreciated by the older person involved. One is the need for occasional reassessment of the older person's functioning in the home to determine if the person can safely continue at the same level of independence. Another consideration is the reevaluation of driving ability. In one family situation an 87-year-old woman had driven a car for years and felt she was perfectly safe. As the years progressed, however, her son felt that his mother's ability to drive safely had seriously deteriorated. He commented, "Mother aims her car in the general direction of town; when people see her coming they head for the side streets." The hyperbole is obvious, but the fact remained that the older woman's eyesight and response time had been decreasing, traffic had been increasing, and her shrinking stature (4'7") further limited her ability to see. A decidedly independent woman, she became irate when her son suggested that she voluntarily stop driving. The issue was later resolved by an outside source when her son felt obligated to inform the Division of Motor Vehicles that in his estimation his mother was no longer capable of operating a motor vehicle safely. The agency requested the mother to come in for an eye-and-road test. She was unable to pass the examination and her license was not renewed. There is no doubt this action struck a severe blow to this woman's sense of independence, but it was necessary to protect her life and those of other members of the community.

A helpful measure that is used by many older people is the buddy system. Many times an older person who lives alone becomes ill or injured suddenly and may lie without assistance for hours or days. Under a buddy system, friends call each other two or three times a day at specified times. If the phone is not answered, the caller telephones a neighbor, the police, or some other designated person to check on the "buddy" who has not responded.

All these preventive measures have their merits, but for various reasons not all are workable or achievable in every situation. The most optimistic and realistic approach is to assess the situation and determine what is best and most workable within the existing conditions.

Abuse and Neglect. Family violence has been in existence since ancient times, but it is only recently that abuse of older adults has been acknowledged by the health care community (Hirst and Miller 1986). Reporting of elder abuse has been sorely lacking. Correct emergency management of those victims requires recognition of abuse and neglect, knowledge of strategies of intervention, and support by the team. Satisfactory resolution is facilitated by focusing on the needs of the patient rather than on the failures of the abuser.

Both the possible victim and caregiver need to be assessed. Assessment of the victim should include a psychosocial as well as a physical assessment. The victim may have a history of frequent visits to the emergency department. Physical signs may include multiple bruises, fractures, and lacerations and abrasions in various stages of healing. Cluster bruises around the face suggest battering. Head injuries may be present from hair pulling. Most often, however, the abuse is more subtle and takes the form of physical neglect as manifested by malnutrition, dehydration, poor hygiene, and inappropriate clothing for current weather conditions (O'Malley and Fulmer 1985). Psychosocially, the victim may be withdrawn or aggressive, demonstrate infantile behavior, display poor social interactions, and express ambivalence toward the family.

Assessment is not easy because it is often hard to distinguish some symptoms of abuse from the debilitation that is produced by illness. An example is a case of a 72-year-old female admitted to the emergency department. She was a poststroke patient with partial right hemiparesis. She appeared quite debilitated and did not speak. Her daughter, who had cared for her since her stroke, stated that her mother had recently become less cooperative, refusing to eat and spitting food when it was offered. The daughter said she was concerned that her mother would starve if something was not done. The patient was found to have several problems. She demonstrated significant dehydration and had some pulmonary infiltrates suggestive of pneumonia. She also had some suspicious bruising patterns just above her knees and on the bottoms of her feet. Bruises on the left knee were worse than on the right partially paralyzed leg.

There was speculation as to how such patterns could be created. One explanation for the bruises was abuse. If it was abuse, it was conjectured that the knees could have been held down firmly by a hand while the bottoms of the feet were being struck. The bruises were more prominent on the left knee because the left leg was stronger than the right as a result of the stroke. The daughter was not able to give adequate explanation for the bruises. The patient was admitted to the hospital for her dehydration and pneumonia. Because abuse was suspected, the case was reported to Adult Protective Services. The patient was also referred to the gerontological clinical nurse specialist for in-hospital following and case management. The nurse specialist worked with the hospital social service department and Adult Protective Services to assess the family situation and begin appropriate discharge planning.

Not all situations are dealt with as effectively. One limited study discussed recognizing and reporting of elder abuse. Problems identified in the study ranged from not wanting to get involved because of potential lengthy court appearances to inability to recognize signs of abuse (Clark-Daniels, Daniels, and Baumhover 1990). Several tools have been developed to assess older people and abuse. Ferguson and Beck's (1983) tool is called H.A.L.F., which is an acronym for four factors that have the potential for contributing to abuse of older persons: *(1) H*ealth status of the older patient, *(2) A*dult's attitude toward aging, *(3) L*iving arrangements, and *(4) F*inances. O'Malley and Fulmer (1985) suggested that anyone over 60 years of age should be assessed to help the staff develop more consistent reporting and better assessment of high-risk cases.

Intervention has its limitations because the older victim has the right to reject any attempts at resolution. If there is a risk of imminent harm because of neglect, hospitalization may be warranted. This action provides an advantage to the health care team by allowing more time for complete identification of needs and arrangement for necessary services. Because the patient has the right to refuse services, health care workers must often accept solutions they consider suboptimal or even unsatisfactory. It is still important, however, to keep negotiating so that both the victim and the abusers recognize that help is available. See chapter 22 for a more detailed discussion of maltreatment of older adults.

NURSING PROCESS

Nursing practice, no matter who the patient or what the setting, is defined by the American Nurses' Association as "the diagnosis and treatment of human responses to actual or potential health problems" (American Nurses' Association 1980). The framework for this practice is the nursing process: assessment, diagnosis, planning, intervention, and evaluation. To be effective in giving care to the older patient in the emergency department, the nurse must have a broad knowledge base in nursing as well as specific familiarity with the characteristics of the older adult.

Assessment

The diagnosis and management of the older client's problems are not always easy. Many older people have more than one chronic illness. For example, a patient admitted to the emergency department may have pneumonia or trauma superimposed on diabetes or cardiovascular disease or both. Multiple diagnoses of this type make assessment and treatment more difficult. The symptoms of such illnesses or disease processes may also be viewed as "just old age," thus complicating data collection.

Altered Response to Illness. An additional factor to be considered during assessment is the older patient's altered reaction to illness and pain. Severe infection in older people may not produce such expected symptoms as elevated temperature and increased pulse and respiration. Even the white blood cell count will generally not be as highly elevated as one would expect. Instead the patient may manifest tiredness, loss of appetite, general malaise, or confusion.

In most hospitals the patient arrives at the triage (sorting) desk of the emergency department. Patients are initially interviewed and by quick and limited assessment the patient's tentative diagnosis and present status are determined. On the basis of this information the triage nurse assigns the patient to the appropriate division within the emergency department and determines whether the patient's condition requires immediate or delayed attention. Consider the following situations.

A 55-year-old man arrived at the triage desk complaining of nausea, weakness, shortness of breath, and severe midchest pain radiating to the neck and left arm. Additionally, his color was ashen and he was diaphoretic. He had had a previous myocardial infarction and a continuing history of angina pectoris. Considering these symptoms and history, the knowledgeable triage nurse had to assume—until proven otherwise—that the patient was having another myocardial infarction and transfer him to the major medicine department for immediate attention.

Contrast the above patient with an 82-year-old man who was brought to the emergency department by his granddaughter. Although normally alert he had begun to display some mild confusion earlier in the day. He did not have nor had he complained of pain or shortness of breath. His respirations were somewhat elevated and he had an occasional nonproductive cough. The patient had no weakness and the results of a brief neurological examination were essentially negative except for the mild confusion. Obviously more evidence had to be gathered because of the vagueness of the symptoms. The less astute nurse might have taken the symptoms at face value, thought the gentleman was developing a cold and that his confusion was a result of "just old age," and on that basis triaged him for delayed treatment in the minor medicine division. As it was later discovered, this older gentleman had in fact suffered a silent myocardial infarction (no pain) and his symptoms were the result of developing heart failure. This example points up the need to develop an inquisitive attitude and maintain a high level of suspicion regarding the symptomatology in the older adult.

The nurse working with older adults must recognize that there is more than one cause for a symptom, thereby avoiding the pitfall of assuming that what "appears obvious" is accurate. Because of the decrease in pain perception that comes with age, it is not uncommon that the only symptoms an older patient may show initially with a myocardial infarction may be shortness of breath with rales and wheezes in the lungs. In the absence of the pain response the symptoms are related to the heart failure resulting when the damaged myocardium can no longer pump the blood effectively. In a young person the stimulus of pain is quick and intense, causing the person to withdraw quickly and seek relief. The older person may not perceive pain as intensely. Discomfort may be minimal or absent even in circumstances in which one would expect severe pain. The absence of pain in such serious conditions as myocardial infarction and cholecystitis could delay diagnosis until severe damage or even death is the result.

In another example an 84-year-old man was brought to the emergency department somewhat unwillingly by his wife and daughter. For the thirty-six hours before his admission he had been experiencing chest pain, nausea, and weakness. Although he did not feel well, his spirits were good. His wife was relieved to get him to the emergency department and hoped the physician would admit him to the hospital.

When he was admitted to the major medicine department, it was found that his blood pressure was low and his pulse was rapid, irregular, and weak. The electrocardiogram indicated a severe myocardial infarction. An intravenous infusion was started and medication was given to stabilize his irritable myocardium. The wife was informed of her husband's condition while he was being transferred to the coronary care unit where a cardiologist was waiting. Minutes after his transfer, the patient sustained a cardiac arrest and resuscitation proved unsuccessful. This man did not seek medical care earlier because his pain "didn't seem that bad." He also thought it would go away after a while, because, in his words, "After all, I am 84 years old." This situation gives another example where the triage nurse might have made an error in assessment if she had allowed the patient's cheerfulness to distract her from his true condition.

In assessing older adults, the nurse should be aware of the possibility of blurring or vagueness of symptoms. Sometimes the problem is that the patient is unable to describe the symptoms accurately or adequately. Because of these limitations, it is important for the nurse to be aware of significant changes and the needs of the older patient in the emergency department setting.

The Nursing History. Assessment means compiling the most complete data base this situation allows. To assure accuracy and thoroughness, the nurse must

take into account the special problems or needs of the older patient. Demonstrating respect will help in establishing rapport and gaining the patient's cooperation. Calling patients by title and last name is more respectful than calling them by their first name or calling them nothing at all. Touch can convey concern and reassurance, especially if they are anxious (Ripeckyi 1984). Taking everything at a slower pace is of utmost importance. Haste on the nurse's part may be interpreted as rudeness and a lack of concern and caring. It can also confuse the patient if questions are asked in such quick succession that the patient is not given adequate time to complete answers before thinking about the next question.

Rambling Historian. The nurse must be able to detect important data mixed with reminiscences. Some patients have great difficulty in adhering to the sequential progression of their symptoms when relating personal history. This problem occurs with people of all ages at times, but many older people tend to be more easily sidetracked. For example:

NURSE: What brings you to the emergency room, Mr. S.?

MR. S.: Well, I got this pain here [pointing to his epigastrium].

NURSE: How long have you had this pain?

MR. S.: Can't rightly recall. . . . You know I've had this stomach trouble on and off since 1931. 'Course, you know, I was much younger then. Really didn't ever think much about it back then. Those were the days. I'd gotten married and times were tough—the Depression, you know. You're probably too young to know about the Depression.

This kind of verbal wandering could have many causes. It may be the result of confusion, recent memory loss, word association, loneliness, or a way to establish oneself as a person of worth or to express concerns (West, Bondy, and Hutchinson 1991). For example, a nurse asked Mrs. Spicer who managed her money. The patient appeared to go off on a tangent and began to speak very positively about herself. After awhile the nurse asked, "Why won't you tell me who manages your money?" The patient replied, "I had to tell you about me so you wouldn't think less of me." The patient needed to paint a picture of a person of inherent worth before admitting financial dependence. In any case the nurse should gently help the patient get back on the subject without cutting him or her off or being condescending.

Medication History. A vital part of the health history in the emergency department is determining what medications the patient is taking and how and why they are taking them. This is especially true of older people, who have a higher incidence of chronic diseases and who are often taking multiple prescription medications.

The nurse should keep in mind that many older clients tend to rely heavily on over-the-counter medicines. Questions about these medicines should not be overlooked, because older clients might not think of patent or over-the-counter medicines as drugs. Compliance with prescription directions among older adults is a common problem. It cannot be assumed that because a bottle is labeled with directions to take the medication three times daily that the client takes it as instructed. Many simply take a medicine "when I need it." Or else they will say, "The medicine is too expensive, so I only take one a day and it lasts longer," or "I really don't like to take medicine; I don't want to have to depend on it," or "I don't take that one because it makes me feel bad." The nurse often has difficulty deciding what medications the patient actually has been taking. An effective way of determining how often medicines have been taken is to do a pill count. Check the prescription for the date it was filled, how many were dispensed, and frequency of dose. Calculate how many should have been taken, subtract that number from the total, and compare to how many actually remain. Time after time one hears older clients identify their medications by saying, "I take a little blue water pill and then a pink one for my heart. Then I take one that I have to drink with milk because it burns my stomach." Because patients often do not know names and dosages of their prescriptions and because only each patient knows what he/she really is taking, it is best to have someone bring in all the bottles of medicines (prescription and nonprescription) from the home. Sometimes the misuse of drugs is the cause of emergency admission, either because of the combination of drugs and their reactions or because the client was not taking them as prescribed.

Sensory Changes That Affect History Taking. Sensory deficits are often detrimental to obtaining an accurate history. Such deficits cause some symptoms to go unnoticed by the patient or may cause miscommunication of information by the patient. If hearing is decreased, the patient may pretend to hear and then answer questions incorrectly. Moving to a quieter area and speaking directly to the patient with slow, distinct speech in short sentences can enhance the patient's hearing (Herr 1991). Ask one-part rather than two-part questions. If the patient does not appear to hear a question, do not increase volume and do not repeat the question. Rather, rephrase the question because the patient may have difficulty understanding certain consonants. Do not chew gum when speaking to the patient because this can confuse a patient who relies on lip reading (Summers 1991). If the patient uses a hearing aid, the nurse should determine if it is functioning. If the aid is not being worn or is not functioning, it is helpful to use a bell-type stethoscope in the client's ears while the nurse speaks clearly (but not loudly). If the patient is totally deaf, an interpreter skilled in sign language may be needed. The need for such an interpreter seldom arises, however, since an older person who has lost hearing gradually will probably not have learned sign language. An alphabet board used in conjunction with gestures may be used to assist communication. The nurse must make sure the patient hears and understands, because erroneous information could be harmful. If any doubt exists, the nurse should ask the patient to repeat what was said. The family, if available, can usually assist by validating or adding to the health history.

Visual losses also cause problems in obtaining an accurate health history. For example, normal stools may be reported, when in reality the patient simply has not been able to see well enough to note abnormalities. The client may be unaware that a fine rash has developed or that the color of the urine is abnormal. On more than one occasion, an older patient has been brought to the emergency department by a family member because of burns from a heating pad that the patient had neither felt nor seen.

Overall, the older patient can probably be expected to show some loss in sensory perception. The nurse should assess these losses and consider them while completing the data base; otherwise, some vitally important information may be overlooked. It is equally imperative that the nurse not assume that every older client has some debilitating sensory loss. Stereotyping is a constant pitfall when working with older people.

Nursing Diagnoses

Nursing diagnoses are made based on data collected during assessment. Lloyd (1984), using Marjory Gordon's classification system for nursing diagnoses, has identified those diagnoses that have relevance for older people in an emergency setting as shown in Table 13-4.

Planning and Interventions

Following categorization of the patient's health problems by nursing diagnosis, behavioral goals or expected patient outcomes that demonstrate resolution of those health problems are established. Interventions are then planned to achieve the desired patient outcomes (Lloyd 1984). Because the health care problems of older adults are multiple and complex, they cannot be resolved in the short span of an emergency department visit. The care of older adults in the emergency department often achieves only the short-term aspects of the planned outcomes (Lloyd 1984).

Priority of patient problems is done immediately upon admission to the emergency department. This differentiates those patients with problems of a life-threatening nature, requiring immediate attention, from those with problems of a less critical or long-term nature (Lloyd 1984). One format for determining priority of problems is Maslow's hierarchy of needs (Maslow 1954):

- Physiologic well-being
- Safety and security
- Love and belonging
- Self-esteem
- Self-actualization

Physiologic Well-Being. The older patient must be monitored carefully for evidence of hypoxia. The signs of anemia, common to older ill people, should be assessed. The potential blood loss in patients with multiple trauma may be significant. Any volume deficit when combined with the increased work load on

the heart from lying in bed can prove hazardous to the patient. A period of moderate hypoxia is found in a significant number of patients with long-bone fractures. The most likely cause is thought to be fat embolism. Other suspected factors are posttraumatic pulmonary microthromboemboli and general anesthesia, if it is administered before the patient has had adequate fluid and blood replacement (Martin 1977). Martin stated that pulmonary emboli can be found in 80–90 percent of cases of long-bone fractures, especially if they have not been immobilized. Clinically detectable fat emboli, however, occur in only 1–5 percent of the cases.

The older patient may be further traumatized by caregivers when they are performing life-saving procedures. In situations such as cardiopulmonary resuscitation, injury may be unavoidable. Ribs may be fractured and/or the chest wall bruised. Care should be taken to apply adequate pressure during chest compressions while keeping in mind that the resiliency of the chest wall is practically nil. It is not advisable to use an automatic cardiac compression device (Thumper) on older patients. The potential for injury is much greater than with manual compressions. After being revived, the patient should be assessed for these potential injuries.

Traumatized older adults are prone to suffer irreversible shock, apparently because of the reduced blood flow resulting from cardiovascular changes. Normally there is also a decrease in kidney tubular function. In trauma and shock there is an even further decrease in blood flow and function, which greatly contributes to permanent kidney damage. The overly zealous administration of intravenous fluids to rectify this problem may quickly overwhelm the cardiovascular system and the patient may die from pulmonary edema. Close monitoring of intravenous fluids for older patients must be observed to prevent circulatory overload.

Reduced lung elasticity is another factor to consider. Hypoxia can occur quickly if respirations are shallow as a result of pain or sedation. Because of this problem, the emergency nurse should be alert to the need for coughing, deep breathing, and turning of the older patient even if the patient has been in the department for only a short time.

Many older patients have high sensitivity and low tolerance to drugs. Therefore dosages should generally be less than for younger adults of the same

Table 13–4   Functional Health Patterns and Associated Nursing
Diagnoses Common to Older Adults in an
Emergency Setting

I.   Health Perception-Health Management Pattern
   A.   Health management deficit
   B.   Potential for physical injury
   C.   Noncompliance

II.   Nutritional-Metabolic Pattern
   A.   Fluid volume deficit
   B.   Nutritional deficit
   C.   Impaired skin integrity

III.   Elimination Pattern
   A.   Constipation
   B.   Urinary incontinence

IV.   Activity-Exercise Pattern
   A.   Decreased activity tolerance
   B.   Ineffective airway clearance
   C.   Ineffective breathing pattern
   D.   Decreased cardiac output
   E.   Potential for joint contractures
   F.   Impaired physical mobility
   G.   Self-care deficit
   H.   Chronic alteration in tissue perfusion

V.   Cognitive-Perceptual Pattern
   A.   Cognitive impairment
   B.   Pain
   C.   Uncompensated sensory deficit

VI.   Sleep-Rest Pattern
   A.   Sleep pattern disturbance

VII.   Self-Perception/Self-Concept Pattern
   A.   Anxiety
   B.   Reactive depression

VIII.   Role-Relationship Pattern
   A.   Dysfunctional grieving
   B.   Social isolation
   C.   Translocation syndrome
   D.   Impaired verbal communication

IX.   Coping-Stress Tolerance Pattern

weight. Even then the patients should be observed closely for signs of overdose or intolerance, especially after the administration of depressant or narcotic medications.

Safety and Security. Apart from saving lives, the single most important function of the nurse dealing with the older patient in a crisis situation is to modify, as much as possible, the trauma the patient is experiencing.

Preventing Further Injury. A number of interventions are applicable in the emergency setting to protect the older patient from injury. Stretchers should always be in their lowest position and siderails up. Placing the patient in an area close to the nurses' station is better for observing and hearing the patient. Leaving cubicle curtains open, when appropriate, provides a better view of the patient and lets the patient see the personnel. The patient should be allowed to wear his/her glasses and hearing aid. Being able to see and hear enhances comfort in a new environment.

Allowing a relative or friend to stay with the patient has many benefits. Patients feel more secure having someone they know at their side. A relative or friend will help to maintain the patient's mental orientation. It is well known that removing older people from their familiar environment causes disorientation and confusion, sometimes to a frightening degree. Having another person close by further enhances safety because the patient is less likely to try to get out of bed unattended if a relative is there to meet needs and to remind the patient to stay in bed. Also, having a visitor while waiting on tests and examinations decreases loneliness and helps the time go by faster.

A call button should be placed within easy reach of the patient and the patient should be instructed on its use each time the nurse sees the patient. If there are no call buttons available and the patient cannot be positioned close to the nurses' station, a small bell may serve the patient's needs. If the patient is confused, it is better to have someone at the bedside monitoring the patient than to apply restraints. Restraints often distress the patients and cause them to be agitated.

Comfort Measures. Older adults tend to become chilled very easily. The nurse should cover the patient with blankets as well as a sheet. When being transported by wheelchair, the patient should be draped with a blanket to avoid becoming chilled while being taken through breezy hospital corridors.

It is necessary to anticipate patient needs and responses related to certain treatments. If a patient has been given an enema or a diuretic, it is important that a bedpan, portable commode, or a bathroom be readily accessible. If urgency is experienced and there is no one around to help, the patient may fall while trying to get out of bed or may become embarrassed if he or she loses control.

Older patients have longer stays in the emergency department (Lowenstein et al. 1986). Additionally, older people often are arthritic and have limited mobility. Being confined for long periods of time on hard, narrow, uncomfortable stretchers can produce pain as well as pressure areas. Frequent position changes prevent severe discomfort and decrease the possibility of pain and stiffness. Slide boards can be used to move patients from one surface to another, such as from stretcher to X-ray table. Their use eliminates the possibility of pulling patients across sheets.

Anticipating what is to be done, the nurse can prevent unnecessary inconvenience to the patient. Occasionally additional blood has to be drawn on patients when a consultant orders more laboratory work. Drawing an additional tube of blood during the initial venipuncture often prevents the need for a second venipuncture. If a patient voids, the specimen should be saved in case a urine analysis may be ordered.

Love and Belonging

Consideration of Family. Not only must the patient's needs be considered but also those of significant others. An older woman was brought to the emergency department after a motor vehicle accident. Because she was not severely injured, she was to be discharged. Just before her dismissal her husband was brought to the hospital after being notified of the accident. He was extremely distraught about his wife's accident and wanted to see her. The nurse who was caring for the woman informed her husband that he could not enter the patient area to see his wife, but he assured the gentlemen that his wife was just fine and was dressing for dismissal. The nurse denied permission to the husband because *(1)* visitors were not allowed in the treatment area when it was busy (and it was busy at that time) and *(2)* the nurse knew the patient to be in satisfactory condition and thought the husband should take the nurse's word for it. The flaw in the nurse's reasoning was that rules are enacted to provide safe, quality care to patients and to ensure a smoothly functioning organization. Rules are not cast in stone and should be reasonably flexible. The husband was not questioning the nurse's credibility or judgment; he merely needed the opportunity to spend a private moment with his wife to see for himself that his spouse was safe.

Self-Esteem. Human touch is an effective supportive measure because it can bring a sense of security and understanding, thus decreasing the loneliness the patient may feel. A good example of this approach is that of an 83-year-old woman who was brought to the emergency department because she was constipated. The efforts made at home combined with the procedures employed in the emergency department for relieving the impaction left the woman uncomfortable and extremely tired. The traumatic situation caused her to seek the security she had known as a child and she began crying and calling for her "mama." She was not really confused, as might be concluded from this behavior; she was just calling out for comfort. The nurse responded by holding the patient in her arms and soon the patient was able to relax and stop crying.

Modesty is very important to the older patient, so the nurse should be sure that gowns are properly fastened and that the patient is adequately covered. Modesty should not be forgotten during physical examinations, which can be done without totally exposing the patient.

Patients' Personal Possessions. All people define their territory by filling it with collections of personal possessions, thereby establishing it as their own. Possessions often take on a special meaning for older people because they now possess less of other things that in our culture nurture self-esteem, such as jobs, recognition, success, social involvement, power, and wealth. For this reason the nurse should make every effort to keep from stripping the older patient of all possessions upon admission to the emergency department. The older woman, for example, should be allowed to keep her purse within reach.

Older people not only have favorite possessions but often favorite pieces of clothing. For example, an older woman was admitted to the emergency department with a possible fractured hip. She was wearing a girdle. The most logical way to remove it was to cut it off. She gave permission by saying that the girdle was old and that she had several new ones at home. From this comment the nurse assumed that the loss of this article was not of great importance to the patient. No so, because after a pause the woman followed her initial statement by saying, "I have so many new ones, but I like this one best." The girdle still had to be cut off, but the nurse took a little extra time and care to cut along the seam so that the girdle could be saved and perhaps sewn and worn again. It did not take much more time to cut along the seam and this action served two purposes. The woman did not lose her "favorite girdle" and the nurse's action formed a bond of understanding and appreciation between the patient and the nurse. The act of taking care of something of value to the patient conveyed to the patient the nurse's concern for her personally. Obviously there are situations where there is not time to cut along a seam neatly to save an article of clothing, but when there is time, the nurse should be sensitive to this type of need and act accordingly. Also, nurses should consider that many older patients are on fixed or limited incomes and cannot readily replace a coat or jacket that has to be cut off.

Respect for Patient Worth. Rushing, impatience, and inattentiveness can be upsetting to anyone, but they probably have a more devastating effect on older patients because by virtue of age and disabilities they have less autonomy and power. Through no fault of their own, older patients may no longer move as fast physically or mentally. If the nurse expresses impatience with the patient's slowness or is not attentive, the patient may feel very unimportant. An example of this is an 87-year-old woman who was brought to the emergency department by ambulance with a tentative diagnosis of stroke. Upon examination the physician began talking to the patient's daughter as though the patient was not there. The patient appeared alert and was talking sensibly. But as part of his examination, the physician tried to ascertain the patient's degree of orientation by asking, "Who is the president of the United States?" The patient struggled with the question. She could tell the physician the president's wife's name. She continued to try to remember but the physician went on to speak to the daughter again as if the patient was not there. He told the daughter that the patient has experienced a transient ischemia attack rather than a stroke. Because of the patient's improved status, she was capable of understanding what the physician was saying but he did not offer her any explanation about her condition. He then left the room. In this situation the patient felt rushed while she was struggling with the answer. The physician did not wait for her to answer and began speaking directly to the daughter.

Patient Education. There are problems that cannot be solved through education, but many behaviors can be changed if the patient is convinced of the value of change. For this reason it is important that the educational experience be tailored to the learning process of the older adult and made meaningful by relating the information to the patient's activities of daily living. Patient and family education must also be adapted in the emergency department because of the limits of the visit. Teaching methods also must be modified to compensate for functional deficits. These methods include allowing extra time for instruction, writing out after-care instructions, using illustrations and demonstrations if the patient cannot read, relating the instructions to the patient's daily routine, using simple terminology, emphasizing areas of particular concern, and involving family members if possible (Lloyd 1984).

Evaluation

Evaluation of effectiveness of the nursing process is difficult because of the briefness and discontinuity of the emergency service. In some hospitals, a call-back system is used. The purposes of the call-back are to *(1)* find out how the patient is feeling since the visit, *(2)* determine the patient's compliance with the after-care instructions, *(3)* ask if any other problems have arisen, and *(4)* determine the patient's satisfaction with the care received during the visit. This evaluation procedure is not possible in every hospital. Each institution must set up evaluation procedures tailored to the setting and volume (Lloyd 1984). Follow-up is crucial if the patient was referred to a community resource. The purpose is to make sure that he/she has been able to contact the agency.

THE FUTURE OF EMERGENCY CARE OF OLDER ADULTS

Emergency departments have been an integral part of hospitals for many years, but the practice of emergency medicine as a specialty is still in its developmental stages. The same can be said for the practice of geriatric medicine. For these reasons the literature is limited on information on the care of the geriatric patient in emergency settings. At most, one can find bits of information or suggestions on the care of older adults tucked away within the contents of articles dealing with specific disease processes or traumatic disruptions. Most books on emergency medicine or emergency nursing discuss with great thoroughness the legalities, traumas, and diseases of emergency care. Almost every textbook has at least one chapter devoted to emergency care of infants and children because the pediatric specialty has clearly identified the unique characteristics and needs of the child and infant and has established care based on this knowledge. There is almost never such a chapter dealing specifically with emergency care of older adults. The fields of physiology, psychology, and sociology have identified many of the developmental changes and needs of older people. But as yet, practitioners in the fields of geriatric medicine, emergency medicine, and emergency nursing have not investigated the ramifications of this knowledge or applied it in any thorough way to the practice of emergency geriatric care. As an indication of this lack of knowledge about the special needs of older people, a general practice physician answered a question about emergency care of older adults by saying, "They can die quickly"—but he did not elaborate. Another physician did not see any significant differences in treating older people because "you treat the problem no matter who has it."

Only through further exploration and study can the specific needs of older people in the emergency setting be identified, thus providing a basis for improved care. A clear beginning in this area would be to determine the knowledge of emergency department personnel regarding older adults and their needs. To what extent do emergency nurses understand the normal physiologic changes that come with old age? To what degree do these people modify their assessment techniques based upon differences and needs of older adults? Psychologists and sociologists have identified developmental changes, needs, and crises of aging, but evidently few have related these changes to the care of older people in emergency settings. What are the attitudes of emergency personnel toward older adults? How are their attitudes reflected in the care they give? What approaches are most effective in bolstering the security and self-worth of these patients when they are in a high-stress area such as the emergency department? What use has been made of and how effective are the services of the hospital chaplain? Only through research can such data from other disciplines be applied and tested to develop the specific body of knowledge needed to give high-quality care to the older patient in the emergency setting.

SUMMARY

The use of emergency services by older adults has been increasing in recent years. They use the emergency department for primary care, emergent and urgent care, and for entry into acute or long-term health care agencies. Some older people use the emergency departments of hospitals because they are not aware of appropriate community services where they could receive needed care. Also, Medicare pays for emergency outpatient services. Some of the common conditions for which older patients receive emergency services are hyperthermia, hypothermia, burns, acute confusional states, accidents (especially falls), constipation and abuse or neglect (including criminal assaults).

The nursing process is utilized in the emergency department as in all other areas of nursing. The assessment phase is very important but sometimes difficult because older people often have altered responses to illness, e.g., different or vague symptoms, and they are not always able to give a complete or clear nursing history. The nurse should obtain exact data about medicines older patients have been taking because they often take multiple prescription and over-the-counter drugs, which may be causing or affecting their current illness.

After the assessment has been completed and the nursing diagnoses determined, intervention measures can be given relative priorities based on Maslow's hierarchy of needs: physiologic well-being, safety and security, love and belonging, self-esteem, and self-actualization. Many of the emergency treatments for older people are the same as for other patients. However, the nurse must realize that the older person's decreased ability to react to stress and adapt can increase the threat to life and independence. Therefore even a minor disruption may have more severe ramifications for them than for younger patients.

Although physiologic well-being and sustaining life have first priority, the older patient should also be made to feel as safe, secure, and comfortable as possible while in the emergency department. Family or friends can help provide support for the older patient *while* receiving emergency care. The patient and family should be given clear instructions regarding home care, if the patient is to be discharged. This is also an excellent time to teach patients how to prevent accidents from occurring in the future, if appropriate. The older person's experience in the emergency department will obviously add stress, but with kindness, respect, and competency, the experience can reinforce the physical health, self-worth, and ultimately the human dignity of the individual.

STUDY QUESTIONS

1. State three reasons for emergency department visits by older people.

2. List the most common conditions for which older patients seek emergency care.

3. Why is assessment of older adults difficult in an emergency department?

4. List several of the nursing diagnoses common to older people in emergency department settings.

5. Which category of Maslow's needs has the greatest priority in emergency care of older adults? Give examples.

6. What are some age-related hazards for older patients in the emergency department?

7. How can family and friends be helpful to older patients receiving emergency care?

8. What can emergency department personnel do to show respect for the dignity and worth of older patients in the emergency department?

9. Describe one method of evaluating the care older patients have received in emergency departments.

10. Is it realistic to expect patient education to occur in the emergency department? Explain.

REFERENCES

American Nurses' Association. 1980. *Nursing—A Social Policy Statement*. Kansas City, MO: American Nurses' Association.

Bobb, J.K. 1988. Trauma in the elderly. In *Trauma Nursing: From Resuscitation through Rehabilitation*, edited by V.D. Cardona, P.D. Hurn, P.J. Bastnagel-Mason, A.M. Scanlon-Schilpp, and S.W. Veise-Berry. Philadelphia: W.B. Saunders Co.

Boswick, Jr., J.A., J.W. Martyn, and A.L. Schultz. 1986. Hypothermia: Not just a winter problem. *Patient Care*. 20(18):84–116.

Britt, L.D., W.H. Dascombe, and A. Rodriquez. 1991. New horizons in management of hypothermia and frostbite injury. *Surgical Clinics of North America* 71(2):345–70.

Clark-Daniels, C.L., R.S. Daniels, and L.A. Baumhover. 1990. Abuse and neglect of the elderly: Are emergency department personnel aware of mandatory reporting laws? *Ann Emerg Med* 19(9):970–76.

Copeland, C.E. 1986. Burns in the aged. In *Geriatric Emergencies*, edited by R.L. Judd, C.G. Warner, and M.A. Shaffer. Rockville: Aspen Publications.

Dunne, M.L. and R.W. Strauss. 1986. Approach to the elderly patient. In *Geriatric Emergencies*, edited by R.L. Judd, C.G. Warner, and M.A. Shaffer. Rockville: Aspen Publications.

Exton-Smith, A. 1977. Clinical manifestations. In *Care of the Elderly: Meeting the Challenge of Dependency*, edited by A. Exton-Smith and J. Evans. New York: Grune and Stratton.

Ferguson, D. and C. Beck. 1983. H.A.L.F.—A tool to assess elder abuse within the family. *Geriatric Nursing* 4(5):301–4.

Grigsby, J.W. 1986. Surgical and traumatic emergencies. In *Geriatric Emergencies*, edited by R.L. Judd, C.G. Warner and M.A. Shaffer. Rockville: Aspen Publications.

Heckman, J.D. and R.P. Williams. 1986. Orthopedic emergencies. In *Geriatric Emergencies*, edited by R.L. Judd, C.G. Warner and M.A. Shaffer. Rockville: Aspen Publications.

Hirst, S.P. and J. Miller. 1986. The abused elderly. *Journal of Psychosocial Nursing* 24(10):28–34.

Judd, R.L. and M.M. Dinep. 1986. Environmental Emergencies. In *Geriatric Emergencies*, edited by R.L. Judd, C.G. Warner, and M.A. Shaffer. Rockville: Aspen Publications.

Kane, R.L., J.G. Ouslander, and I.B. Abrass. 1989. *Essentials of Clinical Geriatrics*. 2d ed. New York: McGraw-Hill.

Kenny, T. 1990. Erosion of individuality in care of elderly people in the hospital: An alternative approach. *Journal of Advanced Nursing* 15(5):571–76.

Kravitz, M. 1988. Thermal injuries. In *Trauma Nursing: From Resuscitation through Rehabilitation*, edited by V.D. Cardona, P.D. Hurn, M. Bastnagel-Mason, A.M. Scanlo-Schilpp, and S.W. Veise-Berry. Philadelphia: W.B. Saunders Co.

Lloyd, M. 1984. The role of the emergency department nurse in geriatric emergency care. In *Handbook of Geriatric Emergency Care*, edited by L.B. Wilson, S.P. Simson, and C.R. Baxter. Baltimore: University Park Press.

Lowenstein, S., C.A. Crescenzi, D.C. Kern, and K. Steel. 1986. Care of the elderly in the emergency department. *Ann Emerg Med* 15(5):528–35.

Martin, V. 1977. Hypoxaemia in elderly patients suffering from fractured neck of the femur. *Anaesthesia* 32:852–67.

Maslow, A.H. 1954. *Motivation and Personality*. New York: Harper and Row.

McDonald, A.J. and S.T. Abrahams. 1990. Social emergencies in the elderly. *Emergency Clinics of North America* 8(2):443–59.

O'Malley, T.A. and T.T. Fulmer. 1985. Abuse and neglect. In *Emergency Problems in the Elderly*, edited by E.P. Hoffer. New Jersey: Medical Economics Books.

Oreskovich, M.R., J.D. Howard, M.K. Copass, and

C.J. Carrico. 1984. Geriatric trauma: Injury patterns and outcome. *Journal of Trauma* 24(7):565–72.

O'Seipel, M.M. 1986. Hypothermia as a threat to the elderly. *Health and Social Work* Fall:286–90.

Pemberton, J. 1989. Chronic constipation: Matching type to treatment. *Contemporary Internal Medicine* September:64–70.

Reed, G. and R.J. Anderson. 1984. Environmental heat illness and hypothermia. In *Handbook of Geriatric Emergency Care*, edited by L.B. Wilson, S.P. Simson, and C.R. Baxter. Baltimore: University Park Press.

Ripeckyi, A. 1984. Psychiatric assessment. In *Handbook of Geriatric Emergency Care*, edited by L.B. Wilson, S.P. Simson, and C.R. Baxter. Baltimore: University Park Press.

Schrier, R.W. 1990. *Geriatric Medicine*. Philadelphia: W.B. Saunders.

Strauch, G.O. 1986. Approach to multiple system injury. In *Geriatric Emergencies*, edited by R.L. Judd, C.G. Warner, and M.A. Shaffer. Rockville: Aspen Publications.

Summers, P. 1991. August 18 interview at Harris Methodist Fort Worth Hospital. Fort Worth, TX.

West, M., E. Bondy, and S. Hutchinson. 1991. Interviewing institutionalized elders: Threats to validity. *Image* 23(3):171–76.

Wilson, L.B., S.P. Simson, and C.R. Baxter, eds. 1984. *Handbook of Geriatric Emergency Care*. Baltimore: University Park Press.

14 Perioperative Care

Mildred O. Hogstel
Mary Taylor-Martof

CHAPTER OUTLINE

FOCUS

The focus of this chapter is the nursing care of the older patient during the preoperative, operative, post-operative, and convalescent periods of surgery.

OBJECTIVES

1. Evaluate the risks of older patients for surgery.

2. Explore the components of the preoperative phase of nursing care in older patients.

3. Identify common problems that should be assessed during the preoperative phase.

4. Explain how medications being taken by older people can affect the operative and postoperative periods.

5. Discuss how the physical preparation of older patients may differ from that of younger adults.

6. Identify risks to older patients during surgery and how problems can be prevented.

7. Identify common postoperative complications in older patients according to body systems.

8. Evaluate nursing care to prevent postoperative complications.

9. Relate the concept of discharge planning to the surgical experience.

10. Explain the important components of convalescence after surgery.

Many older patients, even those in their 70s, 80s, and 90s, tolerate elective surgery quite well *if* they have carefully planned effective pre- and postoperative nursing care. In fact the preoperative and postoperative phases often are more critical and perhaps more dangerous than the surgery itself. No longer is age a major factor in deciding whether or not surgery should be planned if there is a need for it to prolong life, make living more comfortable, or both. Goal priorities may differ. Maintaining autonomy and relief of pain could take priority over prolonging life (Keating and Lubin 1990). Often, however, older people do not tolerate emergency or long complicated surgery as well as younger people because of their decreased ability to adapt to physical and psychologic stress. Morbidity and mortality rates for the very old (over age 90) who require surgery are much higher than for those in the young-old group (ages 70–75) (Jackson 1988).

Several years ago one of the authors cared for a patient who had a transurethral resection of the prostate gland after having had a urinary retention catheter in place off and on for twelve years because of benign prostatic hypertrophy. The family and physician probably thought that he would not tolerate surgery well at age 90. However, at age 102 he finally had the transurethral resection with spinal anesthesia. The morning after surgery he was sitting up in bed eating bacon and eggs and reading the newspaper. Because his overall condition was good, he tolerated the surgery very well. Another older patient, age 79, recovered well after having had three major operations within a period of one week. Many people in their 90s have successful cataract surgery with local anesthesia on an outpatient basis. There also have been recent newspaper reports of patients ages 105 and 108 who tolerated major surgery well.

Ambulatory or day surgery for older adults is increasing. At one time it was believed that day surgery was too great a risk for older people but now the ambulatory setting may be "the one of choice" (Dean 1987). One research study showed that the incidence of serious complications was low for this type of surgery (Frisch, Groom, Sequin, Edgar, and Pepler 1990). In another study, outpatients were just as satisfied with the care they received as patients admitted to the hospital for surgery (Gamotis, Dearmon, Doolittle, and Price 1988). Older people who do not have cardiovascular disease, are physically active, and are not confused can easily utilize this type of service. According to Crawford (1985), some of the advantages of outpatient surgery are *(1)* less chance of complications such as pneumonia, *(2)* less trauma than hospitalization, *(3)* less foreign environment, *(4)* reduced cost, and *(5)* more contact with family or friends. The types of surgery older patients often have on an outpatient basis are "cataract extractions, hernia repairs, microlaryngoscopy with laser applications, pacemaker battery changes, cystoscopies, multiple tooth extractions, hammer toe corrections, and removal of orthopedic hardware" (Crawford 1985).

Careful assessment and preparation are very important in day surgery. Cognitive assessment is especially important when the older patient has ambulatory surgery. The reasons are *(1)* to ensure that perioperative instructions are carried out and *(2)* to facilitate communication between the patient and physician or anesthetist (Kupferer, Uebele, and Levin 1988). Accurate communication between the patient and health professionals is essential when the patient is conscious and must follow instructions. Cognitive assessment should include memory, intelligence, thinking, learning ability, and problem solving (Jackson 1989; Kupferer et al. 1988). Kupferer et al. offered some practical and efficient ways to do this assessment but stressed that the assessment should be stopped (and the incident documented) if the patient showed signs of being offended. [The reader is referred to Kupferer et al. (1988) for some practical ways to enhance cognitive functioning for the older adult having ambulatory surgery.]

PREOPERATIVE PHASE

Upon admission to the hospital the older patient should be made to feel welcome, nursing staff should introduce themselves, and explanations about equipment and procedures should be clear and repeated if necessary. The patient should be allowed all the time needed to remain as independent as possible while undressing and getting oriented to the room and new environment (Jackson 1989; Kupferer et al. 1988). The older adult may need more time to move and to process and integrate information.

The primary goal of preoperative nursing care is to place the patient in the best possible condition for surgery through careful assessment and thorough preparation. Some of the factors that contribute most to a good state for successful surgery are

- careful total assessment

- good nutritional status

- adequate hydration

- control of related physical problems

- evaluation and adaptation of recent medication regimen

- physical preparation

- psychologic preparation and explanations about what to expect during and after surgery

Careful Total Assessment

Baseline data on all body systems is important for comparison with data obtained from the postoperative assessment. It will be important to differentiate the common changes caused by the aging process from pathophysiology and to understand how these common changes influence pathology. (The reader is directed to the postoperative section for discussion of assessment by systems.) Jackson (1989) suggests that the preoperative assessment should include the skin (an index to postoperative and drug complications), the emotions (depression means the patient will be at high risk for surgery), the home environment, ability to perform activities of daily living, the family's competence to provide care following discharge, and range of motion. Stiff necks or fragile teeth could influence intubation; weakened, painful, or stiff joints need special support and positioning during the intraoperative period (Jackson 1989). Communication of important findings to all members of the perioperative team is essential.

Good Nutritional Status and Adequate Hydration

Some older people—especially those who live alone, those who have denture problems, and those who have limited financial resources—often do not eat as many nutritious foods as they should. According to S.N. Walker and Love (1987, 262) "nutrition depletion impairs their ability to withstand surgery." Recent weight loss and laboratory values, especially hemoglobin and hematocrit, should be noted on admission and reported to the physician if abnormal. If the patient's condition does not contraindicate it, a well-balanced nutritious general diet including full liquids should be taken up until the period of fasting for surgery. Fluid intake and output should be measured and recorded from the time of admission, especially in emergency situations, since urinary output helps to determine degree of hydration (Jackson 1988). When warranted, fluid and electrolytes should be replaced by intravenous therapy.

Control of Related Physical Problems

Many older patients have multiple chronic health problems, perhaps in addition to the condition for which surgery is needed. The most common chronic health problems of older adults are

- arthritis
- hypertension
- circulatory problems
- cataracts and/or glaucoma
- presbycusis
- osteoporosis
- urinary tract infections

While the physician or surgeon will be aware of complications of these conditions that might affect anesthesia and surgery, the nurse should also recognize how these conditions will affect the care of the surgical patient during the total perioperative period. Nursing implications related to these conditions will be discussed where applicable.

Evaluation and Adaptation of Recent Medication Regimen

Because of the presence of many of the chronic diseases listed above, the older patient is likely to be taking numerous medications, both prescription and over-the-counter. Therefore, during the nursing history, the nurse needs to assess exactly which drugs the patient has been taking.

Medications that may have been taken routinely and that may cause complications during the perioperative period are

- aspirin (may increase bleeding)
- antidepressants (may lower blood pressure during anesthesia) (Foster 1986)
- any medication with anticholinergic effects (increases the potential for confusion) (Jackson 1989)
- steroids (suppress immunity)
- nonsteroidal anti-inflammatory drugs (increase the risk of stress ulcers and displace other drugs from blood proteins)

- bromide in medications like Sominex (can accumulate and produce signs or symptoms of dementia) (Carruth and Ross 1990)

Several specific types of medications need to be continued during the surgical experience in order to maintain vital functioning. Some of these are

- steroids (to prevent cardiovascular collapse)

- cardiac drugs (especially digitalis preparations, calcium-channel blockers, and nitroglycerin)

- antihypertensives ["must be continued up until the time of surgery to prevent rebound hypertension during surgery" (Foster 1986, 61)]

- miotics (for glaucoma)

- insulin (for diabetes)

Physical Preparation

If the skin needs to be shaved, special care should be taken to prevent trauma. There is diminished hair growth in older adults, especially in the pubic and axillary regions, and the skin is likely to be dry, thin, fragile, and wrinkled, making shaving more difficult and subject to trauma. The skin should not be shaved unless absolutely necessary because traumatized skin causes a higher risk for infection after surgery. The patient may need assistance with a partial bath the evening before surgery. Although a total bath with soap may not be needed, the operative site (especially the umbilicus if abdominal surgery is planned), face, hands, genital area, and feet should be bathed. Although large amounts of a lubricating lotion are normally used on dry aging skin, lotion should not be used on the patient's skin before surgery because it will more likely retain bacteria. Good oral hygiene is important to prevent infection of the mouth and lips because insertion of an endotracheal tube for anesthesia and oxygen may cause some trauma. Elastic stockings may be ordered for the lower legs to help prevent postoperative embolism, which is a particular threat to older patients.

If enemas are ordered before surgery, they should be given the night before, when possible, or several hours before morning surgery. There may be incomplete results due to the relaxation of abdominal wall muscles resulting in involuntary expulsion of feces on the operating table, which will cause contamination and possible infection. Laxatives should not be given in the twenty-four to forty-eight hours before surgery because of the possibility of delayed results. If a urinary retention catheter is not inserted, the patient should be asked to void immediately before going to the operating room. However, if the surgery is expected to be long, a catheter is usually inserted because the size and holding capacity of the bladder decreases in old age.

Some anesthesiologists prefer that dentures be left in place to help the oxygen mask, if used, fit the face better. If possible, dentures, glasses, and hearing aids should not be removed until the patient is ready to be anesthetized to prevent any possible embarrassment or difficulty in communication the patient might experience. If the patient remains conscious, these items should remain with the patient throughout the perioperative period. When general anesthesia is used, the items should be returned before the patient goes to the postanesthesia unit (Jackson 1989).

Preoperative medications immediately before surgery are "usually not ordered in the elderly" (Foster 1986, 65). If they are, they should be given earlier than in younger adults because of delayed absorption due to decreased circulation. Morphine sulfate should never be used as a part of the preoperative medication in patients age 65 or older because of its severe side effects and because it may cause complications in other existing chronic health problems. Neither barbiturates nor hydroxyzine (Vistaril) should be given to older patients because of their adverse effects. Fat-soluble drugs may be stored in the excess body fat of older adults. When these drugs are released from their storage sites, they could interact with anesthetics or other central nervous system depressants.

If it is necessary to give a sedative or hypnotic the evening before surgery, there are several choices. A short-acting drug is preferred so that it will not cause a cumulative effect as a result of the anesthetic being given the next day or interfere with the need to give postoperative medications for pain. Also, a long-acting sedative could cause increased postoperative disorientation and amnesia and hinder the recovery process. Temazepam (Restoril), triazolam (Halcion), and flurazepam (Dalmane) have been widely used for older adults in the past but they are not recommended now (Wolfe et al. 1988). Oxazepam (Serax) is considered safer (Wolfe et al. 1988). Other drugs recommended preoperatively include diphenhydramine, paraldehyde, chloral hydrate, and glutethimide (Matteson and McConnell 1988). The lowest range of safe dosage is usually ordered for each drug used, especially in the old-old (85 years of age and older).

A nurse or responsible family member should remain with the patient after the preoperative medication has been given because of the possibility of temporary confusion or disorientation as a result of the medication. Even though the bed rails are raised, older patients who are even slightly confused very frequently attempt to crawl out the foot of the bed or over the rails. In one study of older hospitalized patients (Lund and Sheafor 1985), it was found that the peak times for falling were from 3:00 P.M. to 7:00 P.M. and from 3:00 A.M. to 7:00 A.M. Of seventy-six patients who fell, 37 percent were taking sedatives and 26 percent were taking hypnotics. Although this study found that having had preoperative medications was one of the low-risk rather than high-risk factors for falling, it was assumed that patients receiving preoperative medications were under close staff supervision.

Psychologic Preparation and Teaching

As with all surgical patients, the older adult should be informed about what to expect, especially in the immediate preoperative, operative, and postoperative phases. Some older people never have been hospitalized and need explanations and support. The nurse should listen attentively, allow the patient time to respond, and speak a little lower, slower, and clearer than normal. Sometimes nurses try to do everything for older patients, thus increasing their feelings of dependency and decreased self-worth.

The nurse should assess if the patient is able to see, read, and understand any informed consent forms that he or she is required to sign for treatment, surgery, or anesthesia. Older patients should keep their glasses near so that "they can read lips and facial expressions and consent forms. Some hospitals have large print consent forms for elderly patients" (M.L. Walker 1986). Some older people are reluctant to question physicians or nurses, assuming that they know what is best, although this is changing with an increasing number of informed, assertive, and active

older adults. It is, of course, the surgeon's responsibility to explain the benefits and risks of surgery, but the nurse has a responsibility to determine if the patient understands what the surgeon has explained. The nurse also does the routine preoperative teaching about what to expect before, during, and after surgery. It is important, however, not to *overtell*, because some patients really are not interested in all of the details about what to expect as long as they have trust in their surgeon and nurse and feel fairly comfortable with the situation. If the patient is confused, disoriented, or otherwise unable to give informed consent, the nearest relative or legal guardian should be asked to do so.

Older patients have most of the same fears about surgery as younger patients, such as the fear of loss of control, pain, separation from family, fear of disfigurement, fear of death, and fear of the loss of a body part (Foster 1986). In one study of ninety persons over age 65 who had surgery, some of the fears identified were *(1)* fear of procedures; *(2)* "fear of one's capacity to tolerate pain"; *(3)* fear of acting like a "baby"; *(4)* fear of rejection due to the possible loss of body integrity; *(5)* fear of death; and *(6)* fear of leaving the hospital (Neugent 1981, 70–71). An additional fear, particularly of those who are facing major surgery for cancer or a fractured hip, for example, is that the surgery will increase their dependence and that they will no longer be able to live independently in their own home. Older people in their 80s and 90s often are able to function quite well independently *until* a major surgery or illness occurs. The physical and psychologic stress of surgery makes it difficult for the older adult to return to a normal level of functioning. Dependency often brings on the fear of increased reliance on other family members or nursing home admission.

Preoperative teaching should include the usual explanations about the immediate postoperative period such as the need for and how to perform deep breathing, coughing, and dorsiflexion and plantar flexion exercises. All explanations should be in a clear and concise manner, taking cues from the patient about how much or how little he or she really has a need and desire to know. Explanations and support should also be given to family members, who may be very anxious about the safety and outcome of the surgery because of the patient's age.

Transfer to Surgery

The older patient should be transferred *carefully* and *slowly* from bed to stretcher to operating table in order to prevent hypotension, muscle or joint discomfort, skin injury, and psychologic trauma. Data from the range-of-motion assessment should be clearly communicated to those responsible for the transfer. Orderlies should be taught the importance of moving patients slowly and that "dumping" them in a rapid manner can cause serious problems.

INTRAOPERATIVE PHASE

Constant observation and support should be continued for the older patient in the holding area, if there is one, or wherever the patient remains until entering the operating room.

The temperature of the surgical suite is usually kept below normal, primarily for the benefit of the personnel, but also because patients are covered with several drapes during surgery and they may become too warm. However, older patients need to be protected from hypothermia both before and during surgery. They are at high risk for hypothermia from decreased metabolism and a normally lower body temperature as well as the effect of the anesthetic agent. According to Potter and Perry (1989, 197), "a temperature of 35°C (95°F) orally is not unusual for an elderly person in cold weather." Therefore it is important to keep the older patient adequately covered in the holding area and the operating room, uncovering him/her only for a minimal amount of time for positioning and skin preparation.

After the patient is transferred to the operating table and anesthetized, the circulating nurse and other members of the surgical team should carefully place the patient in the required position. Dean (1987, 5) stated that "OR table-chairs should be tiltable, padded, and adjustable to account for individual needs." In fact, placing the operating table in a semi-Fowler's position may make the patient more comfortable, especially if a local anesthetic is being used. The position used should allow "for maximal respiratory exchange while affording optimal incisional accessibility" (Dean 1987, 6).

The patient's legs and arms should be moved slowly and carefully. With an older woman who has marked osteoporosis, turning the patient to the lateral position for kidney surgery or positioning legs in lithotomy position for vaginal surgery could cause a fracture of the femoral head or strain on the lumbar spine unless extreme caution is taken. For the lateral position, the trunk should be turned as a log; for the lithotomy position, both knees should be flexed at the same time and then placed in the lithotomy position. The arms, fingers, legs, and feet should be checked to be sure that they are not cramped in an unusual position or touching metal on the operating table. Skin pressed against a metal object for several hours during surgery could cause trauma, bruising, and ulcers very easily because of the thinness and fragility of the skin and poor circulation to the extremities. All extremities and exposed skin surfaces should be carefully checked before the sterile drapes are applied.

The skin should be carefully cleaned and prepped, using the solution that is least likely to cause continued irritation. Adequate cleaning with soap and water or an antiseptic solution such as pHisoHex probably causes less damage to aging skin than iodine-type solutions such as Betadine or Povidone. Paper tape is best to use on aging skin, and it should be used sparingly (Dean 1987, 6).

A combination of anesthetic agents is usually used in order to provide light and safe anesthesia for the older patient. Local or spinal anesthesia is often used if possible. Spinal anesthesia lessens the risk of respiratory problems so common with older surgical patients, but may increase the risk of hypotension (Jackson 1989). Most older patients tolerate general anesthetics such as nitrous oxide, which provides "more analgesia than unconsciousness," rapid induction and recovery, and is "void of hazardous occurrences." However, nitrous oxide "does have some cardiac depressant effects" (Hercules 1987, 286). The synthetic opiate narcotic fentanyl (Sublimaze) may be given intravenously. When combined with droperidol (Inapsine) or diazepam (Valium), the patient is in a "state in which there is tranquilization with little cortical depression. The client has decreased motor activity, decreased anxiety, and a feeling of indifference. The ability to respond to commands remains" (Hercules 1987, 287). This type of anesthesia is especially useful for short operations or diagnostic procedures, but the patient's vital signs must be carefully observed. Sublimaze may have a delayed postoperative effect causing respiratory depression one to three hours following surgery. It is common practice to decrease the first postoperative dose of an analgesic by one-half when Sublimaze has been used for anesthesia.

If the patient has received some type of regional, local, or spinal anesthesia and is awake, all of the surgical team should be careful in their conversation. It is important to recognize that loss of hearing does occur with age in some individuals, but it should not be assumed that all older patients have difficulty hearing. The anesthesiologist or the circulating nurse should periodically speak with the patient to determine his or her condition, concerns, and questions.

Jackson (1989) had several suggestions related to positioning during the intraoperative period. For one, the preoperative assessment of range of motion should be used as a guide for positioning. It might be necessary to consult an orthopedic specialist for the proper placement of artificial limbs (when it is necessary for them to accompany the patient). Finally, when one position has been maintained for any extended period of time, this should be documented and communicated to the rest of the health care team. This last measure will aid in preventing pressure ulcers as well as joint deformities.

POSTOPERATIVE PHASE

The nurse responsible for the patient during the postoperative period should understand not only the physiology and pathophysiology involved in the systems of the body but also the changes produced in these systems by the natural process of aging (described in chapter 3). It is only through such understanding that the nurse will be able to recognize the changes caused by pathology. Further, it is important to know that the aging process makes the patient more vulnerable to certain potential complications of surgery.

Body Systems

Most authorities agree that biologic age (judged by such things as physical appearance, blood pressure, cardiovascular status, and respiratory status) is a better indicator than chronologic age (number of years lived) of where the person stands in the aging process (Cote and Lapointe 1985). Further, each

body system of any individual will vary from the other body systems in its rate of aging. It is for all of these reasons that a recommendation is made to begin this phase of nursing care with a systems assessment (an abbreviated form of the physical assessment). A guide for such is shown in Table 14-1. This guide is intended to be comprehensive. It can be modified to expedite the postoperative assessment as needed. Additional information to assist with planning, implementing, and evaluating care of the older individual follows.

Respiratory Care. The highest priority for the older adult, as for a patient of any age, is maintaining a patent airway. In addition, preventing respiratory complications—postoperative complications to which the older adult is especially prone—receives a high priority.

Patent Airway. A patent airway is maintained by proper positioning, preventing aspiration, and keeping the airways clear of secretions. The head of an unconscious patient should be turned to the side to prevent aspiration. Adequate support should be provided for the head to prevent hyperextension and rotation, both of which will interfere with circulation in the vertebral arteries (Jackson 1989). However, the head needs to be somewhat extended to prevent blockage of the airway by the tongue. The older adult is prone to aspirate due to poor muscle tone, a decrease in airway reflexes (Burden 1989), and a high gastric pH, so prevention of emesis is especially important. However, an antiemetic is given only when necessary and even then a drug should be selected that will not depress the central nervous system. Alternative suctioning is important because the older patient already has increased closure of airways (Matteson and McConnell 1988).

Preventing Hypoxia. The older patient has a low tolerance for even a minor obstruction of the airways for several reasons, all of them related to changes in the respiratory system caused by the aging process. The alveoli tend to enlarge, atrophy, and lose some of their capillaries (Matteson and McConnell 1988; McCance and Huether 1990). The patient has not only a decreased alveolar surface but also less support for the airways. As in the patient with emphysema the airways of the older adult will tend to close when the pressure in them is decreased by low tidal volumes (Matteson and McConnell 1988). Chest wall compliance may be decreased by structural changes and respiratory muscles may be weakened. Both of these changes would interfere with ventilation.

Ventilation is facilitated best by a sitting position. The supine position also aggravates the already-existing mismatch between ventilation and perfusion (Matteson and McConnell 1988). Although the partial pressure of carbon dioxide in arterial blood ($paCO_2$) is affected very little, the partial pressure of oxygen (paO_2) drops steadily with age (Cote and Lapointe 1985; McCance and Heuther 1990). McCance and Huether (1990) gave a formula to help determine the maximum paO_2 that an older patient can attain: Multiply the age of the individual by .3 and subtract the product from 100 (optimal paO_2).

For example, a patient age 90 could not attain a paO_2 greater than 73:

$$.3 \times 90 = 27$$
$$100 - 27 = 73$$

Other factors that increase the older adult's vulnerability to hypoxia include decreased cardiac output [deceased by 40 percent in healthy old people, according to Cote and Lapointe (1985)] and a tendency for anemia. The older client has no margin for further compromise of the ability to deliver oxygen to tissues. It may be necessary to administer oxygen routinely to the older adult, being careful not to depress respirations when the patient has chronic obstructive lung disease. Further, any change in mental status (restlessness, delirium) should be considered a possible sign of hypoxia.

Table 14-1 Systems Assessment

Respiratory: Respiratory rate and rhythm. Breath sounds, adventitious sounds. Arterial blood gases (ABGs). Airway. Inspired oxygen concentration ($F1O_2$)—type of oxygen therapy, liter flow. Chest tubes—setup, drainage, presence of oscillation. Medications before and during surgery (including anesthetic). Any objective or subjective signs/symptoms (sputum or cough). Color of nail beds.

Cardiovascular: Warmth of skin. Heart rate and rhythm. Blood pressure. Heart sounds. ECG. Peripheral pulses and circulation checks as indicated. Capillary refill. Signs/symptoms. Distention of neck veins. Homan's sign.

Urinary: Changes in weight. Skin turgor. Voiding—amount and characteristics of urine. Drains. Electrolyte values. Data from intake and output. IVs—site, type, needle size, amount to be absorbed, and rate. Signs/symptoms.

Nervous: Pupils equally round and reactive to light and accommodation. Orientation. Levels of consciousness. Responses (follows commands, moves all extremities). Glasgow coma scale (when needed). Signs/symptoms. Gag reflex. Pain—full description

Temperature Regulation: Temperature. Shivering, perspiring.

Wound: Incisions, dressings. Any devices or equipment.

Safety: Needs. Emotional state. Side rails. Call light. Other measures as needed—restraints.

Gastrointestinal: Bowel sounds. Nausea or vomiting. Taking fluids—tolerance. Tubes—type, placement verified, amount and characteristics of drainage. Abdomen—distention, tenderness. Signs/symptoms.

Musculoskeletal: Condition—stiffness, contractures.

Skin: Pressure areas. General condition.

Source: This suggested guide for a systems assessment has been adapted from one developed by C. Stephenson. 1985. *Texas Christian University-Harris College of Nursing Senior I Course Manual.* Unpublished manuscript. Fort Worth, TX. Texas Christian University, Harris College of Nursing. Used with permission.

Preventing Atelectasis and Hypostatic Pneumonia. Atelectasis and possibly hypostatic pneumonia would be other ways of compromising ability to oxygenate the tissues. Therefore, preventing atelectasis has even greater significance in the care of the older patient. Other problems include a weakened cough reflex, decreased ciliary movement, and decreased protection of airways by the mucous coat (Michaels and Stephenson 1985). The patient should be positioned so that ventilation is facilitated (allowing expansion of the rib cage and descent of the diaphragm). Special precautions should be taken to prevent excessive depression of the central nervous system. The "stirring-up" regimen should start as soon as the vital signs start to stabilize. Turning every two hours and early ambulation will be essential. A special technique for deep breathing and coughing may be necessary. One such technique is to encourage maximal inhalation and holding this position for a count of three; coughing then occurs during slow exhalation. Chest physical therapy, postural drainage, incentive spirometry, and intermittent positive pressure breathing may be necessary. Matteson and McConnell (1988) recommend that the nurse compare data from preoperative pulmonary function studies with postoperative values for vital capacity, tidal volume, expiratory reserve volume, and inspiratory reserve volume.

Cardiovascular Care. It is logical to deduce that all the factors that make older people prone to hypoxia will also make them highly susceptible to myocardial ischemia. Cote and Lapointe (1985) maintain that myocardial infarction is one of the more common causes of death postoperatively in older people. This potentially fatal complication is difficult to detect because the vital signs may not change as much (the heart has less reserve) and because the pain may be naturally dulled because of the process of aging. If an unsuspecting nurse were to give an analgesic for vague and nonspecific pain caused by cardiac ischemia, the problem could be greatly exaggerated by further respiratory depression. Further, any semblance of the Valsalva maneuver must be avoided because such a maneuver would decrease venous return to the heart and compromise cardiac output (and coronary perfusion) even more.

The vital signs for the postoperative geriatric patient need to be taken more frequently and evaluated more carefully, not only because they may take longer to stabilize, but also because many of the most dangerous complications encountered by the patient in the postoperative period are associated with the cardiovascular system and may be detected by a change in the vital signs. Some such complications might be hemorrhage, shock, arrhythmias, congestive heart failure, and pulmonary embolus (following thrombophlebitis). Because the blood vessels are less able to constrict, hemorrhage and shock are more likely. These complications are also more likely for several reasons related to clotting (Jackson 1989). Older people usually have a decrease in blood proteins (clotting factors included). In addition, poor nutrition (if present) would send clotting factors (including calcium) even lower. Liver function (including formation of many clotting factors) might also be depressed. Dehydration and decreased cardiac output make shock an even greater possibility. Recent medications, sedation, electrolyte imbalance, hypoxia, and changes in the cardiac conducting system of the older adult increase susceptibility to arrhythmias (Jackson 1989). Congestive heart failure could result from the inability of the heart (with low cardiac reserve) to keep up with the additional demands made on it by the stress of surgery. Also, dehydration, decreased muscle tone, drop in cardiac output, and the restrictions placed on physical activity make thrombophlebitis an even greater threat for these patients. Indeed, pulmonary embolism may be the most frequent cause of death postoperatively in this age group. Prevention of thrombophlebitis is described in Table 14-2. Some studies, like the Baltimore Longitudinal Study on Aging, are reporting that older adults who are physically fit do not have a significant change in cardiac output (McCance and Huether 1990). More studies are needed to evaluate the effects of physical fitness on aging, a process that definitely affects the perioperative care of older adults.

Care Related to the Urinary System. Several changes in the urinary system predispose the older individual to postoperative complications. This system has the major responsibility for maintaining the internal milieu. This fact, combined with selected changes in the endocrine system, makes older patients especially prone to fluid, electrolyte, and acid-base imbalances.

Retention of Urine. Retention of urine postoperatively is more common in older patients. Weakened muscles, decreased sensitivity to neurologic stimuli for

Table 14–2 Prevention of Thrombophlebitis

1. Have client exercise ankles and legs (actively, if possible) every hour.

2. Use antiembolism stockings.

3. Avoid pressure under the knees (clients should *not* cross legs; pillows or other objects should *not* be placed under the knees).

4. Check neurovascular signs (color, temperature, movement, sensation, and circulation) in both legs frequently.

5. Check both calves frequently for signs/symptoms of thrombophlebitis (redness, heat, swelling, pain, or positive Homan's sign).

6. If necessary, measure both calves daily.

7. Begin ambulating as soon as possible.

8. Continue active exercise within restrictions imposed by client's condition.

voiding, and a side effect of anticholinergic medication (when it is used) contribute to this problem. In addition, men are likely to have some prostatic hypertrophy. Nurses will need to apply all of the knowledge and skill acquired in dealing with urinary retention, remembering that assuring privacy and assisting men to stand are two important nursing interventions. Catheterization should be postponed as long as possible because the older adult has decreased immunity (McCance and Huether 1990).

Acute Renal Failure. The amount of water contained in the body of older adults drops from 60 percent to 50 percent of the total body weight. Therefore they will have a decreased volume in the plasma compartment. Because they have a decreased volume in this compartment, they may be more apt to develop acute renal failure for two reasons: (1) diminished renal blood flow (could be due to other causes as well) and (2) increased concentration of excreted drugs in the tubule of the nephrons. The increased concentration of drugs is more likely to damage the tubule. Both diminished renal blood flow and damaged tubules are major causes of acute renal failure (McCance and Huether 1990). Both could lead to loss of nephrons in individuals who have already lost many to the aging process (McCance and Huether 1990). Nonsteroidal anti-inflammatory drugs may deprive the patient of essential prostaglandins that protect from renal failure (Beck 1990).

The urinary output should be monitored carefully to be certain that it stays close to 30 ml per hour. If a retention catheter is necessary for such monitoring, nurses need to remember that this patient is also more susceptible to infection due to suppression of immunity.

Fluid, Electrolyte, and Acid-Base Imbalances. The kidneys are major guardians of body chemistry, three of the more important parameters of which are fluid, electrolyte, and acid-base balance. These parameters will be affected by the decrease in renal function produced by aging. They will also be affected by changes in the respiratory and other systems related to intake and elimination.

The decrease in plasma volume mentioned earlier makes some older patients more likely to develop hypovolemia; third space collection of fluid will compound this tendency (Jackson 1989). Others may be at higher risk for hypervolemia and its sequela, pulmonary edema. This is due to the potential for an excess of antidiuretic hormone (ADH) and aldosterone following surgery. The stress of the surgical procedure, pain, the anesthetics, and many other drugs likely to be given during the perioperative period increase the serum levels of these sodium- and fluid-retaining hormones. An excess of these hormones and a decreased ability of the cardiovascular system to expand (due to the changes of arteriosclerosis) would make the older adult prone to hypervolemia.

Nurses will want to maintain careful records of intake and output and assess them regularly. Further, when the specific gravity of the urine is used as an indicator of fluid balance, it is necessary to remember that the ability to concentrate urine decreases with aging (McCance and Huether 1990). Therefore the specific gravity will tend to be low even when the patient is not hypervolemic.

Because electrolytes are dissolved in the body fluids and because the kidneys can no longer reabsorb or secrete electrolytes as well, electrolyte imbalances are more likely. The same applies to acid-base imbalances because hydrogen ions (whose concentration makes up acid-base balance) are part of the electrolyte system. More specifically, acid-base imbalances occur primarily because the kidneys lose their ability to secrete ammonia, a major way by which excess hydrogen ions are eliminated from the body. Prevention of both electrolyte and acid-base imbalances is especially important because not only are they more difficult to correct but also because they could cause life-threatening arrhythmias.

Care Related to the Nervous System. Two problems related to the nervous system will be discussed. The first—confusion—is one encountered frequently in the older adult during the postoperative period (M.A. Williams, Campbell, Raynor, Mlynarczyk, and Ward 1985). The second—pain—is one common to all postoperative patients but managed differently in the older adult.

Confusion. Many factors, only some of which are related to the physiologic changes produced by aging, contribute to production of confusion in older adults. Distortion in perception may be related to decreased functioning of all the special senses. Memory may be impaired not only physiologically but also psychologically due to depression, which is common in this age group. However, the largest contributor may be a slowing of the ability to integrate (M.K. Williams et al. 1979) not only information but also functions within the body itself. Also, many of the changes in mental status may be related to the side effects and interactions of the many drugs usually consumed by people in this age group.

One researcher (M.K. Williams et al. 1979) reported that the best predictors of postoperative confusion in this age group are mental status at time of admission, being male, age (the greater the age, the more likely confusion), decreased postoperative mobility, presence of urinary problems, and being without watches or television. Certainly, if confusion is present, the highest priority will be to rule out hypoxia and fluid, electrolyte, or acid-base imbalances. Other nursing interventions found to be helpful with this problem include good orientation (includes preoperative preparation), clarifying communication, correcting sensory deficits, explaining everything being done for the patient (including the reason for doing it), continuity of care (having the same nurse assigned to the patient), preventing hypoxia (to the brain), good hydration, limiting sensory input, providing a safe and ordered environment, and using drugs wisely (M.A. Williams, Campbell, Raynor, Mlynarczyk, and Ward 1985). Jackson (1989) recommends that a family member accompany a confused patient to the operating room. Use of restraints is not recommended in a population where hypertension is one of the most common problems encountered preoperatively (Cote and Lapointe 1985). Some other alternatives to restraints include the use of touch, calling the patient by name, gently helping to refocus, allowing participation in decision making (when appropriate), and giving much orientation and explanation.

Pain. In general the rules for administering analgesics postoperatively to older clients are clear

- Do not medicate until necessary.

- Give the lowest dose possible to be effective.

- Increase intervals between medications.

- Combine narcotics with nonnarcotic analgesics such as acetaminophen.

In addition, older adults often have a change in sensitivity to medications, being less sensitive to some and more sensitive to others. One family of medications to which they are usually more sensitive is the central nervous system depressants. This will become a special problem postoperatively because of the increased percent of body fat. Many anesthetics will be stored in depots in this body fat, only to be released into circulation at a later time (when they could interact with analgesics or other central nervous system depressants). Nurses in the postoperative period must note the preoperative assessment of medications, those administered during surgery, and those administered in the postanesthesia unit.

Obviously, the nurse caring for an older patient postoperatively will want to use relaxation techniques, back rubs, hot tea, guided imagery and other measures to promote comfort and decrease pain so that medication can be kept at a minimum. Finally, if respirations should be depressed by narcotics, naloxone hydrochloride (Narcan) can be administered as a narcotic antagonist.

At the same time, one should remember that people in this age group probably have a greater tolerance for pain and may be afraid to ask for medication (especially when afraid of addiction). Facial expressions and body language may be more accurate indicators of pain.

Care Related to Temperature Regulation. Older people cannot regulate their body temperatures as well as the young can. They cannot lower temperature as well because they have decreased ability to perspire and because they have a decreased capacity to dilate their peripheral vessels (for heat loss). They also have a diminished capacity to increase body temperature because they cannot shiver (shivering produces heat) or constrict peripheral blood vessels (to conserve heat). Hypothermia is the most likely problem to be encountered in the postoperative period (Jackson 1989). The low temperature is related to the cool environment of operating rooms and to a decrease in metabolism and other effects of anesthesia. It is important to keep the patient warm and to check the temperature frequently. It is also important to recognize that this decreased ability to regulate body temperature could mean that the temperature could remain normal or even be subnormal in the presence of infection.

Care Related to Body Defense Mechanisms. Because a decreased reserve or decreased ability to adjust to stress exists in all body systems of older adults, virtually all signs or symptoms of infection could be masked. For example the cardiovascular system might be incapable of elevating the pulse, the white count could remain normal, and the cardinal signs of inflammation (including pain) could be suppressed. The inflammatory reaction as well as the immune response are both dampened and more slowly reactive. Both of the responses (to any antigen) will be depressed even further if the client has received steroids for treatment of arthritic conditions. Even though infections may be masked, it is more important to detect them in older patients. An infection could easily be the event initiating a chain reaction ending fatally for the patient. Such an infection is most likely to occur in the respiratory tract, the urinary system, or the surgical wound.

Complications of Wound Healing. Wounds of older people heal just as they do in any other patient, except that healing occurs at a slower pace and complications are more likely. Everything a nurse does to promote healing and prevent infection of wounds is even more important in this age group. Complications should be anticipated if health status is poor. This should be reflected by abnormal lab values (the CBC, blood chemistry and proteins, BUN, creatinine, liver function and coagulation studies, urinalysis) and other signs or symptoms. When coagulation studies are prolonged, hemostasis will be more of a problem, and excessive bleeding could interfere with healing. Some common complications of this healing process include keloid or fistula formation, scarring, wound herniation, dehiscence, and evisceration. The last two complications create an emergency situation; an early sign and warning that they are apt to occur is an increase in serous drainage. When wound healing progresses normally, wound rehabilitation and movement to prevent directly related contractures may begin after two weeks. Otherwise, this phase of recovery may be delayed.

Prevention of pressure ulcers is another important component of postoperative care. These ulcers may form in six to twelve hours. Many of the factors that contribute to prolonged wound healing predispose the older adult to them. The ears and balding heads of these patients should be included in the regular inspection of pressure areas.

Care Related to the Gastrointestinal System. Two problems surface as being significantly different for the older adult and directly related to the gastrointestinal system. These problems are paralytic ileus and constipation.

Paralytic Ileus. Paralytic ileus is likely to be prolonged because all motility within the gastrointestinal system is slowed by the aging process. Fluid and electrolyte balance need to be maintained intravenously until bowel sounds are detected. After this the patient can be started on clear liquids. When liquids are tolerated well enough to maintain fluid balance, intravenous therapy may be discontinued. The diet is then progressed, at a slower rate than usual, to what is normal for the patient. In addition, older people tolerate frequent, small feedings better than three large meals a day. Authorities seem to disagree as to whether it is better to offer the heaviest meal at mid-day or as the last meal of the day. Advocates of the last meal of the day maintain that the patient is less likely to awaken hungry; others maintain that a heavy evening meal is not conducive to sleep. Eating is sometimes a problem for older individuals because of dentures or bad teeth or because all of the senses tend to become dulled with age. Favorite foods, which the patient knows are easily digested, and spicy foods (unless contraindicated) are to be encouraged. These patients may also wish to use salt and sugar (if not contraindicated).

Constipation. As implied before, immobility is an even greater hazard for this age group than for others. Constipation is one of the more innocuous complications of immobility. Older people are more prone to develop constipation not only because gastrointestinal motility has been slowed but also because muscle tone in general has deteriorated and because they are less sensitive to the urge to defecate. In addition to the usual care related to this problem, a daily stool softener and a mild laxative may be needed after surgery.

Musculoskeletal Care. Not only is there a loss of muscle tone in the body, but joints and muscles tend to stiffen, especially when immobilized. It is important to assist older people (as needed) when they ambulate and to remember that they must move slowly and more carefully. The presence of osteoporosis will compound the likelihood of serious injury from falling. It is also important to remember that contractures develop more easily in this age group (because of a decrease in the number of elastic fibers in muscles). Therefore extra effort may be needed to prevent contractures.

Providing Physical and Emotional Safety. Physical safety is maintained, as it is for all patients, by keeping side rails up (when appropriate), keeping the call cord within reach, and doing whatever is necessary to protect the individual from injury. Emotional safety can be provided by recognizing the importance of needs and feelings (in treating the whole person) and dealing with them appropriately on an individual basis.

DISCHARGE PLANNING

Discharge planning begins the day of admission. But the nurse responsible for discharging the patient following surgery makes certain that six broad areas of patient teaching have been covered: diet, medications, activity, wound care, signs and symptoms to report, and return appointments. Essentials of good nutrition, knowledge of special diets, and prevention of constipation should be covered under diet. Dosage, times (related to daily events), actions, side effects, adverse reactions, toxicity, and interactions of medications should be written in large print. In addition, ability to open containers and availability of funds for purchasing medications should be assessed.

The patient should be taught to be as active as tolerated, taking frequent rest periods and avoiding long auto trips. The patient and/or a significant other should provide a return demonstration of any treatment procedures such as dressing changes. Dressings should not get wet during the bath, but showers are recommended when the patient goes home with staples. Care of drainage tubes or other special equipment is also important. Patients should know whom to call about wound redness, pain, or drainage, and elevated temperature or other signs or symptoms of infection.

Finally, the patient should have the return appointment in writing. In most cases, a responsible significant other needs to be included in the discharge teaching. (See chapter 16 for further discussion of discharge planning.)

CONVALESCENCE

Some form of assistance is usually needed for the older adult when discharged from the hospital. In addition, convalescence is likely to be prolonged. The patient may need to go to an extended care facility or nursing home with rehabilitation services for a period of time. Physical therapy, a special nutritious diet, speech therapy, and other such services may be needed on a daily basis. If the patient goes home, resources within the community will probably be needed (see chapters 20 and 21). In addition, the nurse needs to work with the family to help them adjust to the patient's care. An example of such a patient is Mrs. D. Howell, a 72-year-old woman who had been hospitalized for amputation of her right leg. Before discharge, her home was made as accident proof as possible and a bedroom was arranged for her on the first floor. Both the patient and her daughter were taught to care for her stump and her diabetes. Arrangements were made for a home health nurse to visit regularly, and transportation to and from the clinic was provided by an agency in the community.

SUMMARY

Although older people are at higher risk than younger individuals for complications during and after surgery, they tolerate elective surgery well if they are in good general physical condition and they have excellent pre- and postoperative nursing care. Preoperative preparation is very important and should include a careful assessment of body systems, the home environment, and ability to perform activities of daily living. Other factors that help to contribute to a successful outcome are good nutritional status, adequate hydration, control of related physical problems such as hypertension, adaptation to recent drug therapy and preoperative preparation and teaching.

Careful choice and administration of preoperative medications is essential because they can affect the anesthesia and immediate postoperative recovery period. While local and spinal anesthesia are probably safest for older patients, they tolerate general anesthetic agents (such as nitrous oxide) well, especially if the surgery is relatively short. The surgical staff also needs to take special precautions while moving, positioning, and cleaning and applying dressings to the skin of older patients.

Nurses caring for the older adult postoperatively need to understand not only the physiology and pathophysiology involved in the body systems but also the changes produced by the normal process of aging. This understanding is essential if they are to detect early signs or symptoms produced by pathology. In addition, many of the changes related to aging make these patients especially vulnerable to postoperative complications. Further, any undetected complication could cause a chain reaction that would affect the other body systems and possibly end unfavorably for the patient. It is for these reasons that a thorough and regular postoperative assessment of body systems is recommended for these patients.

The respiratory system receives highest priority because of the importance of maintaining a patent airway in this age group. Preventing hypoxia and hy-postatic pneumonia are almost equally important. The vital signs may need to be monitored more frequently and for a longer period of time to detect pathologic changes in the cardiovascular system. Frequent and potentially fatal complications related to this system and associated with this age group include myocardial infarction, congestive heart failure, and pulmonary embolism following thrombophlebitis. Changes in the urinary systems of older adults cause them to be prone to urinary retention and acute renal failure. When these changes are combined with changes in the endocrine system, the patient is also more likely to develop fluid, electrolyte, and acid-base imbalances.

A problem frequently encountered in the older adult, but not usually to a great extent in other postoperative patients, is confusion. Authorities agree that good orientation and explanation of everything being done are helpful in preventing and treating this problem. Effective management of pain will require that the nurse use a variety of nursing skills to promote comfort and relieve pain and have full knowledge of how drug use is modified by aging.

Postoperative patients are likely to have subnormal temperatures following surgery. It is especially important to keep older people warm because they cannot regulate their body temperatures as well.

Signs and symptoms of infection will be especially difficult to detect because virtually all of them may be decreased by the aging process. Regardless of this, it is even more important to detect infection early in these clients because infection could easily be the event to initiate a fatal chain reaction. Many of the same mechanisms decreasing the signs and symptoms of infection also prolong wound healing and, in addition, make the older client more vulnerable to the complications of such healing.

Prolonged paralytic ileus and constipation are encountered frequently in the older individual, partly because gastrointestinal motility slows with aging. Another important aspect of care is planning for stiffened muscles and joints when ambulating, and preventing further deterioration of these areas when the patient is resting. Convalesce is apt to take four to six months and will probably require some form of follow-up care.

STUDY QUESTIONS

1. Identify the kinds of surgery that older patients do not tolerate well.

2. What are the major fears of older patients facing surgery?

3. Name several medications that should not be given to older patients.

4. Is day surgery useful for older patients? Explain.

5. Discuss the major physical and psychologic aspects of preoperative nursing care for older adults.

6. Rank the three highest priorities of care for the older postoperative patient.

7. Why is the older client prone to the development of myocardial infarction postoperatively? What can the nurse do to prevent it?

8. Why are hemorrhage, shock, renal failure, and confusion more likely in the older adult? How can they be prevented?

9. How is the management of pain different for older adults?

10. Why is prevention of infection a special problem for this age group?

11. Describe discharge planning for the older surgical patient.

REFERENCES

Beck, L.H. 1990. Perioperative renal fluid, and electrolyte management. In *Clinics of Geriatric Medicine*, edited L.H. Beck. Philadelphia: Saunders.

Brown, L.L. 1985. Anesthesia in the geriatric patient. *Clinics in Plastic Surgery* 12(1):51–60.

Burden, N. 1989. Handle with care: The geriatric patient in the ambulatory surgery environment. *Journal of Post Anesthesia Nursing* 4(1):27–31.

Carruth, A.K. and B.J. Boss. 1990. More than they bargained for: Adverse drug effects. *Journal of Gerontological Nursing* 16(2):27–30.

Cote, J. and P. Lapointe. 1985. Anesthetic management for the elderly patient. *Canadian Anesthetists Society Journal* 32(2):188–91.

Crawford, F.J. 1985. Ambulatory surgery. *AORN Journal* 41(2):356–59.

Dean, A.F. 1987. The aging surgical patient: Historical overview, implications, and nursing care. *Perioperative Nursing Quarterly* 3(1):1–7.

Foster, C.G. 1986. The surgical experience. In *Medical-Surgical Nursing*, edited by S.L. Patrick, S. Woods, R.F. Craven, J.S. Rokosky, and P.M. Bruno. Philadelphia: J.B. Lippincott.

Frisch, S.R., L.E. Groom, E. Sequin, L.J. Edgar, and C.J. Pepler. 1990. Ambulatory surgery: A study of patients' and helpers' experiences. *AORN Journal* 52(5):1000–1009.

Gamotis, P.B., V.C. Dearmon, N.O. Doolittle, and S.C. Price. 1988. Inpatient vs. outpatient satisfaction: A research study. *AORN Journal* 47(6):1421–22, 1424–25.

Hercules, P.R. 1987. Client during surgery. In *Medical-Surgical Nursing*. 2d ed., edited by S.M. Lewis and I.C. Collier. New York: McGraw-Hill.

Jackson, M.F. 1988. High risk surgical patients. *Journal of Gerontological Nursing* 14(1):8–15.

Jackson, M.F. 1989. Elder care: Implications of surgery in very elderly patients. *AORN Journal* 50(4):859–69.

Keating, H.J. and M.F. Lubin. 1990. Perioperative responsibilities of the physician/geriatrician. In *Clinics in Geriatric Medicine*, edited by H.J. Keating. Philadelphia: Saunders.

Kupferer, S.S., J.H. Uebele, and D.F. Levin. 1988. Geriatric ambulatory surgery patients: Assessing cognitive functions. *AORN Journal* 47(3):752–55, 758–62, 764–66.

Lund, C. and M.L. Sheafor. 1985. Is your patient about to fall? *Journal of Gerontological Nursing* 11(4):35–41.

Matteson, M.A. and E.S. McConnell. 1988. *Gerontological Nursing*. Philadelphia, PA: Saunders.

McCance, K.L. and S.E. Huether. 1990. *Pathophysiology: The Biologic Basis for Disease in Adults and Children*. St. Louis, MO: C.V. Mosby.

Michaels, D. and C. Stephenson. 1985. Pulmonary problems. In *Home Nursing Care for the Elderly*, edited by M. Hogstel. Bowie, MD: Brady Communications.

Neugent, M.C. 1981. Social and emotional needs of geriatric surgery patients. *Social Work in Health Care* 6(4):69-75.

Potter, P.A. and A. Perry. 1989. *Fundamentals of Nursing.* St. Louis: C.V. Mosby.

Walker, M.L. 1986. Growing old. *AORN Journal* 43(4):887–90.

Walker, S.N. and C.W. Love. 1987. Preoperative client. In *Medical-Surgical Nursing,* edited by S.M. Lewis and I.C. Collier. New York: McGraw-Hill.

Williams, M.A., E.B. Campbell, W.J. Raynor, S.M. Mlynarczyk, and S.E. Ward. 1985. Reducing acute confusional states in elderly patients with hip fractures. *Research in Nursing and Health* 8(4):329–37.

Williams, M.K., J.R. Holloway, M.C. Winn, M.O. Walanin, M.L. Lawler, C.R. Westwick, and M.H. Chin. 1979. Nursing activities and acute confusional states. *Nurs Res* 28(1):25–35.

Wolfe, S.M., L. Fugate, E.P. Hulstrand, and L.E. Kaminoto. 1988. *Worst Pills Best Pills.* Washington, DC: Public Citizen Health Research Group.

15

The Critically Ill Older Patient

Carol A. Stephenson

CHAPTER OUTLINE

FOCUS

With the advances in technology and the vastly greater number of older people, the older population in critical care units is increasing significantly. Although there are many similarities in caring for the older adult who is critically ill and for a younger adult with a similar physical diagnosis, there are also many differences. This chapter reviews these differences and their application in nursing practice to ensure that optimal care is provided to each critically ill older patient.

OBJECTIVES

1. Describe the increasing significance of the relationship of an aging population to the population of patients in critical care units.

2. Evaluate methods to facilitate the adjustment and adaptation of older adults to their status as critical care patients.

3. Discuss behavioral manifestations that may suggest attitudes of helplessness, hopelessness, or powerlessness in the older critically ill patient and discuss appropriate nursing interventions.

4. Compare possible alterations in adaptability and flexibility in the older adult related to serious illness and relate to appropriate nursing actions.

5. Acknowledge the older adult's need for privacy, respect, and territory and describe appropriate nursing interventions related to these needs.

6. Apply methods of patient teaching to the critically ill older adult.

7. Relate the concept of ICU syndrome and sensory overload to the older adult and describe appropriate nursing interventions to prevent these from occurring or to relieve them.

8. Discuss nursing assessment, decision making, and interventions related to the individual physiological and sensory alterations of the older critically ill adult.

Although more and more older people are staying healthier longer than in previous years, many are not. In fact, older adults are the predominant population of our hospitals. This trend will continue. Statistically, older people accounted for 33 percent of hospital stays and 44 percent of the total hospital inpatient days of care in 1988. While the average length of a hospital stay was 5.3 days for those under 65 years old, those older than 65 had an average hospital stay of 8.9 days (American Association of Retired Persons 1991) Also, elders are more likely to be readmitted to hospitals during the same year than are younger persons. In former years those over age 65 were often excluded from critical care units solely because of age. Now age is not an exclusion for even the most complex problems. Intensive care unit (ICU) mortality is, however, still age-related. Older adults have more problems and recuperate more slowly than younger ICU patients. Older patients are not heterogenous, however. Each patient must be assessed and managed on an individual basis (Fulmer and Walker 1990; El-Sherif 1986).

Although statistics are unavailable, it is well known that a large percentage of the population of critical care units are older adults. Until recently little has been taught in nursing schools or written in the nursing literature specifically related to the care of the critically ill older person. In order to provide optimal care for critically ill older adults, nurses must become knowledgeable about the similarities and differences between these older patients and their younger patients. Earlier chapters in this text discuss specific descriptions of the physiologic and psychologic changes in aging as well as emergency care and the use of drugs and medications. All of the materials in this text apply and should be carefully considered by those nurses caring for critically ill older patients. This chapter is devoted to other specific suggestions for nursing care of these patients.

NURSING CARE RELATED TO PSYCHOSOCIAL NEEDS

Admission

When an older person is admitted to a critical care unit, his or her physiologic status is often so tenuous that his or her life hangs in the balance. The extraordinary amount of attention that must be paid to physical care in the critical care unit can negate or postpone attention to psychosocial needs. This situation is unfortunate because early attention to psychosocial needs may prevent or minimize maladaptive responses to hospitalization such as confusion, disorientation, loss of reality, fear, anxiety, and hostility. Adjustment and adaptation to hospitalization can be facilitated if the older person's psychosocial needs are recognized and attended to from the time of the hospital admission. The patient and family members need support, nonthreatening explanations, and nursing interventions to promote the psychological comfort of the older person in the hospital setting.

The time of admission to the hospital and especially to the critical care unit is a stressful and upsetting time for anyone. The older patient is no exception. If the patient is being admitted from a long-term care facility, nurses in that facility should send all information possible to the hospital staff—not only about the patient's physical condition but also about the psychologic status and what measures have been found to ease the patient's anxiety in the past. If this information is not sent from the long-term care facility or if there are questions, the acute care nurse should contact the long-term care nurse and discuss the patient. If the patient is being admitted directly from home, the critical care nurses should seek this type of information if it is not readily available.

If the patient is able to participate in discussion at the time of admission, it is also important for the nurse to inquire what the hospitalization means to the patient, what he/she expects to happen as a result of it, and any questions or fears he/she might have. Many critically ill patients are too ill to participate in a prolonged interview at the time of admission. In this case, the admission interview should be divided into two or more sessions. It is preferable to obtain the information directly from the patient if possible. This action shows respect for the patient and will elicit more definitive information than that given by someone else. The nurse should not allow family members to interrupt or speak for the patient who is capable of speaking for himself. It is unfortunate when caregivers and family members speak *over* instead of *to* the patient. If the patient is unable to be interviewed, the nurse could show respect by asking permission to interview a family member in the patient's presence.

Rapid role change is one problem that often accompanies admission to the critical care unit. This role change is traumatic to any patient but is particularly so to older patients who are constantly struggling to maintain control of their lives. There is much dependency on the nursing staff during the early stages of a critical illness. The patient often fears that independence will not be regained, that dependence will be a lifelong norm from now on, or that death will occur. For example, the ventilator-dependent patient may not understand that the ventilator is only to support respirations while the body recovers and that it is intended to be temporary only. It is essential that the nursing staff make a special effort to assure older patients that everything possible is being done to bring them to their previous level of wellness or coping and that the dependent role is, it is hoped, only temporary.

Older patients may be mistakenly viewed by the nursing staff as experienced patients. This is not necessarily true (Ferrell and Ferrell 1990). It should not be assumed that any patients *know* the patient role or that they are experienced in coping with that role or with pain. Admission explanations and orientation should assume that the patient does not know the routine and is not oriented to the hospital or critical care unit. The explanations should be repeated and reinforced as often as necessary. Some older persons have not experienced severe pain and have developed few methods to cope with it. Others who have coped with pain and discomfort may or may not have discovered effective coping methods. Observations of the patient for pain-related behaviors such as facial grimaces and agitation are useful to some extent for all patients and especially so for those who are cognitively unable to express themselves. Some, however, will not show these signs because they do not have the energy to do so (Ferrell and Ferrell 1990) or because they have chronic pain and their manifestations of pain have been altered accordingly. Others may cope in ways that lead them to report even severe discomfort infrequently. The nurse, therefore, may be misled to believe that less pain is present than is actually the case. The nurse should inquire carefully about what the patient is feeling and make no assumptions based only on nonverbal behavior. The meaning of all behavioral cues should be validated with the patient before these cues are acted upon. If possible, the patient should participate in the decisions about what action will be taken related to the pain.

Helplessness, Hopelessness, Powerlessness

The role change and the loss of independence or control that result from acute illness can lead to feelings of helplessness, hopelessness, or powerlessness. Hopelessness has been defined as a "feeling of entrapment, a sense of the impossible, of things being beyond one's capabilities" (Gioiella and Bevil 1985, 538). The person who feels hopeless has no energy available for coping and sees no reason to expect things to improve or even to wish that they would improve. This patient may either visualize no future or see a radically altered future. The patient may also believe that because of the illness, all control of the future has been lost. Powerlessness is described as a "perceived lack of personal control of events in a given situation" (Gioiella and Bevil 1985, 538–39). Helplessness relates closely to powerlessness and hopelessness. In this case, the patient feels that what he/she does in the situation will not make a difference anyway.

The behavioral manifestations of helplessness, hopelessness, and powerlessness are very similar. The patient may regress or be passive, uncooperative, noncompliant, dependent, angry, frustrated, depressed, hostile, or withdrawn. The nurse should be alert to behavioral signs of helplessness, hopelessness, and powerlessness in order to intervene as appropriately as possible. In the case of apparent hopelessness, the nurse should not try to give false hope. All too often, patients receive a figurative pat on the head and false reassurances rather than acknowledgement that the situation is real, serious, and very threatening. To assist the patient to deal with hopelessness, the nurse should attempt to determine what the patient believes to be true about the illness and about the future. The nurse can then use that information in discussion that is directed at aiding the patient to see both the realistic and hopeful aspects of the illness or situation. The discussion should acknowledge that the patient's feelings are real and understandable. It will also be helpful if the nurse investigates what support persons are important to the patient and enlists the aid of these persons in providing support. Some other possible ways to foster hope might be to describe other patients who have overcome similar situations, to ask those who have overcome similar problems to visit, and to develop a trusting relationship with the patient, to reinforce reality, to help the patient set attainable goals (Gioiella and Bevil 1985, 539), and to enlist the aid of a social worker or other appropriate person in solving problems and planning for the future. The patient's success in meeting each goal should be recognized and reinforced because a feeling of success is one of the most important factors in achieving a sense of hope, power, and control.

Occasionally it is helpful for the patient to be allowed to be passive, dependent and even depressed for a period of time, especially during an acute illness. When a person is extremely ill, there may be no energy to spare for psychologic coping or decision making. In other situations it is important to strive for the patient to have as much control and decision-making power in the situation as possible. The nurse can make an effort to offer as many choices as possible and be certain that the patient is included in all care-related decisions. When this is done, however, it is important to recognize that the patient has a right to make a different decision than the one the health care team might make. As one postoperative patient said, "I don't know why they are asking me to make these decisions—I can't think clearly, I don't have any energy, and I need to have decisions made for me right now." Before asking patients to make decisions, it is helpful to validate whether they wish to do so at the time. Once the patient makes a decision, that decision should be respected and carried out.

The older patient who feels helpless or powerless may be noncompliant because he/she believes that no effort on his/her part, including taking medication or treatment, will make a difference in the outcome of the illness. In this case it takes a great deal of effort to aid a patient to understand that his or her own behavior can make a difference. Sometimes, the nurse never knows which efforts are most convincing, so the nurse must continue trying.

Decreased Adaptability

The older person is less adaptable than a younger person in a variety of ways. When the older person is ill, there is less energy available to be flexible and adaptable to the situation than ordinarily is true or than a younger person might have. The older patient may or may not have had previous experiences with illness that affect the ability to adapt. For some the fact that they have had much illness may cause them to be more passive, more angry, more dependent, or to exhibit any number of other reactions that have been conditioned by past experiences. For the person who has been relatively healthy, adaptation to illness may be easier or more difficult. Mary, for example, has been extremely healthy and active all her life. Mary believed that if she stayed active, she would never be subject to the usual problems that often accompany the aging process. At age 85 she did her exercises daily and would proudly show anyone how she could bend over and place the flat of her hands on the floor. At age 90 she had several physical problems although none was major, and she was placed in a boarding home especially for older adults. She complained constantly about how ill she was and how awful it was to get old. She refused to socialize or interact with the other residents, all of whom were younger than herself, because she "had nothing in common with those old people." She visited her physician regularly, telling him how ill she was and begging for medication that would "fix" it. She was hospitalized several times for investigation of her complaints. Mary still held out hope that if the health care team would just give her the proper treatment, she would be "well," which she defined as feeling the way she did in her 60s. Mary became an extremely angry and hostile person. When Mary had a stroke and was placed in a nursing home, she refused to eat, often feigned unconsciousness, and finally died.

There are a variety of other reasons why older persons lose their flexibility. Their friends become ill and die, so they have a sense of loss. They may have financial reverses, and they lose roles that are important to them as they retire and their family structure changes. If the person is struggling to retain some sense of self and some control, this may result in inappropriate or inflexible behavior. The nurses who care for these patients should be sensitive to cues that will help them identify particular needs and to select appropriate interventions to meet patient needs for control while encouraging flexibility and adaptability.

Other patients may appear to be inflexible or uncooperative because of fear, misunderstanding of illness, and lack of attention to basic psychosocial needs. Mrs. Brown was such a patient. At age 65 she had had COPD for several years but had never experienced an episode of respiratory failure. She believed that she would remain as she was in a stage of coping well with her physical problem. Mrs. Brown contracted an acute respiratory infection that led to her hospitalization and subsequent respiratory arrest. She awoke in the critical care unit on mechanical ventilation with an oral endotracheal tube in place. Her response was extremely frustrating to her nurse. She fought and squirmed constantly, got her wrist restraints loose, and pulled at her endotracheal tube. She tried very hard to communicate and when the nurse did not understand her immediately, she would throw whatever she could reach at the nurse. The nurses were reluctant to medicate her with the ordered morphine or diazepam in the belief that she would not need the ventilator if she were not sedated.

This is the situation that greeted a nurse as she came on duty. The nurse, who was highly experienced in both the care of older adults and the care of patients on ventilators, started her shift by talking with Mrs. Brown. When a person cannot communicate, it is helpful to use a technique known as *mirroring* the feelings. After the nurse introduced herself, she commented that she had heard that Mrs. Brown seemed to have a hard time coping with her situation. When the patient nodded her agreement, the nurse commented that it must be extremely frightening to wake up in the intensive care unit (ICU) with all of the lines and especially the tube in her mouth. Mrs. Brown agreed and the nurse continued, stating that the inability to talk would be frustrating for her and she thought it probably was for Mrs. Brown also. As the patient nodded eagerly, the nurse assured her that such fear and frustration were normal and understandable. After more discussion on this point, the nurse approached the fear that many patients who are on mechanical ventilators have: that there is no hope of discontinuing the ventilator and that they will always be in this condition for the rest of their lives. Mrs. Brown was very eager to indicate that she indeed felt this way. The nurse carefully explained that the ventilator was simply a type of therapy to keep her breathing while she recovered from her infection. She also explained that when the situation improved and she was able to breathe on her own, which for her was anticipated to be a very short time, they would be able to remove the

ventilator. They had more discussion of this point and then the nurse did her initial assessment for the shift. Mrs. Brown cooperated more than she had for any of the other nurses.

During the shift, the nurse was careful to answer Mrs. Brown's call light promptly and spend time trying to understand her needs. When Mrs. Brown appeared to be upset by her communication difficulty, the nurse reminded her that she was trying too and was also frustrated. She would then encourage Mrs. Brown to work together with her to solve the communication difficulties. The nurse also was alert to Mrs. Brown's other personal needs. The nurse used the intravenous diazepam judiciously, always explaining that this was a medicine to help Mrs. Brown relax and tolerate the things that were happening to her.

Besides attending to comfort needs and using touch frequently, the nurse noted nonverbal cues that indicated Mrs. Brown wanted more closeness with her husband during the visiting period. When the nurse asked her directly if she wanted him to sit on the bed with her, she nodded enthusiastically. The nurse repositioned Mrs. Brown in the bed so that there was extra room on one side, lowered the side rail, and encouraged Mr. Brown to sit on the bed. He sat beside her, leaning over with his chest against hers and holding her in his arms as the nurse left the room and closed the door. From that point on, both Mr. and Mrs. Brown seemed more satisfied with her care. She spent more time resting and sleeping; there was less fighting against the ventilator and intravenous lines and fewer incidents of agitation and frustration.

Many older persons appear to be inflexible simply because they have spent so many years developing habits and rituals, daily life patterns, likes, and dislikes. They are often used to a great deal of structure in their lives. The fact that they have structure gives them security for daily living. The nurse can spend time with the patient and family asking specific questions to discover what rituals, patterns, likes, and dislikes are especially important for the patient. Once the nurse has this information, then as many of the important aspects of the daily life pattern as possible should be incorporated into the patient's life in the critical care unit. For example, if the patient usually takes a bath at bedtime, then reads or watches television, and finally falls asleep in the same position each night, the nurse could follow the entire ritual in preparing the patient for sleep. Along with following the patient's established rituals, the nurse should strive for the hospital environment to be as stable as possible. Transfers to other locations should be done as infrequently as possible. The same nurse should care for the patient each day in order to establish stability and trust. The nurse should show a sincere interest in the patient and family as individuals so that nursing care can be individualized as much as possible.

Privacy, Respect, Territory

All persons need privacy, respect, and territory to call their own. This is especially true for the older person. All three of these are often totally lost upon admission to the critical care unit. Older persons seem especially sensitive to the loss of privacy and dignity. In the critical care unit there is often little recourse as to who enters the room, what body parts are exposed and when, what personal questions are asked, and what treatment is given and when. The caregivers should be diligent in their efforts to assure privacy and dignity. This can be accomplished by knocking before entering the room, screening the patient well before exposing the body, and exposing body parts as little as possible. It is not unusual to find two nurses bathing an older gentleman who lies stripped naked in the bed between them. That is a terribly demeaning experience for anyone. Even the person who is apparently unresponsive should be kept covered and should be addressed with dignity. Even unresponsive patients can hear, understand, feel, and think. They often wake up and are able to tell their caregivers exactly what each said and did.

A very simple way to preserve the patient's dignity is to use respectful forms of address. A nurse should not address an older patient by the first name without permission. One gentleman explained the need for respectful address very explicitly. A retired minister, he said, "Miss, you can call me Mr. _____, you can call me Dr. _____, you can call me Pastor _____, or you can call me 'sir.' You may NOT call me 'George' or 'dearie.' What would people think?"

Another simple way to demonstrate respect for privacy is to be certain that the patient is not exposed or asked personal questions in the presence of visi-

tors or others who have no real need to be there at the time. The nurse should also encourage the family to show respect for the patient. It is not especially uncommon for a family to sit by the bedside of a dying patient and make disparaging remarks or argue about their inheritance. One older woman took care of this problem for her family. She was unconscious and lay day after day while her relatives sat in the room discussing and disputing their inheritance. Only her teenage granddaughter interacted with the woman. She came after school every day, combed her grandmother's hair, applied lotion to her skin, told her about school, and told her she loved her. One day the woman regained consciousness, called her attorney, and changed her will. She died within forty-eight hours after the will was completed. The granddaughter inherited everything. When the family behavior is inappropriate, the nurse should discuss the situation with them *outside* the patient's room.

Critically ill patients often lack territory to call their own because the space around the bed is full of ventilators, intravenous pumps, monitoring equipment, and other equipment. Often that equipment infringes to the point where it even shares the bed with the patient. Everyone needs some space to call one's own, but the patient may have none. This can be a major stress that leads to anger, hostility, and lack of cooperation with caregivers (Gioiella and Bevil 1985). If possible, the nurse should find a way to give patients some space that can be controlled only by them. The space may be very small, but if personal photos or whatever is important to the patients can be arranged satisfactorily and not disturbed by anyone, it can relieve some of the stress. It can also be very helpful to place a relatively recent photo of the patient prominently in the room. This can help staff to visualize the patient at his or her best and assist them to relate to the patient in a more personal manner.

Teaching

Most older patients are unable to concentrate on learning while they are critically ill. This may be due to memory impairment, confusion caused by drugs or disease, pain, anxiety, lowered level of consciousness, fatigue, or other factors. However, some teaching is usually essential. The nurse should confine any teaching efforts to things the patient needs to know at that time and that will ease apprehension, improve cooperation, or reduce stress and aid coping. This teaching includes frequent explanations of what is being done and why, explanations of equipment, discussion and demonstration of how much the patient can move about in spite of the equipment, and what the alarms do and do not mean. The critical care area is not the time for extended teaching about how to take medications at home, for example, although it may be the time for the social service personnel to begin preliminary discharge planning with the family. Teaching episodes should be brief—less than fifteen minutes—and should be done using terminology that the patient understands. The times for teaching should be chosen so that the patient is as awake, comfortable, and as pain free as possible and when distractions are at a minimum. All of these factors will enhance the patient's ability to understand and retain the material being taught.

ICU Syndrome

It is not unusual for older patients to develop an ICU psychosis when they are in an intensive care setting for more than a day or two. This may develop so gradually that it is not recognized until it is extensive, or it may develop more suddenly. The manifestations could include inappropriate behavior, disorientation, illusions, and hallucinations. Many factors are thought to cause this syndrome. The interaction of medications and fluid and electrolyte imbalances combined with the stresses of physical illness and discomfort, an unfamiliar environment, and absence of or alteration in the usual light-dark cycle could cause it. Another factor that contributes to ICU psychosis is sleep deprivation. Frequently, nurses are so busy giving care that they do not notice how little sleep the patient is getting. Sleep is essential, not only for physical healing, but also for energy renewal and reorientation. The person who has had adequate sleep is less likely to be fatigued, disoriented, or irritable than the person who has had inadequate sleep. Procedures should be grouped as much as possible in order to allow for uninterrupted rest periods. Nonessential procedures should be omitted when the patient is sleeping. At night, the unit should be dark and quiet so that the sleep environment is as natural as possible. The nurse should seek to find out what the

patient's normal presleep ritual is and follow it as previously described.

Sensory overload or deprivation can be a factor in ICU psychosis, or it can be an added stressor for the patient and use up energy that should be directed toward coping and healing. Sensory overload consists of multiple stimuli or unusual and poorly understood stimuli that continually infringe on the patient's consciousness. If the critical care unit is an open one, the proliferation of sights and noises can be quite intense. Even if the patient has a private room within the unit, there can be sensory overload because of alarms, other sounds, equipment, and voices that are unfamiliar and continuous or startling. It is important that there be as much freedom from distressing sights and sounds as possible. A private room is preferable to an open ward, and voices should be kept low, especially when the patient is sleeping. Any alarms, sights, and noises should be explained in such a way that the patient is not frightened. For example, the ECG monitor might sound an alarm simply because the leads are loosened on the chest or the ventilator might sound an alarm because the patient coughs. If the patient is able to talk, he/she should be invited to discuss the sights and sounds of the unit and ask questions so that these can be explained to his/her satisfaction. When patients are unable to talk, writing, letter boards, picture boards or the mirror technique may be used.

Sensory monotony or sensory underload can also be a problem to the critical care patient. Frequently, this is not due to the lack of sounds, but to a sound being continuous over a long period of time so that it becomes very monotonous. This can be either annoying or hypnotic to the point where the patient begins to block this and other incoming sounds from awareness. As a result the patient may not listen to the sounds he/she should be hearing.

A source of sensory monotony and frustration to many older patients is the television set. Often, the television set in the hospital room is left on constantly in the hope that it will stimulate the patient. Actually, some older persons watch very little television when they are well and consider the noise an annoyance. When the television is left on in the room and they have no ability to turn it off, the situation may be extremely stressful and frustrating. The patient who finds such sounds annoying may ignore them or may use up a great deal of energy being frustrated. If the nurse wishes to use auditory stimulation for the patient, it is good first to ascertain what sounds are preferred. Some may prefer listening to a certain radio station. Others may prefer certain specific television shows. Some may do better with tapes of family voices. Whatever auditory stimulation is chosen, it should be used only intermittently and not constantly. Attention should be paid to choosing programs and times for listening that are usually preferred by the patient. If the patient is able, the control of the radio or TV should be up to the patient and not the nurse.

Sensory Losses

The person with altered sight or hearing may have more difficulty than others in processing or interpreting the sights and sounds of the critical care unit. If the person cannot distinguish sound well, he/she may be enveloped in a monotonously silent situation, or sounds might be distorted and misinterpreted. Persons may appear withdrawn or react inappropriately to stimuli because they do not hear the words correctly or do not hear some of them at all. Misinterpretation of stimuli can lead to feelings of fright in older people. If they are startled or frightened, they often strike out in self-defense. Caregivers should speak to the patient upon entering the room and avoid startling movements, approaching the patient from behind, or making other motions that could be perceived as threatening (Gray-Vickrey 1987). If the person has a hearing aid, it should be worn during the most acute phases of illness even if the patient appears unresponsive. Hearing has been documented to be the last sense to be lost in many cases. The patient should have every possible chance to hear what is going on around him/her. If a conscious person has a hearing loss, it is important to validate that he/she has heard and understood what is said in conversation.

Many older persons have partial loss of sight, which can be associated with both misperception of the environment and with falls. If the patient usually wears glasses, they should be worn during acute illness. It is important that the patient be able to recognize individuals and to see the environment as well as possible. Other common visual problems of older adults include reduced sensitivity to light, increased sensitivity to glare, reduced ability to adapt to changes in the level of available light, and altered color vision. Rooms of older people should be well lighted during the day, and have good night lights, but without glare. Having surgical permits and other printed information that is given to patients in large print with large uncluttered illustrations can be extremely helpful (Eliopoulos 1989).

Other senses can be affected as well. Smell and taste may be affected by aging or by drugs or disease. Some diseases rob the patient of the ability to eat normally. Sometimes this condition is temporary and sometimes it is not. When a person is unable to eat, one of the most basic sensations and/or pleasures has been lost. One older cancer patient had lost most of his intestinal tract to the disease. He was in the hospital being maintained on hyperalimentation. At one point in his care some food commercials were on television. A sympathetic nurse used his nonverbal response to the commercials as a cue to ask him how he felt about his inability to eat. He seemed to be relieved to have a sympathetic ear as he discussed his feelings of frustration and loss.

Taste and appetite may be affected by the character of the food and the patient's ability to eat it. Dentures should be in place for meals and for their cosmetic value except when they are being cleaned, at night, or for procedures. A pureed diet should be avoided if possible because it is not appetizing to most people. A diet of easily chewed foods such as bread, cooked vegetables, baked chicken, custard, and ice cream, is usually accepted much more readily.

Social and sensory stimulation are affected in a variety of ways by critical illness. The patient still needs touch, stroking, and interaction in as normal a fashion as possible. The nurse can aid the person a great deal by stroking and touching appropriately. If it is possible, the patient could be taken outside to enjoy pleasant weather and good company. If this is not possible, the family should relate to the patient as normally as possible within the critical care unit. They should be encouraged to touch the patient, to hold a hand, comb the hair, stroke the skin, or whatever interaction is normal and appropriate for them. In many instances, this can be carried further by allowing and encouraging the family to participate in the physical care of the patient. This type of care gives the patient a sense of being supported by loved ones and gives the family a sense of aiding in the person's recovery. One very easy way that the family can assist is to help the patient eat, if he/she is able to eat.

The nurse caring for the older patient should be alert to signs of isolation, withdrawal, boredom, and sensory misinterpretation. One sign of withdrawal that is easily missed is sleeping too much (Gioiella and Bevil 1985). Sleep is a common method of withdrawal or of dealing with problems. Certainly a very ill person needs a great deal of rest in order to recover, but sleeping excessively could be a sign of withdrawal or of dealing inappropriately with problems and stresses.

NURSING CARE RELATED TO PHYSICAL DIFFERENCES

The physical changes that are normal in aging are well documented earlier in this book. When any physical differences are noted in an older person, it is important to do a careful assessment and not just attribute them to aging.

The Presence of Chronic Illness

Older persons who are critically ill tend to be quite sick, often with multiple acute and chronic problems. Living with a chronic problem seems to be the norm for many older people. About four out of five older persons have at least one chronic disease. About 86 percent have multiple chronic conditions (Christ and Hohloch 1988). When a person with chronic problems becomes acutely ill, the acute illness may exacerbate the effects of the chronic disease, while the chronic disease complicates treatment and recovery from acute illness. The problem for both patient and health care team becomes quite complex when several acute and chronic illnesses are found together in a single patient.

Altered Response to Disease

The acutely ill older person often has physical signs and symptoms that are different from those experienced by younger persons. The older patient may have a history that is atypical for the illness that is present. The differences may be due to blunted reac-

tions caused by neurologic disorders or other diseases, or to alterations in the ability of the body organs to react in the same manner as when the person was younger. Ongoing medication therapy may also mask reaction to disease.

Body temperature is a prime example of the differences in physical signs in older adults. Normally the body temperature of older people is well below the normal of 98.6°F. One study has shown a mean body temperature of 97.7°F in well persons over the age of 65. Therefore a temperature of 98.6°F might indicate an early illness in these persons. Older people are twice as prone to nosocomial infections, particularly those of the respiratory and urinary tracts, than are younger persons. Any temperature in an older person that is above 98.6°F should arouse suspicion and be investigated. Any fever may be masked by medications the older adult is taking for other conditions, such as aspirin, acetaminophen, steroids, and nonsteroidal anti-inflammatory agents (Schoemick et al. 1991).

Infection is a prime example of altered symptoms of disease in older adults. While cough, fever, and other classic signs of infection may occur in the older adult, they often do not. The presenting signs of infection may be a major change in mental status or activity or an exacerbation of an underlying condition such as chronic obstructive pulmonary disease (COPD), congestive heart failure, or diabetes mellitus. Nonspecific signs of infection in the older adult may include symptoms of dehydration and elevated lab studies such as white blood count, blood urea nitrogen (BUN), sodium, and chloride (Schoemick et al. 1991). A further problem is that once an older person acquires an infection, there is an increased risk of acquiring other infections as well. A superinfection is most likely on the fourth or fifth day of treatment for an infection in the older person who has a debilitating condition. Some infections continue for a long time. Abnormal gut flora may remain in the apparently successfully treated patient for months or even years (Maas et al. 1991).

The older person who has pneumonia may have a low-grade fever and decreased level of consciousness but no chest pain or cough. The older person who develops sepsis may not show the high fever that is common in acute sepsis. Indeed, the body temperature may be low along with hypotension, tachycardia, and a cold, clammy skin. The person with cellulitis may have a local erythema, edema, and tenderness without a fever or even an apparent point of entry for the problem (Schoemick et al. 1991). Problems other than infection also present in unusual ways. The only manifestation of peptic ulcer disease may be blood in the stool; there may be no epigastric pain. The older person who has a myocardial infarction may have a *silent* but very large myocardial infarction with the only signs being agitation or changes in the level of consciousness.

Another problem is that people tend to accept a wide range of symptoms as normal for aging and thus not report them. One extreme example of this was a 45-year-old woman who was referred to a pulmonary clinic after she was found to have serious obstructive airway disease during a spirometry test at a shopping center health fair. A four-pack-a-day smoker for many years, she had already given up hiking and other activities with her children and had left the housework to them. She attributed these changes in her activity level to "getting old."

A related physical change in older adults is that they are more prone to discomfort from chilling and hypothermia. These patients need to be kept warm whether in bed or out of bed. In the acute care area, examination rooms, diagnostic study areas, and patient rooms need to be kept warm. The patient should be well covered and not kept waiting in cool areas for examinations, diagnostic tests, or treatment. Warmth will be facilitated if the patient is dressed in layers and a cap is provided. Having the patient well nourished will also promote the ability to stay warm. But alcohol should be avoided as it promotes vasodilation and increases heat loss from the body.

Behavioral Changes Due to Physical Problems

One physical change that is frequently observed in the acutely ill older person is a change in behavior. Unfortunately the changes of normal aging are often intertwined with changes due to disease, fever, nutritional deficit, fluid and electrolyte imbalance, or drug interaction or toxicity. The person may be withdrawn or confused or, in extreme cases, appear to be psychotic when there is a specific, correctable cause for the behavior alteration.

When a patient is confused or combative or has other mentation problems, continued tactile stimula-

tion (touch) may be helpful. The nurse should touch the patient and encourage family members and significant others to do the same. They should talk with the patient, frequently providing reorientation to reality, such as name, date, and who is present. Unless the patient is in danger of harming self or someone else, restraints should not be used. These only increase agitation and disorientation (Gioiella and Bevil 1985).

Reactions to Medications

One of the most common correctable causes of behavior change in older adults is multiple medication therapy. The multiple medications that are commonly taken by older people can interact, or the patient may develop toxicity or abnormal responses. For example, confusion, weakness, lethargy, and abnormal behavior may be mistaken for a chronic organic mental disorder or Alzheimer's disease rather than a medication problem. Often, the first or only major sign of an adverse medication reaction is a change in the sensorium. When these symptoms occur, the person may be medicated for the new symptoms and thus have more medications in the body to interact. Some medications that are well known to cause adverse behavior include antihypertensives, dopamine agonists such as haloperidol (Haldol), steroids, tranquilizers, cimetidine (Tagamet), anticonvulsants, and digoxin. The more sudden and severe the change in behavior, the more likely it can be restored to normal by prompt intervention (Goldenberg and Chiverton 1984).

When the older person exhibits behavioral changes, it is important to look for a cause. Interviewing the family about whether the patient has had similar problems with medications in the past can be very useful. Mrs. Jones was a gentle, mild-mannered, older woman who broke her hip. She became extremely combative and unruly in the emergency department. This behavior continued into the next day, causing her and her caregivers to have an extremely difficult time. Finally one nurse noticed that she seemed to become calm as her meperidine (Demerol) wore off and then became agitated again after the next dose of the analgesic. The nurse discussed this observation with the family and found that Mrs. Jones had had a similar reaction to diazepam (Valium) several years earlier. The problem was resolved after her analgesic medication was changed. She was again cooperative and rational.

As documented earlier in this text, the older body reacts somewhat differently to drugs than the younger body. Among the reasons for these differences are differences in the proportions of lean body mass and fat and differences in percentage of body fluids. Because of these differences the nurse who administers medication to the older adult should be alert for drug toxicity. Older persons tend to metabolize medications more slowly, so the usual adult dose may be too much for them. Even if the blood levels of a drug indicate a safe therapeutic level, the person may still have adverse symptoms. Medication toxicity can be further worsened by liver or renal disorders, dehydration, and reduced intestinal motility (Todd 1985). For example, because there is less lean body mass to accept it, a higher than normal amount of gentamicin stays in the blood of older people. This then causes the person to be more susceptible to gentamicin toxicity. The use of diuretics in older adults could lead to dehydration, which exacerbates the problem of lower total body water and increases dehydration. The nurse who administers diuretics to older persons, therefore, must be especially observant for the signs of dehydration, hypokalemia, hypovolemia, or otherwise altered fluid and electrolyte balance. Because the signs of drug toxicity may vary from the usual expected symptoms in older adults, nurses should regard even the slightest symptom of toxicity as serious. Symptoms of toxicity of many drugs tend to be more *behavioral* than in younger persons *until the toxic reaction becomes extremely serious.* If an older person is taking a new drug and develops new symptoms, drug toxicity should be considered as the possible reason (Todd 1985). Sometimes, the patient is on a medication for a time before adverse symptoms develop. Therefore even if the patient is not on new drugs, often the most effective treatment for new behavioral problems is discontinuing all drugs.

Changes in gastrointestinal motility can have a profound effect on the levels of drugs that are absorbed in the gastrointestinal tract. If a drug stays in the stomach too long or is absorbed too slowly, its level in the body may be lower than expected. For other drugs that are absorbed in the intestinal tract, a prolonged stay in the intestines can result in a higher than normal level of the drug in the body (Todd

1985). A classic example of a drug whose blood level is greatly dependent on intestinal motility is digitalis (Burggraf and Stanley 1989).

The ability of the liver and kidneys to metabolize and excrete drugs diminishes as a person ages. As a result, the effects of drugs such as tranquilizers or hypnotics tend to last longer and the patient who receives these drugs may be left with a hangover. Other drugs also have longer-lasting effects and a higher toxic potential due to reduced excretion. The nurse should be aware that this might happen and observe the patient for the signs of toxicity and overdosage. Because of slowed excretion, the doses of certain drugs for the older adult may need to be only one-half to one-third of the normal adult dose (Todd 1985). The use of sedative and hypnotic drugs to promote sleep in older adults is often not effective. Their use can lead to drowsiness during the day, delirium, night terrors, agitation, confusion, and incontinence. Sometimes the nurse can promote restful sleep by offering one or two ounces of wine or sherry or one or two tablets of acetaminophen at bedtime (Gray-Vickrey 1987). These could be used in combination with backrubs, warm baths, or other usual nighttime rituals. The patient should not receive caffeine-containing beverages at bedtime.

Anticholinergic drugs such as ephedrine can be very problematic to older men because these drugs can increase the effects of prostatic hypertrophy and result in urinary retention. Hence it is better for older men to avoid taking any medications that include ephedrine. Atropine has similar effects. If it must be taken, the patient should be checked carefully for ability to void after the medication has been administered. It is helpful to instruct the man to void immediately before taking a dose of ephedrine, so that while the drug level is peaking, retention will be less of a problem (Esberger and Hughes 1989). As a person ages, salivary gland responses to stimuli such as food are less than normal. As a result the mouth of the older person is often dry and sore. When the person takes drugs such as anticholinergics, tricyclic antidepressants, or phenothiazines, their side effects will add to the parched-mouth problem. This excessive drying of the mouth could lead to periodontal disease, dental caries, mucosal ulcerations, and superinfections. Efforts to stimulate salivary flow with mechanisms such as gum chewing or hard candy may not be effective. Several interventions can aid the patient who has an excessively dry mouth. Frequent rinsing with tepid clear water is safe and easy. Teeth should be flossed and brushed gently to prevent gum disease or caries. There are some substitute saliva preparations available. Oral hygiene should be a priority for patients in the critical care unit. Excellent oral hygiene not only promotes comfort, but also prevents later complications of the mouth and oral mucosa.

Antihypertensives are drugs that can be problematic in anyone of any age. In the older person whose vascular system has lost some of its elasticity and resilience, the vasodilation produced by antihypertensive drugs can result in postural hypotension, dizziness, and fainting when the patient changes position too quickly. In extreme cases the patient could have a cerebrovascular accident because of sudden lack of blood flow to the brain (Hamilton 1987). The older person who is taking antihypertensives should be monitored carefully and should be taught to avoid situations that precipitate postural hypotension. These patients should learn to change position slowly; to avoid long, hot baths; to avoid alcohol intake (which is a vasodilator); and to have a cool-down period after exercise so that the vessels regain their normal tone and size.

Immobility

Acutely ill older adults are much more prone to the hazards of immobility than are other patients. These effects of immobility include thrombi, hypostatic pneumonia, skin breakdown, contractures, and constipation. The risk of thrombi and emboli is greatly increased in older adults by coexisting conditions including urinary calculi, atherosclerosis, diabetes, varicosities, and peripheral neuropathy. Prevention of phlebitis and emboli includes careful positioning to prevent pressure on a limb, the use of support hose, elevating the legs when sitting, frequent movement and exercise, and sometimes low-dose heparin (Pomerantz 1982).

Even when a person is acutely ill, it is important to turn and move the patient as early and as often as possible to promote comfort and prevent contractures and atelectasis. An incentive spirometer will help to keep the alveoli open in those who are able to use it. An egg create or other type of protective mattress should be used during the period of immobility. If the patient cannot be turned completely, he/she should be rotated frequently from side to side as far as possible. The danger of dehydration in patients who are placed on *Clinitron* beds should be a constant consideration. This is due to the constant circulation of warm dry air in the bed and around the patient (Bristow, Goldfarb, and Green 1987). Passive range-of-motion exercises should be started on the first day of the illness. In order to avoid foot drop, the bedfast patient should wear high-top tennis shoes or foam boots. The shoes and socks should be removed three times daily and the feet thoroughly dried and exercised. Footboards are generally not helpful. Hand splints will be helpful for some patients.

Careful skin care should be given at every opportunity. Harsh soaps and alcohol should not be used in the care of older skin because of their drying effect. The patient's skin should be kept clean and dry at all times. Skin lotions and creams should be applied to all dry and reddened areas of the skin several times a day. If the skin is particularly fragile or is sensitive to tape, the use of tape on the skin should be avoided as much as possible. Even the use of paper tape may not be enough to prevent skin tears. Stockinette or roller bandages may be used on the extremities instead of tape. Stockinette or fishnet may be enough to hold dressings in place on the trunk.

A careful record of bowel movements should be kept and the patient checked for impaction when it is indicated. Appropriate nursing care measures should be used to prevent impaction.

Safety

Safety and protection from injury are major considerations in the care of older patients in the critical care unit. When turning or moving an older patient, great care should be taken to prevent injury. Because older people are prone to osteoporosis, their bones fracture easily. Shoulder and hip joints have reduced muscle tone and can be dislocated easily if there is sufficient pull on them. A hip or shoulder joint could be dislocated if the caregiver pulls on arms or legs or positions the person so that the weight of an arm or leg pulls on the joint. Arms should be well supported on pillows. Legs should be carefully positioned so that skin does not touch skin or the bedrails.

Maintaining Fluid Balance

The fluid balance of the critically ill older person is much more precarious than that of the younger adult. Therefore maintenance of an adequate fluid intake, while avoiding fluid overload, is essential. A diminished fluid intake and the resulting dehydration can cause an altered mental status. Fluids should be within easy reach of the older patient who is able to get them for himself. Otherwise, fluids should be offered at frequent intervals. Many older people will drink only small amounts of fluid at a time, so fluid should be given often. Giving fluids only at mealtime is not adequate.

The older patient is at special risk of dehydration and renal damage when iodine-containing dyes are given for tests. If the patient must fast or has compromised renal function before receiving such a dye, intravenous fluids should be used to maintain hydration. If enemas are necessary as a preparation for studies of the gastrointestinal tract, the patient may become hydrated and electrolytes depleted. This patient should receive intravenous fluids containing potassium during the period of preparation for the examination; the number of enemas limited (Beare and Myers 1990). In one study, 54 percent of the patients over age 72 experienced orthostatic hypotension, confusion, or some other change in mental status after a single diagnostic test. In the same group, 11 percent of the patients studied fell sometime after the test. The nurse should monitor patients who are being prepared for tests very carefully, checking the fluid and electrolyte balance often, keeping the bed low and the siderails up, and assisting the patient in getting up until at least twenty-four hours after the test (Gray-Vickrey 1987). Once the test is completed, the nurse should be aware of the character of stools if barium has been administered. Constipation may prevent the adequate elimination of the barium and necessitate the use of a mild laxative.

If a patient has been dehydrated, there may be some changes as rehydration is accomplished. For example, a person who had normal hemoglobin and hematocrit values on admission may have decreased values as rehydration occurs. A person who is in the early stages of heart failure may not be symptomatic if dehydrated. However, when the patient is rehydrated and the heart is unable to handle the added fluid load, a full-blown heart failure crisis may occur.

Even pneumonia may not show up very well on an Xray if the patient is dehydrated. Once rehydration is done, however, the infiltrates may show clearly.

Nutrition

A high proportion of older adults who are admitted to the hospital are malnourished. Critical illness further depletes nutritional status. Good nutrition is essential not only to healing, but also to survival. At least half of those who need nutritional support in the hospital are older patients. As a result an early nutritional assessment can be a key tool in patient management.

Although the nutritional assessment will probably be done by a dietitian or a metabolic support team, the nurse has important responsibilities related to nutrition. The patient should be weighed daily at the same time each day on the same scale and under the same circumstances. Calorie counts, if ordered, should be done completely and carefully. It is important that patients not be placed on such restrictive diets that they will not eat. A slightly more liberal diet that is palatable will be much more helpful to the patient. Dentures should be in place and the diet should be dental soft rather than pureed. Mealtimes should be pleasant and may be made more so by the presence of significant others, food brought from home, or group meals. The patient should be as comfortable and pain-free as possible at mealtime. If oral supplements are used, they should be timed so that they do not interfere with mealtime. Patients should be allowed to choose the supplement they like best as well as the method of serving it. If tube feedings are given, small-bore tubes should be used because they are more comfortable than the larger ones. One hundred milliliters of water should be administered through the tube every four hours, both to provide the body requirement for free water and to keep the tube clear. A continuous feeding will not keep the tube clear. Patients should be fed only in the upright position, and tube placement should be checked at least three times daily with an air bolus to prevent aspiration. Patients who cannot take nourishment via the gastrointestinal tract will need hyperalimentation. There is much special care associated with this nutritional method. Older patients are especially prone to the complications of catheter sepsis, hyperglycemia, hypoglycemia, and fluid overload. Those with renal or liver disease are also prone to protein overload.

Confusion

Confusion is a frequent by-product of hospitalization in older persons. It is estimated that it occurs in up to 80 percent of hospitalized older adults and that up to one-third of those affected may die. Further it is estimated that the more severely ill the older person is, the more severe may be the acute confusion. Unfortunately, up to 70 percent of patients who become acutely confused in the hospital are not recognized as confused by physicians or nurses because cognitive function is haphazardly and incompletely assessed; the difference between disorientation or agitation and acute confusion is unrecognized. Acute confusion is often correctable because it is a sign of a physical or pathologic condition (Foreman 1990).

Agitation or disorientation often is not due to pathology but may be caused by such factors as sleep deprivation, an unfamiliar environment, fewer and shorter interactions with family members, lack of time-and-place indicators such as clocks and calendars, sensory overload or sensory deprivation, advanced age, and extreme physical or psychological stress. Acute confusion, on the other hand, may be caused by a wide variety of physical conditions and stressors such as hypoxemia, hypercapnia, dehydration, prolonged pump or anesthesia times, intraoperative hypotension, postoperative hypothermia, toxicity from impaired hepatic and/or renal function, polypharmacy, folate deficiency, hyponatremia, hypokalemia, hyperglycemia, or other major pathophysiologic alterations (Foreman 1990).

Those older persons who have chronic illness or polypharmacy or who have just been admitted or have just had surgery are especially high risks for acute confusion. They need systematic assessment and surveillance. This assessment should go further than the usual notation of presence or absence of disorientation, which is not synonymous with acute confusion. Several options for systematic assessment are available and have been summarized by Foreman (1990). One of those is a confusion rating scale consisting of behaviors that indicate impaired cognitive function. It is useful for those with subtle manifestations of acute confusion or those with rapidly changing mental status. Such a scale evaluates disorientation to time, place, or person; inappropriate communication or behavior; and hallucinations or delusional behav-

ior. These behaviors are rated on a three-point scale as often as necessary, somewhat similar to the use of the Glasgow Coma Scale rating system (Williams, Ward, and Campbell 1988). The patient's physical state, laboratory tests, medications, and other data should be studied in an attempt to identify the cause of the confusion. When the underlying cause of the confusion has been identified, it should be corrected as soon and as completely as possible. In addition, the nurse should provide symptomatic and supportive measures, such as restoring the patient's sense of control, relieving pain, and promoting physical and mental activity (Lipowski 1980).

Overmedication or polypharmacy is a special source of confusion. Medications for older patients must be started at low doses and titrated upward to achieve maximum results while minimizing adverse effects. Bezon (1991) developed an excellent tool for doing a comprehensive assessment of multimedication therapy, risks, and reactions.

Cardiac Risks

There are a variety of changes in the cardiovascular system with aging. Atherosclerosis is the most common pathologic process affecting perfusion in older adults; smoking is an important compounding factor (Maas et al. 1991). As a person ages, the number of cardiac pacer cells decreases. The early diastolic filling rate severely decreases over age 65, while the late diastolic filling rate increases and the aorta stiffens. These changes lead to a prolonged relaxation phase and an increase in cardiac work load (Fulmer and Walker 1990). There are EKG changes associated with these physiologic changes. The P-R interval is prolonged to 0.22 seconds for the upper limit of normal; there may be reduced QRS amplitude; there may be alterations in the R wave and ST segment. These alterations cause a loss of specificity in EKG diagnosis, but alterations should not be overlooked. The prolonged P-R interval favors the development of re-entry dysrhythmias. Sinus dysrhythmias and bradycardia may lead to syncope, dizziness, palpitations, and/or weakness. These problems may cause falls or unexplained accidents (Burggraf and Stanley 1989). The normal heart rate for an older person is low at rest (may be as low as fifty beats/minute), elevates slowly in response to increased demands, and takes longer to return to baseline after an elevation. There is a reduced cardiac output and stroke volume (Maas et al. 1991).

The tools that are currently used for assessing cardiac output have not been adapted or tested on older patients, but surveillance, monitoring, and physical assessment are not any less critical (Maas et al. 1991). The signs and symptoms of heart failure take longer to detect and may reflect more serious conditions. Rather than the classic signs, the older person may display nonspecific signs of poor cerebral perfusion such as somnolence, confusion, or weakness. The aging heart is less able to compensate for rapid fluid shifts, so intravenous therapy should be carefully controlled (Fulmer and Walker 1990).

Physical or mental stress or strenuous activity causes an increase in body oxygen demands. The cardiovascular problems of aging cause sudden demands for more oxygen anywhere in the body to be poorly tolerated. There is therefore a poor response to stress or activity. Whatever tachycardia occurs is not as great as in younger persons and takes longer to return to baseline (Maas et al. 1991). Conditioning is important to keep muscles functioning optimally and requiring less oxygen per unit of work. Older persons should therefore be up and moving as much as possible. Bed rest hastens deconditioning and increases cardiac work load. The heart may be unable to meet the oxygen demands of deconditioned muscles.

Older persons tend to have high blood pressure and low blood volume. The baroreceptors do not react quickly when the person changes position. These factors predispose to hypovolemia, make fluid balance more critical, cause a tendency toward postural hypotension and falling, and cause errors in sitting and standing blood pressures if the pressure is taken too soon after the position change. Many physicians do not treat high blood pressure in older adults until it is about 180/90–95. When it is treated, the pressure should be lowered slowly and precautions taken against falls and other adverse effects. If the blood pressure drop is over 20 mm Hg or the diastolic pressure under 100 when sitting or standing, the patient is at high risk for dizziness and falls (Maas et al. 1991; Burggraf and Stanley 1989).

Aaronson et al. describe a variety of precautions that may be used to prevent falls in those with postural hypotension.

Respiratory Risks

The respiratory effects of aging are often difficult to separate from other factors that affect respiration. In general, aging predisposes one to premature airway closure and poorly ventilated or underventilated alveoli, hypoxemia, less-efficient matching of ventilation and perfusion, blunted responses to hypoxia, hypercapnia, other demands on breathing, and lowered defenses: cough effort, respiratory muscle strength, less ciliary action, and less protection for aspiration. There is an increased risk of barotrauma due to mechanical ventilation or intermittent positive pressure ventilation (IPPB). There is also a high risk of ventilator dependence. The patient who is lying in a recumbent position for long periods of time is extremely vulnerable to atelectasis and hypostatic pneumonia. Oversedation is another high risk in older adults, as it reduces respiratory drive and tidal volume. Older people are much more likely to develop postoperative respiratory complications (especially pneumonia and pulmonary embolus) than are younger persons (Maas et al. 1991; Burggraf and Stanley 1989; Fulmer and Walker 1990).

Excellent pulmonary hygiene is therefore critical to older patients. The nurse should turn, cough, deep breathe, and ambulate acutely ill elders as much as possible. If the patients sit up to eat or during tube feedings, they are less likely to aspirate. Ventilators and IPPB should be used with caution and with careful attention to breath sounds and other indicators of barotrauma. Ambulating and moving older patients may be problematic because some breathlessness is common for them, even in the absence of respiratory disease. Younger persons use the abdominal muscles and diaphragm to facilitate deeper respirations when demanded. Older persons commonly use these muscles for routine breathing and have thus lost their reserve for periods of demand. If respiratory disease is present, the breathlessness may be more pronounced. Patients are often reluctant to move and be active because of their fear of breathlessness and dyspnea (Maas et al. 1991; Burggraf and Stanley 1989).

SUMMARY

The study of ways in which the care of the critically ill older adult differs from the care of other acutely ill patients is in its infancy. There is still much to be learned regarding the care of the critically ill older adult. The differences encompass all areas of physiology and psychology and all areas of nursing care. The major problem is that the older patient who is acutely ill often has multiple serious problems that may present differently and need different management implications than the same problems in other older adults. Care of the seriously ill older adult requires a highly knowledgeable and skilled multidisciplinary team and a great deal of individualization of care for the needs of the particular patient.

STUDY QUESTIONS

1. Approximately what proportion of the population of acute care hospitals is made up of older adults?

2. Describe some common maladaptive responses of older adults at the time of hospital admission. Discuss related nursing interventions.

3. Relate the concepts of role, control, helplessness, and powerlessness to the needs of the acutely ill older person.

4. Discuss a method by which the nurse can adapt care to an older person's decreased flexibility and need for routine.

5. Evaluate important concepts relating to the educational needs of the acutely ill older person.

6. List implications of sudden behavioral changes in the older patient.

7. Compare methods of appropriately providing sensory stimulation to the acutely ill older person.

8. Identify common sensory losses of older adults and cite appropriate nursing interventions for each in the critical care unit.

9. Describe at least five ways in which older adults respond differently physiologically to disease than do younger persons.

10. Cite at least four common problems related to medication therapy of the critically ill older adult.

REFERENCES

Aaronson, L., W. Carlon-Wolfe, and S. Schoener. 1991. Pressures that fall on rising: Ways to control postural hypotension. *Geriatric Nursing* 12(2):67.

American Association of Retired Persons. 1991. *A Profile of Older Americans*. PF3049 (1291). D996. Washington, DC: United States Department of Health and Human Services.

Beare, P.G. and J.L. Myers. 1990. *Principles and Practice of Adult Health Nursing*. St. Louis: C.V. Mosby.

Bezon, J. 1991. Approaching drug regimens with a therapeutic dose of suspicion. *Geriatric Nursing* 12(4):180–82.

Bristow, J.V., E.H. Goldfarb, and M. Green. 1987. Clinitron therapy: Is it effective? *Geriatric Nursing* 8(2):120–24.

Burggraf, V. and M. Stanley. 1989. *Nursing the El-*derly. A Care Plan Approach*. Philadelphia: J.B. Lippincott.

Christ, M.A. and F. J. Hohloch. 1988. *Gerontologic Nursing: A Study and Learning Tool*. Springhouse, PA: Springhouse.

Ebersole, P. and P. Hess. 1990. *Toward Health Aging: Human Needs and Nursing Response*. St. Louis: C.V. Mosby.

Eliopoulos, C. 1989. *Gerontological Nursing*. 2d ed. Philadelphia: J.B. Lippincott.

El-Sherif, C. 1986. A unit for the acutely ill. *Geriatric Nursing* 7(3):130–32.

Ferrell, B.R. and B.A. Ferrell. 1990. Easing the pain. *Geriatric Nursing* 11(4):175–78.

Foreman, D. 1990. Complexities of acute confusion. *Geriatric Nursing* 11(3):136–39.

Fulmer, T.T. and M.K. Walker. 1990. Lessons from

the elder boom in ICUs. *Geriatric Nursing* 11(3):120–21.

Gioiella, E.C. and C.W. Bevil, eds. 1985. *Nursing Care of the Aging Client: Promoting Healthy Adaptation.* Norwalk, CT: Appleton-Century-Crofts.

Goldenberg, and P. Chiverton. 1984. Assessing behavior: The nurse's mental status exam. *Geriatric Nursing* 5(2):94–98.

Gray-Vickrey, M. 1987. Color them special. *Nursing '87* 17(5):59–62.

Hamilton, H.K., ed. 1987. *Nursing '87 Drug Handbook.* Springhouse, PA: Springhouse.

Lichtenstein, V. 1982. Nutritional management. *Geriatric Nursing* 3(6):386–91.

Lipowski, A.J. 1980. *Delirium: Acute Brain Failure in Man.* Springfield, IL: C.C. Thomas Publisher.

Maas, M., K.C. Buckwalter, and M. Hardy. 1991. *Nursing Diagnoses and Interventions for the Elderly.* New York: Addison-Wesley Nursing.

Pomerantz, R. 1982. Considerations in the physician's approach. *Geriatric Nursing* 3(5):311–14.

Schoemick, L., P. Katz, and T. Beam. 1991. The many guises of infection. *Geriatric Nursing* 12(5):223–24.

Todd, B. 1985. *Medicating the Elderly* (video). New York: American Journal of Nursing Co.

Williams, M.A., S.E. Ward and E.B. Campbell. 1988. Confusion: Testing versus observation. *Journal of Gerontological Nursing* 14(1):25–30.

16 Patient Education and Discharge Planning

Marta A. Browning
Elaine L. Gross

CHAPTER OUTLINE

FOCUS

The primary focus of this chapter is the role of the nurse as teacher. The process of teaching/learning and the relationship of the nurse-teacher and the client-learner as they interact in this process are essential. Topics appropriate for client learning and specific strategies to enhance learning among older adults are described. The process of discharge planning and case management in all settings is one area where teaching/learning is essential.

OBJECTIVES

1. Identify the rationale for the role of the nurse as teacher.

2. Analyze the basic elements in the teaching/learning process.

3. Describe the elements to be included in assessment of the client-learner.

4. Identify learning needs of older adults.

5. List specific topics appropriate for inclusion in health education for older adults for both health promotion and illness management.

6. Describe teaching strategies that enhance learning among older adults.

7. Analyze the concept of discharge planning.

8. Review the role of the members of the interdisciplinary health care team in the process of discharge planning.

9. Explain the role of the nurse in case management.

10. Differentiate case management and managed care.

TEACHING AND LEARNING

Teaching is a major priority of the nurse, second only to saving and sustaining life. For many nurses the concept of the nurse as educator is secondary as daily responsibilities may center exclusively around the performance of technical procedures and the administration of medications. However, no function of the nurse is more significant or meaningful for clients and families than the transfer of information and skills that decrease anxiety, promote informed choices, and/or lead to self-care mastery.

Teaching and learning comprise a continuous, interactive, and reciprocal process that occurs in an interpersonal exchange between client and nurse. When implemented with good will and conscious intent, the process enhances the self-esteem of both individuals. Client teaching is one of the most richly rewarding of all nursing functions. It is caring in action. The nurse provides information and teaches skills to clients, encouraging them to achieve mastery and competence in the management of their own health care needs. In return, clients teach the nurse creative ways of applying the information presented; new ways of adapting familiar skills; innovative coping styles; the power of courage, faith and persistence; and the validity of old or traditional ways of evaluating the efficacy of new technologies. Insights provided by clients allow nurses to enrich their repertoire of health care strategies. Workable suggestions can be passed from client to client through the nurse.

Teaching and learning with older adults are especially rewarding experiences. When implemented effectively, the teaching/learning exchange between nurse and client in this population group is one of equals. Older adults have much experience, wisdom, and insight to exchange for the information and skill development provided by the nurse. As a group, older adults are appreciative, receptive, attentive, and warm towards their nurse-teachers. They are conscientious and diligent and try to meet the expectations of the professionals who take the time to teach them. In short, they are ideal students. If treated with sensitivity, consideration, and patience, older adult clients will reward their nurses by participating in the negotiation regarding learning priorities and will accept relevant portions of education offered by the nurse. These same learners also will offer valuable lessons of their own to the practitioners who are open enough to receive them.

RATIONALE FOR THE ROLE OF THE NURSE AS CLIENT EDUCATOR

Teaching, as a function of the nurse, is identified in state nurse practice acts and in nursing Standards of Practice suggested by the American Nurses' Association. Hospitalized clients are entitled to information and education detailed in the Patients' Bill of Rights as mandated by the American Hospital Association since 1972. Also, many third-party payors (e.g., Medicare) identify client teaching performed by nurses as a covered service that is reimbursable. Finally, since the prospective payment system (PPS) based on diagnosis related groups (DRGs) was instituted by the Health Care Financing Administration (HCFA) in 1983, emphasis has been placed on timely and effective teaching as a means to promote early discharge from acute care institutions. Thus the inclusion of client teaching in hospital discharge planning protocols is mandated by the Joint Commission on Accreditation of Healthcare Organizations (JCAHO) (*How to Teach Patients* 1989).

Control of escalating health care costs has now become a major focus of the health care industry. Early discharge of Medicare patients from acute care institutions (prompted by prospective payment, increased insurance deductibles, transfer of procedures once done only in acute care institutions to ambulatory care settings such as medi- and surgicenters, emphasis on health promotion and healthy lifestyle activities, and other measures to cap costs) has forced clients and their family caregivers to become involved in self-care activities. Tasks once performed only by professionals in intensive care and step-down units are now expected to be performed by clients and caregivers at home. A list of such procedures could easily function as a curriculum outline for skills-related laboratories in professional nursing programs, see Table 16-1. Older adults currently account for 31 percent of total health care expenditures and for 42 percent of all days of care in the hospital (Weinrich, Boyd, and

Table 16–1 Technical Medical Procedures Commonly Performed at Home by Client and/or Caregiver

---

Monitoring temperature, pulse, and respiration

Monitoring blood pressure

Oxygen therapy

Inhalation therapy using nebulizers, inhalers, and ventilators

Management of feeding tubes (nasogastric, gastrostomy)

Provision of total parenteral nutrition/intravenous hyperalimentation

Management of ostomies (colostomies/ileostomies)

Management of tracheostomies

Management of urinary catheters and drainage devices/nephrostomy tubes

Peritoneal dialysis

Medication administration

    Intravenous

    Parenteral

    Oral

    Topical

Chemotherapy administration

Pain control (medications, TENS)

Application of hot/cold treatments

Wound care and dressing

Blood glucose monitoring

Chest physiotherapy/postural drainage

Active and passive range-of-motion exercises

Implementation of therapeutic diets

Collection of laboratory specimens

Application and use of assistive devices (e.g., braces, splints, reachers, walkers, wheelchairs, lifts)

Cast care

Infection control (e.g., AIDS)

Management of dying individual

Nussbaum 1989). Twenty-five percent of aged hospitalized individuals are readmitted at least two times within twelve months of their discharge date (Johnson 1989). Readmissions are frequently due to failure to comply with medication or treatment regimens, resulting in an inability to control unstable medical conditions. As many as 8 percent of older adults are homebound due to illness (Folden 1990). As many as 15 percent of older adults suffer severe cognitive impairment that impacts their ability to perform activities of daily living, yet three-fourths of these individuals live at home (Gilles 1986). Also, according to the National Association for Home Care (NAHC), over a million and a half chronically ill older adults annually require skilled professional services from nurses and other allied health professionals under the Medicare home care benefit. Thus health education is needed by hundreds of thousands of older adults to promote health, prevent illness, maintain or enhance the quality of life, and delay costly hospitalization and readmission.

However, clients and caregivers often become casualties of fragmented or nonexistent discharge planning. Johnson (1989) found that nurses place little or only moderate value on discharge planning. Nurses in this study viewed their major priority as physical care of the client and seldom took advantage of the time taken to perform procedures to simultaneously teach these same procedures to the clients under their care. Teaching was viewed by the nurses as a totally separate function from patient care. It was placed low on the priority list of nursing activities, superseded by the demands of technical activities. On the other hand, the clients in Johnson's study rated the teaching component of discharge planning as very important. They wanted to know about diet, medications, treatments, and referrals to community resources. They also wanted their families to be involved in the patient education process. In Johnson's study, comments such as these were common among patients:

- "If I can take care of myself, I can live at home. If I can't do it, I will have to go to a nursing home."

- "I don't understand the instructions they gave me."

- "I know she explained it to me once but I am not sure what she meant."

- "They gave me a list of instructions as they wheeled me out the door. I never had time to ask questions."

Professional caregivers—nurses, physicians, and allied health professionals—become upset when dealing with passive or dependent clients and are quick to label them uncooperative and noncompliant. However, the system in which the professionals practice is not structured in a way that promotes collaboration or partnerships between older adults and professionals through the transfer of learning. There is usually little planning related to client education. The implementation of poorly planned teaching strategies do not produce desired client responses. Professional caregivers are often inaccessible, unavailable, or unresponsive to clients' requests for assistance. Since the advent of DRGs and the push to early discharge, older adults are often placed in new roles and given awesome responsibilities (e.g., irrigating Hickman lines, managing home intravenous antibiotic therapy, providing tracheostomy care, and performing blood glucose monitoring) with only cursory training. They are then criticized for inadequate performance and labeled as noncompliant with medical and nursing regimens. Professionals are usually unaware of the contribution they have made to client noncompliance through their failure to plan, structure, and implement experiences that will foster learning and ensure client competence. In addition, professionals often fail to recognize that knowledge is power and that they may receive secondary gains when the client is maintained in a powerless, dependent state by their failure to transfer sufficient knowledge to enable independence and freedom from their care.

One underlying problem is the professional's failure to understand that *telling* is not *teaching* nor does it sufficiently transfer knowledge from one individual to another. The research of Lipetz, Bussigel, Bannerman, and Risley (1990) revealed that 58 percent of their sample of physicians and nurses indicated that the patient's lack of interest in changing behavior is frequently an impediment to patient education; 77 percent indicated that the patient's lack of interest in learning skills was frequently or sometimes an impediment. In exploring these assumptions further, the researchers found real differences in what constituted patient teaching between physicians and nurses. Nurses viewed patient teaching as an activity that requires specific planning, execution, and follow-up. Physician respondents, on the other hand, equated patient education with the process of informed consent, giving a diagnosis, and providing instructions for taking medications or self-care. Physicians did not view education as a process, but rather viewed each contact with patients as an educational one.

Rendon, Davis, Gioiella, and Tranzillo (1986) stated that "our society believes that human beings have a right to know, to be informed, and to be taught. These rights are known as the 'rights to well-being or needs fulfillment rights'." These authors noted that nurses do not respond to these rights in an equalitarian manner across the life span. Preference is given to children and middle-aged adults when teaching or providing information. Older adults are often erroneously perceived to be too old to learn or incapable of understanding new information. Rendon et al. noted that our high-tech society devalues older adults and may ultimately deprive them of their "right to know" by placing barriers to their access to information. They stated that age-related changes in the client require modification of teaching strategies on the part of the nurse. They further stated that "negative stereotypes concerning the elderly and a lack of sound gerontological knowledge have prevented nurses from employing teaching strategies that would enhance elderly clients' knowledge and use of health related information" (33).

Professional nurses who practice in home care and community health invariably find clients and caregivers at home on the first or second day after hospital discharge confused, frightened, and bewildered. Most of the time the client has been discharged with several sets of instructions. More often than not, elements of each set of instructions are in conflict or contradictory to the others. If the clients were taught self-care skills in the acute care institution, the learning has not transferred to the home setting where adaptations must often be made in the use of equipment or supplies. These clients and their caregivers face the raw fear that failure to perform the expected tasks may result in death, injury, or rehospitalization of the client. If this fear cannot be translated into mastery and competence, the client's caregiving system will break down when confronted with the strain of twenty-four-hour responsibility for providing total care. Thus the client will be admitted to an acute or long-term care institution.

BASIC ELEMENTS OF THE TEACHING/LEARNING PROCESS

Teaching

Teaching is defined by Redman (1988, 9) as "any interpersonal influence aimed at changing the way in which other persons will behave." Redman further defined teaching as "activities by which the teacher helps the student to learn" and "communication specially structured and sequenced to produce learning" (1988, 9). Teaching is defined by Cheeseman and Selekman (1987, 2) as a "collaborative process that involves communication between the nurse and the patient. Its goal is to add to the patient's knowledge base so he can improve or maintain his health and comfort."

Learning

Learning is a change in human disposition or capability and is represented by a change in behavior (Kozier, Erb and Oliveri 1991). Learning theories are classified into two broad categories: behavioristic and cognitive. Behavioristic theories describe learning as conditioning or reinforcement of behaviors. Cognitive theories describe learning as the development of insights or understandings that provide a potential guide for behavior. According to cognitive theorists, learning may occur with or without a change in behavior (Redman 1988). Thus the process of teaching/learning is interactive but learning may or may not result in a change in behavior.

Learning is dynamic and fluid and takes place over time. The total process of learning and remembering requires apprehending (noting or perceiving, paying attention, and coding of a stimulus), acquiring (ascertaining personal relevance and assigning a unique code), and sharing and retrieving information (Huckabay, 1980). For learning to take place, a stimulus must be perceived by the senses, interpreted or attended by the learner, briefly stored and coded in primary memory, and then stored in secondary memory (Rendon, Davis, Gioiella, and Tranzillo 1986). Thus the process of learning requires establishing memory that involves receiving input, then coding and storing it. According to Gilles (1986, 357), "meaningful information put in 'digestible' form (encoded) is assigned a specific location in long-term memory (storage) and later is found and returned to focused attention (retrieval)."

Distinctions should be made between sensory memory, primary (short-term) memory, and secondary (long-term) memory. Sensory memory is a temporary perceptual holding system that retains images and sounds for one to two seconds until perceptual images fade or are replaced by the continuing input of new stimuli. Primary (short-term) memory can be called working memory and holds information selected from sensory memory for active attention and further processing. The capacity of primary memory is seven (plus or minus two) pieces of information that are retained no longer than thirty seconds. At the end of this time it is either forgotten or transferred to long-term memory. The capacity of primary (short-term) memory can be increased by "chunking" or categorizing information to be held at the center of attention. Secondary (long-term) memory is a holding system for information that has been selected from primary memory for permanent storage. In long-term memory each piece of information is coded and cross-filed in several ways—acoustically, visually, and in terms of meaning. Thus retrieval is facilitated and can be cued in several ways (Gilles 1986). "Of all sensory information perceived by an individual, that which is related to current needs and interests is selected, transferred to primary or short-term memory where it is 'rehearsed' and 'chunked,' and transferred to secondary or long-term memory where it is hooked to related, previously learned information" (Gilles 1986, 358). Information in long-term memory does not decay but may be unavailable for retrieval if inappropriately tagged for storage or not logically a part of the searching procedure taking place during an effort of recall.

Health care providers have long associated learning with client compliance. Many health care providers judge learning to have occurred when clients recognize and accept the need to learn, expend the energy to learn, and follow through with appropriate behaviors that reflect the learning (Kozier et al. 1991). Clients are said to be in compliance with health care regimens when they learn and implement information or procedures as they are taught by the health care provider.

Learning also has been closely associated with change theory as proposed by Kurt Lewin. Lewin described change as having three basic stages: unfreezing, moving, and refreezing. During the unfreezing stage, the client becomes aware of the need to change and is motivated to establish change. In the moving stage, information is gathered, the change is planned and started, and reinforcement for the change is sought. Finally, refreezing occurs and the individual involved in the change integrates the change into his or her own value system and the change is stabilized in the person's behavior (Kozier et al. 1991).

ASSESSMENT OF THE CLIENT-LEARNER

For the purpose of this chapter, the "client" is used to encompass both the individual client/patient and the individuals comprising his or her caregiving network.

Common Physical Changes that Impact Learning

Both clients and older adult members of their caregiving systems are affected by physical changes that accompany aging. (These changes are covered in detail in chapter 3.) The effective nurse-teacher must be aware of these changes and adopt teaching strategies that minimize their negative impact on learning. Health care providers often overlook the effect that physical and physiological changes have on the ability of the older adult to apprehend or perceive stimuli, to process and encode messages, and to store and retrieve information from long-term memory. Therefore they are surprised when older adults do not respond to their teaching strategies and instructional materials in the same manner as younger or middle-aged clients. As a result of unexpected or less-than-favorable responses to teaching, health care providers erroneously assume older adults to be incapable of learning; stimuli may simply need to be presented in an alternate manner.

Changes in the senses create the first barrier to learning. If stimuli are never received, they cannot be encoded to subsequently serve as stimuli for behavior change. Obviously, gross changes such as blindness or deafness will prove a significant barrier to the receipt of stimuli. However, more subtle changes that occur in aging are also of substantive concern in learning. Alterations in hearing—e.g., an inability to discriminate sounds; an inability to distinguish words with *S, Z, T, F,* and *G*; loss of high-frequency sounds; decreased sound conduction; decreased ability to filter background noise; decreased ability to comprehend speech as speech rate and pace increase—impair the effectiveness of spoken lessons. Visual changes—e.g., decreased depth perception, loss of accommodation of the lens, loss of peripheral vision, fading of colors, inability to discriminate colors (for example blue, green, and violet), decreased visual acuity and discrimination of fine visual detail, and inability to adjust to glare—may render the perusal of printed material a frustrating mystery rather than an illuminating and edifying experience (Weinrich, Boyd, and Nussbaum 1989).

Similarly, decreases in smell, touch, taste, and control of body thermoregulation can block routes of sensory stimulation available to the teacher or alter the quality of messages received. Also, alterations in sensation may make it difficult for older adults to perform some types of skills promoted by the nurse-teacher. (For example: teaching a diabetic to monitor the color of his/her chem strips will be ineffective if he/she cannot discriminate color; teaching an older adult to monitor the signs of impending urinary tract infection will be ineffective if he/she cannot smell the foul odor of his/her urine; teaching an older adult to test the temperature of bath water may be dangerous if peripheral neuropathies are present and the client does not own a bath thermometer.)

The older adult's attention span may be altered both by normal physical changes that accompany aging and by the symptoms of chronic disease. The loss of muscle tone in the perineal floor for women and benign prostatic hypertrophy in men can lead to increased frequency, urgency in voiding, and episodes of incontinence that interrupt concentration and attention. Alterations in thermoregulation can cause older adults to chill and can distract them from learning activities in drafty or cold environments. Pain interferes with concentration and many standard medications can alter or impair thought processes and sensory messages. Altered sleep-rest cycles and decreased blood to the pulmonary circulation can lead to fatigue and abbreviate attention span. Finally, alteration in muscle tone, decreased fine-motor coordination, and diminished rate and magnitude of reflex responses may lengthen the time required to perform skills that once were performed quickly (Rendon, Davis, Gioiella, and Tranzillo 1986; Weinrich, Boyd, and Nussbaum 1989).

The nurse-teacher must be aware of the client's requirement for assistive devices such as eyeglasses, hearing aids, pain control pumps, walkers, wheelchairs, braces, canes, and portable oxygen. The relationship that these devices have to sustaining the client's functional ability must be recognized. When such devices are required, the nurse-teacher must ensure that the client has them and that they are in working order, or learning will be less effective.

Cognitive Changes and Learning

Many cognitive losses in older adults are the result of common age-related changes. Memory may be affected by decreased brain transmission of acetylcholine and other imbalances in neurotransmitters. Pathological states also may impair learning and memory. The presence of toxins, nutritional deficits, circulatory inadequacy, and degeneration in nerve-cell structure and organization can lead to mild or severe deterioration of cerebral functioning (Gilles 1986). Depression also can alter the ability to learn and remember and, in severe forms, may mimic components of organic brain pathology. Assessment instruments such as the Mini Mental State Examination, the Geriatric Depression Scale, and the FROMJE test may be useful for the nurse in assessing alteration in cognitive functioning (Kane and Kane 1981).

In general, older adults may have a greater decrement in recall memory than in recognition memory on newly learned material; may have a decrease in short-term or primary memory; may require more trials on initial learning to transfer learning to long-term or secondary memory; may learn better when material is relevant and its contents are rehearsed frequently; may have a decreased ability to concentrate; and may require an increased reaction time when presented with a stimulus (Kim 1989; Weinrich, Boyd, and Nussbaum 1989). Older adults experience a decrease in fluid intelligence (basic components of information processing and reasoning: mechanics of intellectual functioning) but compensate with an increase in crystallized intelligence (content and contextual elaboration of reasoning and knowledge: pragmatics of intelligence) (Theis 1991).

Position of Learning in Client's Life Priorities

The nurse who is planning health education for chronically ill older adults must carefully assess the rank that health education and learning will be given on the client's scale of life priorities. Unfortunately health care providers often overlook the tremendous amount of time consumed by clients and their caregivers in the management of many chronic-illness conditions. For example, a client with end-stage chronic pulmonary disease may require three to four hours in the morning to bathe, dress, and eat breakfast; two to three hours per day for nebulizer and other breathing treatments; two hours a day for toileting and rest breaks in between; and one hour for taking medications. When time and energy are focused on survival and carrying out the most basic activities of daily living, little time remains for attending to the demands of learning. In addition, a caregiver who is exhausted by the daily demands of twenty-four-hour caregiving may view the suggestions of the nurse as just one more burden, particularly if such suggestions will alter caregiving routines that are well established and are functioning, however minimally. In planning learning activities for the overburdened client and/or caregiving network, careful assessment of daily routines should be performed. Information and skills taught should be adapted and integrated to cause the least disruption or change that is consistent with maintaining client safety. Clients should be laden with the need to incorporate new information only if it will lighten the overall caregiving burden or appreciably improve the older adult's or caregiver's quality of life. Therefore nurses should recognize when to refrain from teaching even though they may possess valuable information.

Coping Styles and Learning

Clients respond to illness in stages. In some stages of adaptation to illness they will be more amenable to health education efforts by the nurse than in others. Shortly after diagnosis, the client may be in a state of denial regarding the diagnosis or the implications that the diagnosis may have for alterations in life-

style. Attempts to teach about self-care at this time may be vigorously resisted or passively ignored. As the client develops awareness of the significance of the illness in his or her life, feelings of anger, fear, self-blame, and frustration may be negatively projected onto others including health care providers. Teaching will be difficult in this atmosphere of hostility and will not be absorbed when the client is overwhelmed with fear, either real or imagined.

When the client gains some measure of acceptance of the disease process, a reorganization of the approach to illness may take place. At this time, the client will begin to ask questions about his or her condition, though these initial concerns may not be shared with significant others in the client's life. As successful adaptation to management of the disease process evolves, the client may display a series of positive coping responses. These may include: increased ability to express emotions and feelings about the disease, seeking information about the condition, seeking help and support from those who have the same or related conditions, accepting help and/or actively seeking support from significant others, and becoming more independent in decision making and implementation of technical procedures required to manage the disease. When these positive adaptive responses are manifest, teaching by health care providers is most apt to prove effective (*How to Teach Patients* 1989).

Nurses also need to recognize the impact that classical coping mechanisms such as anxiety, denial, rationalization, displacement, conversion, regression, and projection have on the receptivity of older adults to learning. For example: mild anxiety is a stimulus to learning but 4+ anxiety blocks even the simplest instructions; denial serves as a stone wall to learning; regression may require that initial teaching be highly structured until more mature responses allow unstructured teaching that can involve the client actively in decision making.

Locus of Control and Learning

Individuals are described as possessing an external or internal locus of control. Persons with an *external locus of control* perceive events (such as illness) as the result of luck, chance, or fate; lacking predictability; or under the control of powerful others, some of whom may be supernatural. These individuals may believe that they have little control over their lives and therefore may be passive participants in health education efforts. They may exhibite "learned inflexibility," which can be described as a complex of orientations to social reality that includes a strong belief in external conformity, rigidity, mistrust, and a limited range of available behaviors to use in coping situations. Such individuals may respond best to highly structured client education, the health care provider as authority figure, and strong support groups who act as a source of external control.

Persons who exhibit *internal locus of control* view events as contingent on their own behavior. Internally-oriented individuals will respond best to learning situations that offer multiple options for management of chronic conditions, allow a great deal of participation in decision making, place a strong emphasis on personal responsibility and action, and promote accountability of the individual for treatment outcomes. Internally-oriented individuals may find security in establishing a safety net by planning for future events in their illness trajectory so that they can control changes as they occur and manage the alterations in functional ability that result (Dimond and Jones 1983).

Chronic Disease and Learning

Nurses who are teaching older adults to manage chronic illness must assess the type of illness and the long-term prognosis of the individual client. The type and stage of a disease condition will have important implications for teaching. For example, an otherwise healthy older adult with pneumonia who has an excellent prognosis and no sequelae may need fairly simple health education. Client instruction may be limited to information regarding management of the current illness (e.g., rest, fluids, diet, antipyretic and antibiotic use, infection control) and prevention of future episodes (e.g., flu, immunizations, avoidance of exposure to infected individuals, maintenance of a healthy lifestyle).

Education related to ongoing chronic illness will be dependent on whether the condition is stable, progressive, or intermittent. Individuals whose chronic condition has stabilized may require little instruction regarding lifestyle changes. However, if the maintenance of stability is dependent on adherence to med-

ical regimens, greater emphasis must be placed on acquiring information and skills to assure compliance. Chronic illness characterized by slow, progressive deterioration of functioning may require long-term planning of educational strategies. Individuals with an external locus of control may need educational efforts directed towards symptoms only as they arise. Persons with an internal locus of control may wish to plan coping strategies in advance across the entire trajectory of the illness. Chronic illnesses that are marked by unpredictable exacerbations followed by remissions may require intense educational efforts directed toward prevention of exacerbations and/or extension of the length of remissions.

Older adults and their caregivers who must manage the sequelae of chronic disease are committed for a long haul. They must develop a certain degree of medical sophistication regarding the illness to negotiate appropriate treatment plans. They must learn strategies that will enable them to adhere to the treatment plan and must develop satisfaction with management of the disease rather than a cure. For these individuals the major task is to maintain control of symptoms of illness in order to function at an acceptable level in the social arena. Nurse-educator efforts will need to be directed toward management of client and caregiver anxieties, grief over loss, and provision of strategies for dealing with symptom exacerbation or crisis. Nurses must incorporate caregivers in teaching and recognize that caregivers are instrumental in recognizing or validating client symptoms, deciding what to do in relation to symptoms, encouraging adherence to plans of treatment (or fostering deviation from them), and providing direct care to the client (Dimond and Jones 1983).

Education directed toward management of chronic disease states deviates from classical health education directed towards the ill who manifest *sick role* behavior. In traditional *sick role* behavior, described by Parsons, the client is not viewed as responsible for the disease condition, is exempt from normal social role obligations during the period of illness, is obligated to do what can be done to restore health, and is obligated to seek and accept professional care (Dimond and Jones 1983). Therefore health professionals expect and exact compliance from individuals manifesting the sick role during a period of transient illness. However, the chronic illnesses typically manifested by older adults are not transient; their presence is permanent. Therefore the sick-role paradigm of client management is not applicable to individuals with chronic disease and differs in three major ways. First, chronically ill older adults are not totally exempt from social obligations. They are excused from social participation only selectively and may not be totally excused until the chronic illness is far advanced or terminal. Second, in acute illness the obligation to seek and accept treatment is a given. In chronic illness the need of the individual to seek or accept treatment must be carefully balanced by considerations of human dignity and impact on quality of life. Clients must be allowed to decide whether the cost of the treatment will be too great in social or psychological terms, is compatible with the individual's value system, and can be integrated into lifestyle preferences. Thus nurses must recognize that the client may learn about illness management but that no obvious behavior change may occur or the resulting behavior change may not be the one expected or desired by the nurse-teacher. Finally, in chronic illness, the *sick role* demand for compliance with health care regimens may need to be suspended. Total adherence may foster a dependency on professional caregivers that is not ultimately productive for the person with a chronic disease (Dimond and Jones 1983). Dimond and Jones described the management of chronic illness in the following manner:

> The client with chronic illness is to a large extent the manager of his care, making the day-to-day decisions to modify the medical regimen to fit personal needs and preferences and to ameliorate symptoms as they arise. The client is not simply compliant but follows the therapeutic regimen because it makes sense (p. 42). In chronic illness, usual role performance may be only partially resumed after the acute stage of the illness; motivation to get well is an inappropriate expectation in the presence of irreversible pathology; considerations of quality of life may outweigh the obligation to seek treatment; and compliance with medical advice can only be a partial expectation when the client and family are the major managers of illness (p. 42).

Therefore nurse-teachers working with the chronically ill older adult must be prepared to *negotiate* learning priorities and must acknowledge that selective acceptance of health education may be a sign of healthy coping. Blind compliance is not an appropriate expectation.

Learning Styles

Individuals have preferred methods of learning, though these are sometimes influenced by intelligence and education. Visual learners learn best by seeing or reading what is being taught; auditory learners learn best by listening to education information; and tactile or psychomotor learners perform best by doing. It is important to ask older clients how they learn the best in order to plan appropriate learning activities and teaching strategies. When planning for group teaching, it is important that presentations incorporate strategies directed toward all three learning styles (*How to Teach Patients* 1989).

Literacy and Learning

Twenty-three million American adults may not be able to understand what health professionals are saying and may be functionally illiterate. It is estimated that one out of every five American adults lacks the literary skill (reading at or above the fifth grade level) to function in today's society and that 33.9 percent of the population is only marginally competent (Doak, Doak, and Root 1985).

Today's older adults may be particularly disadvantaged in relation to literacy skills. Many were reared in agrarian sectors of the nation and were able to complete only minimal schooling in order to be available for the demands of farm work. Others were educated sufficiently to participate in a simpler society but their levels of literacy and numeracy have not kept pace with the explosion of technology and information. Literacy and numeracy used to be assessed by determining the number of grades completed by clients, but this is an unpredictable measure at best. Literacy may be impacted by the quality of schooling, policies regarding social promotion, and inability to diagnose and treat dyslexias in earlier times. Older adults suffering from limited literacy and numeracy are often very intelligent and have spent a lifetime compensating for and concealing the fact that they cannot read, understand what is read, and/or compute. Comments such as "I forgot my glasses," "I want my husband to see this first," or "Would you read this for me? My eyes are tired" should be a cue to the nurse-teacher that literacy may be a problem (Doak, Doak, and Root 1985).

Clients with low levels of literacy suffer from some of the following problems which have significant impact on teaching strategies adopted by the nurse:

- Slowed or retarded information processing

- Impaired ability to process images and symbols

- Failure to recognize word if letters are handwritten rather than printed

- Inability to comprehend meaning of words read

- Limited vocabulary may lead to an inability to articulate concerns, ask or respond to questions, and/or convey information in a concise and sequential manner

- Inability to understand that abbreviations are a type of shorthand for other words or phrases

- Impaired ability to process generalized information such as principles for action or to draw inferences from examples

- Information is absorbed only if personalized to the client's specific situation

- Reluctance to ask questions or clarify information for fear of being thought stupid

- Inability to handle abstractions or to sort information into related groupings

- *Literal* interpretation of instructions (e.g. instructions to "force fluids" may result in the caregiver choking a client who tries to resist swallowing)

(Doak, Doak and Root 1985, pp. 5-9)

Nurses should explore the use of such strategies as the CLOZE technique, listening tests, and word recognition tests such as the Wide Range Achievement Test (WRAT) to identify literacy levels in older adult clients (Strieff 1986). In the absence of the use of such direct measures of literacy, nurses can use the techniques of comprehension restatement, teaching strategies involving multiple senses, and definitive questioning to verify follow-up actions and enhance learning. In comprehension restatement, the client is asked to read or listen to health care information and is then asked to restate that information in his or her own words (orally or in writing). When possible, clients should be presented with the same information in several ways and by the stimulation of multiple senses. For example, material can be presented by videotape, orally reviewed with the client, demonstrated, and documented in a written pamphlet. Demonstration and return demonstration are very effective techniques to use with low-literacy older adults. Many of these individuals are quite intelligent and can readily memorize a procedure if it is demonstrated several times. During the return demonstration the nurse can correct errors in performance and clarify instructions that have been misunderstood. At the conclusion of teaching sessions, nurse-teachers can use definitive questioning to verify understanding and ability to apply knowledge. A statement and a question will assist in this process: "Now tell me what you have learned," followed by "What are you to do?" (Doak, Doak, and Root 1985).

Health education materials should be evaluated for literacy level and readability. There are more than forty formulas for assessing the degree of difficulty of written materials, most of which focus on difficulty of the vocabulary and average sentence length. Two of the poplar formulas are SMOG testing and the Fry Readability Formula (Strieff 1986). Nurses who work with older adults are strongly urged to learn about these formulas through such books as *Teaching Patients with Low Literacy Skills* by Doak, Doak, and Root or by collaborating with education specialists or professional health educators in the selection and/or development of health education materials and presentations.

The authors work with older adults, minority (both native born and new immigrant) who are poor and reside in inner city neighborhoods in Philadelphia, Pennsylvania. The application of readability formulas and implementation of teaching strategies directed toward low-literacy problems have made a marked improvement in learning and behavior change on the part of their clients. In areas where large numbers of recent immigrants reside, such strategies are vital since individuals who are learning or use English as a second language experience the same difficulty with literacy as native born non-readers. Finally, low-literacy teaching strategies are also useful with older adults who are ill and have shortened attention spans, with those who are experiencing changes in memory or cognition, and those fatigued by the burden of constant caregiving.

Information Conflict:
Overload and Learning

Prior to teaching, nurse-teachers need to assess what information the client and caregiver have already been given and who provided that information. The nurse needs to determine the value placed on the information by the client, the level of respect the client has for the information and/or the individual who provided it, and, if there is more than one source of information, whether messages are consistent and in accordance with accepted health care practices. Older adults usually have several sets of instructions from several health care providers (e.g., physician specialist, physician internist, nurse, dietitian, pharmacist, and/or physical therapist). This is especially true if they have been hospitalized or receive outpatient services in a large medical center that is also a teaching institution.

Information received from these sources also must be reconciled with instructions given by the neighborhood or family physician, folk practitioners, spiritual advisors, and relative or friends who exert influence and in whom the client may place great faith. A thorough assessment of the client's chief complaint and the belief system surrounding the management of his or her condition is essential before health instruction is planned by the nurse. (See chapter 7, "Psychosocial Assessment"; Appendix B; Psychosocial Assessment Guide, section II.)

IDENTIFICATION OF
LEARNING NEEDS

Identification of learning needs is a joint responsibility involving both the client and the nurse-teacher. Teaching strategies should be developed to address learning needs based on client priorities, national health goals, and/or anticipatory guidance related to

the management of illness. Table 16-2 and 16-3 identify specific topics that may be presented in health education sessions.

Client Priorities

Health care providers must assess the client's priorities in identifying and sequencing learning activities. Health care practitioners are often academically sophisticated and far removed from the process of initial skill development. Therefore they may be unaware of basic behaviors or issues that may prove threatening to the client or members of the caregiving system. For example, a client who has a profound fear of blood will have difficulty performing blood sugar screening tests. In addition health care professions are often surprised to discover how divergent the client's priorities are from their own. For example, the nurse-teacher may be geared up to teach a newly diagnosed diabetic the entire outline presented in Table 16–2, Health Education Topics for Older Adults Managing A Specific Illness. However, the client's burning question might be "How am I going to get to my daughter's house since the doctor told me I can't drive until my blood sugar stops fluctuating?" or "How can I follow this diet when I don't have a refrigerator to store food?" The authors find it useful to briefly outline the range of topics that will need to be learned by the client to master specific self-care or health promotion activities and then follow this overview with these questions:

- "I have reviewed quite a number of topics with you, how did you hope that I would be able to help you?"

- "What would you like to learn about your illness (or promoting your own health)?"

- "What would you like to work on first?"

- "What would like to work on this session?"

The nurse's teaching priorities should take precedence over the client's prioritization of learning needs in only one instance—when the client *must* learn some critical element or skill to save or sustain his or her life until the next teaching-learning session. Forcing of the professional's priorities on the client will seldom be warranted. In almost all nurse-teacher/client-learner interactions the nurse's

Table 16–2 Health Education Topics for Older Adults Managing a Specific Illness

- Risk factors
- Anatomy and physiology of the disease condition
- Causes of the disorder
- Symptoms associated with the disorder
- Prognosis
- Treatment

  Tests and procedures for ongoing management of recovery of symptom control

  Medications

  Diet

  Activity and exercise

  Use of equipment and supplies

  Lifestyle changes required
- Self-care, self-management responsibilities
- Caregiver training and support groups
- Prevention of complications
- Identification and plan for management of potential crises
- Professional or community resources available for assistance
- Financing of acute and rehabilitative services
- Prevention of reoccurrence of disorder or exacerbation of symptoms

Table 16–3 Health Education Topics for Health Promotion in Older Adults

I. Components of a healthy lifestyle

II. Prevention of disease and disorder

III. Maintenance and promotion of physical health

   A. Diet

   B. Exercise

   C. Smoking cessation

   D. Rest and sleep

   E. Prevention health practices

     1. Immunizations

     2. Cancer screening (mammography, Pap smears, sigmoidoscopy, prostate screening, skin cancer evaluation)

     3. Vision evaluation

     4. Monitoring of high blood pressure

     5. Control of stress incontinence

     6. Depression screening

     7. Prevention of osteoporosis (exercise, calcium supplements, hormone replacement therapy)

     8. Safe sex practices

(Table continued)

IV. Stress management

   A. Relaxation techniques

   B. Breathing exercises

   C. Positive self-talk

   D. Use of humor

   E. Assertiveness training

   F. Guided imagery

   G. Visualization

V. Preparation for and/or management of retirement

   A. Development of leisure skills

   B. Integration of part-time employment with retirement benefits

   C. Continuing education opportunities

   D. Budgeting and managing expenses on a reduced income

   E. Evaluating and accessing alternative living arrangements

VI. Developing and using social support networks

   A. Managing relationships with siblings, children, and grandchildren

   B. Establishing and/or expanding friendship networks

   C. Establishing and/or participating in caregiving networks

VII. Developing independent management skills

   A. For woman: social participation as a widow

     1. Financial management

     2. Simple household maintenance

     3. Hiring and managing repairmen

     4. Simple car maintenance

   B. For men: social participation as a widower

     1. Food shopping

     2. Meal planning and preparation

     3. Laundry management

     4. Social networking

     5. Health care management

VIII. Changes in normal aging

   A. Anatomical

   B. Physiological

   C. Psychological

     1. Compensatory techniques to reduce impact of changes

IX. Adapting activities of daily living (ADL) to maintain functional ability

X. Planning for life transitions

XI. Managing bereavement and loss

XII. Educated consumption of health services

    A. Accessing health services

    B. Identifying types of providers

    C. Types of health care services available

    D. Criteria for selection

    E. Evaluation of quality

    F. Expectations of providers

    G. Limitations of health services

    H. Obtaining second opinions

    I. Changing health care providers

    J. Managing the services of multiple providers

    K. Assisting family members or friends to utilize health services

    L. Communication and relationships with young health care practitioners

XIII. Financing health care

XIV. Identification and use of community resources to meet health and social needs

XV. Legal issues

    A. Living wills

    B. Powers of Attorney

    C. Court-appointed guardians

XVI. Safety

    A. Crime prevention

    B. Accident prevention

        1. Falls

        2. Burns

        3. Choking

        4. Poisoning: medication misuse

    C. Motor vehicle safety

    D. Physical and emotional maltreatment of older persons

XVII. Updates on current health issues

    A. Current health problems/discoveries as they impact seniors

    B. Issues as they affect younger family members

XVIII. Mentorship of the younger generation

    A. Whom to mentor

    B. How to mentor

    C. Pleasures to be gained from mentoring

    D. Intergenerational relationships

priorities can be easily subordinated to the client's identified needs. The nurse-teacher does not eliminate his or her own priorities; they are simply renumbered or resequenced in their order of presentation.

National Health Care Goals

The nursing profession participates in meeting the nation's health care goals. Therefore nurses who work with older adults must plan learning activities that are directed toward the national health care goals established in the Surgeon General's report, *Healthy People 2000: National Health Promotion and Disease and Prevention Objectives* (Department of Health and Human Services 1990). Three broad health goals for the nation's population are to be achieved by the turn of the century: increase the span of healthy life, reduce health disparities, and achieve access to preventive health services for all Americans. The nation's health goals as they are applied to the specific needs of older adults indicate that health education efforts need to be directed toward

- Increasing the years of healthy life by enhancing the ability to perform activities of daily living (ADLs) into late life (beyond age 85).

- Preventing the major causes of death (heart disease, cancer, stroke, chronic obstructive pulmonary disease, pneumonia, and influenza) in the older adult age group.

- Preventing chronic problems such as arthritis, osteoporosis, incontinence, visual and hearing impairments, and dementia.

- Enabling older adults with disabilities to preserve function and prevent further disability.

- Increasing life expectancy by the promotion of smoking cessation, good nutrition, and reduction of sodium intake.

- Delaying physiological decline by reversing patterns of inactivity and promoting regular, moderate physical activity and exercise. Increased physical activity among aging clients is seen as the key to reducing the incidence of coronary artery disease, hypertension, non-insulin dependent diabetes, colon cancer, depression and anxiety.

Furthermore, physical activity in older adults increases bone mineral content; reduces the risk for osteoporotic fractures; maintains appropriate body weight; increases longevity; and improves balance coordination, and strength, which may also reduce the incidence of falls. Exercise is also closely associated with the maintenance of functional independence into later life.

- Promoting preventive health activities and encouraging the use of preventive health services.

- Establishing and maintaining social support networks to prevent social isolation—a risk factor for disease, depression, and suicide—and reduced functional independence.

Table 16-3 identified some health promotion topics that may aid in meeting national health care goals.

Anticipatory Guidance Related to Management of Illness

Nurses should be attuned to learning needs of older adults who must cope with acute or chronic illness. Suitable topics for health education for these individuals were enumerated in Table 16-2. Anticipatory guidance, judiciously provided during both acute and chronic illness trajectories, will serve to allay anxiety, promote competence and mastery, prevent complications and disability, and delay or forestall hospitalization. Lubkin (1986), adapting the work of Strauss, Corbin, Fagerhaugh, Glazer, Maines, Suczek, and Weiner, has identified seven tasks of the chronically ill.

1. *Carrying out the medical regimen*—learning to manage the process, timing, energy expenditure, and discomfort required to implement the regimen.

2. *Controlling symptoms*—learning to plan ahead, modify the environment, and plan activities in order to remain symptom free.

3. *Preventing and managing crisis*—learning to identify crises, preventing their occurrence, and developing strategies for their management when they occur.

4. *Reordering time*—learning to adjust schedules and allocate time to manage health care regimens along with other life experiences.

5. *Adjusting to changes in the course of the disease*—learning to deal with predictable and unpredictable situations/symptoms and adapting to deterioration.

6. *Preventing social isolation*—learning to interact socially with the altered identity caused by the illness and preventing self-withdrawal or the withdrawal of others.

7. *Normalizing*—learning to hide disabilities and manage or compensate for symptoms in order to be treated as normal by others.

Nurses should direct learning activities for chronically ill older adults toward achieving these tasks required of the chronically ill.

TEACHING STRATEGIES TO ENHANCE LEARNING EFFECTIVENESS AMONG OLDER ADULTS

Older adults are ideal students. However, changes in physical and psychological functioning that accompany aging require that careful attention be given to teaching strategies used by the nurse-teacher to transfer information or skills to the client-learner. Gerogogy involves strategies that have proven effective in enhancing learning among older adults.

Provide Sufficient Time for Implementation of the Teaching/Learning Process

Nurse-teachers must first direct attention toward an essential component of the teaching/learning process: time. It takes time for the nurse to assess the needs of the learner, negotiate teaching priorities and define goals of learning with the client, identify teaching strategies required to enhance learning, prepare and/or select appropriate instructional materials, teach, evaluate the learning that results from teaching, correct errors in learning, revise teaching strategies as required, and teach again. It takes time for the client-learner to apprehend and process information, code and store stimuli, retrieve relevant portions of material learned for application, recognize the needs for behavior change, rehearse or practice behaviors required for change, and incorporate change as a part of his or her own value or behavioral system. Time

for the teaching/learning process is lengthened when the learner is distracted by psychological stress, physical disability, cognitive impairment, and/or low-level literacy or numeracy.

In reality the structure of the current health care environment allows little time for teaching. Clients being seen by primary health care providers in offices and outpatient clinics are routinely scheduled for fifteen-minute appointments. Standard scheduling procedure in many of these settings is to double-book appointments in order to assure an adequate flow of clients to meet fiscal goals. Therefore if all clients appear as appointed, their actual appointment times shrink to some smaller proportion of fifteen minutes. Alternately, the clients may be kept waiting an inordinate period of time until the health care professional can catch up with the backlog of clients waiting to be seen. When this happens, the provider and client interact in an environment of pressure and haste and activities are restricted to those surrounding diagnosis and treatment, not health education.

In inpatient settings, clients fare little better. Nurses often care for large numbers of clients. Times that could be set aside for client teaching are often interrupted by the pace of activities. (e.g., tests, procedures, treatments, medication administration, expert consultations, and examinations) that drive the schedules of modern acute care institutions. In addition the average length of stay for an older adult in the hospital is 8.9 days (American Association of Retired Persons and Administration on Aging 1991). The illness that precipitated an acute care admission may render the client too ill to attend to learning needs during the major portion of the hospitalization period. If teaching is instituted, it may have to wait until the last couple of days of the hospitalization when discharge is imminent. Therefore nurse-teachers may have no opportunity to validate that learning has occurred or to revise teaching strategies that were ineffective.

Professional health care providers—nurses and physicians—recognize their responsibility to provide health care information. But they often fail to examine the structural impossibility of doing so in the environments in which most practice. Given constraints of time, most of these professionals provide health information via pamphlets and written handouts that require a self-directed, literate client with an internal locus of control for the teaching strategy to prove productive.

Therefore the primary decision to be made by the nurse is whether sufficient time is available for an effective teaching/learning program to be instituted in his or her practice setting. Is there time for assessment of clients? priority setting? preparation of instructional materials? design of learning activities? the nurse-teacher/client-learner interaction? client learning assimilation? If not, the nurse should institute changes in the institutional structure that permit effective teaching and learning to occur. If changes in the institutional structure are not possible, nurses should look for alternate ways to meet the education needs of clients. Perhaps they should be referred to the visiting nurse who may have more time for instruction and will be able to teach the client and caregivers in their own home. The nurse also may wish to consider the use of nursing students, who have more time to spend with clients, as client educators. Frequently, client teaching is an expectation of their educational program and much time can be spent on the preparation and execution of teaching projects under the supervision of faculty members. Nurses may also be able to secure the assistance of institutional professional health educators and nurse clinical specialists to augment client education activities.

Reinforce the Hope that Self-Care is Attainable

The attitude of the nurse-teacher working with older adults is a critical element in the teaching/learning process. Older adults are more cautious in problem-solving situations and are less willing to take risks than are younger individuals (Lancaster and Simpson 1988). Kim (1989,43) stated that "fear of being wrong or fear of failure may cause the elderly not to respond in a doubtful situation." Resnick (1991, 19) stated that "elderly individuals are sensitive to their decreased abilities and do not want to look bad in front of others." She noted that fear of failing can be expressed through increased anxiety and/or resistance to risk taking. Resnick also warned that older individuals desperately need to seek approval for trying and that disapproval of their efforts can prove devastating. These characteristics couple with what

the authors have observed to be self-induced, unrealistic expectations for achievement to create a crisis in confidence for older clients.

Older adults, because they are adults and not children, erroneously believe that they should be able to learn and remember something after hearing it only once. They hesitate to ask questions or request repetition of material for fear of appearing stupid. Often, because the health care provider has allowed only enough time to teach or tell the material once, the teacher becomes impatient when clarification or elaboration is requested. Therefore the provider unintentionally projects the message "What's the matter with you? Are you stupid? I already told you how to do it." Older adults guard dignity and self-esteem zealously. Fears surrounding a perceived inability to learn caused by their own (or provider-induced) unrealistic expectations, can destroy the self-confidence of older learners and cause withdrawal, apathy, and noncompliance. In order for learning to occur, one must believe that he or she can accomplish the goals that have been established.

Therefore it is of paramount importance that the nurse-teacher approach the client with an attitude of optimistic expectancy and calm certainty (Rendon, Davis, Gioiella, and Tranzillo 1986) about their ability to master required skills if given enough time and the proper structure for learning. It is helpful to tell clients that when in school, the nurse learned to perform *X* (the task at hand) with the help of instructors but that it took time and a number of trials before being able to achieve mastery. Therefore the nurse should establish time lines that are significantly longer than it will actually take for the client to learn and process the information. For example, if a newly diagnosed diabetic must learn to draw up and self-administer insulin, a goal is set for task mastery at one month from the date that teaching commences. If the client masters self-administration in ten days, he or she is praised for being an incredibly fast learner. Caring is providing hope and empowerment. Nurse-teachers who have performed an accurate assessment of learner needs can fulfill the client's hope for achieving mastery in self-care by structuring learning activities that make learning conceptually and physically possible. This can *rarely* be done in one teaching/learning session.

Use Domains of Learning to Suggest Appropriate Teaching Strategies

Learning behaviors fall into three domains: cognitive, psychomotor, and affective. Behaviors in the cognitive domain of learning primarily reflect intellectual abilities; behaviors in the psychomotor domain reflect tasks accomplished through physical or motor activities; and behaviors in the affective domain are reflected in feelings, attitudes, and values. A fourth domain of learning—the perceptual domain—has been proposed. Behaviors in this domain would reflect ability to extract information from stimuli impinging on the sense organs; but this domain has not yet been as well developed as the preceding three (Redman 1988; *How to Teach Patients* 1989). Behaviors in the three principal domains of learning are arranged in hierarchies (called taxonomies) from simple to complex. Complex learning behaviors must be built on mastery of the behaviors that preceded them, Table 16-4 briefly summarizes the three major behavioral learning hierarchies.

After global learning priorities are identified with the client, the nurse must establish specific objectives

Table 16–4   Brief Summary of Behavioral Hierarchy of Learning Domains

Domain of Learning	Learning Behavior	Manifestation of Behavior
Cognitive	Knowledge (simplest)	defines
		describes
		identifies
		lists
		names
		selects
		reproduces
	Comprehension	explains
		gives examples
		paraphrases
		rewrites
		summarizes
		predicts
		generalizes
	Application	demonstrates
		manipulates
		prepares
		shows
		solves
		uses
		computes
		changes
	Analysis	diagrams
		discriminates
		differentiates

(Table continued)

Domain of Learning	Learning Behavior	Manifestation of Behavior
	Analysis (cont'd)	separates
		subdivides
		illustrates
	Synthesis	combines
		compiles
		composes
		creates
		modifies
		plans
		reorganizes
	Evaluation	compares
	(most complex)	concludes
		interprets
		justifies
		supports
Affective	Receiving	asks
	(simplest)	chooses
		locates
		names
		replies
		follows
		points to
	Responding	answers
		assists
		discusses
		helps
		performs
		practices
		reads
		recites
		selects
		writes
		completes
		describes
		follows
		initiates
		joins
		works
		arranges
		combines
	Valuing	completes
		describes
		follows
		initiates

Domain of Learning	Learning Behavior	Manifestation of Behavior
	Valuing (cont'd)	joins
		shares
		works
	Organization	arranges
		combines
		completes
		explains
		integrates
		organizes
		relates
		synthesizes
	Characterization by value (most complex)	acts
		influences
		performs
		proposes
		qualifies
		questions
		solves
		verifies
Psychomotor	Perception (simplest)	describes
		chooses
		isolates
		distinguishes
		identifies
		selects
	Set	reacts
		responds
		shows
		volunteers
		displays
		begins
	Guided response	assembles
		builds
		calibrates
		constructs
		dismantles
		manipulates
		measures

(Table continued)

Domain of Learning	Learning Behavior	Manifestation of Behavior
	Mechanism	(see guided response)
	Complex overt response	(see guided response)
	Adaptation	adapts
		changes
		reorganizes
		revises
		varies
	Origination (most complex)	arranges
		combines
		creates
		designs
		originates

Table constructed using material from Redman, 1988, p. 79; Springhouse 1989, p. 22; Cheeseman and Selekman, 1987, pp. 10-11.

for teaching/learning activities. The nurse-teacher must ask the question, "What behavior change do I want to see in the client as a result of learning?" The domains of learning, their associated learning behaviors, and manifestations of those behaviors are used to identify specific learning objectives for the client in behavioral terms. For example, if the broad learning goal established by a nurse-teacher and client-learner is for the client to learn the self-administration of insulin, the nurse might use some of the following as specific behavioral learning objectives:

At the conclusion of the teaching sessions, the client will be able to:

- Identify the parts of an insulin syringe. (Knowledge: Cognitive learning domain)

- Identify the dose scale on the syringe. (Knowledge: Cognitive learning domain)

- Read the label on the insulin bottle. (Responding: Affective domain)

- Prepare insulin for withdrawal from bottle by rolling bottle between the palms. (Application: Cognitive domain)

- Describe the amount of insulin dose to be withdrawn from the bottle. (Knowledge: Cognitive domain)

- Demonstrate withdrawal of insulin from bottle into the syringe. (Application: Cognitive domain; Set: Psychomotor domain)

Teaching strategies must subsequently be selected that will enable the client-learner to meet the behavioral learning objectives. Learning is believed to occur only when a behavioral change is manifest (the behavior change may not be in the direction that the nurse-teacher has anticipated). Teaching strategies are evaluated on the basis of the learner's ability to achieve the behavioral learning objectives. When the objectives are not met, the nurse-teacher must revise the teaching strategies used and attempt to present the information or skill in another way that will prove more effective. Teaching thus becomes a process of trial and revision until the right combination of teaching strategies is found that enables the client to reach the behavioral learning objectives.

Learning objectives also serve as a road map that gives the client an overview of what needs to be accomplished and the steps to be taken to reach the desired goal. Older adults take a problem-solving approach to learning and will not invest time and energy in tasks that are considered meaningless, irrelevant, or appear to be "nonsense" (Kim 1989; Resnick 1991; Picariello 1986; Rendon, Davis, Gioiella, and Tranzillo 1986). To facilitate coding and storage in long-term memory, tasks should have practical value, relate to the ability to maintain daily functional ability, and be taught in a way that renders them immediately applicable (Resnick 1991). Behavioral learning objectives outline a pattern that has overall meaning. They allow older adults to see how the steps in the learning process relate to what has gone before and to what must come after. Therefore individual learning activities or objectives are less apt to be isolated and abandoned. Construction and sequencing of behavioral learning objectives also helps the nurse assure that learning activities progress from simple to complex within the hierarchies of the learning domains. Finally, since older adults tend to be achievement oriented (Resnick 1991), behavioral learning objectives serve as a type of checkoff list to measure progress toward goal achievement.

Use Concepts of Mentorship as a Basis for the Teacher/Learner Relationship

Adult learners are self-directed, use a reservoir of life experience as a basis for new learning, can translate and interpret information for immediate application, focus on problem solving, and expect to participate actively in planning and implementing learning activities. Therefore the nurse-teacher who attempts to exert and hold total power and control over the older adult client's learning activities is doomed to failure as a teacher.

The appropriate relationship between the nurse-teacher and client-learner is a modification and adaptation of a role generally assigned to senior adults themselves—the role of mentor. Older adults have in the past mentored or are currently mentoring younger individuals. It is a role that many readily assume or that is assigned to them by virtue of experience, wisdom, or expertise. They are amused and delighted when younger health professionals explain the teacher/learner relationship between them as a temporary reversal in mentorship roles. Normally the older adult is the mentor; the younger adult, the protégé. Temporarily, for the teaching/learning interval, the roles will be inverted and the younger professional will become the mentor; the older adult the protégé. The use of the concept of mentorship, by its very nature, implies a successful outcome. The protégé is viewed as having great potential that simply needs to be developed. The ultimate goal of any mentorship is that the protégé will become equally or more successful than the mentor.

Hamilton (1990) described a mentor as the accomplished, more experienced professional who extends to a protégé on a one-to-one basis advice, teaching, sponsorship, guidance, and assistance directed toward establishment of a chosen profession. Adapted to the teaching/learning situation, the goal of the mentor is to establish the older adult in self-management of health care needs. According to Hamilton, the mentor

- believes in the protégé and helps the protégé to believe in himself or herself.

- enhances skills and knowledge of the protégé.

- provides counsel and support in times of stress.

- provides encouragement during risk-taking endeavors.

- is a practical helper.

- is crucial to the protégé in supporting and facilitating goal attainment.

- is a creator of competence.

Hamilton further described mentorship as a temporary relationship that ends with a shift in the balance of power. In the beginning the novice (in this case, the learner) is uncertain, is hesitant, is open to suggestions, and challenges little. As the relationship evolves and the protégé gains a better sense of his or her own capacity for autonomous decision making, the relationship is more of a mutual give-and-take experience. It is at this point that the relationship may terminate because goals have been met or a transition may be made from the mentor-protégé dyad to a collegial or interactive relationship.

Control the Environment to Prevent Distractions

The nurse-teacher must be sensitive to the impact that the teaching/learning environment may have on the older adult's ability to learn. Teaching should be done in rooms that are brightly lit. Great care should be taken to eliminate glare; light sources should shine from behind the learner. When available, natural light may enhance visual acuity. Soft white bulbs may prove effective if electric light is used. Seating should be comfortable and arranged so that the teacher and any instructional aids are clearly visible. Avoid making the room completely dark for audiovisual presentations, slow the pace of slide presentations, and use black slides for breaks between slides to facilitate visual accommodation to changes from dark to bright light. Observe safety precautions with the electrical cords used for audiovisual equipment (Weinrich, Boyd, and Nussbaum 1989; Picariello 1986).

The nurse should eliminate all extraneous and distracting noises in and around the teaching environment to compensate for older persons' hearing losses and decreased ability to filter background noises. The nurse-teacher should face the learner and avoid covering the mouth while speaking. Female teachers should consider wearing bright lipstick to assist learners who may need to lip read. Voice pitch should be kept low since older adults have difficulty with high-pitched sounds; consideration should be given to using a microphone when teaching groups. Learners using hearing aids should be positioned within four feet of the teacher and should be given time to turn and/or adjust hearing aids before teaching commences. Room temperature should be carefully monitored and the room should be kept free of drafts (Weinrich, Boyd, and Nussbaum 1989; Picariello 1986).

Pace Teaching Activities So that Learning Can Occur

Pacing is important in teaching older adults and may mean the difference between whether stimuli are ap-

prehended or ignored. Since processing of stimuli may be diminished due to both normal changes of aging and/or disease conditions, the speed of instruction should be slowed and the time allowed for response to stimuli should be extended. Studies show that both healthy and hospitalized older adults benefit more from instruction that is self-paced or slow-paced, e.g., delivered at 106 words per minute versus the normal 159 words per minute. Self-paced responses to learning conditions prove to be superior to either slow-paced or normal-paced learning conditions. Older clients work best at their own speed; if rushed, their learning performance may be poor even when they know the material (Kim 1989).

In addition to the speed of instruction, nurses should give consideration to the quantity of information to be presented and the length of time for teaching sessions. Older adults with painful conditions, stiffness of joints, or urinary urgency will find it difficult to listen to teaching for long periods of time. Information should be broken into small digestible units focusing on a limited number of concepts or actions in a single session. Organizing teaching material into smaller units enhances not only perceiving and acquiring but the coding and storing of information. Teaching sessions should provide frequent stretch and rest-room breaks and should be planned to start and end well within the energy continuum of the learner(s). Since older adults frequently do not hydrate themselves adequately due to a decreased sense of thirst, liquid refreshments might be appropriately offered during breaks in teaching sessions (Weinrich, Boyd, and Nussbaum 1989; Rendon, Davis, Gioiella, and Tranzillo 1986).

Use Techniques that Enhance Memory

Learning can be enhanced by teaching techniques that tag information for easy storage and/or retrieval from long-term memory. Some of these learning strategies include:

- *Mediational or imaging techniques*—encouraging clients to form mental images of the words or items they wish to remember or to link mental images or visual pictures to concepts they wish to retain. Learning occurs more readily if these images are self-generated by the client as opposed to being generated by the teacher (Kim 1989; Gilles 1986).

- *Digital grouping or "chunking"*—dividing material into seven (plus or minus two) bits of information for easy retention. Phone numbers are an example of chunking.

- *Associative or mnemonic techniques*—learning can be enhanced by the use of jingles, paired associations, rhymes, and acronyms (letters that spell a word, each letter of which triggers the memory to recall a vital bit of information). For example, a client might use the word lamb to remind her to take her Lasix in the *a.m.*—morning—after her bath (Johnson and Gueldner 1989).

- *Repetition and overlearning*—the teacher or student can repeat material two or three times within a ten to fifteen minute period to reinforce learning. Older adults may require several repetitions to absorb and store newly learned materials in long-term memory (Gilles 1986).

- *Rehearsing and self-talk*—this technique involves guiding oneself through a difficult task with internal self-talk (Gilles 1986).

- *Sensory stimulation*—material should be presented in several ways to stimulate as many senses as possible (e.g., hearing, sight, and touch). Stimulation of multiple senses is especially important if the older adult is suffering from diminished sensory functioning or has specific types of sensory impairment.

- *Restatement and rewriting*—learners restate or rewrite information in their own words. This technique is particularly effective with low-literacy learners or for all older adults who are trying to learn the steps in procedures.

- *Demonstration and return demonstration*—watching and listening followed by doing stimulates three of the senses and is an excellent way to ensure that stimuli are coded and stored in long-term memory.

- *Analogies and examples*—older adults may have a diminished ability to perform abstract thinking. Therefore analogies and examples should be used to illustrate and clarify concepts.

- *Summary and review*—learning sessions should be concluded with a summary and review of the key points that were covered. Learning is enhanced if the client-learner does the summarization in his or her own words.

Prime the Learner for Selectively Attending to Stimuli

No individual can attend and process all of the stimuli that bombard the nervous system. All learners selectively attend and apprehend stimuli for processing and storage in long-term memory. Older adults may have difficulty filtering and screening stimuli; there is some indication that some individuals are easily distracted by too much detail or suffer from a diminished ability to sort information (Kim 1989). Learning in older adults can be facilitated if nurse-teachers prepare or prime the client-learner to pay particular attention to key or critical elements that will be presented during the teaching session or are covered in written handouts. One method of instituting this technique is to state, "During this presentation, I want you to pay attention to three things:. . . ." or "During this presentation I want you to find the answers to four questions: . . ." For example, if the topic to be discussed is the use of medication, the questions might be:

- "What is the purpose of this medicine?"

- "How much do I take?"

- "What will it do for me?"

- "What do I do if I have side effects?"

Advanced organizers serve as headers or clues to focus the learner's attention to what is coming, enable them to filter out extraneous material, and ensure that essential material is perceived. If several concepts are to be presented, advanced organizers should be used for each concept (Doak, Doak, and Root 1985; Redman 1988). Redman (1988, 142) presented the following outline using advanced organizers as a sample of priming a learner to receive information related to diagnosis and prognosis:

"I am going to tell you:
What is wrong with you
What tests we are going to carry out
What I think will happen to you
What treatment you will need
What you must do to help yourself"

Priming for selective attention should be done any time handouts are used, particularly if they are used in lieu of interpersonal interaction. The nurse should tell the older adult why the written material has been selected for his/her use and what to specifically look for in regards to content. Sometimes the nurse may wish to use a colored marker to highlight material that is particularly critical to learner success. When written materials are used, the nurse should make them interactive by giving the older adult an assignment to complete and return to the nurse for the focus of joint discussion. Learning is enhanced when the learner is an active participant rather than a passive observer. For example, the client-learner may be asked to read a pamphlet and list three questions about the content to discuss with the nurse during the next nurse-client encounter. Alternately, the client may be asked to carry out some activity as detailed in the pamphlet, such as weekly aerobic exercise. When the client comes for the next teaching session, he or she may bring an activity log that documents the type of exercise that was done, the days on which it was done, and the length of time spent on each activity. Written materials are useless if the older adult is not coached regarding their use or significance and if questions on their content are not requested and evaluated.

Provide Liberal Amounts of Reinforcement and Praise

All learners need to have a sense of how they are progressing. Reinforcement on performance is essential. Praise is the most powerful form of reinforcement and serves as an incentive for continued or improved performance. Nurses should try to find at least one element to praise in every teaching/learning interaction. Usually there are many opportunities for positive reinforcement if the nurse is observant and pays attention to the little successes in performance as well as the overall picture. If the learner is experiencing great difficulty in achieving goals and success is slow in coming, praise is even more essential, and opportunities for providing it may be harder for the nurse to identify. If performance itself is not good, praise can be directed toward the older adult's willingness to attend teaching sessions and attempt learning activities. In extreme cases if no behaviors can be found worthy of praise among the teaching/learning activities, then initial offerings of positive reinforce-

ment may need to be directed toward personal attributes of the older person. An example might be, "I'm so glad to see you today. Your beautiful smile makes me glad that I could be here today to share health information with you."

Contract for Change

Learners need support and encouragement as they try or practice changes in behavior. This is particularly true for older adults who may be making changes in lifelong habits and/or lifestyle activities. Goals for behavior change should be realistic, measurable, positive, time-dated, written, rewardable, and evaluated (Redman 1988). For example:

- *Realistic*: "Is this goal realistic for you?"

- *Measurable*: "How often do you do this?" "Specifically, how will you do this?"

- *Positive*: "What strengths do you have that will help you to do *X*?"

- *Time-Dated*: "When will you start?" "How often will you do this during the next week?"

- *Written*: "Let's write down the goals you discussed."

- *Rewardable*: "When you accomplish this, how will you reward yourself?"

- *Evaluated*: "How do you plan to measure your success?" "Can you share your achievement with anyone else?"

Contracts are particularly useful in defining actions for older adults and in obtaining a commitment for risk taking from them. They are also helpful in measuring progress towards goals.

Use New Technologies to Enhance Learning

Nurses should incorporate videotapes, audiotapes, and computers into teaching activities when possible and appropriate. Audiotapes can be used by the nurse-teacher to record health information and/or personalize instructions for the client-learner. One effective technique is to record the nurse as he or she is providing instructions and then the restatement of the instructions in the client's own words. The client can then use the taped instructions at home as a stimulus or reinforcement for memory. Audiotapes are particularly useful for low-literacy learners and for older adults who have difficulty reading due to visual impairment. Audiotapes can also be used as a method for clients to list questions or concerns they wish to raise with the primary health provider on the next office visit. Tapes can also be used by some clients with deteriorating conditions. They can provide instructions to caregivers or significant others regarding personal preferences and wishes prior to an anticipated diminished ability to communicate or make appropriate decisions (Browning and Gross 1991).

Nurses should take advantage of personal computers as an adjunct to the preparation of personalized teaching materials. Personal computers can be used to prepare personalized instructions for client learners, see Figure 16-1, or to create handouts or learning materials that can be used over time with a succession of older individuals.

When designing printed materials, visual changes in aging should be considered. Use 24-26 point type and serif letters; provide high contrast between background and foreground (e.g., black on white or beige); avoid the use of dark colors on dark backgrounds; avoid using blue, green, or violet type; and use color to create depth perception. Images and letters should have crisp edges (photocopying sometimes blurs borders and images) and shiny paper (which produces glare) should be avoided. Ornate type faces with fancy italics are difficult for older adults to read. Free or white space around letters and words and a line length no longer than five or six inches enhance readability (American Association of Retired Persons 1986).

Computer-assisted-instruction (CAI) and Interactive Video Disc (IVD) technologies hold much promise for client instruction. These new technologies have not yet had their potential for client education fully explored. While these technologies may not be the nurse's first choice of method to deliver client instruction, they have the advantage of providing self-paced instruction.

A wide spectrum of health teaching is currently provided via videotape. Nurses should familiarize themselves with those designed for or capable of adaptation to the needs of older adults. Many are available for rental from local video outlets for a small fee or are free when checked out from the local public library. Videotapes are also available from the American Association of Retired Persons (AARP) and cover such topics as prevention of elder abuse, long-term care options, hearing problems, dietary programs, over-the-counter medication safety, and women's health issues. Another source of videotapes is "Audiovisuals on Aging" published by the Association for Gerontology in Higher Education in Washington, DC.

The use of teaching models is an excellent way to enhance the learning of older adults, especially those with low literacy. Models are an excellent way to give learners an opportunity to practice hands-on skills before actually having to perform them. Models are available to practice techniques for giving injections, drawing medications into syringes, mixing insulins, performing wound care, practicing breast self-examination, caring for Hickman catheters, port-a-caths or urinary catheters, and illustrating anatomical structure and function. The actual performance of a skill reinforces any verbal instruction that has been given and allows the teacher to correct errors in perception or performance. Through the practice of skills caregivers gain confidence, develop psychomotor coordination, and learn from mistakes made on something other than a living person.

A DREAM FOR THE FUTURE

What if health care providers working with older adults could establish learning resource centers in central locations, completely stocked with learning aids and staffed by nurse-teachers and health educators? What if health care providers could write a self-care prescription for health education, see Figure 16-2, like they do for treatments and medications? What if health education was a reimbursable and high-priority function of nurses? Nurses working with other nurses and older adult advocates could make such a dream a reality (Browning and Gross 1991).

DISCHARGE PLANNING AND CASE MANAGEMENT

Contemporary nurses are busy and often overworked. During a single year they bear significant responsibilities for the health, well-being, and survival of large numbers of individuals. Direct client care is delivered in high-pressure environments with limited resources and according to a myriad of regulations (institutional, regional, federal) that render meeting the real human high-touch or practical daily needs of clients virtually impossible. In the process of juggling and fulfilling multiple responsibilities to multiple authorities (including clients and their families), nurses often forget that their impact on clients, while significant (maybe even crucial), is transitory. Nurses cannot remain with the client and family system forever. The nature of their relationship is transitional. The nurse's role is to provide temporary support and guidance for those confronting major lifestyle changes and to supply them with the resources and skills that will enable them to return to the real life they have chosen. All of this must be accomplished in a limited period of time.

Nurses must not lose sight of the time-limited nature of the nurse-client relationship. If the client and his or her family are to become self-sufficient in the management of their own health care needs, this abbreviated interlude of professional caregiving must

---

1. Your next appointment is on June 18, 1993

2. Bring all of your medicines with you

3. Bring a list of questions you want me to answer about your care.

Figure 16–1 Personalized instructions for client learner

Name of patient: _____

In order to care for yourself (your spouse, your friend, your mother/father, your brother/sister, etc.), you will need to learn the following:

To gain the skills you need, between now and your next appointment with me I would like for you to:

___ Work with the visiting nurse (occupational therapist, physical therapist, speech therapist, nutritionist, etc.) who will come to your home and teach you the skills we have identified.

Watch the VHS tape _____(title)_____ _(#)_ times. You may:

___ Check this tape out at the county library.

___ Purchase the tape from _____.

___ Borrow the tape from our office.

___ View the tape in the learning resource center located

_____.

___ View the tape at one of the senior centers listed here:

___ Complete the computer-assisted instruction (CAI) titled _____.
Bring your final printout with you. You may use the computer center resources located:

___ In our office

___ In the learning resource center located

___ In the county library

___ In one of the senior centers listed here:

(Figure continued)

Figure 16–2 Self care prescription

___ Write instructions in your own words describing how you are (or will)
_____ (self-care activity) _____ .

___ Call (health professional) on (date) to report on your progress learning (self-care activity).

___ Practice _____ (self-care activity) _____ and be prepared to show me how
you do it during your appointment scheduled on _____ (date) _____ .

___ Make a list of at least __(#)__ questions you want me to answer about your illness/condition and/or
the self-care activities you are trying to learn.

___ Bring the following things with you on your next visit:

    ___ All of your medicines

    ___ The names and phone numbers of your other doctors

    ___ Instructions you have received from (other health care providers).

    ___ Insurance cards

    ___ _____ (Type) _____ specimens

Other instructions:

Signature: _____ (Name of professional) _____

be carefully fulfilled by the nurse in collaboration with other health care providers. Control of health care management and decision making must be transferred back to the client and family in a timely manner. The key to this transfer lies in careful discharge planning, which starts during the initial psychosocial assessment and continues through the discharge process.

Discharge Planning

Discharge planning is the process of ensuring continuity of care (Corkery 1989). Continuity of care is defined as a coordinated process of activities that involves the client and health care provider. They work together to facilitate the transition of health care from one institution, agency, or individual to another (Haddock 1991). Ideally the objective of discharge planning is to create and sequentially provide varying levels of health care services. These will move the client and family system from a state of dependency on health care providers to independence in the management of health care activities and decisions. Discharge planning should provide a variety of resources for clients and families and allow them to choose those most compatible with their unique needs. Discharge planning may involve teaching clients and their families how to manage their own health care needs and resources and/or providing referral to a variety of institutions, agencies, or individual providers who can provide a continuum of support services until independence is feasible. For some older adults and/or their caregiving systems, independent health care management will prove impossible. For this small number, appropriate discharge planning will facilitate entry into long-term care institutions where continuous professional caregiving can be provided.

Discharge planning is the development of a specific, preferably written, plan that answers the following questions:

1. Where is the client going when he or she leaves the current professional caregiving system?

2. What is the client's current functional (ability to manage activities of daily living [ADLs] and instrumental activities of daily living [IADLs]),

physical, and mental status? What medications and treatments will be required after discharge? What is the nature of the client's support system?

3. Based on the above, what type of health or social service needs does the client currently have?

4. Who will provide continued care for the client or family system that meets the identified needs? (Family? Other health care institutions? Community agencies? Individual health care providers?)

5. What type of teaching has been done with the client and/or family? What was their response to the teaching activities? What remains to be taught before self-care mastery can be attained? Who is available and capable of learning the information and/or skills that will be required? Who is best suited to teach what is needed?

6. What equipment and/or supplies will be needed by the client and/or family to achieve self-care?

7. What referrals are appropriate for this client? Does the client meet the eligibility criteria for access to these health or social services? What are the financial implications of referral?

8. What choices were presented to the client and/or family? Which ones were chosen? Why?

9. If referrals were made, who made them? Who received them? What information was transmitted to facilitate the integration of the client into the new caregiving system or service?

10. Who will assume responsibility for coordinating follow-up care? (Family? Physician? Case manager?)

Discharge planning should be implemented in all professional caregiving settings: hospitals, rehabilitation centers, intermediate care facilities, and home care agencies. It is also appropriate when clients are transferred from one level of service to another within an institution (e.g., intensive care unit to medical-surgical floor) or from one program to another (e.g., inpatient psychiatric facility to community mental health center).

Participants in Discharge Planning. Discharge planning involves a holistic examination of client needs. Selection of relevant health care options is dependent on developing an accurate understanding of client and family needs and the strengths and limitations they bring to bear in meeting those needs. Effective discharge planning is also dependent on determining what the patient and family want from health care providers and on resolving conflicting goals (if present) of the client and family members. Discharge planning is a multidisciplinary process. Holistic assessment requires ideas from the client, family, physician, nurses, social workers, therapists (physical, occupational, and speech), nutritionists, pharmacists, utilization of quality-assurance personnel, clergy or spiritual advisors, and significant others in the client's life. Referrals that assure continuity of care also are multidisciplinary in nature as they are made to a wide variety of professional providers and social service and health care agencies (e.g., home health agencies, senior centers, respite care centers, adult day-care centers, and Meals on Wheels). (See chapters 20 and 21 for details regarding these services.)

Legal, Economic, and Quality-of-Life Bases for Discharge Planning. In 1982 a prospective method of reimbursement was introduced to control the escalating cost of health care in the United States. This cost-containment measure was initially instituted in the Medicare program. The installation of DRGs shifted the fiscal reward system from lengthy hospital stays and maximum use of cost-reimbursed services to a reward system based on provision of a limited number of reasonable services delivered with maximum efficiency within a clearly defined time limit. Thus the ability to maintain operating budgets or to make a profit suddenly depended on moving older adults through acute care hospitals quickly, delivering only the services that were profitable. High-technology services, once provided only in the hospital, were transferred to the community or home setting to be managed by clients and caregivers under the supervision of community-based physicians, nurses, and allied health professionals. Private insurers rapidly followed the lead of the federal government in cost containment. Today effective discharge planning that efficiently moves clients through the health care system while maintaining a high quality of health care is critical to an institution's fiscal health and survival in the marketplace (Browning 1992).

Discharge planning services are now mandated for hospitals and other health care institutions by a variety of laws, regulations, and standards of practice. These mandates are required by some of the following: Heinz-Stark Bill, 1986, Medicare Quality Protection Act; the Joint Commission of Accreditation of Health Care Organizations (JCAHO); the American Hospital Association; and the American Nurses' Association Standards of Practice (Browning 1992).

Fiscally-induced expedited discharges place frail elders at risk for postdischarge difficulties and increase the potential for costly readmission (Haddock 1991). Currently, older adults account for 31 percent of total national health care expenditures and 42 percent of all days of care in hospitals (Weinrich, Boyd, and Nussbuam 1989). They comprise over half of the census on medical-surgical units; their length of stay averages 8.9 days, 3.6 days longer than persons under 65 years of age (American Association of Retired Persons and Administration on Aging 1991). Twenty-five percent of older persons are readmitted to the hospital at least two times within twelve months of their discharge date (Johnson 1989). Therefore there are major human and economic imperatives for instituting effective discharge-planning procedures.

Effective discharge planning is associated with improved health status and increased health satisfaction in older clients. Haddock (1991, 10) stated that this enhanced satisfaction is important because it "creates an emotional tone that can augment patient teaching, increase acceptance of care, positively influence future relations with the health care system . . . [and] has the potential to affect the accreditation, reputation, and profitability of a health agency."

Though discharge-planning services are mandated by regulation, there is little uniformity in their development or application from institution to institution. Naylor's (1990) study of hospitalized older adults revealed that 85 percent of the clients were considered high-risk and in need of discharge planning, but only 20 percent received these services. Researchers evaluate the current quality of discharge planning as poor. They recognize that its low-priority ranking among health professionals results in delayed and inadequate assessment and fragmented implementation of continuing care services after discharge. Johnson's (1989) study of fifty pairs of older clients and their nurses on two medical units revealed that nurses viewed discharge planning as an activity secondary in importance to meeting the physical needs of their clients. Nurses indicated that lack of preparation in gerontology, large client loads, and a shortage of nursing staff contributed to their avoidance of discharge-planning activities. In contrast the clients in the study ranked discharge-planning activities as "extremely" or "very" important to them. They stressed a need to have their families included in discharge-planning activities and expressed displeasure at being given little or no opportunity to ask questions, clarify instructions, or demonstrate mastery of self-care activities prior to discharge. They were particularly frustrated by what has been jokingly termed "elevator teaching"—the tendency of health care providers to dispense instructions as the client is being wheeled onto the elevator in preparation for exodus from the health care facility.

Health care clinicians and administrators (Wilson, Deeves, Clancy, and Schnitt 1991; Haddock 1991; Esper 1988) emphasized that effective discharge planning must involve multidisciplinary collaboration and be the result of a structured assessment, uniformly applied. Discharge-planning programs should include: program policies and procedures, written job descriptions for discharge planners and liaison personnel, client screening assessment instruments with a multidisciplinary focus, focused assessment protocols applied at the time of admission and throughout the time of service to alert providers to high levels of postdischarge risk, postdischarge evaluation of effectiveness of interventions and follow-up referrals, and annual evaluations of the entire institutional discharge planning process.

The Role of the Nurse in Discharge Planning. Nurses may perform one or more roles in the discharge-planning process. They may serve as primary nurses who identify the high-risk clients and initiate the discharge plan and/or refer the client to an individual specified by the institution as a discharge planner. Professional providers designated as discharge planners are usually nurses or social workers who specialize in the identification of health and social service resources and have developed a high degree of skill in counseling other professionals, clients, and their families about access to and utilization of these services. Finally, nurses may function as liaison nurses for home care agencies. These specialized nurses assist discharge planners in facilitating the transfer of identified clients from institutional to home-based care. They are employed by home health agencies that have contracts with the institution to expedite discharge and to assure that medical care (often complex and highly specialized) and client and family education for self-care, which commenced in the institution, are continued in the home after discharge. These nurses make rounds to evaluate the clients identified for referral by the institutional discharge planner or other members of the professional staff. They also determine whether the client's condition can be safely managed at home and whether he or she qualifies for home care services.

Research by Drew, Diordi, and Gilles (1988) provided evidence that discharge planners and home health liaisons may differ in their ultimate goals for client service. Discharge planners may see their primary responsibility as assisting the clients toward a plan of continuing care that includes very precise means and techniques to support that care. Therefore they tend to give very specific information regarding agencies and community resources to contact. In contrast to the specificity of referral sources supplied by discharge planners, home health nurses focus holistically on sustaining primary care in the home and integrating physical care and health teaching to promote client and family independence. Home health nurses tend to focus on family concerns and emphasize the important role of the family in meeting the actual demands of caregiving needs. Discharge planners and home health liaisons agree that older adults selected for nursing home placement are those who need intensive skilled care, who have significant recurring medical problems, and are lacking support systems. However, the researchers found that discharge planners are more likely (68 percent) than home health liaisons (54 percent) to refer the older person to a nursing home.

Functions. Nurses who function as staff or primary nurses participate in the discharge planning process by: identifying clients who will need postinstitutional care; teaching self-care activities to clients and their families; obtaining consults from nurse clinical specialists regarding specialized discharge needs; obtaining physicians' orders for referral to other professional disciplines, the discharge-planning department, or community resources; participating in multidisciplinary rounds; ensuring that clients are discharged with sufficient medication and/or medical supplies to last until such services can be secured outside the institution; providing information for discharge planners to use in the preparation of written referrals to other agencies or institutions; and writing discharge-planning summaries (Browning 1992).

Nurses who function as designated discharge planners perform the following functions: direct and coordinate institutional discharge-planning activities; conduct multidisciplinary discharge-planning rounds; educate professional staff, clients, and families regarding discharge-planning responsibilities; interview clients for evaluation of discharge-planning needs; make referrals to other institutions, agencies, or providers for continuing care; evaluate institutional admission, discharge, or transfer lists to identify potential clients who may require discharge-planning services but have not yet been re-

Table 16–5　Risk Factors that Warrant Evaluation for Referral of Older Adults to Discharge Planning Programs

1. Client and/or family requests help and seeks discharge planning services.
2. Inability to perform ADLs or IADLs.
3. Older adult lives alone.
4. Client is above 80 years of age.
5. Client has had repeated acute care or emergency room admissions.
6. Client is poor or near poor.
7. Older person is a member of a minority group.
8. Older person uses English as a second language.
9. Address is distant from health care services.
10. Client suffers from confusion or altered mental status.
11. Older adult has a history of substance abuse.
12. Multiple medications have been ordered.
13. Client has sensory impairment.
14. History of falls or accidents.
15. Client will need assistive or adaptive devices.
16. Family support system is uncertain, uninterested, or physically distant.
17. Family is in conflict with the client or with one another regarding goals and management of care.
18. Caregiver is advanced in age or suffers from chronic illness.
19. Caregiver is very young (e.g., a teenager or young child).
20. Client's endurance is limited.
21. Client's medical condition is unstable or deteriorating.
22. Self-care regimen will include performance of technical medical or nursing procedures (e.g., catheter care; injections; monitoring of blood glucose; maintenance of central lines, intravenous antibiotic, or parenteral nutrition).
23. Condition will require pain control and pain management.
24. Client has questionable hydration status.

(Table continued)

25. Client has inadequate twenty-four-hour dietary recalls, poor appetite, or is on a special diet (e.g., diabetic diet, renal diet).

26. Client has problems with bowel or bladder elimination.

27. Communication is impaired (e.g., aphasia, tracheostomy).

28 Client has no telephone.

29. Availability of transportation is limited.

30. Coping ability of the client or family is uncertain or questionable.

31. Depression is present in client and/or caregiver. (Assessment using depression screening inventories should be done.)

32. Client has a history of recent or cumulative losses or has had a recent change in lifestyle.

33. Current clinical condition precipitates a change in social roles of the client and/or caregiver.

34. Elder abuse or neglect is suspected.

35. Older adult lives in a high-crime neighborhood.

36. Response to teaching by client and/or family is passive, poor, or uncertain.

37. Condition requires adaptation of the home environment or requires support systems beyond the normal range of family caregiver means.

38. Many physicians are involved in the client's care.

39. Client has expressed dislike for one or more of his or her physicians.

40. Client and/or family openly expresses doubt about the ability to perform self-care activities or to sustain them over time.

41. Prognosis is terminal and the client and/or family wish death to occur at home.

Adapted from M.A. Browning. 1992. Discharge planning. In *Clinical Manual of Gerontological Nursing*, edited by M.O. Hogstel. St. Louis, MO: Mosby Year Book. p. 259.

---

ferred; collaborate with physicians to secure ordered services; participate on institutional utilization and quality-assurance committees; order durable medical equipment and/or disposable medical supplies; coordinate and obtain authorization for services from third-party payors; develop policies, procedures, and protocols for the discharge-planning program; maintain records and documentation; evaluate discharge-planning services; and finally, coordinate discharge planning with quality-assurance efforts within the institution (Browning 1992).

Identification of Older Adults at High Risk Who Require Discharge Planning Services. Table 16-5 provides a list of the kinds of clients who may be at significant risk and may require a thorough evaluation for discharge-planning services.

Case Management

Case management is related to discharge planning because it is a system of identifying and coordinating services based on client need. Just as in discharge planning, the psychosocial assessment is the vehicle for identifying needed services and the basis for strategic planning to integrate the identified services into the client's lifestyle.

The term "case management" is applied in a multiplicity of ways. It is often difficult to define in today's health care environment since it is often confused with the concept of "managed care." Case management, when used to refer to the coordination of services, is not new to nursing. Community health and visiting nurses have been coordinating services for clients and their families since the last century.

Contemporary clinicians, such as nurse practitioners, also have case management functions. However, concepts of case management are expanding in the broad community beyond nursing. Case management has now become a serious issue for health care financing organizations and professional providers in many disciplines who are trying to plan community-based long-term care for today's and future older populations.

Case management seeks to provide an array of both home-based and other-based long-term care services that will enable the older adult to remain in his or her own community. The goals of case management include: prevention and reduction of premature institutionalization, enhanced quality of life for caregivers, reduction in caregiver burden, enhanced continuity of care, reduced barriers to health care services, and a reduction in expenditures for long-term care by both clients and insurers (federal and private) (Green 1989).

From 1982 to 1985 a national test of the implications of expanded financing for expanded home care was conducted in ten communities through the National Channeling Demonstration Project. The channeling projects sought to substitute case managed care at home for care in a nursing home, thereby reducing long-term care costs and improving the quality of life for older adults and their families who participated (Kemper 1990). Five case management sites within the project were extensively analyzed: the Long-Term Care Project of North San Diego County, the New York City Home Care Project, the South Carolina Community Long-Term Care Project, and the On Look Community and Project Open (Green 1989). Clients served by these projects were disabled older adults at risk of nursing home placement. They were provided with expanded home care services that included personal care (e.g., bathing, toileting, or feeding), supportive care (e.g., help with house cleaning, meal preparation, shopping), traditional home health care, and community supportive care (e.g., transportation, home delivered meals, and adult day care). Individualized care plans or programs of service were developed. Case managers determined client eligibility, performed needs assessments, developed the plan of care, coordinated service delivery, advocated for the clients in the health care delivery system, implemented quality-assurance protocols, negotiated contracts with providers of service, and authorized payments to providers for services rendered. The channeling projects, contrary to expectations, did not reduce the costs of service to the frail older population nor did they prevent the admission of some clients to nursing homes. They did result in an increased satisfaction with life among clients and caregivers, increased confidence in the care received, and a reduction in previously unmet health care needs. The channeling demonstrations also illustrated the potential for such systems to control quality of service through the power of the nurse, to reduce costs of services through negotiation and contracting, and to manage the costs of service by controlling the matrix of services provided (Kemper 1990).

In *Nursing's Agenda for Health Care Reform* (National League for Nursing 1991), the nursing profession advocates expansion of case-managed health care. The nursing profession defines case management as a system rooted in the client-provider relationship. The allegiance of the provider is to the client. Acting as advocates, providers are to provide both direct care and negotiate with other service systems on behalf of the clients. The goal of case management, as defined by nursing, is to make health care less fragmented and more holistic for those individuals with complex health care needs.

Managed care, in contrast, is directed more toward the needs of insurers and the payors of large insurance premiums, such as big business. The goals of managed health care are to reduce the need for health care services, reduce the variations in practice patterns among providers, and create significant financial incentives for beneficiaries to use providers and follow procedures or protocols established by the insurer (Frieden 1991).

SUMMARY

Nurses have a professional obligation to provide educational services for older adults that will enable them to achieve competence in the prevention of illness, maintenance of health, and control of acute or chronic illness. Contrary to popular opinion embedded in cultural myths such as "you can't teach an old dog new tricks," older adults are receptive and committed learners. However, common physical and mental changes that may be caused by the aging process or by chronic illness require a modification of teaching strategies to enable sensory stimuli to be processed and stored in and retrieved from memory. The relationship formed between the nurse and the client during the teaching/learning interval is critical and is most effective if the nurse presents as a mentor rather than as an authority figure. The key to enhanced learning in older adults is careful identification of learning needs and negotiated sequencing of learning activities based on the client's priorities. If the teaching/learning interval is structured around an interpersonal nurse-client relationship that is interactive and reciprocal, nurses will *learn* as much or more from their clients as what they *teach* them. Thus health education will be one of the most deeply satisfying and personally rewarding of all nursing activities.

Discharge planning begins during the assessment phase on admission to any health service and continues until the patient is discharged to another setting. It is essential that discharge planning focus on an interdisciplinary approach so that the client may benefit from all services that are available. The teaching/learning process continues from admission until discharge.

STUDY QUESTIONS

1. Why does the nurse have a responsibility to teach older clients?

2. What is teaching? What is learning?

3. How do teaching and learning impact behavior change?

4. Explain the mental processes involved in learning and remembering.

5. What components should the nurse assess in evaluating the needs of the client-learner?

6. How does the nurse identify the learning needs of older adult clients?

7. What health education topics are appropriate for *(a)* hospitalized older adults, *(b)* chronically ill older adults, and *(c)* well older adults requiring instruction in health promotion?

8. Identify teaching strategies suggested to enhance learning in older adults.

9. What do nurses gain professionally and personally from participating in client education?

10. Discuss the role of the nurse in discharge-planning activities.

REFERENCES

American Association of Retired Persons. 1986. *Truth about Aging: Guidelines for Accurate Communication.* Washington, DC: American Association for Retired Persons.

American Association of Retired Persons and Administration on Aging. 1991. *A Profile of Older Americans.* Washington, DC: United States Department of Health and Human Services.

Browning, M.A. 1992. Discharge planning. In *Clinical Manual of Gerontological Nursing,* edited by M.O. Hogstel. St. Louis, MO: Mosby–Year Book.

Cheeseman, G.S., and J. Selekman. 1987. *Patient Teaching Manual.* Springhouse, PA: Springhouse Corporation.

Corkery, E. 1989. Discharge planning and home health care: What every staff nurse should know. *Orthopaedic Nursing* 8(6):18–27.

Department of Health and Human Services: Public Health Service. 1990. *Healthy People 2000: National Health Promotion and Disease Objectives.* (DHHS Publication No. (PHS) 91-50212). Washington, DC: United States Government Printing Office.

Dimond, M. and S.L. Jones. 1983. *Chronic Illness Across the Life Span.* Norwalk, CT: Appleton-Century-Crofts.

Doak, C.C., L.G. Doak, and J.H. Root. 1985. *Teaching Patients with Low Literacy Skills.* Philadelphia: J.B. Lippincott Co.

Drew, L.A., D. Biordi, and D.A. Gilles. 1988. How discharge planners and home health nurses view their patients. *Nursing Management* 19(4)66–70.

Esper, P.S. 1988. Discharge planning—A quality assurance approach. *Nursing Management* 19(10):66–68.

Folden, S.L. 1990. On the inside looking out: Perceptions of the homebound. *Journal of Gerontological Nursing* 16(1):9–14.

Frieden, J. 1991. What's ahead for managed care? *Business and Health* 9(13):43–49.

Gilles, D.E. 1986. Patients suffering from memory loss can be taught self-care. *Geriatric Nursing* 7(5):357–61.

Green, J.H. 1989. Long-term home care research. *Nursing and Health Care* 10(3):139–43.

Haddock, K.S. 1991. Characteristics of effective discharge planning programs for the frail elderly. *Journal of Gerontological Nursing* 17(7):10–14.

Hamilton, M.S. 1990. Mentorhood. In *Contemporary Leadership Behavior*, edited by E. Hein and M.J. Nicholson. Glenview, IL: Scott, Foresman and Co.

How to Teach Patients. 1989. Springhouse, PA: Springhouse Corporation.

Huckabay, L.M.D. 1980. *Conditions of Learning and Instruction in Nursing.* St. Louis, MO: The C.V. Mosby Company.

Johnson, J. 1989. Where's discharge planning on your list? *Geriatric Nursing* 10(3):148.

Johnston, L. and S.H. Gueldner. 1989. Using mnemonics to boost memory in the elderly. *Journal of Gerontological Nursing* 15(8):22–25.

Kane, R.A. and R.L. Kane. 1981. *Assessing the Elderly.* Lexington, Massachusetts: D.C. Heath and Company.

Kemper, P. 1990. Case management agency systems of administering long-term care: Evidence from the channeling demonstration. *The Gerontologist* 30(6):187–24.

Kim, K. 1989. Patient education. In *Nursing the Elderly: A Care Plan Approach*, edited by V. Burggraf and M. Stanley. Philadelphia: J.B. Lippincott Co.

Kozier, B., G. Erb., and R. Olivieri. 1991. *Fundamentals of Nursing: Concepts, Process and Practice.* Redwood City, CA: Addison-Wesley.

Lancaster, J. and K.R. Simpson. 1988. Psychologic changes. In *Nursing Care of the Older Adult*, 2d ed., edited by M.O. Hogstel.

Lipetz, M., M.N. Bussigel, J. Bannerman and B. Risley. 1990. What is wrong with patient education programs? *Nursing Outlook* (July/Aug):184–89.

Lubkin, I.M. 1986. *Chronic Illness: Impact and Interventions.* Boston: Jones and Bartlett Publishers, Inc.

National League for Nursing. 1991. *Nursing's Agenda for Health Care Reform* (PR-3 220M, June). New York, NY: National League for Nursing.

Naylor, M. 1990. Comprehensive discharge planning for hospitalized elderly: A pilot study. *Nursing Research* 39(3):156–61.

Picariello, G. 1986. A guide for teaching elders. *Geriatric Nursing* 7(1):38–39.

Redman, B.K. 1988. *The Process of Patient Education*, 6th ed. St. Louis: C.V. Mosby Co.

Rendon, D., D.K. Davis, E.C. Gioiella, and M.S. Tranzillo. 1986. The right to know: The right to be taught. *Journal of Gerontological Nursing* 12(12):33–37.

Resnick, B.M. 1991. Geriatric motivation: Clinically helping the elderly to comply. *Journal of Gerontological Nursing* 17(5):17–20.

Strieff, L.D. 1986. Can clients understand our instructions? *Image* 18(2):48–52.

Theis, S.L. 1991. Using previous knowledge to teach elderly clients. *Journal of Gerontological Nursing* 17(8):34–37.

Weinrich, S.P., M. Boyd, and J. Nussbaum. 1989. Continuing education: Adapting strategies to teach the elderly. *Journal of Gerontological Nursing* 15(11):17–21.

Wilson, E.B., M.E. Deeves, C. Clancy, and A. Schnitt. 1991. Take a fresh look at discharge planning. *Geriatric Nursing* 12(1):23–25.

17 Nursing Home Care

Mildred O. Hogstel

FOCUS

This chapter provides an overview of the nursing home environment and the role of the nurse in providing safe and effective care in that environment.

OBJECTIVES

1. Identify the type of persons who most commonly need nursing home care.
2. Identify factors that should be considered in helping families choose a nursing home.
3. Discuss how nursing home care is financed.
4. Evaluate the important factors to consider when admitting a new resident to a nursing home.
5. Discuss the rights of nursing home residents.
6. Evaluate the requirements and problems of OBRA of 1987.
7. Discuss the use and misuse of physical and chemical restraints.
8. Analyze the common medical emergencies among older residents in nursing homes.
9. Identify the types of residents who are especially high-risk for falling.
10. Plan nursing interventions for the most common long-term care problems of residents.
11. Discuss the role of the Director of Nursing in the nursing home setting.

Appreciation is expressed to Vera Phillips for her assistance with this chapter.

12. Analyze the use of case management in nursing homes.

13. Identify the need for in-service education and research in nursing homes.

The lifestyle of older adults has changed considerably since the 1950s. The life expectancy of individuals has continued to increase. The Social Security system and private pensions have not produced security for older adults. Modern medical science has produced an older generation with multiple chronic conditions and disabilities.

Approximately 5% of the over-65 age group resides in long-term health care facilities, with the percentage "ranging from 1% for persons 65–74 years to 5% for persons 75–84 years and 25% for persons 85+" (*A Profile of Older Americans*, 1991).

In this chapter the term *nursing homes* refers to long-term health care facilities that provide inpatient care for older adults who are convalescing from surgery or illness and who require nursing supervision and medical care. As discussed here, the nursing home does not refer to an institution that provides custodial care.

CLASSIFICATION OF NURSING HOMES

Many nursing homes are an integral part of life-care retirement centers. These planned living centers for older adults allow them to remain active and independent in a protected environment. Older adults may have their own homes, apartments, or several rooms in an apartment complex. As they pass through various stages of diminished health, they may move into the nursing home facility that is part of the retirement living center. These centers are privately owned, church-sponsored, fraternal, or union-planned retirement communities.

Private ownership of nursing homes is the most common form of proprietorship. Many health care corporations own chains of nursing homes in various parts of the United States. Nursing homes are also classified as "for profit" or "nonprofit" homes. State mental hospitals also admit older adults whose be-

havior is so disruptive that nursing home care is not advisable.

The staff of each nursing home decides the type of older adults who will be admitted. Some facilities admit only private paying residents with any kind of condition or problem. Other facilities admit residents who receive Medicaid* assistance and are, therefore, classified into specific categories.

Long-term health care facilities that receive Medicaid funds are classified as Nursing Facilities (N.F.). Nursing Facilities provide services to older adults who require institutionalization and nursing care directed by registered nurses or licensed vocational or practical nurses. These older adults need assistance with medications and a protective environment. All nursing homes that receive Medicare funds are classified as Skilled Nursing Facilities (S.N.F.), and provide more skilled nursing care, such as tube feedings and sterile dressings.

All nursing homes provide twenty-four-hour care seven days a week by licensed nurses. The Director of Nurses is a registered nurse and a registered nurse is on duty during the daytime seven days a week and is on call during evening and night hours.

Private paying residents may be admitted to any facility, but Medicaid certifies the level of care for their recipients. Many nursing homes combine services but keep residents who need less care separated from the skilled nursing section. As the nursing needs of older adults change, they are transferred to the other nursing section within the nursing home.

DESCRIPTION OF RESIDENTS IN NURSING HOMES

The typical older adult who becomes a resident in a nursing home is usually a woman who is over 65 years of age. She has two or more chronic conditions

---

*Medicaid is a federally funded, state-operated and administered program that provides medical benefits for certain low-income people who are in need of health care.

that have produced functional disability, such as limited mobility and incontinence. There may be psychologic changes, especially related to memory. Older adults who are no longer able to be independent for a twenty-four-hour period and have no support system from family or friends are referred for nursing home care. Age is not as important as general physical and psychologic condition.

Families of nursing home residents many times are the middle-aged families of older adults and are having problems managing their own living situations. Too often when the word *son* or *daughter* is mentioned by an older adult, a young person is pictured; in reality, these sons and daughters are no longer young themselves. Extended families need assistance in making plans for family members who are becoming less independent and require alternative living situations. Many times the role change is sudden and the son or daughter assumes the role of responsible party without any previous preparation or plan.

Husbands and wives may be admitted together, as a couple, to nursing homes. Perhaps only one member requires nursing care, but the other member decides to be admitted also to maintain a relationship that has existed for many years. Another factor that precipitates the move may be that the caregiver in the home is no longer able to care for the spouse. The health of each one will determine how long the two may occupy the same room in the nursing home.

Men are in the minority in a nursing home, partly because men do not live as long as women. However, sometimes a surviving husband is no longer able to maintain his own living arrangements independently after the death of his wife, or he needs nursing care. Childless older people and single people are faced with problems different from those who have families. Brothers, sisters, and other family members often come to the assistance of these people who have found it necessary to be admitted to a nursing home. Friends may be the only source of assistance some older people have as the years pass. These friends are often unable or unwilling to assume responsibility for the older person and alternative living arrangements have to be considered.

The federal prospective payment system (PPS-diagnostic related groups) implemented in 1983 also has affected the type of residents in nursing homes. Because older residents on Medicare are being discharged "quicker and sicker" from hospitals, the acuity level of nursing home residents has increased. Langer, Drinka, and Voeks (1991, 16) noted that there is a "shift in location of death from the hospital to the nursing home, and higher numbers of required nursing procedures suggests that more seriously ill residents are being cared for in nursing homes." Nursing homes are now caring for residents with tracheostomies, oxygen, and intravenous fluids and medications as well as gastrostomy feedings and cystostomy catheters. Some nursing homes also are opening units for ventilator-dependent residents and providing chemotherapy. This change in type of residents in nursing homes has also emphasized the need for an increase in the quantity and quality of nursing staff (Harron and Schaeffer 1986).

Most Common Medical Diagnoses of Nursing Home Residents

Older people tend to have more than one or two medical diagnoses when they are admitted to a nursing home. Cardiovascular problems and congestive heart disease are major reasons for admission. Coronary thrombosis and cerebrovascular accidents change active older adults into people who can no longer care for themselves. Many older people are admitted to nursing homes for a period of prolonged convalescence after surgery. Surgery for malignancies may be particularly devastating to older people, who are then never able to return home again.

Orthopedic problems are prevalent. Arthritis and osteoporosis are crippling conditions that prevent independence in the activities of daily living. Fractures are common and require a long period of recovery. Elective surgery for knee or hip replacement requires long periods of convalescence and daily physical therapy. Older adults with diabetes, blindness, glaucoma, and emphysema require supervised environments. Hypertension, a common problem of many older people, often adds to the complications of other conditions. There are various mental health problems, such as organic mental disorders, severe confusion, and depression, that require nursing home care. The number of residents diagnosed as having dementia of the Alzheimer's type also is increasing. Many older adults are admitted to nursing homes because they no longer can live alone and still follow prescribed medications and diet. All older adults who are admitted to nursing homes must be under the supervision of their private medical doctor or a staff physician.

SELECTION OF A NURSING HOME

Many times older people and their families have not thought about a nursing home until this suggestion is made to them by the family physician. Few older people make plans to enter a nursing home. The thought of being admitted to a nursing home means "giving up" for many older adults, because they think they will have to surrender all their rights to make decisions for themselves.

An older person's ability to be independent, health of spouse, personal health, and income often change drastically within a short time. The need for nursing home care may require a sudden and traumatic decision. For example, an older adult may be admitted to a hospital for treatment of an acute or chronic condition. The utilization review committee of the hospital decides when discharge is appropriate under Medicare regulations (the Prospective Payment System). The shortened period of hospitalization does not allow most older adults to recover and return to their former living environment. Many times, they will not be able to resume independent living because of their conditions, so the family must make decisions regarding posthospital care. Usually the first realization that a nursing home will be needed is startling to the entire family. Social service departments in acute care hospitals help families plan for and secure placement in a nursing home.

The time involved in seeking a nursing home often does not allow the family and the older adults to make decisions together. In one situation the daughter, who was a nurse, was confident that it would be easy to find just the right nursing home. But she found that many of them did not have vacancies or she was told that a vacancy was expected any day but not immediately. Some hospitals provide a computerized nursing home placement service to the entire community. Information about the availability of vacant beds by type of home and location can be determined by one telephone call. This service can be very helpful to families who have to make such decisions in a short time.

In communities where there are extended care facilities, some of which are approved by Medicare, older people may go to these facilities for a time. Acceptance into these facilities depends on the need for this type of care. Rehabilitative care, the need for dressings, and physical therapy are considered reasons for extended care. These services are not always available to every community, or bed space may not be available.

How does one find the right nursing home? The physician may suggest certain nursing homes because they are convenient to visit. Perhaps the physician has many residents in a particular home and believes the care that is provided there is good. The family's church is also a good source of information regarding nursing homes. A nursing home should be selected so that it is convenient for family members to visit frequently. One 91-year-old man admitted his wife to a nursing home easily accessible to his home through neighborhood streets so that he would not have to drive on freeways or other highly congested roads. Friends can also make suggestions about good nursing homes, perhaps from their personal experiences with family members in these homes.

Evaluating the Home by a Personal Visit

Several facilities should be visited before a decision is made to place a loved one in a nursing home. There are many pamphlets and booklets available with checklists to help families evaluate and select nursing homes. Often these can be obtained from agencies such as the local Area Agency on Aging or the Mental Health Association. The family is fortunate if they can make a selection from among several homes. It is important that as many members of the family as possible make the visit. There tends to be less conflict among the family members about the decision if each member has seen what facilities are available. If the older adult is able, he or she should visit the nursing homes with the family. One member of the family is usually designated the responsible party to handle all the necessary arrangements.

Tour of the Facilities

A tour of the nursing home is a must. The family should observe the activities of the residents and the personnel who are caring for the residents. Is there a rush to close doors as if something is being concealed? It is helpful to stop and talk to one or two of the residents who are in the halls or in the activity room.

One or two of the rooms should be inspected. What furnishings are provided? May the family bring a favorite chair, television, radio, or pictures? May the family provide colorful sheets and blankets and be responsible for the laundry of the bed clothing? How much space is there in the room? The space between the beds should be at least thirty-six inches. Is there space for a wheelchair?

What about roommates? How many share a bathroom? Are there provisions for married couples? In rooms with double occupancy are screens or curtains provided for the privacy of each individual? What are the bathing facilities? How many doors will the personnel open to show the facilities?

Is there an activity or social director and is there an activity room? What projects are the residents doing? May the family assist in the activities? Are bed residents kept in bed or are they sitting up in wheelchairs during the day if their physical conditions allow? How much freedom do the residents have in the nursing home? May they walk or wheel themselves about and visit with other residents?

What types of clothing are the residents wearing? Are they dressed and wearing shoes or slippers? Perhaps they are wearing jacket restraints. This is a good opportunity to ask the reasons for the restraints.

Where do the residents receive their meals? If physical conditions permit, may the residents eat in the dining room? Is there a charge for special foods? Who plans the meals? Is there a registered dietitian employed by the nursing home? One nursing home administrator makes it a policy to have a member of the staff eat the regular food that is served to the residents at each mealtime; a different staff member performs this function each day. May the family bring food to the resident if the food is allowed on the resident's diet?

What are the visiting hours? If physical condition permits and there is physician's approval, may the resident visit outside the home? May the resident remain out overnight? Medicaid restricts the length of time a resident may remain out of the home. The length of time is usually seventy-two hours.

Is the older adult allowed to smoke? Safety rules are very strict. Fire restrictions limit smoking to certain areas and all smoking must be done under supervision. No smoking is allowed in residents' rooms. Residents are not allowed to keep cigarettes or matches in their possession. Individual resident's smoking supplies are not used by other residents or by the staff. Visitors to the nursing home also have to follow the restrictions on smoking in designated areas only.

Are the residents allowed to write letters and make telephone calls? Do they receive their own mail and will someone help them read it? Families should inquire about the activities that are available in the nursing home. What programs are offered? Are there movies? Do people from the community present programs? Are the residents allowed to plan programs? Do the residents participate in community projects such as stuffing envelopes for a charitable agency or making gifts for day-care centers?

Are religious services available for the residents? Are there Bible study programs? Are the services of a beautician and barber available?

After a tour of the facility the family and older adult should ask other questions. They should ask to meet the nursing director. One question that is asked repeatedly of nursing personnel is: Will you telephone me if something happens to my mother or father? This question so often depicts the feelings family members have about nursing homes. Will the physician be notified? In the event of a medical problem, will the resident be able to remain in the nursing home or must he or she be transferred to the hospital? What happens to the personal laundry of the residents? The family may elect to do the laundry. What about money or valuables? Adequate information about these concerns should be given to families.

While the family and the older adult inspect the nursing home, one observation can be made without any questioning. Is there an odor? If there is no detectable offensive odor, the family might ask how the odors are controlled. There should not be a strong odor of disinfectants either.

The family and the older adult should never be pressured into making a decision quickly. They should have the opportunity to talk about the nursing home among themselves and perhaps return later on for another visit. Visiting hours or mealtimes afford the family an opportunity to see another side of life in the nursing home.

Financial Arrangements

When families visit a nursing home, one question is foremost in their thoughts. Can we afford this kind of care? At least one nursing home administrator has observed that it is better to discuss finances first instead of talking around the subject. Usually it will be a staff member in the administrative office who will receive the inquiry about the home. During this interview, the staff member should obtain information about family finances. The business staff has the necessary information to assist families in making financial arrangements.

If finances are not a problem, the resident will be admitted as a private pay resident. However, financial arrangements are available through several sources. The majority of older people and their families do not realize that Medicare does not pay for nursing home care except for a limited number of days and only if the resident needs specialized care such as physical therapy after a fracture. One of the major problems facing older people is the potentiality of having to pay for long-term care in a nursing home for many years. Some insurance companies provide insurance that will pay for long-term nursing home care. It is very important, however, that older people and their families study the costs and benefits of these insurance plans before investing in one of them. If older adults receive Social Security benefits or a small pension, this amount can be supplemented by Medicaid. The administrative staff of the nursing facility has this type of information available and will give family members instructions about how to apply for assistance. Application for Medicaid assistance is made at the local level by the resident or by the family member who is responsible for the financial arrangements. Medicaid approval is granted based on financial standing, including bank accounts, real estate, and personal income of the resident. If Medicaid assistance is approved, a certificate of need is granted and payments are made to the nursing home to supplement the payments made by the resident.

If the older adult is accepted for Medicaid assistance, the monthly Social Security check will be paid to the resident or to the responsible family member. The resident or family retains a certain portion of the check, which can be used for clothing and personal supplies for the resident. Medicaid payments supplement the money received from the family to pay for the services at the nursing home. The daily rate of charge for nursing home care is determined by state regulations when residents are on Medicaid. Medicaid will pay for needed prescription drugs for each recipient. Pharmacists work closely with physicians and families to provide direct billing to the Medicaid office for payment of these prescription drugs. The nursing home is responsible for furnishing commonly prescribed drugs such as aspirin, antacids, and laxatives, as well as supplies such as nasal gastric tubes, urinary catheters, drainage bags, dressings, and tube feedings, to residents who qualify for Medicaid assistance.

Medicaid funds are paid only to nursing homes that meet Medicaid standards. Physicians' services must be paid by the family. Reimbursement for these fees is applied for through Medicare or Medicaid. Physicians must bill Medicare directly. Standard fees are authorized for physicians' services. In some situations the income of older adults changes during the years or their savings may be reduced to such a small amount that they will qualify for Medicaid assistance later.

ADMISSION TO A NURSING HOME

If the decision is made to admit the older adult to a nursing home, the necessary forms must be completed. Physicians' orders must be received when the resident is admitted to the nursing home. A history and physical examination are required. If the older adult is transferred from a hospital to the nursing home, a summary of the hospital stay is needed. Every form that is signed by the responsible party should be completed in duplicate and copies retained by the family. Upon completion of the forms, the nursing home has entered into an agreement with the family and the rights and responsibilities of the nursing home and the family have been agreed upon. Nursing homes furnish information on the "Resident Bill of Rights," a major component of the Omnibus Budget Reconciliation Act (OBRA) of 1987. Many nursing homes have an enlarged copy of this Bill of Rights framed and displayed in a prominent place in the lobby of the nursing home. The family has the freedom to select the pharmacy to be used. Medical care and supervision are furnished by the admitting physician. Information is also collected regarding the name of the resident's dentist and which ambulance service is preferred.

Preparing the Resident for Admission

The family will be faced with the responsibility of telling the resident that he or she must be moved to a nursing home. What does such a change really mean to older adults? As they have been growing older, they have been faced with one loss after another. Now the move to a nursing home may represent a further loss: it will mean separation from loved ones and perhaps rejection by the family. Complete honesty between the resident and the family is by far the best way. Families should explain that in the nursing home needed nursing care can be given, and at the present time this is the kind of care required. Only promises that can be kept should be made to the older adult. There is no reason why the family cannot admit that they too are unhappy about the decision that has had to be made. Families should avoid statements such as "You will like it there." The older adult should also know that there are other homes he or she might move to if the one selected is not satisfactory.

Helping the Family Cope

Nursing home personnel should understand that family members will have many feelings of guilt when admitting a member of their family to a nursing home. Unexpressed thoughts such as, "I have failed Mother" or "Am I doing the right thing?" sometimes produce behavior in family members that is difficult to understand.

When a resident is admitted, nursing home personnel can follow certain guidelines that will help ease the burden on the family. The personnel should accept whatever behavior is exhibited and avoid forming negative opinions about the family. During the first few days the family "moves in." Unless contraindicated they should be allowed to assist in the care of the resident. Personnel should be prepared to answer the same questions over and over again, and to listen to family members when they discuss the likes and dislikes of the resident. Explanations of certain activities are important. The care of the resident should be planned with the family. When a resident is admitted, the nursing home is really taking in the whole family, the neighbors, and the church. It often helps if one or two family members are asked to eat a meal initially with the resident and other residents in the nursing home. During the first few days, 70–80 percent of the care is actually geared for the family, although nursing home personnel generally are more prepared to care for the resident. It is important that a trusting relationship be established between the resident, the family, and the staff. If the family is comfortable with the staff, the family will feel comfortable leaving their loved one with the nursing home staff.

Accommodations and roommates within a nursing home are not always satisfactory. Should there be dissatisfaction with either, it is often not possible to move the newly admitted resident at once. Perhaps the source of dissatisfaction is not the roommate but the fact of admission to the home. Residents who are unhappy about their new status may complain about many other things instead, often making the other family members feel guilty.

The effect of relocation, or movement from home or hospital to nursing home, has been studied extensively since the 1950s when it was believed that moving an older person from one environment to another increased the emotional stress for that person. Research in the 1960s proposed "that the emotional stress of relocation may precipitate rather traumatic consequences, such as death" (Burnette 1986, 8). Research in the 1970s showed that dissatisfaction was more prevalent than death and that the person's response was based on control of events. For example, if there was a careful orientation to the new environment, there was less chance for a decrease in mental status. To dispel some of the loneliness, favorite objects that belong to the resident may be brought in to make the living arrangements more pleasing. Family pictures also lessen the feelings of loneliness. The environment should be manipulated in such a way that the resident views a part of the room as his or her own. If the room is shared with another person, space needs should be clearly defined. Caregivers must be careful to avoid using perfume or powder that belongs to one resident on another resident. Personnel who enter a resident's room should ask permission to look in a drawer or open a closet. These precautions are especially important if the resident has failing vision or memory. Many older people become suspicious when they cannot see what someone is doing in their room. Perhaps a bulletin board close to the bedside with pictures and cards will bring loved ones into better focus for the older resident. Pictures can be changed frequently. Older people like calendars and clocks; the reminder of the date and day provide orientation to day and time. Color-coordinated curtains and bedspreads can be used.

The Process of Admission

As soon as possible after the resident has been admitted to the nursing home and if his or her condition permits, a personal history should be taken. If at all possible the resident should be the information giver. Parts of the history are obtained by the nurse, the dietitian, the social worker, and the aide who will be caring for the resident. The more active the resident is in this interview, the more personalized the care will be. An early introduction to the staff may lessen the resident's feelings of loneliness and helplessness. Staff should remember that first impressions are very important.

The personal belongings of the older adult are very important. Staff members should be aware of all the articles that are brought with the resident. Adequate identification of all belongings is important. The resident should be assisted in unpacking clothing and personal items. Bedside stands, dresser drawers, and closet space for the resident should be well identified and marked. If clothing is labeled with the resident's name, the label should not be in clear view; it should be placed on the facing or hem.

An admission physical and mental status assessment are essential. To lessen the fear of the examination, the personnel involved should provide privacy and an adequate explanation. The professional nurse and the aide should share the admission procedure so that both know the physical capabilities and limitations of the resident.

The nurse should be prepared for expressions of grief and sorrow from the resident during the admission process. The resident's freedom to express feelings is important at this time. The nurse should accept the feelings and not overreact to the words.

STANDARDS AND QUALITY OF CARE

Licensure

Licensure of the home is required by the state Department of Health. Licensure denotes that the nursing home has maintained specific minimal standards and is frequently inspected for observance of fire and safety codes, sanitation standards, health codes, and the maintenance of approved methods of purchasing and preparing foods. Guidelines for licensure are legislated at both the federal and state levels. Certain state agencies are designated as licensing agencies for long-term health care facilities. The title of the agency varies from state to state, but its function is to oversee the care of older adults in nursing homes. These standards cover building construction, number of qualified personnel, maintenance of health standards, operation of the home in compliance with medical and nursing standards, and the number of older adults who can be cared for within the facility. The state is the licensing agency; private pay homes are also licensed by the state agency. The inability of the home to maintain minimal standards could mean that the home will lose its license. Minor infractions must be corrected within a thirty-day period. The level of care provided to the residents is also considered a part of the licensing process.

The administrator must have a current state license as a nursing home administrator. State laws define the type and number of hours of education the administrator must have to qualify for licensure. The successful completion of state licensing examinations is required before licensure is approved. Yearly relicensure is granted upon the submission of proof of attendance at workshops or seminars related to nursing home administration. Many nursing homes have several employees who are licensed as administrators. Registered nurses and licensed vocational or practical nurses must have current licenses. All employees are required to have current health cards issued by the local health department and based on state standards. Personnel are especially screened for tuberculosis and sexually transmitted diseases.

Accreditation

Voluntary accreditation may be received from the Joint Commission on Accreditation of HealthCare Organizations (JCAHO). The bed capacity of the nursing home will determine whether this type of accreditation is sought. Nursing homes are usually members of state and local nursing home associations. Membership in the American Health Care Association or the American Association of Homes for the Aging is also available.

Nursing Home Reform

The Omnibus Budget Reconciliation Act (OBRA) of 1987, implemented on October 1, 1990, came about as a result of the efforts of a number of national organizations, such as the American Nurses' Association (ANA), the American Association of Retired Persons (AARP), and the National Citizens Coalition for Nursing Home Reform (NCCNHR) (Strumpf, Evans, and Schwartz 1990). The major requirements of this federal legislation are listed in Table 17-1. While all of these regulations are important, the major ones will be discussed.

Staffing. Staffing regulations include at least one registered nurse during the day shift seven days a week. [Although most nursing homes previously had at least one registered nurse, it was not required in an intermediate care facility (ICF), now called a nursing facility (NF).] Also, a licensed nurse (LVN/LPN) is required on site twenty-four hours a day. A social worker is required if the home has 121 or more beds. A major change has been the increased amount of education for nurse aides. They must have a minimum of seventy-five hours of training within the first four months of employment and pass written and clinical tests. All nurse aides who have met these requirements must be listed on a state registry and an employer must check this registry before employing them. The intent of this regulation is to be sure that the nurse aides have been certified regarding training and testing and that they have not been convicted of a felony or other wrongdoing.

While training and testing for nurse aides has progressed well in most areas after a slow start, meeting the requirement for registered nurses has been more difficult because of the severe shortage of nurses in this country.

Admission Assessment. Another section of the OBRA regulations relates to quality of care (see Table 17-1). These include a comprehensive admission assessment of each resident by a registered nurse, written care plans based on a comprehensive assessment, and quality assessment and assurance committees. These regulations have been easier to implement because many of them were already in place.

Restraints. Greatly needed but more difficult to implement was the need to justify the use of both physical and chemical restraints. Too many restraints had

---

Table 17–1 Federal Omnibus Budget Reconciliation Act (OBRA) (passed by Congress in 1987)

Summary of Requirements (effective 10/1/90) with OBRA 1990 Additions

A. Staffing
1. RN (at least one) eight hours a day, seven days a week (waiver available).
2. LVN/LPN twenty-four hours a day, seven days a week (waiver available).
3. Social worker (at least one) if 121 or more beds.
4. Nurse aides must have seventy-five hours of training within first four months of employment.
5. Must check state registry before hiring nurse aides.

B. Quality of care
1. Comprehensive admission assessment by RN within 14 days of admission.
2. Written care plans after comprehensive assessment.
3. Quality assessment and assurance committees required.
4. Must justify medical need for physical and chemical restraints.
5. Cannot admit mentally ill or retarded unless certified by state as needing such care.

C. Other
1. Residents' rights are all important.
2. Patient Self Determination Act must be discussed with patient and/or family.

been used in nursing homes, primarily for the convenience of the staff though stating that they were for the safety of residents. Most research has demonstrated that the use of restraints does not prevent falls (Gross et al. 1990). Nurses have always known that physical restraints are a last resort, must be specifically ordered by the physician, and actually require more nurse time because of the need to assess the resident frequently to prevent complications.

The new regulations stated that restraints should only be used if needed for the medical benefit of the resident (e.g., for a resident who might pull out a nasogastric feeding tube if not restrained). Restraints should not be used to keep a resident who can walk from being ambulatory [e.g., a resident with a diagnosis of dementia of the Alzheimer's type (DAT); he/she needs to walk]. The initial interpretation of these regulations caused some nursing homes to remove all restraints because they were receiving deficiencies from state inspectors. Consequently, some resident falls with serious complications occurred. Recent changes in the federal guidelines have eased this problem somewhat. The number of restraint-reduced nursing homes is increasing (Coberg, Lynch, and Mavretish, 1991). (Alternatives to restraints are discussed more completely in the "Accidents" section later in this chapter.)

Chemical restraints, primarily psychotropic medications such as sedatives, hypnotics, antianxiety agents, and neuroleptics, also have been used in the past to control the behavior of hyperactive, wandering, agitated residents. The new regulations state that these medications should only be given to residents who require them for a specific diagnosis. This regulation has increased the number of mental status assessments being performed in nursing homes by psychiatrists and geropsychiatric nurses. When appropriate, there is referral for further evaluation and treatment. The outcome has been beneficial because many older people are receiving treatment they might not have received otherwise. Also, the reduced number of psychotropic medications is generally beneficial to the health of the older person; it also saves money.

Mental Illness. Another regulation relates to the fact that persons whose primary medical diagnosis is mental illness or mental retardation should not be in nursing homes. Organic mental disorders, such as Alzheimer's disease, are excluded because they are

physical problems. There are two reasons for this: *(1)* residents cannot receive adequate treatment for mental problems in nursing homes because that is not these institutions' purpose; *(2)* residents with these diagnoses often disturb the other residents. An evaluation program—Pre-Admission Screening and Annual Resident Review (PASARR)—has been used to determine if these residents should be in the nursing home or if they could be cared for more effectively in another setting.

Levels of Care. OBRA (1987) also eliminated the distinction between skilled nursing facilities (SNF) and intermediate care facilities (ICF). Now all nursing homes are referred to as nursing facilities (NF) or skilled nursing facilities (SNF). Another focus was to determine the level of care and thus reimbursement by Medicaid, based on residents' "impairment and disability rather than on medical diagnosis" (Boondas 1991, 311). In addition a comprehensive instrument was developed through research to record health data about residents upon admission, yearly, and whenever there is a change in resident's status. This Minimum Data Set (MDS) is used to assign residents to the appropriate level of care (Morris et al. 1990). This process determines resource requirements for each resident based on that person's individual characteristics and needs (Boondas, 1991). Therefore this case mix classification based on MDS "is a method that will provide a more equitable system of payment, and an improved staffing pattern consistent with the case mix and an improved understanding of care time requirements" (Boondas 1991, 311).

Implementation. Revised guidelines and waivers for many of these regulations have made the nursing home reform law less effective than was originally planned. One major problem is that although the federal government passed the OBRA law in 1987, the exact guidelines for implementing the law were very slow in being distributed and the method of implementation was vague. Some guidelines were only available late in the summer of 1990 before the law was to take full effect in October 1990. Also, the federal government did not provide for additional funding, primarily through Medicaid, to implement many of these requirements. Thus states with major budget problems did not have the Medicaid money available to help nursing homes meet the federal guidelines. Nor do most states have other services or facilities for the treatment and care of chronically mentally ill older adults.

COMMON NURSING CARE CONCERNS

Acute Medical Emergencies

Acute medical emergencies occur among older adults in the nursing home as well as in the community. These emergencies may involve acute illnesses, such as a myocardial infarction or a cerebrovascular accident, or accidents such as falls. See Table 17-2 for symptoms, possible causes, and emergency interventions for the most common medical emergencies.

Immediate assessment and emergency treatment may be provided in the nursing home, but the resident usually will require transfer to a nearby hospital for further evaluation and treatment.

Accidents. The environment should be made safe so that the resident is not injured. A study of incident reports is a good method of determining the most common causes of accidents. Appliances used in assisting the person with walking, such as canes or walkers, should be kept in the same place when not in use so that they may be located quickly. The terrain where the person is likely to walk should be level; inclines or steps should be clearly marked with signs and different colors and should have handrails.

Table 17–2 Common Medical Emergencies among Older Adults in Nursing Homes

Problems	Symptoms	Possible causes	Interventions*
Myocardial infarction (MI) and/or cardiac arrest	Sudden behavior change, e.g., confusion, disorientation, (probably before chest pain, nausea, vomiting, dyspnea, cyanosis, absence of pulse/respiration)	Long-term cardiovascular problems	Initiate CPR if needed (if no "Do Not Resuscitate" order) and call 911 for ambulance.
Choking, obstructed airway, and/or aspiration	Coughing, dyspnea, cyanosis, hand to throat	Past CVA, other neurological damage, edentulous, dysphagia, dilated esophagus	Assess type and degree; suction; Heimlich maneuver (if needed); continue to assess temperature and lung sounds, teach feeding techniques.
Stroke (CVA)	Numbness in extremities, falling, slurred speech, ptosis of eyelids, inability to see	Long-term cardiovascular problems	Assess vital signs, neuro signs (especially pupils), hand grip.

(Table continued)

* The attending physician and at least one family member should be notified as soon as possible in all these situations.

Problems	Symptoms	Possible causes	Interventions
Acute abdominal pain	Severe pain, nausea and vomiting, jaundice, elevated pulse and respiration	Possibly ruptured peptic ulcer or gall bladder, intestinal obstruction or rupture, internal hemorrhage	Assess vital signs and abdomen.
Falls	On floor, overturned wheelchair or chair	Any of the above, postural hypotension, medications (e.g., cardiovascular, psychotropic)	Assess vital signs and possible injuries before moving, especially head and extremities.
Acute closed-angle glaucoma	Sudden severe pain in and around eyes, blurred vision, nausea and vomiting	Chronic open-angle glaucoma	Take to ophthalmologist as soon as possible.
Fever > 99°F**	Increased pulse, respiration, dehydration, dry lips, sunken eye sockets, decreased urination, decreased appetite	Infection, possibly infection of urinary tract or upper respiratory tract, including pneumonia	Call physician for further diagnostic tests and/or orders.

**Note that 99°F (rather than 101°F) should be referred for further evaluation because of the normal lower body temperature in older adults.

Dangerous equipment and substances should be kept behind locked doors (Heim 1986; Ridder 1985). In many incidents of falls it is impossible to determine how the accident occurred.

Hernandez and Miller (1986) reported that most falls occur on the 11 P.M. to 7 A.M. shift, before and after shift change, and in the resident's room or bathroom. However, Gross et al. (1990, 22) found that most falls occurred "between 8:00 A.M. and 5:00 P.M. with peaks at 10:00 A.M. and noon" and that most "falls occurred in patients' rooms." Each institution should identify its residents at high-risk for falling and plan specific measures for prevention in their nursing care plans, see Figure 17-1. Residents at highest-risk for falling are

1. those who are taking medications that affect the central nervous system

2. those who have elimination problems

3. those who are disoriented or confused

4. those who have impaired gait

5. those who have had a previous fall

6. those who want to be independent but are not able to walk safely alone

7. those who are using orthopedic devices

Berryman et al. (1989, 200) developed a Predisposition for Falling Assessment Guide that "measures 10 factors: age, mental status, number of days in hospital, bowel and bladder incontinence, history of falling, uncompensated visual impairment, ambulatory status (confinement to a chair), drop in systolic blood pressure, gait and balance abnormalities, and classification of medicines."

Other than side rails and restraints, preventive measures to consider are

1. Keeping the door to the high-risk resident's room open at all times and reminding all staff to look in the room as they walk by.

Figure 17–1 Institutional assessment of older residents who are at high-risk for falling

Name _____ Room # _____ Age _____

Factor	Assessment
1. Previous falls	No _____ Yes _____ Number _____ Reason _____ Outcome _____
2. Recent admission (one to two weeks)	Yes* _____ No _____
3. Mental status a. Orientation	Person* if ø _____ Place* if ø _____ Time _____
b. Memory	Immediate* if ø _____ Recent* if ø _____ Remote _____
c. Diagnosis of mental impairment	Yes* _____ No _____
4. Ambulation/devices	Alone _____ With assistance* _____ Instability of gait * _____ Cane* _____ Walker _____ Wheelchair* _____

5. Elimination	Urine: continent _____ incontinent* _____
	       frequency* _____ urgency* _____
	Feces: continent _____ incontinent* _____
	       diarrhea* _____

6. Vision	Acute _____ Limited* _____ Blind* _____ Cataracts* (without surgery) _____ Glaucoma* _____ Macular degeneration* _____

(Figure continued)

7. Hearing	Acute _____ Limited _____
	Severely limited* _____
8. Medications* Affecting ambulation, blood pressure, mental status	Drug　　　　　　Dose　　　　　　Time
9. Psychological factors	Attempts to ambulate independently* _____
	Uncooperative* _____ Agitated* _____
10. Physical factors	Age* (if >80) _____ Male _____ Female* _____
	Caucasian* _____ Black _____ Hispanic _____
	Height* (if <5'5") _____ Poor balance* _____
	Dizzy* _____ Cardiovascular problems* _____
	Neurological problems* _____
Total number of risk factors	_____

Initiate the high-risk for falling intervention program (given here) for any resident with *any* one or more of the categories marked with an *. The greater the number of *s, the greater the risk.

1. Label the rooms of high-risk residents so they are obvious to staff but not visitors.

2. Keep the door open as much as possible and have all staff look in the room each time they walk by.

3. Check the resident at least every fifteen to twenty minutes twenty-four hours a day.

4. Attach the signal cord to the resident's gown so light or buzzer will come on when it is pulled out of wall when the resident tries to get out of bed. Label lights of high-risk residents' rooms at the nurses' station (red or orange).

5. Answer the signal light or buzzer as soon as possible.

6. Anticipate and meet elimination needs (especially in the early morning and between 10 P.M. and 6 A.M.).

7. Locate the resident in a room as close to the nurses' station as possible.

8. Stagger breaks for personnel so that the unit is well covered at all times.

9. Use families and volunteers (if available) on the units during feeding and medication time because many falls occur when nursing staff are busy.

(Figure continued)

10. Locate the resident in a room with a television monitor if possible.

11. Use restraints, if ordered, as a last resort and follow institutional policy regarding observing and releasing intervals.

12. Display posters with these guidelines in the nurses' station and lounge.

13. Provide in-service training on these guidelines for all staff at routine intervals.

Figure 17-1 was compiled from E. Berryman, D. Gaskin, A. Jones, F. Tolley, and J. Macmullen, 1989, "Point by point: Predicting elders' falls," *Geriatric Nursing* 10(4):199–201; Y.T. Gross, Y. Shimamoto, C.L. Rose, and B. Frank, 1990, "Monitoring risk factors," *Journal of Gerontological Nursing* 16(6):20–25; M. Hernandez and M. Miller, "How to reduce falls." *Geriatric Nursing* 7(2):97–102; and E. Lund and M.L. Sheafor, 1985, "Is your patient about to fall?" *Journal of Gerontological Nursing* 11(4):37–41.

---

2. Keeping the bathroom light on at night if the resident is ambulatory.

3. Anticipating and meeting elimination needs, especially on the night shift.

4. Locating the high-risk resident close to the nurses' station or in a room with a television monitor, if available.

5. Attaching the call cord to the resident's gown so that the light will come on if the cord is pulled out of the wall.

6. Keeping the intercom system open to the resident's room during the night shift so moaning or movement by the resident can be heard.

7. Reminding all staff of the severe problem of accidental falls through in-service education and posters on the unit.

Safety measures should be closely monitored. A resident's poor vision and unsteady gait, as well as unsafe surroundings such as wet floors, dim lights, and furniture in the way, tend to increase the likelihood of accidents. Residents who are able to walk independently should not be restricted just because they might fall, but safety must be maintained in the environment. With adequate supervision, residents should remain mobile for as long as they can.

Nursing home residents sometimes choke on food during mealtimes. Donahue (1990, 7) warns that "all patients should be carefully assessed during meals until they are judged as being at low risk for chok-

ing." Refer to Donahue (1990), Hogstel and Robinson (1989), or Kolodny and Malek (1991) for specific techniques to aid in feeding the older person who has difficulty swallowing. Supervision by the staff while residents are eating in the dining room is a necessity. (The residents' mealtimes are not the best times for the staff to take their own meal breaks.) The Heimlich maneuver for choking can be administered (if needed) to residents who are sitting in chairs or wheelchairs in the dining room. Residents may choke because their swallowing reflex is often depressed; they talk, cough, or laugh frequently while eating; they forget or are unable to chew food adequately; they might eat too quickly in their hurry to return to their favorite television programs. Residents who eat in their own rooms should be checked frequently by the staff to ensure that they do not choke on food. Residents who eat in bed should be kept in a semi-Fowler's position for at least one hour after meals. This prevents regurgitation and possible aspiration of food or fluids, which is common in many older people who have a dilated esophagus or hiatal hernia (Hogstel and Robinson 1989).

Inadequate orientation and supervision of new personnel could cause the unsafe use of whirlpool baths. They might allow the temperature of the water to be too hot or too cold. Because older persons have lower metabolisms and decreased perception of heat and cold, they are more subject to hypothermia and skin injuries when the water is too cold or too hot.

Long-Term Care Problems

Residents in long-term care facilities are vulnerable to many changes in their ability to maintain a constant state of normal functioning. Many diseases from which they suffer are chronic, and even vigorous preventive measures or treatment are unable to prevent deterioration. Common changes of aging will occur, but measures can be taken to help the resident adapt to the aging process and to prevent complications. The nurse encounters a number of common problems related to aging in the process of implementing nursing care in the nursing home.

Skin Problems. The aging process produces many changes in the skin of older adults. Loss of subcutaneous tissue, decreased elasticity, and increased fragility cause many problems. The use of drying powders, too much soap, and immobility lead to skin breakdown. A daily bath does not increase dryness of the skin, as previously thought. Essential areas of the body, such as the face, axillary areas, and genital region, must be bathed as often as needed. Nurse aides are often accustomed to using a large amount of soap when bathing residents; this procedure should be avoided with older adults. Also, older people are not as agile as younger adults and therefore cannot dry their lower extremities, especially their feet, very well. The aides should cleanse and dry the areas between the toes very well, often a difficult process with residents who have contractures or severe arthritis. Older adults are extremely sensitive to temperature changes and require extra warmth when being bathed, a fact that auxiliary personnel may not realize.

The identification of areas that are prone to skin breakdown and special massage of these areas lessen the potential for breakdown. For residents who are bedfast and unable to move independently, a specific schedule of turning every two hours will relieve pressure to sensitive areas. Linens should be changed as soon as possible when they become soiled. The use of alternating air, water, or sand mattresses, egg-crate-shaped foam-rubber mattresses, or sheepskin pads decreases pressure on sensitive areas such as the scapulae, coccyx, sacrum, ischial tuberosities, iliac crests, heels, and ankles. Care should also be taken to protect the sensitive skin and cartilage of the ears when the immobile resident is positioned on the side.

Numerous bruises often can be observed on the skin of older residents, especially those in their 90s and 100s. Gentle handling is essential. It is necessary to obtain assistance from other personnel in turning, moving, or getting residents out of bed when the residents are unable to help themselves. Older residents also bruise themselves. They bump bedrails, wheelchairs, and doors, and even rub their own dry skin vigorously. Short fingernails and thin protective gloves prevent self-inflicted scratches. The extent of any skin breakdown should be described accurately as to appearance, size, and depth. Pressure ulcers should be documented according to stage (Phipps et al. 1984). Daily observations of the treatment and healing process are recorded in the nurses' notes. It is much easier to prevent skin breakdown than to treat the problem areas later.

Bowel and Bladder Control. Physical disabilities often hinder residents from having control over elimination. They may be unable to communicate this need or to go to the bathroom independently. A schedule of bowel and bladder training will assist residents in achieving control or at least remaining dry. New products similar to disposable pants (the term "diaper" should not be used) are available for incontinent adult residents. These products help keep the residents ambulatory and their skin dry and control odors. Cleaning the residents after elimination is essential. To prevent skin breakdown and assist in the control of odors in the nursing home, bed residents should be checked at least every two hours, genital areas should be washed and dried thoroughly (when needed), and linens should be changed often. Very lightly dusted powder or cornstarch can be used in areas that are slightly irritated where skin touches skin, such as in the groin or under the breasts. Powder or cornstarch should not be used directly on the genital area of the woman or man. Soiled linens should be placed in tightly covered containers and emptied frequently. This essential and frequent change of linens demands ample linen supplies.

Immobility and Contractures. Exercises are important for residents who are partially immobile and/or unable to move independently (Benison and Hogstel 1986). The professional nursing staff should teach the nurse aides and show them how to provide normal range of motion during the resident's bath. Proper positioning of residents in bed and in wheelchairs will help maintain range of motion in the joints. Daily activities should be planned to keep the residents as mobile as possible. The social activities director can provide exercise classes for residents, including ball tossing and games that residents in wheelchairs can play. The nursing staff assists in preparing the residents for these activities. Ambulatory residents are encouraged to walk in groups about the halls or outdoors in safe areas.

Residents who have had strokes or fractures require rehabilitative measures to help them become mobile again. Self-help devices need to be checked frequently to assure that the devices are in good repair. Wheelchairs, crutches, and walkers have many parts that wear out and require repair. Realistic goals are set with the residents and the goals are updated frequently. The general goal is to maintain maximum activity. *The concept of rehabilitation to reach maximum potential despite physical problems and handicaps is just as important for the nursing home resident as for residents in other settings.*

Food and Fluid Needs. Appetites change and older people forget that they need to drink fluids. Fluids should be offered to residents at least every two hours when they are checked, turned, or moved by the aides. Dietary restrictions sometimes discourage residents from eating their meals. Suggestions may be made to change some of the foods on their diets. Dietary changes may also be needed because of dentures and mouth problems. Good oral hygiene before and after meals is important and will help make eating more pleasant. Lemon and glycerine are no longer used for mouth care because they are drying to the mucous membranes. Other disposable mouth care products are now available that have a pleasant taste and can be used to cleanse the gums and teeth and keep the mucous membranes of the oral cavity moist. Referral to a dentist may be necessary to correct poorly fitting dentures. Residents who have changes in memory or who forget to eat when meals are served need help in eating. Stiffness in their fingers may prevent residents from opening containers, using silverware, or cutting food. Poor vision may make it impossible for the older resident to see the food that is on the tray. Taste buds may not be as sensitive as they used to be, and therefore appetites are poor. Many residents are on caloric-restricted diets, which also creates problems. Residents must be weighed weekly, because they often secure candies and cookies from other residents, gaining unwanted weight in the process.

General Hygiene. Fingernails should be kept clean and short. Aides are allowed to cut fingernails. Toenails require the attention of a podiatrist or the professional nurse because of the possibility of trauma, which may cause infection and slow healing due to inadequate circulation to the lower extremities. Shaving and hair care are also part of daily care. Residents should be dressed and out of bed most of the day, if at all possible, since self-esteem is enhanced by a feeling of being presentable. Residents should be encouraged to make decisions about the clothing they wish to wear. Many times residents forget to change clothes because they have failing vision or a poor sense of smell.

Changes in Behavior. Regression, hostile behavior, memory loss, disorientation, and confusion are disturbing to the family and the staff. Assessment of the cause of the behavior is essential before the type of nursing intervention is determined. In some communities, a geropsychiatric nursing consultant or multidisciplinary team have made their services available to nursing homes on a regular or emergency basis. They help the nursing home staff plan for and give care to residents who have psychotic episodes or who experience sudden major aggressive or disruptive behavior. This plan can prevent the need to send the resident to a hospital emergency room, which often makes the resident even more aggressive or hostile and where adequate geropsychiatric services usually are not available (Tierney, Cronin, and Scanlon 1986). Methods other than drugs to control or modify behavior should be considered. The techniques of facilitative communication, sensory stimulation, and reality orientation can be used to improve some of these conditions. (See chapters 7, 10, and 16.)

Wandering Behavior. Wandering behavior is a common problem in many nursing homes. Wandering is usually caused by organic factors (e.g., Alzheimer's disease, multi-infarct dementia, or medications) or environmental factors (e.g., over- or understimulation) (Davidhizar and Cosgray 1990). Some nursing home residents have wandered away from the nursing facility, become lost, and been returned to the home by strangers or the police. Others, not as fortunate, have been struck by an automobile or train or found dead alongside a road.

Assess the mental status of all new residents on admission to the nursing facility (see chapter 6) to determine those who might be high-risk for wandering. Davidhizar and Cosgray (1990, 281) recommend using the following interventions with those residents who tend to wander:

- Use "kind firmness."
- Install "waist-high fences" at doors.
- Place a sitting chair by the window.
- Use reality orientation.
- Be sure glasses and hearing devices are in use.
- Decorate the resident's room.
- Assign consistent staff.
- Encourage family visits.
- Use touch if appropriate.
- Plan activities for a short attention span.
- Encourage exercise.
- Use a rocking chair. (Rocking wheel chairs are available.)
- Have a clock and calendar.
- Do not use restraints.

Coberg, Lynch, and Mavretish (1991, 133) recommend to "redirect energies of agitated or wandering patients." They also recommend a wooden lounge chair with an exaggerated downward tilt of the seat back. An enclosed, outside courtyard decorated with tables, chairs, plants, and flowers also allows the wanderer to walk and exercise in a safe and relaxing environment. Buzzers on all unsupervised doors that lead outside alert the staff that a resident has left the building. A number of electronic security systems also are available (Negley, Molla, and Obenchain 1990).

Sexuality in Older People

Obvious sexual behavior in older people is often disturbing to nurses, staff, and visitors in nursing homes.

However, the staff in one nursing home showed exceptional understanding. They personally purchased a double bed for a couple who had recently married and moved to the home. They had both been residents of another home but were asked to leave when they decided to marry. Staff members should discuss the topic freely among themselves. They should have the opportunity to explore their own beliefs about sexuality so that they can learn to accept the sexual behavior of older residents, who are so often thought of as being sexless.

Death and Dying

Caring for a dying resident is stressful for the staff. Older people who have lived many years in a nursing home become, in effect, part of the family. By exploring their feelings about death and dying, staff members may lessen the impact of death of a resident. The policies in each nursing home dictate whether residents are sent to a hospital to die or whether they will remain in the home. Physician decisions, family wishes, and perhaps resident requests also determine whether to move the resident to a hospital. In any case, a skilled nursing home is qualified to care for residents who are dying. In some instances eligible residents receiving hospice services through Medicare are provided care and support by hospice personnel in the nursing home.

ROLE OF THE NURSE

State standards define the minimum requirements for nursing staff in nursing homes. Minimal standards are suggested for the number of residents per nurse. However, the number of nurse aides needed to give adequate nursing care is not clearly defined. A registered nurse must be on call twenty-four hours a day and the home must have a licensed vocational or practical nurse on duty for each shift. Only registered nurses may start intravenous fluids, give intravenous medications, and insert nasal gastric tubes. The director of nursing must be a registered nurse and cannot also function as the in-service coordinator or be responsible for training the aides. Bedside nursing or personal care is provided by nurse aides who must be supervised by licensed personnel. Medications are given only by licensed personnel. There are programs in some states that provide for the certification of medication aides. This type of assignment must be supervised closely. Professional nurses should be alert to legislative proposals that allow such practices and monitor this issue carefully.

The Director of Nursing

The director of nursing is responsible for the nursing care of the residents. The director works closely with administrative personnel to ensure that the standards of nursing care are maintained. The *Standards and Scope of Gerontological Nursing Practice* (see chapter 1), as developed by the American Nurses' Association, should be implemented and maintained by the professional nursing staff. All medications, treatments, and transportation of residents to and from hospitals must be ordered by physicians. A copy of all telephone orders must be forwarded to physicians, signed, and returned to the resident's chart. The director of nursing serves as an important liaison between the resident, family, and physician. Any changes in the condition or treatment of the resident must be reported to the family. A registered nurse who is on call for the skilled nursing facility during the evening or night hours is notified of any changes in the condition of the residents or if any unusual incidents occur. Many times, the registered nurse will need to return to the nursing home to observe and interpret changes in the condition of a resident. Expertise in assessment skills and nursing care are needed in nursing home settings.

The assessment of each resident is the function of the professional and licensed personnel in the nursing home. As mentioned previously, several departments will assist in resident assessment. The professional nurse assesses the residents and identifies their individual problems, abilities, and needs. The assessment of mobility, independence in the activities of daily living, and the degree of assistance required provides a baseline for planning nursing care and assigning staff to care for the residents.

Resident assessment involves a summary of the resident's ability to function physically, emotionally, mentally, and psychosocially. From this assessment, goal-directed therapy is planned for each resident. The prevention of further disabilities and rehabilitation are part of goal-directed therapy. With the use of a summary of the resident assessment, an individual-

ized nursing care plan is prepared for each resident. These summaries are also helpful in evaluating nursing care. Comprehensive nursing care is continued for each resident and the various departments within the nursing home collaborate in this care. Physical therapy and speech therapy services are available within the facility, or the facility may request these services from other health care agencies.

Specialized Nursing Staff

More gerontological clinical nurse specialists (GCNS) and gerontological nurse practitioners (GNP) are needed in nursing homes to provide assistance in assessment, care, planning, interventions, and teaching. They could be employed on a part-time basis or as consultants. National nursing organizations and the nursing home industry need to become more involved in the legislative process and seek additional third-party reimbursement from Medicare and private health insurance companies for these specialists who could improve the quality of life for nursing home residents.

Planning Nursing Care

The staff nurse who is assigned to the unit is responsible for overseeing the care of each resident. There are specific functions for which the professional nurse is responsible. Rehabilitative measures prescribed by the physical therapist will be supervised by the nurse. Each nurse aide is responsible for the care of a specific number of residents. The aide becomes familiar with the likes and dislikes of these residents and is able to manage their environment. One nursing home uses a checklist for the activities of daily living for each resident. Each shift has a checklist for each resident, and the form is a part of the resident's record. This checklist is an excellent guide for the identification of the kind of care each resident requires and is a means of validating that care is actually given.

Monthly resident care plans should be made for each resident. The aide is an important member of the team conference. The dietitian, the social worker, activities director, the registered nurse, and other licensed personnel are included in the conferences. The director of nursing is available for consultation if needed. A regular schedule for team planning permits the aides to meet with the team and to discuss the care needs of their residents each month. Aides have valuable information about their residents and are able to identify problems the residents are experiencing daily. Open lines of communication among the team participants promote improved resident care. Goals for each resident can be established, and the team members who are responsible for the care are able to coordinate the care. The nurses and aides who are responsible for the continued care of the residents on all shifts will receive a summary of the nursing care goals for each resident.

Among the problems that are reported by the aides most frequently are disturbed behavior or difficulties with the daily activities of self-help. If consistent care if provided by all personnel, the residents' behavior problems may be corrected, their memory span may be increased, and their self-help abilities may be maintained. Consistency is a key word in teamwork for all personnel.

The licensed personnel are responsible for making entries in the nurses' notes. Validation of all care is of the utmost importance. Changes in the physical condition of the resident are recorded as well as the time the physician was notified, visits by the physician, new orders, and the time the director of nursing and the family were notified of any changes. Physical and behavioral changes in the residents and the nursing actions initiated are accurately documented in the resident's record. With approval from the licensing agency and the physician, it is possible to do problem-oriented recording of only one phase of the resident's condition daily. The nurses' notes for the entire week will give a complete picture of the status of the resident. Whenever there are changes in the condition of the resident, the chart will reflect these changes. For example, one day of nurses' notes will reflect the self-care activities and the amount of assistance the resident requires. Elimination and skin conditions will be documented on another day. Each day another aspect of the resident is observed: the emotional and psychologic state of the resident, the food and fluid intake, the interaction of the resident with the environment and during social activities, and the mobility of the resident. A weekly summary documentation reflects the diagnoses of the resident, the medication and treatments the resident has re-

ceived, and the effectiveness of the regimen. Changes in the condition of residents in the skilled section of the nursing home are either so minute that it is difficult to notice them or else the changes are so dramatic that problem-oriented documentation is needed.

OTHER PERSONNEL

The nursing home is required to employ a pharmacist as a consultant. A monthly review of all medications is made. The validation of the effectiveness of the medications is a responsibility of the nurse. The pharmacist is available to furnish up-to-date data regarding medications and their effects. The pharmacist is responsible for monitoring or reviewing the system of drug administration for each resident.

A registered dietitian plans the regular menus for the residents as well as special diets. Eating and feeding problems, including likes and dislikes of foods, are considered when the diet is planned. Therapeutic diets such as low-sodium, diabetic, high-protein, bland, and blended diets are planned by the dietitian, who also assists in the evaluation of their effectiveness. The dietitian is responsible for the maintenance of standards in the kitchen.

A medical director is required for each home to provide medical care to those residents who do not have a regular physician, to provide emergency care to residents when needed, and to participate in interdisciplinary meetings and activities.

A social worker is required in all homes with more than 120 beds to counsel with the resident and family regarding concerns and problems related to the resident's total care. The activities director works closely with the nurses and social worker assessing residents' leisure time interests and needs. The activities director plans and directs social activities, religious services, exercise programs, pet therapy, and teaches and supervises crafts to residents.

A number of other persons are employed in the area of environmental services to maintain the equipment, cleanliness, and general operation of the home. In some areas, twenty-four-hour security personnel are employed to protect the residents and visiting family members from possible criminal dangers in the environment.

MANAGEMENT

Case Management

A major trend in health care in the 1990s is evaluation of care based on *resident outcomes*. Accrediting agencies and funding sources, for example, want to know the outcome of goals, plans, nursing procedures, and techniques, not just that these things were done, even though efficiently. The nursing process is an excellent example. There is no need for a nursing care plan unless that plan can be evaluated based on resident outcomes. A case-management system focuses on assessing residents' needs and accessing and coordinating the most efficient available resources that will result in positive resident outcome. Case management involves "admission screening, comprehensive assessment (physical, mental, spiritual, social, economic), multi-disciplinary care planning, arranging and coordinating prescribed services, monitoring the plan and services (e.g., quality assurance and utilization reviews), and periodic re-evaluation of the resident/client" (Wood 1991, 3).

Nursing care in nursing homes traditionally has been task-centered (giving medications, doing treatments, and documenting care), with less emphasis on evaluating resident outcomes as a result of that care. Is the resident less depressed, walking more, eating better, more alert, or participating in more activities as a direct outcome of the planned nursing interventions? These types of questions, although perhaps discussed by staff, often are not answered, written, or reported. It does not matter how well nursing care is given unless the ultimate desired outcome is effective.

A case-management approach, found to be so efficient and cost-effective for community-dwelling older persons, is now being used in some nursing homes. Smith (1991) implemented a case-management system in a nursing home for one year. All licensed nurses in the facility were assigned a specific number of residents. They were responsible "for the assessment, care plan, implementation, and evaluation of care for the assigned cases" (35), with special focus on the residents' priority problems. Although the nurses still maintained other functions (e.g., medication administration), their primary focus was a case manager role. Smith (1991, 38) found that "there was evidence of a significant improvement in the application of the nursing process to achieve pos-

itive patient outcomes" and that "the correlation of the care plan and nursing progress notes provided a means to evaluate patient outcomes based on nursing intervention." She also noted that nursing staff understood the nursing process better, used the nursing care plans to write periodic progress notes, developed a special relationship with residents and their families, and indicated increased job satisfaction. Also, "the participating facility was found in compliance with state and federal regulations in care planning and charting during this project (38)."

Staffing

Health care facilities experience staff turnover, inadequate staffing as a result of illness, a lack of transportation for personnel to the agency, and a demand for nurse aides that is greater than the supply. Staffing is a major problem. Supervisory personnel who are employed in nursing homes for extended periods of time tend to forget that all people do not have the same sense of responsibility to the home. Working conditions are difficult because of staffing problems and the multiple needs of chronically ill residents and their families. It is not easy to manage personnel when there is a large employee turnover.

Orientation and Supervision of Personnel

Orientation to the physical facilities, the staff, and the departments within the facility assists new personnel in becoming a part of the organization. During their first day, new personnel should become acquainted with policies, other personnel, and the role that each member of the staff fills. New employees should not be expected to assume total responsibility for resident care immediately or to perform the same amount of work that will eventually be their assignment. New employees need to become acquainted with the functions of the facility and the responsibilities they will have. They should learn about the kinds of residents who are in nursing homes.

Nurse aides who seek employment in a new institution may have completed courses and received certificates in the care of older adults. This type of training is available through high schools and community colleges. Other facilities elect to train aides who have had little or no experience. Whatever the policy, there must be a well-planned orientation period.

The rights of residents and the confidentiality of resident records must be stressed to new nurse aides. These employees often have not considered the ethical and legal aspects of nursing care.

A study of aging should be part of the orientation process and should be presented frequently in in-service education programs. New aides should understand that their role is a supportive one and that the residents' wishes and needs should be met if at all possible. Supervisory staff members are responsible for assessing and managing residents' problems.

Even though aides may present certificates of training, it is essential that their skills be evaluated by a member of the nursing staff when they give nursing care. A safe practice in one home might not be a safe practice in another home.

Aides with certification of training are usually assigned to another experienced aide to learn about the specific residents and their needs. Licensed personnel are responsible for evaluating the previous experience and training of the aides.

The job description for each employee dictates the amount of training required. Personal care skills should be taught in the classroom and not on the job. Training can consist of various types of instructional media, such as films and slides, and the demonstration and practice of procedures before the aides begin caring for residents. Supervisory nursing personnel should continue to evaluate all aides in their care of residents.

In-Service Education

In-service education is not a substitute for orientation. Many of the same topics should be covered in in-service education programs as in the orientation. These programs should be provided for all personnel, professional or paraprofessional, and should be scheduled at convenient times so that all employees can attend.

Planning in-service education programs is the responsibility of the in-service coordinator. The coordinator should work with supervisory personnel and involve them in the programs. Few programs are for aides only. Staff should especially be provided with the knowledge and skills to care for emergencies (see Table 17-2) when they arise (Duchemin, Clark, and Keeber 1991).

An understanding of the aging process is important. One or two programs on the effects of aging should be presented during the year. Simulated situations in which aides participate in role-playing help them experience the limitations brought on by aging. The discarded glasses of older people can be prepared with colorless nail polish, the lenses made dirty, or the sides clouded so the aides have difficulty seeing. By wearing thick gloves, the aides can experience limitations of the hands and fingers in eating, shaving, or even cleansing themselves after elimination. If the aides experience these limitations, they will have a better understanding of some of the physical restrictions in their older residents. Programs on death and dying are also important. A good question to ask is "What would you like done for you if you were dying?" At the end of the discussion there is generally a good summary of the kind of care the dying resident needs. The in-service coordinator should not present all the programs. Other staff members should share their philosophy and knowledge about caring for the residents.

Some in-service education programs should be concerned with the health and welfare of the personnel. Programs on cancer detection, blood pressure screening, and family planning are of value to the personnel. Special programs on fire prevention, disaster preparedness, and personal health maintenance are also helpful to the personnel and their families.

The professional staff should be alert to the fact that routine and repetitious care for older people who are sick and dependent is not an easy assignment. Many complaints and frustrations are transmitted by residents to aides. The professional staff should be a source of physical and emotional support to the aides. *The need to provide positive reinforcement to aides is important.* The nurse supervisor should help aides express their feelings about particularly difficult residents and recognize that a resident's family may be making it difficult for them to care for the resident.

There are incidents of abuse of residents in nursing homes. Programs should be planned to discuss the legal responsibility of the nursing home and the consequences of the discovery of abuse. The neglect of residents is also a major concern in nursing homes. Aides themselves are able to identify how residents are neglected. The open recognition of these two major concerns tends to lessen the incidence of abuse or neglect.

There are many excellent videotapes and books for nurse aide training. A book should be given to the aides so they can refer to it for information on nursing care. A sense of owning the book, if this is possible, influences the feelings of worth the aides have.

FUTURE NEEDS IN NURSING HOME CARE

Adequate quality staffing in nursing homes is a major concern and will continue to be a problem. There is a special need for more registered nurses. Professional nurses who are skilled in geriatric health assessment and management are needed in the nursing home setting. Financial remuneration for professional nursing services in nursing homes must be competitive with other health care facilities. However, the amount of money spent on health care is not reflected in the salaries of the caregivers in nursing homes. In addition to better salaries, training and recognition programs for staff such as certificates, special awards, length of service awards, and birthday recognition will improve morale. A caring facility must be considerate of its employees if direct resident care is to be improved. Aides often need help with transportation. Many times public transportation is altered or nonexistent on weekends. This problem could be solved if nursing homes would provide transportation for those days. The concept of medication aides is a topic for continuing study and discussion, as is the problem of whether nurse aides should be licensed.

Further studies need to be made on the effect of Medicare's Prospective Payment System (PPS) on nursing homes. Many older adults who are admitted are acutely ill, need more intensive care, and may not be expected to live many weeks. Nursing homes

must plan to provide this type of care. One long-term care facility has implemented an innovative geriatric intensive care unit (GICU). The purpose of this unit is to "provide highly skilled care to residents who are seriously ill and to those. . . requiring special treatment or being clinically complex" (Barnett 1987). After minor structural adaptation, the purchase of additional equipment, and recommendation of staffing changes (including at least one gerontological nurse practitioner), a sixteen-bed unit was opened. Such a unit can help meet the needs of older residents who have been discharged from the hospital but who still need some degree of intensive care. This type of care could also prevent hospitalization of some nursing home residents who become acutely ill for short periods of time.

Many nursing homes are expanding their services to include adult day care, specialized units for residents with Alzheimer's disease, hospice units, special services and care for chronically ill children, and care for residents with AIDS. The nursing facility (home) of the future will be much different and require additional qualified and specialized staff to provide these specialized services.

Nursing schools should plan for more clinical experiences for nursing students in nursing homes. New students are sometimes shocked by this type of experience at first, but with proper orientation and a selection of residents who are not the most difficult, nursing students usually find the experience rewarding. Faculty who have had special preparation in gerontological nursing and who enjoy working with older people are the best role models in these settings. The nursing home is a good setting for student experiences in basic (fundamentals) nursing, the chronic care component of medical-surgical nursing (which needs to be emphasized more), and nursing management.

SUMMARY

Because of multiple chronic disabling diseases and increasing dependence, approximately 5 percent of the older population requires nursing home care at any one time. The majority of nursing homes are privately owned. The acuity level of care needed by nursing home residents is increasing. Older persons and their family members need to select a nursing home carefully. They should evaluate several nursing homes, if possible, and not make the decision in a

hurry. However, often the decision to place an older family member in a nursing home occurs suddenly after a hospitalization for acute illness or an accident.

Admission of an older person to the nursing home is an important process. The resident and the family should be oriented to the nursing home policies and procedures. Financial matters should be discussed early and openly. Most of nursing home care is financed by either private payment or Medicaid.

Nursing homes must be licensed by the state and may be accredited by the Joint Commission for the Accreditation of HealthCare Organizations. The federal Omnibus Budget Reconciliation Act (OBRA) of 1987 and 1990 have had a tremendous impact on the improvement of care in nursing homes.

Initial physical and psychosocial assessment and preparation of a care plan are the responsibility of the professional nurse. The major goal is to maintain and/or improve maximum functioning for each resident. The major nursing care problems in the nursing home are acute care emergencies, such as accidents, and long-term care problems, such as skin care,

bowel and bladder control, complications of immobility, adequate food and fluid intake, changes in behavior, and wandering.

Recruitment, selection, orientation, in-service training, supervision, and evaluation of nursing staff are very important. A case-management system with more emphasis on evaluating resident outcomes is needed. In nursing home settings *caring* rather than *curing* is the key word. Caring cannot be accomplished unless there is a closer examination of nurses' attitudes about aging, knowledge of the aging process, and a commitment to improving the quality of life for older adults.

STUDY QUESTIONS

1. What percentage of the over-65 and over-85 age groups are in nursing homes at any one time?

2. Describe the different types of nursing homes.

3. Describe the demographics of the typical older adult in a nursing home.

4. Give examples of major medical diagnoses of nursing home residents.

5. How has the Prospective Payment System (PPS) for Medicare residents in hospitals affected nursing home admissions and care?

6. What are the major factors to consider in the selection of a nursing home?

7. Evaluate the sources of payment for nursing home care.

8. Differentiate licensure and accreditation.

9. Describe the major requirements of OBRA, 1987.

10. Evaluate the most common medical emergencies that occur in nursing homes. How can they be managed?

11. What are some nursing interventions for the common long-term care problems encountered in a nursing home setting?

12. Name and describe the role of nursing staff in nursing homes.

13. Relate the concept of case management and resident outcomes to nursing homes.

14. Discuss the types and roles of other staff in a nursing home setting.

15. List several ideas for research in nursing home care.

REFERENCES

American Association of Retired Persons. 1991. *A Profile of Older Americans.* (PF 3094 (1291). D996). Washington, DC: United States Department of Health and Human Services.

Barnett, P. 1987. Implementing a geriatric nursing intensive care unit. *Long-Term Care Currents* 10(1):4–5.

Benison, B. and M.O. Hogstel. 1986. Aging and movement therapy: Essential interventions for the immobile elderly. *Journal of Gerontological Nursing* 12(12):8–16.

Berryman, E., D. Gaskin, A. Jones, F. Toolley, and J.

Macmullen. 1989. Point by point: Predicting elders' falls. *Geriatric Nursing* 10(4):199–201.

Boondas, J. 1991. Nursing home resident assessment clarification and focused care. *Nursing and Health Care* 12(6):308–12.

Burnette, K. 1986. Relocation and the elderly. *Journal of Gerontological Nursing* 12(10):6–11.

Coberg, A., D. Lynch, and B. Mavretish. 1991. Harnessing ideas to release restraints. *Geriatric Nursing* 12(3):133–34.

Davidhizar, R. and R. Cosgray. 1990. Helping the wanderer. *Geriatric Nursing* 11(6):280–81.

Donahue, P.A. 1990. When it's hard to swallow. *Journal of Gerontological Nursing* 16(4):6–9.

Duchemin, K., J. Clark, and M. Keeber. 1991. Emergency procedures training program. *Journal of Gerontological Nursing* 17(7):6–9.

Gross, Y.T., Y. Shimamoto, C.L. Rose, and B. Frank. 1990. Monitoring risk factors. *Journal of Gerontological Nursing* 16(6):20–25.

Harron, J. and J. Schaeffer. 1986. DRGs and the intensity of skilled nursing. *Geriatric Nursing* 7(1):31–33.

Heim, K. 1986. Wandering behavior. *Journal of Gerontological Nursing* 12(11):4–7.

Hernandez, M. and J. Miller. 1986. How to reduce falls. *Geriatric Nursing* 7(2):97–102.

Hogstel, M.O. and N. Robinson. 1989. Feeding the frail elderly. *Journal of Gerontological Nursing* 15(3):16–20.

Kolodny, V. and A.M. Malek. 1991. Improving feeding skills. *Journal of Gerontological Nursing* 17(6):20–24.

Langer, E.L., P.J. Drinka, and S. Voeks. 1991. Readmissions and acuity in the nursing home. *Journal of Gerontological Nursing* 17(7):15–19.

Lund, E. and M.L. Sheafor. 1985. Is your patient about to fall? *Journal of Gerontological Nursing* 11(4):37–41.

Morris, J.N., C. Harnes, S.E. Fries, C.D. Phillips, V. Mor, S. Katz, K. Murphy, M.L. Drugouich, and A.S. Friedlob. 1990. Designing the national resident assessment instrument for nursing homes. *The Gerontologist* 30(3):293–307.

Negley, E.N., P.M. Molla, and J. Obenchain. 1990. NO EXIT. The effects of an electronic security system. *Journal of Gerontological Nursing* 16(8):21–25.

Phipps, M., B. Bauman, D. Berner, M. Butler, A. Kalinoski, M. Looby, N. Malacaria, L. Pratt, P. Reiley, M. Sullivan, and J. Vend. 1984. Staging decubitus care. *Am J Nurs* 84(8):999–1003.

Ridder, M. 1985. Nursing update on Alzheimer's disease. *J Neurosurg Nurs* 17(3):190–200.

Smith, J. 1991. Changing traditional nursing home roles to nursing case management. *Journal of Gerontological Nursing* 17(5):32–39.

Strumpf, N.E., L.K. Evans, and D. Schwartz. 1990. Restraint free care: From dream to reality. *Geriatric Nursing* 11(3):122–24.

Tierney, J.C., A. Cronin, and M.K. Scanlon. 1986. . . . And don't send her back! *Am J Nurs* 86(9):1011–14.

Wood, L.A. 1991. Geriatric case management: The time is now. *Journal of Gerontological Nursing* 17(4):3.

18 Nursing Care In the Home

Mira Kirk Nelson

CHAPTER OUTLINE

FOCUS

This chapter is about nursing care of the older adult in the home, adapting the home environment to fit the needs of an older person who has physical limita- tions, the community resources to assist in this care, and the availability of finances to help with the costs of home nursing care.

OBJECTIVES

1. Describe the advantages of home care versus in- stitutional care.

2. Identify differences in assessing older adults in the home versus the clinic/institution setting.

3. Discuss the most frequently reported chronic illnesses among older adults residing in the com- munity or home setting.

4. List the common nursing diagnoses among older people in the home and the nursing interventions for each.

5. Describe adaptations of the home environment that may be needed to enhance the functioning of older adults.

6. Evaluate the types of medical equipment avail- able for use in the home.

7. Discuss financing of home health care services through Medicare, Medicaid, and private pay/in- surance.

Home care refers to that component of comprehen- sive health care in which services are provided to in- dividuals and families in their places of residence for the purpose of promoting, maintaining, or restoring health or minimizing the effect of illness and disabil- ity. Services appropriate to the needs of the client are planned, coordinated, and made available by an agency/institution organized for the delivery of home health care through the use of employed staff, contractual agreements, or a combination of administrative patterns. These services are provided under a plan of care that includes, but is not limited to, medical care, dental care, nursing, physical therapy, speech therapy, occupational therapy, social work, nutrition, homemaker, home health aide, transportation, laboratory services, medical equipment, and supplies (National Association of Home Health Care Agencies 1980). This definition has been generally accepted by a wide variety of health professionals representing national agencies and organizations.

Home health care is seen by many health professionals as a more humanistic approach to the long-term care of older people. Care received in the home provides clients with the positive benefit of an opportunity to maintain control over significant aspects of their lives. Some of the advantages of home care for older individuals as opposed to institutional care are an ability to eat what and when they desire; to wear what they please; to wake and sleep on their own schedules; to sleep in their own beds in familiar surroundings; and to have family members present to provide moral support and therapy.

Assessment of an older adult in the home is different from other nursing practice settings, such as the hospital, clinic, or skilled nursing facility. Nursing personnel in the clinic or hospital setting maintain control over the environment to a large extent. However, in the home the client and family control the environment. The home reflects the client's lifestyle, socioeconomic status, values, culture, and personal preferences. For example, a home visit may reveal family pictures or other memorabilia. A nurse can observe verbal and nonverbal communication patterns among family members in this primary social context.

A home health nurse works with the client and family to achieve client and family care management and independence. Individualized instruction of the client and family become paramount in the nursing process. The home setting offers the home health nurse an opportunity to observe how the older adult copes in familiar surroundings with available resources. The home health nurse also has an opportunity to assess the need of any adaptive devices and structural improvements that will help the older adult function at home. The home becomes a therapeutic environment that is interwoven with the client's

health and requires evaluation while assessing the client's needs (Hashizume 1991).

Home care agencies serve clients needing acute short-term care, clients with chronic disease who need rehabilitation or health maintenance, and terminally ill clients who wish to die at home. The two main criteria used to predict whether or not a client is a good candidate for home care are an adequate and willing support system and an environment conducive to maximum recovery and rehabilitation (Steffl and Eide 1984).

INCREASE IN THE OLDER POPULATION

The United States population is living longer and more people are surviving to the upper age brackets, especially those in their 80s, 90s, and 100s. The increase in the frail older population in conjunction with hospitals' early discharge practices have intensified the need for community-based services, especially home health care.

A large proportion of older people are women who are widowed or living alone. As a result of more rapidly increasing life expectancy for women as compared with men, most older people are women. Currently 95 percent of older people reside at home alone, with a spouse, or with another relative; whereas the remaining 5 percent reside in nursing homes or other institutions.

TYPES OF OLDER PEOPLE NEEDING HOME NURSING CARE

The types of older individuals who need home nursing care can be inferred from the types of services that are available. Many individuals have been recently discharged from the hospital and require nursing care and medical supervision in the home environment. Sophisticated medical treatment, such as intravenous fluid replacement, antibiotic therapy, hemodialysis, enteral and parenteral nutrition, and continuous ambulatory peritoneal dialysis, can be provided in the home. Other clients need rehabilitative services such as physical or speech therapy that can be continued in the home after discharge from the hospital. Other services such as home-delivered meals, homemaker services, and chore services may be needed by the same persons who also need skilled nursing care. Another large group has functional impairments that restrict their ability to shop, cook, or care for their homes (U.S. Congress. Office of Technology Assessment 1985).

Types of Illnesses

Although the aging process does not cause any specific disease, chronic illnesses are more prevalent among older people. Acute illnesses (lasting less than three months) are less common among older adults than the total population. Only 14 percent of noninstitutionalized older adults are free of chronic illnesses. The most frequently reported chronic illnesses among noninstitutionalized older people in 1981 were arthritis (46 percent), hypertension (37 percent), hearing impairment (28 percent), heart conditions (28 percent), vision impairment (12 percent), and arteriosclerosis (12 percent) (Robb 1984a; U.S. Congress. Office of Technology Assessment 1985).

The prevalence of chronic conditions differs between the sexes. Women display considerably higher rates of arthritis and hypertension, slightly higher rates of visual disorders, and slightly less hearing impairment. Heart conditions are similar for both sexes. The prevalence of all chronic conditions except ulcers is higher among the poor (Steffl and Eide 1984).

The health care system will feel the impact of the increasingly older population because one of the normal characteristics of the aging process is an increase in physical limitations and disabilities. The prevalence and severity of chronic conditions and their associated disabilities increase in old age. Among those over age 65, almost two-fifths are unable to carry on a major activity. Among those over age 75, more than two-fifths are unable to carry on a major activity. Beyond age 85, some 60 percent of community-dwelling older people experience activity limitation from a chronic condition; more than one half of these persons are unable to carry on a major activity. Thus the severity of physical and mental limitations from chronic conditions is a critical problem for older adults. The increase in prevalence of dysfunctions among the very old is noticeable for osteoarthritis, heart conditions, hearing and vision impairments, and urinary incontinence.

Community-dwelling older adults have a much lower prevalence of severe limitations and dependency than the institutionalized older population.

While more than 85 percent of noninstitutionalized older adults reported one or more chronic conditions in various surveys over the past twenty years, fewer than half of them reported any degree of limitation because of these conditions. Most older people thus continue to be independent and active members in the community (U.S. Congress. Office of Technology Assessment 1985).

THE HOME HEALTH NURSE

Professional nurses delivering home health care have great responsibilities in the performance of their duties. They must have a clear concept of the scope of professional nursing practice and a desire to promote the role of the nurse in delivering both present and potential services. In addition to possessing desirable credentials of education, preparation, and experience, nurses should possess certain personal traits that would enhance their ability to function in this type of setting.

Personal traits of importance include the ability to make independent decisions on a sound and theoretical scientific knowledge base; the willingness to accept responsibility for one's own actions; the possession of highly developed interpersonal skills with ability to articulate clearly, both orally and in writing; the ability to stay calm in crisis situations; and warm empathetic concern and respect for older people, especially older adults (Browning 1985).

Preparation and Experience

The foremost requirement of home health care nurses is demonstration of professional competency. Home health care nurses evolve from a variety of educational and experience settings that influence the contributions the nurse makes to home health care. Nursing education has the responsibility of producing competent and skilled practitioners. Home health care nurses should be educated to function at a high level of competency so they can be relied upon by their professional colleagues as well as by the community.

The American Nurses' Association and the National League for Nursing advocate that a baccalaureate degree be the minimum level of professional preparation for the community health nurse. At this level, the nurse is capable of practicing as a generalist in community health settings provided that the following curricula are included along with clinical materials (American Nurses' Association, Division of Community Health Nursing 1980): general systems theory; statistics; introductory epidemiology; community assessment; history, principles, and practice of public and community health; knowledge of public health laws; and environmental health and safety.

The specialist in home care is prepared at the master's level and has in-depth knowledge and ability to apply this knowledge to health problems in the community. At this level, preparation requires advanced study in community health nursing theory, advanced clinical skills, public health science, leadership, management, interdisciplinary collaboration, research process, health policy and planning, community organization, dynamics of health politics, and health economics (Garvey and Loque 1988).

MAJOR NURSING DIAGNOSES

Two of the most common nursing diagnoses among the older population are those dealing with incontinence and impaired physical mobility. These problems are particularly difficult for older adults who are being cared for in the home and are often the primary reasons for institutionalization. Incontinence and impaired physical mobility are often regarded as inevitable when growing older and may not even be mentioned to health care professionals by caregivers or clients themselves. However, careful assessment can often uncover factors that contribute to these problems. As a result, interventions for these nursing diagnoses can be planned to improve the quality of daily living for older individuals.

Incontinence

It is difficult to establish prevalence of urinary incontinence among the older population residing in the home. It is estimated that between 10 percent and 20 percent of older persons living at home and close to 50 percent of those living in institutions for long-term care experience urinary incontinence. Urinary incontinence is a costly problem that results in skin irritation, urinary tract infections if managed improperly, and psychosocial difficulties such as isolation, depression, caregiver burden, and nursing home placement. The economic cost of management of the

problem is between 0.5 and 1.5 billion dollars per year or 3–8 percent of the Medicare expenditures in nursing homes (Ouslander 1986).

Urinary incontinence may result from any medical or psychologic condition or drug that interferes with the normal storing and emptying functions of the lower urinary tract. It is closely associated with decreased mental status function and decreased mobility, especially among the nursing home population. Adequate function of the lower urinary tract must be accompanied by sufficient motivation, mental acuity, mobility, and dexterity to anticipate the need for toileting; locate and reach the toilet, commode, or bedpan; and manage clothing. There also must be no environmental or iatrogenic barriers, such as inaccessible toilets or drug side effects.

Ouslander (1986) classifies urinary incontinence clinically as acute or persistent. Acute urinary incontinence is often reversible, and the causes may be remembered by the mnemonic DRIP, which is an acronym for *d*elirium; *r*estricted mobility and *r*etention; *i*nfection, *i*nflammation, and *i*mpaction (fecal); and *p*harmaceuticals and olyuria. The drugs most commonly associated with urinary incontinence are diuretics, sedatives, hypnotics, antipsychotics, anticholinergics, and alpha antagonists. Acute urinary incontinence usually disappears when the underlying cause is treated. Persistent urinary incontinence may be classified as stress, urge, overflow, and functional. The underlying causes may be urologic, neurologic, gynecologic, functional, iatrogenic, environmental, or a combination of these.

Initial assessment data may be collected by the home health nurse. The history should focus on any active medical disorders, medications, and prior genitourinary conditions that might be involved. It is important to determine what triggers the incontinence episodes, such as coughing or laughing (stress), and sensations of fullness with inability to delay voiding (urge). Infections may have such irritating symptoms as frequency, nocturia, urgency, and dysuria. Symptoms of obstruction include hesitancy, interrupted stream, dribbling, and impaired sensation of bladder fullness.

Whereas the pathologic causes for urinary incontinence are often complex and may ultimately require a comprehensive evaluation and medical work-up, the nurse may assess biopsychosocial variables that may provide valuable data to assist in making an accurate medical diagnosis. To help in assessment, the older person or a caregiver should be asked to record the frequency, timing, and amount of continent voidings as well as incontinent episodes. In addition other significant data should be recorded such as pain, burning, itching or pressure, characteristics of urine (odor, color, sediment, or clear), and difficulty starting or stopping urinary stream. The nurse should determine the older person's ability to reach and use the toilet, including management of clothing. Also, assessment means determining which medications the older person may be taking, particularly sedatives, hypnotics, anticholinergics, and diuretics. Vaginal discharge and bowel elimination patterns should be determined, and the client should be checked for fecal impaction if indicated. Many of the common functional and iatrogenic causes for urinary incontinence may be resolved by nursing interventions.

Bladder-Training Procedures. Greengold and Ouslander (1986) described key features of bladder-training programs and the development of a post-indwelling catheter bladder retraining protocol. The protocol can be implemented by visiting nurses in the home setting and may also be used to identify appropriate candidates for the retraining protocol.

Between 25 percent and 50 percent of acutely ill hospitalized older people are treated for their urinary incontinence with an indwelling catheter during some part of their hospitalization. Many of these clients may be discharged with the catheter in place or very soon after it is removed. This removal of an indwelling catheter may cause the older person to again become incontinent and therefore a bladder retraining program may be needed.

The objective of a bladder retraining program is to allow the older individual to restore a normal pattern of voiding and continence. It is indicated for older persons with adequate cognitive function, mobility, dexterity, and self-motivation. Bladder retraining involves a combination of methods, such as the progressive lengthening of time intervals between voiding, triggering and bladder-emptying techniques, intermittent catheterization (if indicated), and adjustments of the timing and amount of fluid intake. This documentation of incontinence is helpful in assessing incontinent individuals as well as monitoring responses to various interventions. The article by Greengold and Ouslander provides a specific bladder-retraining protocol and a thorough explanation of its use.

Impaired Physical Mobility

Mobility of older adults may be limited by a variety of physical ailments, such as paresthesias, hemiplegia, arthritis, neuromotor disturbances, fractures, foot problems, and illnesses that deplete one's energy. Older persons tend to acquire such conditions more frequently, and the effects of impaired physical mobility are more debilitating than they are for younger people (Ebersole and Hess 1990).

Exercise can be used to prevent deterioration and to maintain and improve an individual's functional health status. Physical activity helps older persons adjust to certain physiologic changes and helps maintain bone tissue, flexibility, and work capacity. Exercise has been shown to have a positive influence on psychologic and social well-being (Paillard and Nowak 1985).

Senior Centers, YMCAs, and YWCAs throughout the United States have instituted physical fitness programs in which older adults can maintain or enhance their overall fitness. For those whose mobility is limited, other exercises should be encouraged (Ebersole and Hess 1990).

Exercise Inhibitors. Older people frequently overrate sporadic work, such as "cleaning house." While they may feel tired doing this, they probably have not put their joints through a full range of motion, used all of the large muscle groups, or achieved much (if any) cardiovascular benefit. Many older people believe that need for exercise decreases with age. Evidence shows the need to exercise to maintain functional capacity probably increases with age. Some older people believe they will hurt themselves or have a heart attack if they exercise. The American Academy of Sports Medicine lists only three contraindications: (1) life-threatening conditions such as myocardial infarction, (2) pulmonary embolism, and (3) severe arrhythmias. Without proper exercise, older adults are at great risk for injury and impaired functioning. Some health professionals forget to prescribe exercise for general good health. They may remember to encourage specific exercises such as wall climbing for arthritic shoulders but neglect exercises for other joints and muscles (Johnson-Pawlson and Koshes 1985).

Assessment. An assessment of the cardiovascular, pulmonary, and musculoskeletal systems should be completed, including blood pressure and the heart rate and rhythm. If an endurance program is anticipated, a stress test should be done. A decrease in pulmonary function will signify a lesser exercise capacity. However, even a person with chronic obstructive pulmonary disease (COPD) can exercise for flexibility, muscle strengthening, and mild endurance. Limitations in the musculoskeletal system usually involve joint immobility or neurologic defects. The client's feet and ankles should be observed for any deformity that may inhibit the ability to exercise. Finally, attitudes toward exercise should be assessed. The nurse should determine what types of exercise the client has done and enjoyed in the past.

While a well-rounded program includes exercises, flexibility, muscular strengthening and endurance, and cardiovascular conditioning, even frail older people can participate in exercises for flexibility (stretching) and muscular strengthening.

Interventions. The nurse can suggest participating in a group exercise program, if one is available. If not, or if older persons are homebound, exercises may be tailored to the physical limitations even if they are confined to bed or chair, or if they are ambulatory. The intent should be to maintain flexibility of all joints as much as possible by putting joints through an active range of motion.

ADAPTING THE HOME ENVIRONMENT

A goal of nursing care of older adults in the home is to assist them in maximizing the quality of life in their homes. Assessment of and adaptation of the home environment to enable the older person to reach higher levels of health are essential roles of the home health care nurse.

Opportunities to remain independent in one's home are possible by attention to adaptations, design factors, and behaviors that promote safety and security. Safety is a fundamental issue as persons age and the potential for disabilities becomes greater. Injuries and deaths from falls and fires are the most common dangers to older people living at home. In the United States older people account for one-fourth of all accidental deaths, with falls as the leading cause. Persons over age 65 account for more than two-thirds of all deaths from falls in the United States.

Fire safety is a second major concern in the living environment of older persons. Smoke detectors in strategic locations within the home are vital to the safety of older people and should be installed in kitchens and hallways and adjacent to bedrooms. Hand-held fire extinguishers located in easily accessible areas are an additional safety factor (U.S. Congress. Office of Technology Assessment 1985).

Renovations

A physical therapy visit in the home to assess the living situation is valuable in determining the environmental adaptations that will make client ambulation safer and easier. Recommendations might include structural alterations, such as replacing a porch step with a ramp or remodeling the kitchen and bathroom to increase access to the counters, sink, toilet, or tub. Doorways should be wide enough to permit access to all rooms for persons in a wheelchair. The threshold to the doorway should be flush with the floor and not a barrier to crossing from room to room.

The bathroom is one of the most dangerous places in the home for an older person. The bathroom is a frequent site of falls; the surrounding hard surfaces contribute to the severity of the injuries. Adaptations of the bathroom should include strategically placed and well-anchored grab bars on the inner and end walls of the bathtub and by the toilet. Bathtubs as well as floors should have nonskid surfaces. Other adaptations could be made in the bathroom depending upon the mobility of the older person.

A simple change in the bedroom would be to raise the height of the bed for easier access or egress for older persons with limited joint mobility. Half-side rails can be used to help the client move around in the bed or get in or out of bed. A telephone should be within easy reach from the bed. Other adaptations include rearrangement of furniture to allow easy access to a favorite chair. Persons with joint motion difficulty can be aided by using upholstered chairs with hydraulic or mechanical lift mechanisms under the seat cushions. Scatter rugs in all rooms should be securely anchored or have nonskid backing. Stairways can present problems, particularly for falls, but a physical therapist can teach clients safe methods to ascend and descend. There should be light switches at both the top and the bottom of the stairway. Walkways must be kept clear of water, ice, furniture, clothing, or anything that might become a hazard. Highly waxed floors should be avoided to prevent falls. Adequate lighting should illuminate the surfaces to be viewed, such as the floor, the pathway to the bathroom or kitchen, the front door, and other commonly used areas.

All potential hazards in the environment of an older person need to be eliminated. Modifications to the environment of an older person, especially one with reduced vision, can be a hazard even though they are necessary. The nurse should explain to the client that safety modifications need to be made and to be aware of the changes in the home environment (Thomas 1985; U.S. Congress, Office of Technology Assessment 1985; Tideiksaar 1989).

The American Association of Retired Persons (AARP) (1988) has published an excellent booklet that gives specific details concerning renovations that can be done to make the home safer for an older person. Included in this booklet are suggestions for sources to obtain special grants and loans to assist in paying the cost of the renovations. This publication is highly recommended as a reference for anyone contemplating renovating a home to fit the needs of an older person who experiences physical limitations.

Equipment and Supplies

Many types of equipment and supplies are available to maintain ill or disabled people at home. For a complete listing of the types of equipment and supplies available for home health care, the nurse or the client should consult the many catalogues that are available. A large assortment of equipment and supplies is available from local surgical supply stores and may be rented or purchased as needed. The assortment includes oxygen and respiratory devices; rehabilitation equipment, such as exercise handgrips; and durable medical equipment, including manual or electric hospital beds, manual or electric wheelchairs, hydraulic patient lifts, trapeze bars, walkers, and canes. Bedside commodes, bedpans, urinals, plastic mattress pads, and covers are also available.

Other products that are available include nursing care supplies, such as dressings, pressure cushions, and catheters; drug therapy supplies, such as disposable syringes and intravenous therapy supplies, oxygen concentrator, or needleless insulin injector; nutritional supplies; and home kidney dialysis equipment and supplies (Spradley and Dorsey 1985; Thomas 1985).

Some clients have incontinent problems that require management. Many commercial products are available, but cost, comfort, convenience, and dignity of the client are factors in selecting the means of controlling incontinence. Use of protective garments, such as waterproof pants, disposable undergarments, and pads to absorb urine, enables the client to have improved mobility. Marsupial pants may be preferable to wearing a pad. Marsupial pants have a pocket in the anterior crotch into which an absorbent pad can be placed and easily changed (Ebert 1984).

A variety of self-monitoring devices are available for clients in the home, including blood glucose monitoring, a chemical guaiac test for occult blood in the stool, urine glucose testing, and blood pressure monitoring. By monitoring their own health status, older clients will be able to reduce some of the expense of their medical care as long as they recognize that these are screening devices and any abnormal findings require further evaluation.

Older adults want to remain in their own homes as long as possible in spite of their changing physical status. Use of the various types of equipment and supplies that are available will help the client attain that goal.

Monitoring the safety of a frail older client living alone is necessary. If there are no family members who can check on the client on a regular basis, enlistment of a neighbor or the mail carrier to alert professional help may be possible. An emergency response system can be arranged that will provide service to homebound, frail older persons. This is an automatic monitoring system that links people to emergency medical services when their life or safety is in jeopardy. These services include the installation of the individual monitoring unit; training associated with the use of the system; periodic checking to assure that the unit is functioning properly; equipment maintenance calls; response to the emergency call by medical professional, paraprofessional or volunteer; and follow-up with the client. (See chapter 20 for more information on the use of emergency help systems.)

AVAILABILITY OF COMMUNITY RESOURCES

Community health resources consist of agencies, professionals, or services available to members of a community for purposes of helping them to meet their health-related needs. These resources may provide direct or indirect health care services.

Direct health care services include medical, nursing, and dental care. Indirect services include resources that do not provide direct health care, but provide services that facilitate health care for members of the community. For example, a community referral service could be an indirect resource by referring the individual or family to a particular physician or home health care agency to meet their health needs.

A nurse's knowledge of available resources develops over a period of time while working with families and agencies and identifying needs. Some of the resources, such as hospitals and clinics, are available in most communities. However, it is important to know what other resources exist in the community. Common sources of obtaining listings or directories of resources include the following: *(1)* telephone book and yellow pages; *(2)* hospital social services departments; *(3)* professional societies; *(4)* local, county, and state health departments; *(5)* chambers of commerce; *(6)* the local area agency on aging; and *(7)* other health care providers. A file of these resources should be established and should include data pertinent to specific agencies or individuals, names and phone numbers of contact persons, and satisfaction with services provided. With this information the nurse can compare resources and assist clients in making appropriate selections. Evaluation data are obtained from the resource itself, users of the resource, and the experiences of the nurse and other health professionals (Burgess 1983a).

Referrals

The referral process is a systematic approach that helps clients utilize resources available in the community for the purpose of resolving needs. This is one of the most frequently used skills of the nurse in the home care setting. According to Burgess (1983b), the referral process can be defined as an assessment of referral needs, selection of appropriate resources, determination and implementation of interventions, and evaluation of the interventions for a client or family.

A home health nurse should always be alert to the potential needs of clients for referral to other agencies or health care providers. When the needs of the client cannot be met by the present caregivers, other possible providers are considered. A referral can be initiated by either the nurse or the client. The potential benefits of the referral should be realistically considered by both the nurse and the client. Once the assessment has been completed and the need for a referral has been agreed upon by the nurse and the client, then the selection process to find the proper resource begins.

The nurse must have knowledge of the community and of the resources that are available. Possible resources should be evaluated to determine if they fit within the needs and resources of the family. The resources should be identified and discussed with the client. The client may have suggestions of a resource that has provided satisfactory care in the past. The nurse should evaluate and determine that the referral fits the type of care that is needed and attempt to secure the resource that might provide positive feelings in the client. The client or family members should make the final selection in order to achieve maximum satisfaction with the referral.

Once the choice has been made, there are several ways to implement the referral. The nurse must be aware of the ability of the client or family members to participate in implementing the referral. The least amount of involvement a nurse may have is to give the client the name and phone number of the referral. This client-initiated approach is the simplest if the client has the ability to perform this function.

An intermediate level of involvement by the nurse would be to contact the resource to provide it with information regarding the client. The client must be informed of this action, which can occur before or after an initial contact by the family. Direct contact would allow both agencies to ask questions and clarify any confusion pertaining to the needs and care of the client. The receiving agency would have the benefit of pertinent information regarding the client ahead of time that would help them provide more comprehensive initial care.

A comprehensive level of involvement occurs when the nurse initiates and implements the entire referral without participation of the client or the client's family. This action may be necessary if the client is in some way incapacitated physically or mentally. Under these conditions, every effort should be made to involve the family of the client in making the referral. In some cases legal protection may be needed and obtained through the police department, an official state agency, or the agency's lawyer.

Ongoing evaluation and follow-up are probably the most crucial step in the referral process. Evaluation of the referral is a responsibility of the nurse who initiated the action. This evaluation can be accomplished by consultation with the client to determine if the needs that prompted the referral have been met. During the consultation, the nurse can determine the client's satisfaction with the referral and determine any problems that may have arisen during the process. Through the appropriate application of the referral process, the home health nurse can most effectively help a client meet health needs (Burgess 1983b).

Home Health Care

Home care is a unique setting in which professionals can function interdependently and work together to accomplish the client's care goals. Interdisciplinary collaboration is an integral part of home health nursing. Collaboration is a process of working together using professional and individual skills, knowledge, and philosophy to attain common goals. It requires willingness to share, to listen, and to communicate openly and directly about one's feelings, thoughts, and differences to attain the desired result. Continuity of care in the home setting requires effective collaboration of all members of the interdisciplinary team. Medicare regulations, professional organizations, and state licensing boards dictate the responsibilities and functions of the disciplines in home health care.

The interdisciplinary team consists of a variety of health care providers that are available in the community, although each case will dictate the type of care needed. Each client in the home care program must be under the care of a physician to certify that a medical problem does exist. The physician refers to a doctor of medicine or osteopathy who is legally authorized to practice medicine by a state in which the doctor is performing his/her duties (Garvey and Loque 1988).

Registered nurse responsibilities include the following: *(1)* assessment of the physical, mental, emotional, social, and spiritual needs of the client; *(2)* formulation of the nursing care plan; *(3)* implementation of medical orders; *(4)* direct delivery of client care or supervision of other nursing personnel in the delivery of that care; *(5)* evaluation of care; *(6)* maintenance of written client records; *(7)* health counseling of clients and their families; *(8)* health teaching; and *(9)* collaboration with other members of the health team to meet client needs (Browning 1983).

Licensed practical/vocational nurses (LPN/LVN) are used to care for some of the health problems that do not require the expertise of a professional registered nurse. They assist with physical examinations and carry out nursing and medically prescribed procedures. In most states, LPNs are allowed to give medications. The LPN can make an ongoing assessment of the client's situation and discuss it with the professional nurse who might want to visit the client to make a professional evaluation (Fromer 1983; Henson, Sirles, and Sloan 1984).

Home health aides are used in the home care setting when their level of care is sufficient. However, they are limited in the care they give to clients due to their minimal education requirements and lack of knowledge of skilled care. They give general hygienic care, such as bath, bed change, and mouth care, in addition to feeding clients, transferring clients from bed to chair, taking vital signs, and giving enemas. Continual close contact with the client allows the aide to identify changes in the client's condition and refer any potential problems to the professional staff. Nurse aides work under the supervision of a registered nurse or a licensed vocational nurse.

Physical therapists (PT) are graduates of a baccalaureate or master's level physical therapy program. They provide services that enable clients in the home to improve or maintain their level of functioning, prevent loss of functioning, prevent loss of functional ability, and restore clients to their optimal level of functioning. These goals are accomplished by evaluating the client's neuromuscular and functional abilities and conferring with the client's physician and home health care nurse. The physical therapist gives direct care, which includes strengthening muscles, restoring mobility, controlling spasticity, gait training, and teaching active-passive exercises. The therapist also teaches the client and family the treatment regimen to promote self-care and responsibility. The therapist gives indirect care when serving as a consultant to the staff and shares skills in the specific area of expertise (Garvey and Loque 1988).

Speech-language pathologists (SLP) are certified

by the American Speech-Language-Hearing Association and are prepared at the master's level. They assist people with communication problems related to speech, language, or hearing. The goal of speech therapy is to assist individuals to develop and maintain maximum speech and language ability so they can use these abilities to their optimal level. People who have swallowing and eating problems are assisted also. By consulting with other home health team members, the speech-language pathologist can teach providers of care and family members how to encourage development of the best method of communication for clients.

Occupational therapists (OT) earn baccalaureate degrees and, when registered by the National Occupational Therapy Association, are subsequently referred to as OTRs. They help clients by teaching them to develop and maintain the abilities to perform activities of daily living in their home. Treatment is focused on the client's upper extremities by assisting to restore muscle strength and mobility for functional skills. The occupational therapist evaluates the level of function and ability by testing muscles and joints. The occupational therapist teaches self-care activities and assesses the client's home for safety with possible modifications for removing barriers and provides adaptive equipment when needed. This discipline is a valuable resource in assisting the client to once again become independent in self-care (Garvey and Loque 1988).

The social worker in home health care holds a master's degree in social work (M.S.W.) and assists clients and families with social, emotional, and environmental factors that affect their well-being. Upon returning to their home after a stay in the hospital, clients may find they are unable to cope with their level of functioning and need help to reorganize their lives. Other functions performed include crisis intervention, resource identification and application, and equipment procurement when payment is a problem (Garvey and Loque 1988).

Mobile Dental Units

Mobile dental units are a relatively new concept in home care of older adults. Use of mobile dental units enables the dentist to make the necessary impressions, examine the trial dentures, and deliver the completed product all in the comfortable and discreet surroundings of the client's home. The making of the dentures usually requires at least three appointments over a period of several days. Although this service is available to all, the majority of people who need or wear dentures are older people. A full dental program is also offered, including cleaning, filling, and crown and bridge work.

Mobile dental units provide dental care for older people who are unable or unwilling to drive very far, if at all, and must depend on a friend or relative to provide transportation to a dental appointment. This service provides greater access and convenience to the public, especially older people in the community.

Home-Delivered Meals

Home-delivered meals programs provide nutritious, well-balanced meals to persons in their own homes. Through these programs, persons who are unable to prepare their own meals can have a hot meal brought to them in their own home. While some programs furnish lunch, dinner, and sometimes breakfast, most of them deliver one meal, usually at lunchtime.

The meals are prepared in a central kitchen and are individually served usually in disposable containers and kept in a warming oven while being delivered to the recipients in the community. This arrangement is important to older homebound adults not only because they will receive a hot, nutritious meal every day, but also because they are able to visit with the delivery person, which may be their only contact with another person all day. Need of this program by the homebound may vary from a few weeks during an illness or accident to an indefinite time depending upon the individual situation.

Many of the recipients of home-delivered meals often have diet restrictions as part of their health program. The availability of low-salt, low-fat, and diabetic diets increases the number of persons in the community who can use this service. Service to persons living in multiethnic communities may require more than one type of regular diet.

Many of the home-delivered meal programs are sponsored by the community or the local churches, whereas a few are privately owned. Almost all rely heavily on volunteers who donate their time or money to assist the needy. While clients must purchase the home-delivered meals and many are on limited incomes, the cost of the meal is kept as low as possible. There are many persons who are unable to leave their homes to eat out, to shop, or to prepare meals. Home-delivered meals enable them to remain at home, which otherwise would not be possible (Ebersole and Hess 1990).

Hospice Care

Hospice care can be provided in the home by family members or friends who are taught basic nursing care sufficient for the needs of the dying individual. The hospice staff helps them to learn care techniques and dietary approaches, to give medicines, and to handle the problems that occur when a member of the family is dying. This orientation helps to eliminate much of the anxiety associated with the care and enables the client to die at home (Ebersole and Hess 1990). (See chapter 11 for additional information on hospice care.)

FINANCING HOME NURSING CARE

Home nursing care has experienced the same dramatic increase in costs that has occurred elsewhere in the health care industry. Few home health clients are able to pay cash for all of the home care services they need. Before 1966 most clients paid cash for home health care services. Donations subsidized clients who were unable to pay for these services. Since 1966, third-party health insurance has become a major funding source for home health care services. Federal health insurance programs of Medicare and Medicaid are the predominant funding sources, while private health insurance is gradually expanding its coverage for coordinated home health services.

Medicare

Medicare is a federal health insurance program for people age 65 and older, people of any age with permanent kidney failure, and certain disabled people under age 65. The Health Care Financing Administration (HCFA) of the United States Department of Health and Human Services administers Medicare. The Social Security Administration provides information about the program.

Medicare has two parts: hospital insurance (Part A) and medical insurance (Part B). Hospital insur-ance helps pay for medically necessary services furnished by Medicare-certified hospitals, skilled nursing facilities, home health agencies, and hospices. Medicare medical insurance helps pay for physician services and many other medical services and supplies that are not covered by Part A.

Medicare strictly regulates client eligibility and the kinds of services that are eligible for reimbursement under home care procedures. There are three major Medicare eligibility criteria for home care.

1. The client must be homebound.

2. The client must require skilled care.

3. The client must have a physician's written plan for that skilled care.

The referring physician must certify these requirements for every client in order to receive reimbursement from Medicare.

Homebound can be described as the normal inability to leave home or that leaving home would require a considerable and taxing effort. This inability is usually caused by illness or injury. Clients can remain eligible if they leave home infrequently only for the purpose of receiving medical care. Dependence or insecurity brought on by advanced age does not qualify the person to receive home health care under this definition.

The need for skilled nursing care is the second requirement for Medicare eligibility. This includes the administration of drugs, diagnostic tests, medical supplies, appliances, and rehabilitation services. Initially, Medicare defined skilled nursing care as hands-on nursing for the resolution of the medical condition that qualified the client for services in the home. The definition has since been expanded to include teaching as well as hands-on service, provided the teaching is necessary for the medical resolution of the primary condition.

The third requirement for Medicare eligibility is the plan for care that is to be developed by the physician and used by the nurse as the definitive guide for service given to the client. The plan must involve skilled care services allowable under Medicare (Mundinger 1983). The plan must include the components listed in Table 18-1. The plan must be reviewed at least every sixty days and requires recertification by the physician if the care is to be continued.

Table 18–1   Components of Plan for Home Care Under Medicare

- Types of services required
- Frequency of visits
- Anticipated length of care
- Diagnosis
- Description of the client's functional limitations
- Medications
- Diet
- Activities permitted
- Medical supplies and appliances needed
- Safety of home environment

Medicare Part A pays the full cost of medically necessary home health care for homebound beneficiaries and 80 percent of the approved cost for durable medical equipment supplied under the home health benefit. Coverage includes the intermittent skilled services of a licensed nurse. The services of physical therapists and speech-language pathologists also are covered when they are furnished through a Medicare-certified home health agency. If any of these services are required by homebound clients who are under the care of a physician, Part A can also help pay for other services including part-time or intermittent home health aide and skilled nursing services, occupational therapy, medical social services, and medical supplies. Coverage is also provided for a portion of the cost of durable medical equipment provided under a plan of care set up and overseen by a physician. If a beneficiary qualifies for home health care but does not have Medicare Part A, then Part B pays for all covered home health visits. There is no deductible or coinsurance for home health services. However, the beneficiary or the beneficiary's insurance company must pay the coinsurance of 20 percent of the cost of any durable medical equipment supplied under the home health benefit and all of the other costs not approved by Medicare.

Medicare Part A does not cover physicians' fees (covered under Medicare Part B), full-time nursing care at home, homemaker services, meals delivered to the home, blood transfusions, medications, and biologicals (may be covered under Medicare Part B). When skilled nursing care is not needed, Medicare provides no help at all for a recuperation period at home. Neither Part A nor Part B coverage allows anything toward custodial nursing or cost of medications that can be self-administered. Custodial care includes assistance with such activities as walking, eating, bathing, and taking medications. Such care primarily assists in meeting personal care or housekeeping needs (Health Care Financing Administration 1991).

Medicare beneficiaries certified as terminally ill —i.e., having six months or less to live—may elect to receive hospice care rather than regular Medicare benefits for the terminal illness. Medicare Part A pays for two ninety-day hospice benefit periods, a subsequent period of thirty days, and a subsequent extension of unlimited durations.

Beneficiaries enrolled in a Medicare-certified hospice program receive medical and support services necessary for symptom management and pain relief. When these services—most of which are provided in the beneficiary's home—are furnished by a Medicare-certified facility, the coverage includes: physician's services, nursing care, medical appliances and supplies (including outpatient medications for symptom management and pain relief), short-term inpatient care, counseling, therapies, and home health aide and homemaker services. There is no deductible, but clients must pay limited cost-sharing for outpatient medications and inpatient respite care. In the event the client requires medical services for a condition unrelated to the terminal illness, regular Medicare benefits are available.

Medicare coverage is inadequate in several areas. It fails to cover the greatest need of older adults—

long-term care for chronic diseases and disabilities. It is oriented toward short-term acute illnesses and accidents. Arbitrary limits have been set on the length of time services will be paid and these are unrealistic for the needs of older people. The deductible and coinsurance features of Medicare serve to encourage delay in seeking medical help. Both Part A and Part B of Medicare have a deductible amount that the client must pay. This amount is deducted by Medicare before paying for the cost of the services. Part B of Medicare is usually reimbursed at the rate of 80 percent of usual, customary, and reasonable charges. The remaining 20 percent must be "coinsured" for protection against excessive expense. The costs not paid by Medicare must be paid by the beneficiary or the beneficiary's insurance company. Acquiring Medicare supplemental health insurance is encouraged to cover the costs that Medicare does not pay. In recent years, costs of financing health care have exceeded the national inflation rate. This has caused delays in political decisions to assist older persons in paying for health care services (Ebersole and Hess 1990; Health Care Financing Administration 1991).

Medicaid

Under federal Medicaid guidelines, states are required to provide skilled nursing care and home health aide services and, on an optional basis, other services such as personal care services, physical therapy, speech therapy, hearing therapy, and occupational therapy (U.S. Congress. Office of Technology Assessment 1985). All services or items provided must be ordered by a physician as part of a written plan for the client's care. In most instances, Medicaid home health services must be provided by an agency meeting Medicare certification requirements.

Home health care is for people confined to their homes because of illness or injury who need health services part-time. Any eligible Medicaid recipient may receive up to fifty home visits a year by a nurse or aide from an approved agency. A written recommendation from the physician and approval from the state agency's health insuring agent are required. Some medical supplies and equipment are included when medically necessary. Assistance with bathing, dressing, changing bed linens, and other personal care is covered when medically necessary. Medicaid

may be able to help with transportation to and from a physician, hospital, or other medical provider if transportation is unavailable from a friend, relative, or community resource agency. Medicaid pays for up to three prescriptions a month from pharmacies participating in the program. Medicaid pays only for certain prescription medicines prescribed by a physician. People who qualify for Medicare must use that program's services first (Texas Department Human Services 1990).

Home health care services have not thrived under Medicaid. The reason for poor utilization of these services can be traced to several causes. First, although each state has developed its own health care services under Medicaid, some states have adopted very restrictive policies for clients to receive this care. Several states adopted regulations making home care available only as a posthospital benefit and home health aide services tied to nursing care. Another cause for poor utilization of home health care services is that many states set the reimbursement amount lower than the actual cost of providing these services. Therefore home health agencies are not eager to care for clients with Medicaid coverage only, because they must use agency funds to subsidize part of the cost of providing this service.

Low utilization of home care services under Medicaid is unfortunate. Medicaid has the potential to provide the desired level of home health care. This care can provide persons with health problems an opportunity to maintain an independent lifestyle at home in a safe and health environment (Stewart 1979).

Private Pay/Insurance

Until a few years ago the predominant method of financing health care in the United States was personal or private payment. This method is described as direct consumer payment of health costs. Out-of-pocket payments are made for different reasons. Individuals who have no insurance coverage must pay for health and medical services. Many consumers carry only major medical insurance or have limited coverage or exclusions and must pay the amount that is not covered. The insurance policy may include a deductible amount that must be paid by the insuree before reimbursement begins (Spradley 1985).

Insurance companies underwrite policies aimed at decreasing consumer risk of economic loss from the use of health services. Many of these policies are purchased as a supplement to Medicare. Almost all individual policies bought after age 65 include a waiting period during which prior health problems are not covered. For Medicare supplement policies, this exclusionary period is limited to six months. For other types of policies there is no limitation. Some insurance companies might require a physical examination of the insuree, which may exclude coverage or require higher premiums.

Many of the services not covered by Medicare will not be covered by supplemental policies either, such as routine physical examinations, eyeglasses, dental care, cosmetic surgery, homemaker services, and intermediate and custodial nursing home care. However, there are various types of policies that can help improve the level of protection from catastrophic health costs. The goal in purchasing insurance coverage should not be to have total coverage. Insurance ceases to make sense when the cost is disproportionately large in comparison with the risk.

The Omnibus Budget Reconciliation Act of 1990 (OBRA-90) passed by Congress on November 5, 1990, contains new rules that will significantly impact Medicare supplement insurance policies in the future. To protect consumers from the confusion of comparing these policies, Congress authorized the National Association of Insurance Commissions

(NAIC) to develop ten model Medicare supplement policies to replace the many varied policies on the market. On July 31, 1991 the NAIC finalized the ten model policies shown in Table 18-2. These have been offered by insurance companies as of January 1, 1992. Explanations of the standardized benefits as outlined in the Medicare supplement insurance policies are shown in Table 18-3 (Acordia 1991; United States Congress 1990).

Regulation of the insurance business is a right retained by the states. However, federal legislation continues to dictate how the states should regulate the industry. Regarding these regulations, OBRA-90

- requires a limit of only ten policies.

- gives authority to the United States Secretary of Health and Human Services to approve and monitor state actions regarding Medicare supplement insurance.

- increases federal regulation of the state insurance department.

- reverts control to the federal government if a state fails to conform to the standardization regulations.

These standardized policies have advantages and disadvantages for the older applicants who purchase them (Acordia 1991). Some of these advantages and disadvantages are shown in Table 18-4.

Table 18–2   Standard Medicare Supplement Plans

PLAN A	PLAN B	PLAN C	PLAN D	PLAN E	PLAN F	PLAN G	PLAN H	PLAN I	PLAN J
Basic Benefits	Basic Benefits	Basic Benefits	Basic Benefits	Basic Benefits	Basic Benefits	Basic Benefits	Basic Benefits	Basic Benefits	Basic Benefits
		Skilled Nursing Coinsurance	Skilled Nursing Coinsurance	Skilled Nursing Coinsurance	Skilled Nursing Coinsurance	Skilled Nursing Coinsurance	Skilled Nursing Coinsurance	Skilled Nursing Coinsurance	Skilled Nursing Coinsurance
	Part A Deductible	Part A Deductible	Part A Deductible	Part A Deductible	Part A Deductible	Part A Deductible	Part A Deductible	Part A Deductible	Part A Deductible
		Part B Deductible			Part B Deductible				Part B Deductible
					Part B Excess (100%)	Part B Excess (80%)		Part B Excess (100%)	Part B Excess (100%)
		Foreign Travel Emergency	Foreign Travel Emergency	Foreign Travel Emergency	Foreign Travel Emergency	Foreign Travel Emergency	Foreign Travel Emergency	Foreign Travel Emergency	Foreign Travel Emergency
			At-Home Recovery			At-Home Recovery		At-Home Recovery	At-Home Recovery
							Basic Medications ($1250 Limit)	Basic Medications ($1250 Limit)	Basic Medications ($1250 Limit)
				Preventive Care					Preventive Care

Source: United States Congress. *Omnibus Budget Reconciliation Act of 1990—Public Law 101-508.* Washington, DC: United States Government Printing Office. Reprinted with permission of Acordia Senior Benefits.

Table 18–3   Standardized Benefit Explanations

Basic Benefits—benefits required in all Medicare supplement policies sold after Janury 1, 1992. (See chart below for list.)

Skilled Nursing Coinsurance—the amount per day that Medicare does not pay for day 21–100 in a skilled nursing facility.

Part A Deductible—the amount Medicare does not pay for an inpatient hospital stay per benefit period.

Part B Deductible—the annual amount Medicare will not pay before considering physician or other outpatient services.

Part B Excess—the difference between what Medicare allows and the total legal charge for a service. Under standardization insurers can pay either 80 percent or 100 percent of the difference.

Foreign Travel Emergency—after a $250 deductible, health expenses for emergency care received in the first sixty days of a trip to a foreign country are paid at 80 percent up to a lifetime maximum of $50,000.

At-Home Recovery—covers home health visits when Medicare home health coverage runs out. Maximum payment is $40 per visit and $1600 per year.

Basic Medications—after a $250 deductible, covers 50 percent of prescription medication expenses up to a maximum annual payment of $1250.

Extended Medications—same as the Basic Medication benefit but with an annual maximum payment of $3000.

Preventive Care—provides benefits for an annual physical exam and related tests and Xrays (not covered by Medicare) up to $120 per year.

BASIC BENEFITS—INCLUDED IN ALL PLANS
HOSPITALIZATION

Part A coinsurance plus coverage for 365 additional days after Medicare benefits end.

MEDICARE EXPENSES

Part B co insurance (20 percent of Medicare-approved expenses).

BLOOD

First three pints of blood each year.

Source: United States Congress. *Omnibus Budget Reconciliation Act of 1990—Public Law 101-508.* Washington, DC: United States Government Printing Office. Reprinted with permission of Acordia Senior Benefits.

Table 18-4 Advantages and Disadvantages of Standardized Medi-Gap Policies

Advantages	Disadvantages
• *Guaranteed access* to coverage at age 65 for applicants who apply within the first six months they become eligible for Part B of Medicare • *Protection* from cancellation except in cases of misrepresentation or fraud as long as the premium payments are made • *Credit* for waiting periods whereby the amount of time accumulated toward a pre-existing condition waiting period under one insurer has to be applied to the waiting period required by a new insurer if a customer changes insurance companies • *Protection* from excessive insurance • *Simpler comparisons* of policies	• *Reduced choice* in the benefits contained in the ten policies from the volume and variety available today • *Reduced services* caused by increased competition that will be focused on price rather than services as the insurer's product becomes the same • *Reduced access* to coverage for unhealthy applicants who wait past the six month period they become eligible for Part B of Medicare

Current Medicare-supplement policy holders are not required to change to a standardized policy. Although these policies are still good and will be continued by the insurance companies, only policies that exactly match a standardized model policy can be sold after January 1, 1992 (Acordia 1991).

THE FUTURE OF HOME HEALTH CARE

Home health care as a component of the health care delivery system will continue to grow in the future. The increasingly older population and the prevalence of their chronic conditions will assure the need of an expanded system of home health care.

Two distinct populations of older clients will continue to require home health care services. Clients who have been hospitalized and are recovering from a specific illness will need continuing medical services or convalescent care outside the institution. A second population who experiences deteriorating health or declining self-care abilities is at risk for institutionalization. At present the second group of clients has no access to reimbursable home care until they qualify for one of the services provided by Medicare. These older persons need preventive health care to maintain or upgrade their health status to prevent the need for more expensive institutional care (Mundinger 1983).

The need for well-prepared home care nurses also will continue to increase. There is especially a need

for qualified nurse managers/supervisors who will employ, orient, supervise, and evaluate staff who provide nursing care in the home. Effective and well-managed home health agencies need to employ various types of clinical nurse specialists, such as oncologic, respiratory, and gerontological, to be providers of care, consultants, and teachers of other nursing staff because of the complexity of care clients in the home require. These nurses also need to learn how to give the most comprehensive client and family care possible within the restrictions of Medicare and other insurance reimbursement requirements.

The major expansion in home nursing care also has implications for the professional nursing curriculum, which should provide *all* of their students learning experiences in home nursing care and gerontological nursing.

Changes in government regulations are beginning to eliminate past barriers to the home health care delivery system, although more drastic changes will be necessary to assure quality care for older people who need long-term care in the home.

The status and future of long-term care insurance is changing rapidly. Insurance policies are available to include coverage for care both at a nursing home and at home. Most people would prefer to stay at home than spend their last days in a nursing facility. Older people who desire and can afford to purchase long-term care insurance should study the costs and benefits carefully. They should buy a comprehensive policy that pays for both nursing home and home care that cover a wide range of services with the fewest restrictions (Consumer Reports 1991).

SUMMARY

Home health care provides a variety of services to individuals and families in the home environment for the purpose of enhancing the well-being of the older client. The rapid increase in the older population has brought about a higher demand for home health care.

Nursing, medical, and rehabilitative care can be provided in the home depending upon the needs of the client. The prevalence and severity of chronic conditions and their associated disabilities increase in old age. The most frequently reported chronic illnesses among older adults who reside at home are arthritis, hypertension, hearing impairment, heart conditions, vision impairment, and arteriosclerosis. These illnesses contribute to physical, functional, and mental limitations.

Two of the more common nursing diagnoses that are problems for clients and caregivers alike are incontinence and impaired physical mobility. Incontinence causes psychosocial problems resulting in a decreased quality of life. The economic cost of management of incontinence is an enormous burden for both the client and society. Older persons tend to acquire a variety of physical problems that limit their mobility and can be debilitating. A program of exercise tailored to the client's disabilities can be used to prevent deterioration and enhance the client's health status.

An assessment and adaptation of the home can assist in providing a safe environment where the client can maintain more independence. Adaptations may include major structural changes or simple rearrangement of the furniture. Various types of equipment and supplies are available for rent or purchase to assist older adults who want to remain in their own homes as long as possible despite their physical limitations.

A wide range of community health resources, such as interdisciplinary teams of home health care professionals, home-delivered meals, mobile dental units, and hospice care, can be arranged for depending upon what is available within the community.

Medicare, Medicaid, and private insurance companies provide the financing for most of the health care costs in the United States today. Strict requirements imposed by the federal and state governments regulate eligibility and reimbursement for services available under these programs. The programs are designed for acute care clients and are inadequate for assisting those with chronic diseases and disabilities who need long-term care.

A baccalaureate degree in nursing, which enables the nurse to have the background and specific knowledge to perform in an effective manner, should be the minimum level of professional preparation for nursing in home health care. Empathetic concern and good interpersonal skills enhance the nurse's ability to function in this type of setting. The role of the home health nurse will continue to grow in the future. The increase in the older population will assure the need of an expanded system of home health care.

STUDY QUESTIONS

1. List some of the advantages of home care versus institutional care.

2. Compare assessing an older adult in the home versus the clinic setting.

3. What are the most frequently reported chronic illnesses among noninstitutionalized older adults?

4. What are the two common nursing diagnoses among older people and the nursing interventions for each?

5. Describe some adaptations of the home environment that may be needed for a client with debilitating arthritis.

6. What types of equipment may be rented or purchased for home health care of an older adult?

7. How can the nurse or client locate available community resources needed for home care?

8. Describe criteria that must be met for reimbursement by Medicare, Medicaid, and third-party payors.

9. What educational preparation and skills are desirable for professional nurses working with older clients at home?

REFERENCES

Acordia Senior Benefits. 1991. *Standardization*. Indianapolis, IN: Acordia Senior Benefits.

American Association of Retired Persons. 1988. *The Do-able Renewable Home: Making Your Home Fit Your Needs*. Washington, DC: American Association of Retired Persons.

American Nurses' Association, Division of Community Health Nursing. 1980. *A Conceptual Model of Community Health Nursing*. (Publication No. CH-102M). Kansas City, MO: American Nurses' Association.

Browning, M.A. 1983. An interdisciplinary approach to long-term care. In *Management of Personnel in Long-Term Care*, edited by M.O. Hogstel. Bowie, MD: Robert J. Brady.

Browning, M.A. 1985. Home health care: The nurse's perspective. In *Home Nursing Care for the Elderly*, edited by M.O. Hogstel. Bowie, MD: Brady Communication.

Burgess, W. 1983a. The evaluation of community resources. In *Community Health Nursing—Philosophy, Process, Practice*, edited by W. Burgess and E.C. Ragland. Norwalk, CT: Appleton-Century-Crofts.

Burgess, W. 1983b. The referral process. In *Community Health Nursing Philosophy, Process, Practice*, edited by W. Burgess and E.C. Ragland. Norwalk, CT: Appleton-Century-Crofts.

Consumer Reports. 1991. An empty promise to the elderly? June:425–41.

Ebersole, P. and P. Hess. 1990. *Toward Healthy Aging—Human Needs and Nursing Response*. 3d ed. St. Louis: C.V. Mosby.

Ebert, N.J. 1984. Elimination in the aged. In *The Aged Person and the Nursing Process*, 2d ed., edited by A.G. Yurick, B.E. Spier, S.S. Robb and N.J. Ebert, Norwalk, CT: Appleton-Century-Crofts.

Fromer, M.J. 1983. *Community Health Care and the Nursing Process*. 2d ed. St. Louis: C.V. Mosby.

Garvey, E. and J.H. Loque. 1988. The community health nurse in home health and hospice care. In *Community Health Nursing: Process and Practice for Promoting Health*, edited by M. Stanhope and J. Lancaster. St. Louis: C.V. Mosby.

Greengold, B.A. and J.G. Ouslander. 1986. Bladder retraining: Program for elder patients with post-indwelling catheterization. *Journal of Gerontological Nursing* 12(6):31–35.

Hashizume, S. 1991. Home health care. In *Clinical Gerontological Nursing: A Guide to Advanced Practice*, edited by W.C. Chenitz, J.F. Stone, and S.A. Salisbury. Philadelphia: W.B. Saunders.

Health Care Financing Administration. 1991. *1991 Guide to Health Insurance for People with Medicare*. Baltimore, MD: Health Care Financing Administration.

Henson, C.S., A. Sirles, and R. Sloan. 1984. The community health nurse as family nurse practitioner. In *Community Health Nursing—Process and Practice for Promoting Health*, edited by M. Stanhope and J. Lancaster. St. Louis: C.V. Mosby.

Johnson-Pawlson, J. and R. Koshes. 1985. Exercise is for everyone. *Geriatric Nursing* 6(6):322–25.

Mundinger, M.O. 1983. *Home care Controversy. Too Little, Too Late, Too Costly*. Rockville, MD: Aspen Systems.

National Association of Home Health Agencies. 1980. *Policy Statement on Health Care, 1980*. Washington, DC: National Association of Home Health Agencies.

Ouslander, J.G. 1986. Urinary incontinence: Geriatric challenge. *Diagnosis* 7:42–50.

Paillard, M. and K.B. Nowak. 1985. Use exercise to help older adults. *Journal of Gerontological Nursing* 11(7):36–39.

Robb, S.S. 1984. The elderly in the United States: Numbers, proportions, health status, and use of health services. In *The Aged Person and the Nursing Process*, 2d ed. edited by A.G. Yurick, B.E. Spier, S.S. Robb, and N.J. Ebert, Norwalk, CT: Appleton-Century-Crofts.

Spradley, B.W. 1985. Organization and financing of community health services. In *Community Health Nursing Concepts and Practice*. 2d ed., edited by B.W. Spradley. Boston: Little and Brown.

Spradley, B.W. and B. Dorsey. 1985. Home health care. In *Community Health Nursing Concepts and Practice*, 2d ed., edited by B.W. Spradley. Boston: Little and Brown.

Steffl, B.M. and I. Eide. 1984. Long-term care: Discharge planning, home care, and alternatives. In

Handbook of Gerontological Nursing, edited by B.M. Steffl. New York: Van Nostrand Reinhold.

Stewart, J.E. 1979. *Home Health Care*. St. Louis: C.V. Mosby.

Texas Department of Human Services. 1990. *Medicaid: A User's Guide*. (Stock code 20591-0611). Austin, TX: Texas Department of Human Services.

Thomas, S.D. 1985. Assessing and adapting the home environment. In *Home Nursing Care for the Elderly*, edited by M.O. Hogstel. Bowie, MD: Brady Communications.

Tideiksaar, R. 1989. Home safe home: Practical tips for fall-proofing. *Geriatric Nursing* 10(6):280–84.

United States Congress. Office of Technology Assessment. 1985. *Technology and Aging in America*. (OTA Publication BA-264). Washington, DC: United States Government Printing Office.

United States Congress. 1990. Omnibus Budget Reconciliation Act of 1990. Public Law 101-508. November 5, 1990 (42 USC 1395ss). Part 5 "Medicare Supplemental Insurance Policies," sections 4351–58. Washington, DC: United States Government Printing Offices.

Part 5

SUPPORT SYSTEMS

19 Family Support

Marta Askew Browning
Mildred O. Hogstel

CHAPTER OUTLINE

FOCUS

The focus of this chapter is the role of the family as a source of support for older adults. Emphasis is placed on family dynamics and relationships; family caregiving; and caregiver rewards, burdens, and support.

OBJECTIVES

1. Compare changes in family responsibilities for older adults in 1900 and the 1990s.

2. Discuss the different types of family development related to retirement and old age.

3. Discuss Duvall's stage of family development related to retirement and old age.

4. Define *caregiver* and *caregiving*.

5. Determine the role of men as caregivers.

6. Analyze the positive aspects and major problems in family caregiving for older persons.

7. Compare the advantages and disadvantages of caring for an older family member in the home.

8. Analyze the concept of eldercare in the workplace.

9. List sources of support for family caregivers.

10. Describe the role of the nurse related to family caregiving.

Adult health care in the United States is client/patient centered as opposed to family centered. In the current structure of services and reimbursement the individual is the unit of service whether he or she is in an intensive care unit, is a patient in a medical surgical unit, is enrolled in an outpatient clinic, or is the recipient of home health care. Conferences regarding the patient's condition are held with the patient and with one or two family members who may or may not be representative of the family unit as a whole. Acute care health care providers often view the family as a nonentity encountered only in fleeting moments during visiting hours. Generally little effort is made by staff to discriminate the roles of these family members, their relationships and value to the patient, and utility to the family unit as a whole. Prolonged or meaningful interaction with family members tends to occur only when a member has relieved hospital staff of some caregiving tasks, staff empathy is engendered by an imminent death, or conflict results between family and staff regarding the family's perception that the patient's care is inadequate. Seldom are older adult patients queried about their view of family relationships nor are they specifically asked whether they wish to share decision making with family members. Private and/or critical health care information may be given to everyone, or to no one, or to the wrong one. As a result, anger and hostility between the patient and the family members, between the family and the health care system, and within the family itself may occur. This same myopia toward the family as a unit of service occurs in outpatient clinics, private provider practices, and intermediate and transitional health care facilities. Nursing's persistent focus on the individual obstructs the ability to use the power of the family system on behalf of the patient.

Presently, with the exception of nurses engaged in home health care, community health practice, and family therapy in mental health settings, most nurses do not have the education or experience in dealing with families as a unit of service. Yet in the future if nurses are to expand their participation in the development of meaningful long-term care programs for older adults, the provision of family-centered care is essential. Such care encompasses not only the patient but also the caregiving network that provides the essential core of support enabling older adults to remain functional in their own home and community

settings where they prefer to remain. Nurses must move beyond mere lip service to the value of family, polite greetings given to family members, and brief problem-centered encounters. The profession has a marvelous opportunity to plan a continuum of support and mentorship for caregiving family systems. This support can be accomplished by utilizing the sequential efforts of acute care staff, home health professionals, and adult or gerontological nurse practitioners and clinical specialists. Active involvement with the family on an ongoing basis can be achieved through targeted interventions timed to meet anticipated needs utilizing the appropriate nursing specialist. Nursing support should be visible throughout the cycle of caregiving, not just at the time of diagnosis or at the time of death. The full political clout of the profession should be enlisted to promote long-term care policies that promote the creation and maintenance of family caregiving systems and ensure the health of all members within them.

EXPANSION OF FAMILY CAREGIVING

In the 1980s, contrary to myths, American families did not abandon their frail elders. More than 80 percent of home-based care was provided by family members. While only 5 percent of adults over age 65 resided in nursing homes or other long-term care institutions, more than twice that number were cared for at home by spouses and adult children. At any given time about 10 million adults were providing care to older adults (Baldwin 1990). The ties of love and affection, the bonds of duty and obligation, the values of established ethnic mutual aid systems, changing demographics, and economic constraints all predict the expansion of family caregiving as the nation enters the next century.

Trends

As the older population continues to increase in numbers and age into the late 80s, 90s, and 100s, the role of the family as caregiver will become much more prevalent. Nursing homes, with an average cost of $25,000–$30,000 a year, are not a viable alternative for most older people. Older persons with a limited income who meet specific criteria qualify for nursing home care through the Medicaid program (see chapter 21). Middle-income older people who do not qualify for Medicaid or who do not have long-term care insurance may not be able to afford nursing home care if needed. With major budget problems at the federal, state, and local government levels, Medicaid funding also has its limits. Criteria for nursing home care through Medicaid will probably become more strict. Current estimates of the number of nursing home beds and the cost of those beds for older persons into the early part of the next century are probably conservative. Therefore some families will not have a choice and family care may be the only alternative for them.

Unfortunately most families do not anticipate and plan ahead for contingencies when an older family member becomes ill. Many adult children, even those in their 40s and 50s, tend to assume that their parents or grandparents will always be healthy and independent. Many adult children continue to look to their parents for some kinds of guidance, support, or even financial assistance, perhaps for help with a child in college or purchasing a new home. When the older parents become ill, roles may reverse and the adult child will need to provide guidance, support, and perhaps financial assistance to parents, if the illness and treatment last for many years. The process is often gradual, however, because roles do not change that quickly. The adult child may not feel comfortable suggesting alternatives to a parent or may not even know what to suggest. Older parents may recognize that they need help but are reluctant to ask for or accept assistance from an adult child, especially if they still think of the child as a child.

The suggestion has been made that in the future "the average American woman" will spend seventeen years raising children and eighteen years helping aging parents ["Trading Places," *Newsweek* (July 16, 1990):49]. There are similarities and there are differences in child care and parent care. Children need intense care for several years and then the degree of care decreases as the years go by and the children gradually become more independent. The opposite is true for older parents who are independent and then gradually become dependent over a period of many years. For example, a person with Alzheimer's disease may live for fifteen to twenty years from the time of first symptoms to death. Also, not all people have children, but most all individuals have parents, unless one or the other died at a young

age. A similar issue—dependence versus independence—assumes critical importance in care of individuals on both ends of the age spectrum. Children seek independence as soon as possible and older persons want to maintain independence as long as possible. The health care system must consider and plan for this trend and health care personnel—nurses, physicians, and social workers—need to be made aware of the potential problems and solutions to meet the needs of adult family caregivers.

SHIFTING THE FOCUS FROM THE INDIVIDUAL TO THE FAMILY

Health care appears to be coming full circle. For most of our nation's history, health care was provided in the home by family, friends, and lay healers who were occasionally assisted in their ministrations by physicians. Advances in health care technology and liberal health care financing evolved only in the latter half of the present century. This shifted care from the home to the hospital. While never completely abolishing the role of the family caregiver, the health care delivery system held out the promise that institutions would take over when caregiving demands were untimely, inconvenient, or cumbersome. However, the era of rapid expansion of health care accessibility appears to be drawing to a close. Fiscal constraints are now being imposed to slow the spiralling costs of health care in general and of Medicare in particular. Fear regarding the projected costs of supporting older adults in the next century is sparking the rumblings of intergenerational conflict. Economics and demographics are returning responsibility for eldercare back to the family caregiving network.

Many of today's older adults remember family caregiving of the days of their youth and are shocked by its absence when needed now in their old age. They assumed that the old rule of "caring for one's own" would always apply. Forgotten are the massive societal changes of the last decades and the impact that such changes have had on family caregiving. The younger generation is now called upon to be the caregivers. They are being asked to assume responsibilities for which they most likely have never seen a role model. They always assumed these responsibilities would be carried out by an institution acting in their stead. Health care providers must shift the focus of their practice from narrowly addressing the needs of the older patient to developing assessments, interventions, and evaluations directed toward support of the family system as a whole.

This task is a complex endeavor because it means that nurses must deal with a group of patients—the family system. The nurse will need to recognize and understand the impact that individuals within the system have on one another and on the family system as displayed to the world. If the older adult's family system works together to implement shared values and goals in meeting the needs of aging relatives and friends, then the older adult will find nurturance when beset by the frailty and dependency that often accompany advanced age. However, if a family system cannot be assembled by an older adult, or the one to which he or she belongs is disorganized, overwhelmed, or in conflict over values related to the integration of aging relatives into the network, the outlook for the older adult is uncertain when dependency occurs. When the family system cannot be maintained and its energy channelled into productive efforts on behalf of the aging individual(s), these patients may experience unnecessary institutionalization or premature death. Thus the role of the nurse is to promote creation of vital and dynamic family systems and to provide mentorship as these systems provide the goods and services needed to sustain older persons in the community. Successful family-centered nursing requires an appreciation of family types, family developmental tasks, and the role of reciprocity in family relationships.

Family Types

Families are the structural units that create the center of American society. Changes within the structure of the family system, over time, impact the character of the nation. Older adults live in the same family configurations adopted by the younger generation. Stereotypical beliefs about aging and the assumption that older people live in lonely isolation often prevent health care providers from suggesting the infinite variety of options available to today's older population. They may be part of a nuclear dyad because the children have left home or because they are childless.

Older couples are also apt to live as part of a nuclear family whose children have not yet left home or whose adult children have returned home unable or unwilling to establish an independent household. Older adults and their children may constitute single-parent families as a result of widowhood, divorce, separation, failure to marry, or single parent adoption. Many older adults who were divorced or widowed remarry and live in blended or reconstituted families and function within kinship networks drawn from both old and new family alliances.

Older people may live in a household containing an extended, multigenerational family group, or in a geographical area with a tight kinship network of relatives united by blood or marriage. Still other elders are members of homosexual unions of a serial, transitory nature, or liaisons characterized by long-term monogamous commitment by legal bonds that sometimes include homosexual marriage. Cohabitation as trial marriage, but more often as a measure for protecting dual Social Security incomes while enjoying the benefits of companionship, is fairly frequent. Communal living with a group of friends has been beautifully popularized by the television show "Golden Girls" and is an alluring option for many. Finally, there are the single adults who may live alone but maintain ties with an existing family network or create a new one from friends and carefully selected family members (Ross and Cobb 1990).

Ethnicity may influence who is defined as family and what the particular duties and obligations of family members are. For example, ethnic English and Germans tend to define primary bonding as occurring between parents and their children and confine responsibility for older family members to this parent-child relationship. Italian, Polish, Irish, and African-American ethnics define family as extending beyond the nuclear unit to siblings, cousins, aunts, and uncles; all are expected to participate in family caregiving networks (White-Means and Thornton 1990a).

In addition to blood kin, African-Americans may include *fictive kin* or *parakin* within their family systems. Fictive kin function in the absence of blood relatives or when family relationships are unsatisfactory. These individuals are called *play* siblings, children, or parents. But these *play* relationships are considered equivalent to relationships by blood or marriage and carry with them similar responsibilities. Among African-Americans, identification of children is not always based on biological criteria, as the rearing of the child of another may confer parent status on the one performing the role. Thus foster children, children left by family members, and even white children that she helped raise may all be identified as children by an older African-American woman (Johnson and Barer 1990).

In addition to identifying the types of families and individuals who are included in the family system, the nurse must understand the quality of the relationships and how the older adult functionally perceives and uses family members. In a study of four hundred older adults Connidis and Davies (1990) reported on the relative importance of family members. The results of their research revealed that spouses were viewed more often as companions than confidants and that children were viewed more often as confidants than as companions by those who had children. This research also highlighted the importance of friends as confidants among the previously married and childless. Friends were cited as companions by single, never married, childless women; siblings were identified as confidants. Among never married, childless men, friends were viewed as companions; but these men made greater effort to develop ties to relatives who would serve as confidants than any other group of older adults.

"Although siblings never replace spouses or adult children in the lives of older adults, they do act as confidants, caregivers, and cherished friends. Relationships between brothers and sisters seem to grow progressively stronger in old age and siblings appear to function as a social insurance policy when other sources of social support fail" (Gold 1990, 741). These bonds seem to be especially strong among African-American siblings. In Gold's study of White and Black sibling dyads, themes of loyalty, solidarity, and enduring affection emerged in interviews with Black siblings nearly three times as frequently as they did in interviews with Whites (Gold 1990).

Talbott (1990) stated that the strength and durability of bonds between parents and adult children are well established and that high rates of interaction and aid flow between the generations. However, she noted that studies of social support consistently find no positive effect of contact with adult children on the well-being of their older parents in contrast to a consistent finding of the positive effects on well-being of friends. Her study of the negative side of the relationship between older adult widows and their adult children identified a number of stressors as perceived by the mother. Among these were a strong desire on the part of the mother to remain independent and refrain from bothering her children, fear of bothering children, dissatisfaction with the amount of help received from children, feeling unappreciated and left out, being overprotected by children, making substantial financial sacrifices in order to help children, needing to purchase involvement with children through the provision of instrumental support, and fending off the excessive demands of children for goods and services. Gold (1990) noted that problematic relationships may be the result of a mother's disproportionate giving. Some mothers appear to trade goods and services for emotional rewards from children but the rewards received are inadequate in relation to the items given. Gold further noted that 51 percent of the study subjects noted no negative aspect to their relationships with their children. Even among those citing negative aspects in their relationships, there was great pride in their children and acknowledgement of gifts and services provided by children to the mother.

This brief review highlights the complexity of discerning the types and values of family relationships. It also identifies the importance of friends and the frequency of inclusion of friends in the family network as substitutes for missing family members, as members of a family system the older adult never had or has lost, or as fictive kin. A further adjunct to the nurse's understanding of the family system and its effect on the older adult patient is recognition of the developmental tasks of the older adult family and the relationship of the older adult family to other families within the developmental life cycle.

Developmental Tasks of Families in Retirement and Old Age

Duvall (Ross and Cobb 1990) described family development as progressing through eight stages, Table 19-1. The specific developmental tasks of Stage VIII (Families in Retirement and Old Age) include: confronting the psychological and physical changes of aging, adjusting to retirement from the world of work, adapting to diminished income, coping with altered living arrangements, and managing the loss of and bereavement for a spouse. Satisfactory achievement of the late-life family developmental tasks is not easy. Remarkable individual and family

Table 19–1   Eight Stages of Family Development

Stage I: Beginning Family (the couple establishing themselves as a unit)

Stage II: Early Childbearing (commences with the birth of the first child)

Stage III: Families with Preschoolers

Stage IV: Families with School-Age Children

Stage V: Families with Teenagers

Stage VI: Launching or Empty Nest Families (releasing children as young adults to the world)

Stage VII: Middle-Aged Families (begins when the last child leaves home and extends to retirement)

Stage VIII: Families in Retirement and Old Age

---

unit flexibility and adaptability in patterns of social interaction are required to meet the successive developmental challenges posed for this age group. Mastery of the developmental tasks requires substantial redefinitions of self, of one's marital partner, and of nuclear and extended family relationships.

In addition, the Stage VIII family involves primary and secondary relationships with kith and kin who are involved in expanding family networks of their own, each in its own stage of developmental evolution. Thus each family subunit is deeply involved in its own specific developmental concerns and, depending on the resources and energy consumed by these developmental obligations, may or may not be able to assist other subunits within the larger family network when the need arises. Occasionally developmental needs of one subunit are in direct opposition to the developmental needs of another, and conflict occurs within the family system.

Reciprocity as the Foundation for Caregiving

The Stage VIII family, while coping with new developmental tasks for itself, has lived through the prior stages of family development now being experienced by their significant others. By virtue of this experience, the older adult family often freely offers emotional support (care, empathy, love, nurturing), informational support (information provided to enable problem resolution), instrumental support (help with tasks, finances, and physical acts), and appraisal support (information that enables self-evaluation of performance) (Mercer 1983) to the evolving families and/or the individuals within them. According to the Exchange Theory of Social Interaction (Talbott

1990), which states that individuals seek balance in social exchanges, the provision of support tends to be reciprocated by younger families and usually acts to cement the ties of love and affection. However, the types of support exchanged may be dissimilar. For example, an older adult family may provide a Stage III family (with preschoolers) instrumental support in the form of babysitting. The young family may reciprocate by providing emotional support in the form of providing companionship during visits to the older couple's home. Each family or individual involved in the exchange tends to establish a value for the resource exchanged. In ongoing functional relationships there is both a conscious and unconscious desire of the participants to continue the reciprocity of equivalently valued goods and services for mutual benefit. Reciprocity occurs throughout the entire network of relationships accessed by the older adult family (or individual). It is the foundation of the family's desire to take care of "their own" as a result of exchanged love and affection or as a result of exchanges that demand, at the least, a return based on duty and obligation.

Reciprocity becomes a key issue in caregiving since caregivers within the family system function successfully only as long as reciprocity occurs. When it fails, either between the caregiver and the care recipient or between family caregivers themselves, the family caregiving network begins to crumble. Lack of reciprocity in the exchange of valued forms of support (emotional, informational, instrumental, or appraisal) leads to imbalances in social exchange and the persons involved in such exchanges will react negatively to them.

WHAT IS CAREGIVING?

Pearlin, Mullan, Semple, and Skaff (1990) described *caring* as the affective component of one's commitment to the welfare of another and *caregiving* as the behavioral expression of that commitment. These authors remind readers that caregiving is embedded in ordinary relationships. It refers to particular kinds of actions found in established primary role relationships, such as husband-wife and parent-child. The authors continue on to warn that, under some circumstances, caregiving is transformed from the ordinary exchange of assistance among those in close relationship to one another to an extraordinary and unequally distributed burden. A profound restructuring of relationships occurs when the dependency needs of one partner in the relationship increases. Caregiving, which may previously have been but one component of the total relationship, becomes the dominant, overriding component and expands to occupy the entirety of the social exchange. Reciprocity fades and help and assistance become unidirectional, proceeding only from the caregiver to the recipient.

Thus caregiving occurs in normal reciprocal relationships but may progressively change character. In extreme cases, caregiving may become a unidirectional and negative role in the life of the caregiver. In the final circumstance the caregivers have been described as "invisible victims" (Baldwin 1990, 173) who may as a result of caregiving become care recipients themselves.

The definitions of caregiving are not clear (Barer and Johnson 1990). Caregiving may mean periodic assistance and support to someone who lives alone in his or her own home; it may involve total physical care over a period of twenty-four hours in the caregiver's home; it may mean support and advocacy for someone in an institutional setting. Caregiving in this chapter refers to all of these. For example, caregiving usually involves a variety of tasks and responsibilities, such as those listed in Table 19-2.

Research and literature on family caregiving for older adults have proliferated in the last five years (Barer and Johnson 1990). Much of this literature has related to family caregiving for older family members who have a diagnosis of dementia of the

Table 19–2 Family Caregiving Tasks and Responsibilities

- Providing transportation for health care, shopping, church, and social activities

- Assisting with financial matters, such as paying bills and balancing a checkbook

- Helping with household tasks, such as repairs, cleaning, and laundry

- Assisting with food purchases and/or preparation

- Providing social and psychological support and care (e.g., spending time with the person, listening, recognizing the worth of the person)

- Directing physical care and providing assistance with activities of daily living (bathing, dressing, toileting, and walking)

- Assisting with gaining access to the health care system, coordinating health care services, and accompanying the older person to health care appointments

- Providing direct nursing care (injections, dressings, catheterizations)

- Compensation for sensory deficits (reading for an individual whose vision is impaired, writing for a person with hand tremors, etc.)

- Protecting the individual from harming self or others

- Providing spiritual support (accompany person to church or synagogue, reading religious texts, requesting visits from religious advisor)

Alzheimer's type (DAT) (Reed, Stone, and Neale 1990). While this focus has contributed greatly to the body of knowledge on caregiving, there are many other patient and family situations that are just as tragic and traumatic. But they have not yet received the national and local support and publicity that families dealing with Alzheimer's disease have received. Total care is needed for many other types of conditions, e.g., a paralyzing stroke or severe rheumatoid arthritis, and many other degenerative neurological problems that produce severe agitation, confusion, disorientation, and verbal and physically aggressive behavior. Home health case loads are filled with patients suffering from the debilitating effects of chronic obstructive pulmonary disease, terminal cancer, and end-stage renal disease. In the not-too-distant future, caregivers will provide care to a growing population of older adults who have HIV infection. Whatever the diagnosis, emotional, mental, and behavioral problems probably are more stressful to caregivers than is basic physical care related to activities of daily living.

WHO ARE THE CAREGIVERS?

The caregiver may be a spouse, daughter, son, daughter-in-law, sibling, friend, or other. Selection of family caregivers is a highly individualized process. One person may carry more responsibility than others by virtue of one or more of the following characteristics: only child, only female, most responsible, emotionally closest, geographically closest, or is a member of a helping profession (Green 1991). Seventy-two percent of the 2.2 million unpaid caregivers in the United States are women (Gaynor 1990). While daughters have been the primary caregivers of older parents in the past, more men are becoming involved in caregiving roles. In one study of the caregiver role among 302 older persons (Stoller and Pugliesi 1989) sons and daughters were almost equally represented (27.6 percent each). The authors suggested that perhaps there were more men because many of the older persons in this study had "limited impairment" (233).

In one study of 243 older participants by Stoller (1990) 24.7 percent of the primary helpers were sons (not spouses) and 22.6 percent of the helpers were daughters. Other primary helpers identified were male relative (5.3 percent), female relative (17.7 per-cent), male friend (11.1 percent), and female friend (18.5 percent). So men other than sons become helpers. Fathers more likely had son-helpers (67.6 percent) and mothers more likely had daughter-helpers (55.1 percent). Both men and women helped with household chores and finances, but men were less likely to help with traditional female types of activities such as meals, shopping, or laundry. Stoller (1990) suggested that further research needs to determine whether men are caregivers by choice and willingness or because they are the only family members able and willing to provide the care.

White-Means and Thornton's (1990b) research on labor market choices and home health care provision among employed ethnic caregivers indicates differences in the amount of time spent on daily caregiving tasks. Germans spent 2.45 hours per day; Irish—2.95 hours; English—2.82 hours; and African-Americans—4.2 hours. African-American and English women showed the highest overall average of daily care hours with 4.5 and 3.29 respectively. Irish and African-American men provided the next highest average care hours with 3.19 and 2.88 respectively. The researchers noted that compared to other groups, African-Americans clearly provide more hours of care without the use of substitutes than do other ethnic groups. They postulate that many African-Americans live in extended family groups where other members of the household may perform the routine tasks of family life freeing the caregiver to specialize in eldercare.

Visiting nurses often work with caregivers who are children. At times these children perform assistive, supplemental roles that aid the primary caregiver, such as providing companionship for the patient, assisting with transfers or feeding, or performing errands that would otherwise take the primary caregiver out of the home. However, at other times the role of the child is more central and he or she may be the primary caregiver. For example, an adolescent who was sixteen had already been caring for her mother for over three years. The patient required total care and was bedfast as a result of five strokes. Though she could communicate, she was completely dependent on her two teenaged children (her daughter and a younger son) for care. These two young people balanced the responsibilities of caregiving with mandatory school attendance by rotating school attendance, staggering class schedules, and alternating days of absenteeism. This care was even more remarkable because care had been maintained in this family for almost fifteen years by a series of siblings turning the caregiving responsibilities over to younger siblings as they reached maturity and left the home. More frequently, children are often substitute caregivers in the periods after school before adults return from work. In some of these families the older adult patient is left alone during school hours or the child is kept home from school to provide care if a crisis occurs. The final solution in which youthful caregivers are active is when the family does not speak English. In this case even a very young child (age 8 or 9) may be used as a translator to establish communication between the family and the health care system. Often the author finds that the English-speaking child assumes responsibility for the medication regimen and for instructing the other family members in implementation of the health care provider's instructions.

POSITIVE ASPECTS OF CAREGIVING

While there are many problems associated with caring for an older family member, there are also personal rewards. Adult children begin to renew—or perhaps experience for the first time—a close friend-to-friend relationship with older parents, as opposed to the parent-child relationship of their childhood and adolescent years before they left home. Such experiences can be rewarding to the caregiver as well as to the older parent. Grandchild-grandparent relationships also may be enhanced. These relationships help the children develop a greater understanding of their family heritage and increased respect for older persons.

For some three- and four-generation families who live together, there may be financial rewards because of shared housing and other expenses. A portion of the older person's retirement income may be used for the total family (e.g., for food) with, of course, the complete cooperation and consent of the older person. An older responsible grandchild may provide a few hours of selected care for the older person, perhaps for nominal payment. This plan would help all three generations, the older parent (care), the adult child (respite care), and the grandchild (pocket money). If the older person qualifies as a dependent, the family may benefit from reduced income taxes,

both because of an increased number of dependents in the family as well as deductions for such expenses as medical care, equipment, and supplies.

For those caregivers who do provide extensive, loving, and willing support to an older parent over many years, there should be few if any regrets or feelings of guilt after the parent dies. Some adult children feel guilty during the bereavement period, thinking "I should have done this or I should have done that" or "If only I had. . . ." If the adult child believes and feels that he or she did everything possible for the parent and was still able to maintain a happy, healthy, and productive personal and professional life, there should be no major feelings of regret or guilt during the period of bereavement.

CAREGIVER PROBLEMS AND BURDENS

Caregiving changes things. Lifestyle adjustments are required. At times these adjustments are minor and relatively easy to institute. At other times lifestyle changes are major, reaching the point where they destroy individual family caregivers and ultimately the caregiving network itself. Caregiving involves reciprocity. At times reciprocity cannot exist between the caregiver and the care recipient. However, for the caregiving system to survive, reciprocity must occur in the form of exchanges elsewhere within the family and professional caregiving network. No single individual can constantly give without burning out. Psychological and physical stores must be replenished before they are totally depleted. Therefore caregiving is a risky endeavor. Most caregivers are unaware of the potential hazards when the responsibilities of caregiving are assumed.

Alterations in the Caregiver/Care Recipient Relationship

As dependency needs of the older adult become greater, reciprocity in the relationship is lost and the balance of power in the caregiver/care recipient relationship changes. The care recipient may fear becoming a burden or become threatened by encroaching powerlessness within the relationship. Caregivers may go through a period of mourning for the loss of the relationship that was and feel acute and unexpected sorrow over the relationship that is evolving. When the social interaction between caregiver and care recipient becomes unilateral, the caregiver will be investing more in the relationship than he or she receives. This imbalance will be resented, if not greeted with outright hostility, unless other reciprocal relationships can fill the void.

Caregivers may be confronted with shifts in intimacy that expose them to the most private habits of family and/or friends, such as toileting, bathing, and maintenance of hygiene. Profound disappointment may occur when the care recipient exhibits uncharacteristic, aberrant, or socially unacceptable behavior.

Poorly Defined Caregiver Role

Some caregivers assume their responsibilities willingly but without awareness of the implications of that decision. For others the job evolves insidiously, progressively taking over larger parts of their lives. It may be hard for them to remember when critical transitions occurred or to define the changes involved in subordinating their own needs to those of another. Still other caregivers will have arrived at their position by default because there was simply no one else to do it. They have accepted their assignment, however unwillingly, and are simply trying to execute it within the limits of their resources.

The role of caregiver has no clearly defined job description. Each person faces unknown responsibilities. Because caregivers often are isolated and unable to share information with one another, it may be difficult to identify commonalities in one's own experience with that of others. Tasks of caregivers can be similar, but the process of implementation is unique within each caregiving system. Seldom do caregivers attempt to identify the specific elements of the job and ascertain whether portions of their position description are even appropriate or whether portions can be delegated to others (Green 1991).

Caregivers also experience conflict with others who vie for the principal caregiver role or who serve as caregiver substitutes. Sometimes these are other family members, each of whom wishes to gain the control and decision-making authority often seen as the prerogative of the primary caregiver. Competition may also occur when one family caregiver provides most of the physical care but another is preferred by the older adult as confidant, companion, or principal authority. Caregivers also face competi-

tion from professional health care providers. These providers may undermine the family caregiver's role by overzealous correction of mistakes or by negating information obtained from the caregiver regarding caregiving routines or effective strategies for managing caregiving tasks.

Lack of Knowledge and Preparation

American society is youth oriented. Americans do not study about the process of aging or prepare to live substantial portions of their lives as older people. Advanced age arrives unexpectedly and few adults can distinguish normal from abnormal changes of aging. Thus caregivers may have difficulty discriminating between care-recipient problems that need to be promptly evaluated and those that can safely be ignored.

Visiting nurses are familiar with the panic of caregivers who must administer injections, collect blood specimens, irrigate catheters, and care for Hickman lines. Performance of technical medical skills, taught to professional providers on a one-to-one basis over years of clinical instruction, are now routinely expected of family caregivers with a few hours of instruction. They may have seen the procedure demonstrated only once, have been shown a video in place of direct teaching, or have been given a pamphlet with diagrams to follow. The sane response to these unrealistic expectations is a high degree of insecurity. Caregivers are desperate for instruction and fear that their lack of competence may result in a loved one's death. Even simple caregiving skills such as lifting, bed-chair transfer, and bathing can be overwhelming until one has been shown these skills or has obtained equipment to make the execution of these tasks easier.

Younger and even middle-aged adults may have had little interaction with the health care delivery system and not know how to secure appropriate medical help, rehabilitative services, home health care, or short- or long-term nursing home placement. Once secured, the family may not know how to evaluate the efficacy of such care. Negotiating and coordinating programs such as Medicare, Medicaid, Supplemental Security Income, pension payments, and extended Medicare insurance policies can cause anxiety and stress. Discussions regarding finances between younger adults and their parent or other older adult relatives often commence for the first time. These conversations may be marked by evasiveness on the part of an older adult seeking to avoid disclosure of assets (or lack of assets) and timidity on the part of the caregiver who feels inappropriate exploring this very private realm. Discussions may also have to expand to cover such sensitive topics as wills, living wills, execution of durable powers of attorney, and guardianship to the mutual discomfort of all involved.

Intrafamily Conflict

The potential for conflict is just beneath the surface in most family caregiving networks. Sometimes such conflict is intergenerational between the caregiver and patient or between the patient's spouse and/or siblings and the younger generation caregivers. At other times the conflict occurs between younger contemporaries. Most often these conflicts center around issues of independence versus dependence, goals of caregiving, methods of reaching goals, caregiving values, perceptions of obligations and responsibilities, equitable divisions of labor, and finances.

Caregiving is an intimate, interpersonal process that can reactivate old wounds. Green (1991, 11) stated,

> "History that has been ignored or escaped reawakens and assumes new power when contact between the generations increases. Family events, secrets, and unresolved struggles from decades before demand attention through their silence or when they resurface during conflict. Relationships are then characterized by hypersensitivity or power struggles."

Surveillance and Vigilance

The caregiver frequently gives care twenty-four hours a day if living with the recipient(s) of care. If not in residence the caregiver has assumed responsibility for monitoring certain activities, patterns of activity, or temporal periods of the care recipient's life. The caregiver is involved in constant surveillance efforts to identify and control problematic behaviors of the patient. He/she must remain vigilant to protect the care recipient from harm to himself/herself or to others (Pearlin, Mullan, Semple, and Skaff 1990).

The functions of surveillance and vigilance may lead to a reluctance of caregivers to leave the older person at all for fear that something will happen while they are out of the house.

Social Isolation and Lack of Respite

Many caregiving situations are temporary in nature and have a positive outcome. The older adult(s) become independent and able to engage in the full reciprocity of normal social exchanges. The more problematic caregiving situations do not hold a favorable prognosis. These are characterized by a steady deterioration in the care recipient's condition. Many times the patient progresses from a state of independence in activities of daily living (ADLs) to requiring total around-the-clock care. Early in the caregiving cycle, family and friends rally around both patient and caregiver to provide assistance. Initially, home health and rehabilitation services also are provided as the patient is considered to have potential for rehabilitation; such services are reimbursable by Medicare.

When the responsibilities of caregiving continue day after day, week after week, and month after month, professional provider support services drop out as the patient's condition changes from rehabilitatable to custodial and he or she becomes ineligible for reimbursable services under the Medicare program. All but the most committed family and friends tend to drift away. As patient care requirements increase, few are willing to relieve the caregiver of tasks. In fairness to family and friends, these individuals are often afraid that they lack competence to provide the type of care required or may not have the time to give to the now extensive demands of caregiving. When vigilance and surveillance reach a zenith, the caregiver may be unable to leave the home, resulting in isolation, alienation from others, loss of leisure, lack of respite from caregiving, and physical fatigue. The constant demands of caregiving and an inability to predict an end to the daily grind robs the caregiver of ability to plan for the future and to anticipate a time when things will be better. Isolated, the caregiver may lose perspective; without validation from others, he/she may suffer loss of self-esteem and/or depression.

Role Conflict and Role Overload

Contemporary older adults and their caregivers participate in the options offered by a busy world. Most play multiple roles in the society at large, such as spouse, parent, child, sibling, employer, employee, friend, volunteer, church worker, and professional. Initially, caregivers and care recipients do not drop all external roles. Indeed one of the functions of the caregiver is to see that multiple roles are sustained by the care recipient. For caregivers, juggling multiple roles can result in role strain or role overload. This is especially true when an increasing number of activities must be wedged into smaller amounts of time. Stoller and Pugliese (1989, 235), however, found that "occupying additional roles contributes positively to well-being" of the caregiver, probably because of the additional contacts and support. "Other roles may buffer stresses originating from the caregiver role, provide links to additional resources, or bolster the caregiver's self-concept" (237). Caregivers therefore should continue to be active in the workplace and continue in other roles and activities in the community to the extent possible. The more external contacts, the better the caregiver can cope.

Role conflict and role strain are often greatest for Stage V, VI, and VII families who are approaching mid-life and dealing with complex developmental issues of their own. The adult individuals in these families are often referred to as members of the "sandwich generation." This term refers to middle-aged adult children who have the responsibility of caring for children and grandchildren as well as parents and grandparents. With an increasing number of older people living into their 90s and 100s, there is a greater prevalence of three-, four-, and five-generation families. Sometimes persons from each generation live in one house or at least in one neighborhood or city. Responsibilities related to the simultaneous care of all these persons can be extremely stressful for the adult child in the middle.

Psychological Stress

Caregiving of an older family member, even when direct physical care is not needed, can be very stressful. Examples of situations that can have a psychological impact on the family caregiver are shown in Table 19-3. Some of these behaviors may be manipulative because of a fear of loneliness or death, agitated depression, dementia, or a tendency to become more self-centered in the old-old (over age 85). Whatever the older person's condition or medical diagnosis, he or she often does not have insight into the effects of these behaviors on the caregiver.

Gibeau and Anastas (1989) studied seventy-seven women who were working full-time and who were also primary caregivers for an older family member. They stated that as a result of caregiving they experienced emotional stress (94 percent), sadness (24 percent), and anxiousness. They also noted that "solutions to their problems will have to include a range of resources in the workplace, in the family, and in the community" (37). The fact that most community support services are only available during the day is also a major problem.

Life-long relationships among family members and social support available to the caregiver are probably more important in the degree of stress among caregivers than is the degree of severity of the older person's illness (Morris, Morris, and Britton 1988). Caregiving is much more stressful for those caregivers who have never had a good relationship with the care recipient than for those caregivers who have had a long, close, loving relationship with the care recipient.

People face difficult transitions when a chronic illness is first diagnosed or when decisions suddenly have to be made about living arrangements. Sometimes a period of transition is more difficult than the later time when decisions and adjustments have been made and a routine of caregiving has been instituted, even though caregiving may be more intense in the latter circumstance.

Two of the most common caregiver problems are those of fatigue and depression. Guilt is a major feature of both. The caregiver may feel that he or she cannot provide the type of care needed. However, the amount and type of care needed may be overwhelming, especially if given on a twenty-four hour basis. The caregiver must be helped to realize that one person cannot do everything and that all anyone can expect is to do the best he or she can.

Because of the increasing longevity of many parents (80s, 90s, 100s), many caregivers are themselves getting old (50s, 60s, and 70s). They too may begin to be affected by health problems and tire more easily. Also, they begin to think about the possible

Table 19–3   Examples of Situations Causing Psychological Stress for Caregivers

- An 82-year-old man tells his middle-aged daughter as she leaves for work, "I'll be dead when you get back."

- An 85-year-old woman arrives at her 63-year-old daughter's house every morning at 7:30 A.M. because she is bored at home.

- A 92-year-old woman tells her daughter by telephone that if she does not come to see about her right away, she will call 911 (the local emergency number).

- An 85-year-old man talks constantly from 10 P.M. to 5 A.M., keeping family members awake. (He can sleep all day while they must go to work.)

- A middle-aged woman is responsible for the care of her aging mother and mother-in-law, both of whom are bedfast and being cared for in the caregiver's home.

- An 86-year-old man embarrasses his alert 83-year-old wife and daughter by accusing his wife in front of others of having an affair with another man.

- An 89-year-old woman can no longer write her own checks or balance her own checkbook, but she will not trust her only daughter with signed checks made out to pay bills.

effects of aging on themselves as they care for aging relatives. This can contribute to anxiety and/or depression.

Depression is a major problem for both caregiver and care recipient. Depression is the most common functional psychiatric disorder of older adults (Meyers and Alexopoulas 1988). Estimates of depressed older adult populations in combined community and nursing home settings range from 5 percent to 65 percent (St. Pierre, Craven, and Bruno 1986). A longitudinal study of normal older volunteers resulted in the identification of 30 percent of the sample as suffering from mild depressive symptoms (Meyers and Alexopoulas 1988). Blazer (1986) reported that approximately 15 percent of older adults mention significant depressive symptoms. Parmelee, Katz, and Lawton's (1989) study of 708 older nursing home and congregate apartment residents revealed that 12.4 percent of subjects met the DSM-III-R criteria for major depression, another 30.5 percent of the sample reported less severe but nonetheless marked depressive symptoms. In a survey of 74 home health care patients responding to items on the Geriatric Depression Scale, one of the authors found that 39 percent of the sampled patients had scores compatible with the presence of depression (Brow-

ning 1991). Depression negatively impacts the ability of both patient and caregiver to respond to new situations, to summon energy for caregiving or self-care tasks, to attend to and retain instructions, and to make decisions. Furthermore, depression affects bodily functions, causing alterations in rest and sleep, in nutritional intake and metabolism, in gastrointestinal functions, and in the perception of pain and other somatic symptoms.

In a study of caregiver burden, Stoller and Pugliese (1989) found that caregiver burden caused stress and depression when

- the caregiver and older person lived together.

- personal care assistance was needed.

- the caregiver viewed the health of the older person negatively.

- relationships between the caregiver and older person were not positive.

Psychological stress also occurs as a result of unrealistic expectations. Caregivers may have beliefs about what a "good son" or "good daughter" should do. They may falsely believe that if they were providing care the "right" way, relationships with parents would be smooth and free of difficulties. These caregivers may be vulnerable to a myth that everyone else has control of their situation and has figured out the "right" way to do things and ensure success. The resulting false belief is that the caregiver alone has failed in the task of caregiving (Green 1991). In these cases the caregivers establish an impossibly high standard of performance and are doomed to failure with all of its self-doubt and recriminations.

Caregivers also experience stress when they allow demanding and abusive behavior from the care recipient to go unchallenged. Care recipients, like caregivers, become isolated from social interaction and discourse. In addition they must deal with the frustration of declining capacity, lack of energy, diffuse somatic distresses, pain, and depression. As a result care recipients become irritable and cranky. However, without the constraints and restrictions on behavior imposed in normal social settings, the older person causes increased caregiver stress with erratic cooperation, psychological control, and frank verbal abuse. In public, more restraint in behavior would be shown to one's worst enemy than some care recipients show toward the caregiver. Often the caregiver attributes this behavior to illness and excuses it. In some cases—such as the dementias—the behavior is a result of disease. However, it can also be the result of projected frustration hurled toward the nearest and safest target—sometimes the only available target. Tragically, such behavior reflects a loss of socialization skills and may gradually become a habituated response.

Caregiver Illness

Long-term caregiving appears to exact a toll on the immune system of caregivers. They experience more infections and more stress-related illnesses such as hypertension and heart disease than non-caregivers (Baldwin 1990; Gaynor 1990). Gaynor (1989) described a health-to-illness trajectory in her study of eighty-seven female caregivers. From the first two to twenty-one months of caregiving, study subjects reported no difficulty with health problems. By thirty-two months of caregiving, tranquilizers appeared on medication lists and the use of aspirin for musculo-skeletal complains increased markedly. By month thirty-eight, subjects described themselves as "un-

healthy" (p. 123). They reported the existence of stress-related illnesses such as colitis and hypertension. Until the thirty-sixth month, caregivers negotiated with the care recipient for uninterrupted sleep. After thirty-six months, negotiations regarding rest had ceased and the caregivers' lives revolved completely around the care of the spouse. They also seemed to have ceased caring about their own health. By month fifty, the subjects frequently reported illness and had become passive about health maintenance. They described only two health related activities: resting and taking medicine. Gaynor deduced that a critical transition from health to illness occurred between twenty-four and thirty-two months after the commencement of caregiving.

Financial Strain

Long-term caregiving imposes financial burdens. Families in mid-life are often purchasing a home, financing college educations, and saving for their own retirement. Declining purchasing power has mandated dual earners in households to maintain middle-class lifestyles. Poor families must work long hours at low wages just to survive. The poorest of the poor must stretch public assistance dollars that are steadily shrinking. Unless the care recipient can finance all or most of the goods and services required for care, the family caregiving network will need to subsidize the costs of long-term care. Medication purchases often prove to be the first of the financial shocks as chronically ill adults usually take several prescription medications. Many of the items that facilitate caregiving tasks and make life pleasant for the care recipient prove prohibitively expensive over time. For example, the cost of adult waterproof pants and plastic bed protectors (used to make the management of incontinence easier) and the cost of nutritional supplements (if the older person will not or cannot eat) are not reimbursable insurance benefits. Purchase of such items rapidly outpaces the fiscal resources of families who must also buy medications and pay insurance premiums, deductibles, physicians' uncovered fees, and transportation costs to and from health care facilities. Finally, if caregivers must sacrifice gainful employment to care for a family member, the income lost may place the family unit in a crisis of survival.

NURSING INTERVENTIONS

Nurses need to accept responsibility for designing structural systems that support the family caregiving network. Creation of such systems does not depend on and need not wait for federal government sanction, authorization of third party payors, or institutional restructuring. Eventually each of these will be desirable. But large-scale change is still many years in the future and family caregivers and care recipients need assistance now. Nurses can begin by using resources and other professionals readily available in most practice environments. These resources and attributes include: perceptive assessment skills; collaboration with other professionals (physicians, social workers, physical therapists, occupational therapists, speech-language pathologists, nutritionists, pharmacists, discharge planners, and home health liaison nurses); referral to other nursing colleagues (visiting nurses, adult or gerontological nurse practitioners, and clinical nurse specialists); and knowledge of community resources, particularly those that can be accessed through Area Agencies on Aging or other senior service coordinating groups in the local community.

Creating Primary Interventions

Nurses work with other nurses in defined environments for the purpose of delivering client/patient health care services. Within these environments practitioners develop patterns of care delivery and norms of work. Many patterns of care delivery are mandated by regulators and institutional licensing authorities, such as the Joint Commission for Accreditation of HealthCare Organizations (JCAHO) and the Health Care Financing Administration (HCFA). However, the most important decisions regarding patterns of care and the ones that determine the quality and depth of services are made by the individual and collective action of nurses who work with clients and caregivers day to day. By mutual consent they decide what will be important and become a part of the work norm and what has to be ignored or not given much emphasis.

One of the first decisions to be made by the nursing team is to look for and identify clients who currently or soon will need to become part of a family caregiving system. Nurses must pay attention to the long-term implications of the conditions manifested by their clients whether they are in acute care beds or are being seen in an outpatient setting. Too often nurses focus only on the task of the moment, the current treatment or medication, or resolving immediate crises. Nurses must begin to project client needs two weeks, six months, or a year into the future. Nothing begins to happen for a client until the professional provider activates the system on the client's behalf. For example, consider the long-term care implications for the clients shown in Table 19-4. None of the patients described in Table 19-4 will be capable of self-care when initially discharged from an acute care facility. They will all need assistance with activities of daily living (ADLs) and medical treatments. None of these conditions, in and of themselves, require institutionalization. Given the right support system, all can be managed effectively in the home care setting. However, for effective home care to occur, nurses must identify the high-risk clients early and carefully plan an orderly transition from the acute care bed to the home care living room. Seldom is this first step ever taken. Naylor's (1990) study of hospitalized older adults indicates that 85 percent of the patients needed supportive care following discharge, but only 20 percent of these older adults received discharge-planning services. Therefore the first responsibility of the nurse is to identify the client at risk. Subsequently he or she should collaborate with the family and physician to ensure that appropriate referrals are made to establish a caregiving network.

Nurses should be aware that in many institutions discharge planners and home health liaison nurses are not allowed to approach families with discharge-planning services until they have first been referred by a nurse or physician. Nurses, in conjunction with the physician, should work with the client and family and determine their specific desires before referrals are made. Families may elect to manage client care alone without assistance from home health care professionals. However, they may desire assistance from the acute care staff in learning procedures and techniques that will be required to execute care after discharge.

The nursing team should also make some basic decisions about dealing with families in their professional setting. For example: What kinds of information will be given to family members? Which family

Table 19–4 Examples of Patients Needing Long-Term Caregiving

- An 86-year-old stroke patient with right-sided hemiparesis, impaired communication, and difficulty swallowing

- A 76-year-old patient with chronic obstructive pulmonary disease who suffers severe shortness of breath when dressing, needs continuous oxygen, and suffers confusion and disorientation when stressed

- An 82-year-old woman who suffers from an inflammatory inner ear disorder causing bouts of extreme dizziness and nystagmus

- A 70-year-old cancer patient with a new tracheostomy that will need frequent suctioning and who will be receiving pain control medications and radiation together with chemotherapy

- A 69-year-old new widow who is suffering from depression so severe that, in her self-absorption, she forgets to eat, does not dress, and will not leave home

- An 88-year-old with congestive heart failure and coronary artery disease whose peripheral edema makes walking almost impossible and who becomes short of breath on exertion when talking or eating

- A 90-year-old with pneumonia and anemia who is extremely weak and on a 10 medication regimen

---

members will be given information? Which nurses work best with families and like to teach families caregiving skills? What type of communication systems do members of the acute care staff wish to establish with visiting nurses and outpatient gerontological nurse colleagues? What types of in-service do staff need to improve care for older adults and family systems? How will staff work with discharge planners and home health liaison nurses? Are gerontological clinical specialists or nurse practitioners available for case consultation with the staff? Can these experts be used to demonstrate the delivery of direct care services? How does the staff wish to use the skills of a family caregiver when a client being cared for at home is readmitted to the institution? What courtesies will be offered to family members (coffee, meals, use of the lounge, assistance in locating physicians)?

The staff should periodically spend time clarifying their values related to family support and make group decisions that all can support. This is an internal nursing matter and should not be dependent on directives from some external source.

Assessing the Family System

Health care providers seldom take the time to assess the family system and tend to act on assumptions that

may be erroneous. For example, a 76-year-old farmer was admitted ambulatory to a hospital. Within twenty-four hours he became confused and disoriented and was diagnosed as suffering from severe anemia secondary to previously undiagnosed multiple myeloma. His condition was complicated by the dramatic effects of alcohol withdrawal.

The physician, the nursing staff, and social work staff tried to communicate with the patient's wife who became very anxious and refused to make decisions expected of her. After a number of days of frustrating dialogue between the wife and staff, a niece who happened to be a nurse arrived from out-of-state and was able to clarify the situation. Her aunt was overwhelmed by the hospital setting and was paralyzed with fear over her husband's cancer diagnosis. A simple woman, she functioned well in her home on the farm but the trip into the city placed her in a new environment and provoked tremendous anxiety. Not used to making decisions, she was having difficulty understanding what she was being told and was therefore concerned about the decisions she was being asked to make. One such decision was to give consent for a "Do Not Resuscitate" order. The niece explained that the patient worked closely with his two brothers who owned and managed a series of large farms. She further explained that the patient's older brother might be the most appropriate one to participate in the decision-making process because he held the patient's durable power of attorney. In this case the staff made the assumption that because the wife was the closest living relative, she was the one who would assume legal responsibility for the patient. They were wrong.

Situations such as this occur regularly and create unbelievable chaos leading to dangerous errors in judgment. Nurses should therefore take time to assess and clarify the precise family situation of the older client. First and foremost if he or she is competent, the client should be asked about his/her personal desires regarding management of the family. Who does the client wish to be involved in decisions regarding his/her care? Who does the client wish to be given information about his/her prognosis, treatment, or changes in condition? Does the client want all family to be allowed to visit or does he or she want family visits restricted? Should the client become incapacitated, which family member is authorized to make decisions? When the client is incapacitated, health care providers may wish to talk with several family members in order to identify the power structure and organization of the family before selecting specific family members with whom they will negotiate. It is critical that nurses determine who has legal authority for decision making and whether that individual has the knowledge or skill to execute that authority. For example, in the situation of the farmer, a second niece, abhorred by the family system and normally rarely seen by the client, made lengthy daily visits to the hospital and presented herself to the staff as "almost a daughter" to the patient.

Of more importance to the long-term well-being of the older adult, family assessments help health care providers evaluate the feasibility of constructing a family caregiving network. Potential participants in the network can be identified and their value to the client can be ascertained. In addition such assessments can, from the outset, assist caregivers to define caregiving as a group responsibility and to identify the specific participants in the group effort. Questions related to family assessment are located in Appendix B. However a specialized technique can be used that readily crystallizes family relationships. This technique is family assessment by genogram.

Genograms are based on a systems-theory approach to family structure and are a method of visually illustrating, reducing, ordering, and simplifying material describing complex family interactions. The genogram portrays the family system through time and allows the client to step outside the family system to describe family dynamics and identify how characteristics, role assignments, past history, and patterns of communication affect the current situation (Ross and Cobb 1990). Genograms are an elaboration of a family tree and may be used to give information about the genetic, medical, social, behavioral, and cultural aspects of a family system (Herth 1989). Herth stated that the manner in which the genogram is taken may be more important than the actual data collected. She noted that the interaction between provider and client involves several processes: social interaction, reminiscing, and evolving of self. That the interaction involved during the collection of a genogram may in and of itself have therapeutic value is a chief recommendation for its use according to Herth (1989).

Genograms begin by drawing the basic family structure that includes those considered to be significant others in a diagrammatic family-tree format. The tree can be constructed going back as far as the client remembers or may be abbreviated to more recent generations if time and efficiency demand. After the diagram has been drawn, information is requested regarding each of the individuals identified. Objective information includes the content listed in Table 19-5. As the individuals are described by the older adult, subjective information regarding the strength of emotional bonds, closeness, or distance, should be evaluated and symbolized. The nurse may wish to use color coding for this process. The margins of the genogram may be used to note critical life events, successes, transitions, and losses as they have occurred in relation to the individuals being discussed. Health care providers focus particularly on the nature of relationships with current contemporaries to identify individuals who provide emotional and/or instrumental support and are candidates for membership in the family caregiving network.

Symbols are used in genogram construction. Males are represented by squares and females by circles. Husbands are placed to the left and wives to the right; they are connected by a solid straight line to indicate marriage. The date of their marriage is placed on the solid line connecting them. Other kin are joined similarly by solid lines linking them in their relative relationship to one another. Deceased individuals are indicated by an *X* placed through their square or circle. The older adult client is usually identified by a double square or double circle depending on gender. Families of origin usually appear above the client on the tree and families of procreation beneath. People who are not family members, such as friends, paid companions, or home health aides, but who are closely involved in family life should be included on the genogram. Their squares or circles are connected by a dotted line to the family member(s) to whom they are the closest (Smoyak 1987). Thus symbolic representation follows the familiar pattern seen in the construction of genealogical family trees, see Figure 19-1. However, nurses need not become overly involved in symbolic representation on the genogram. If they wish to develop more complex schematic illustrations, they may refer to the literature in psychiatric and family nursing for detailed instructions. Practically speaking, any mutually agreed upon symbols can be used by the client, family, and nurse to represent relationships for the purpose of discussion.

Construction of genograms also provides nurses with other valuable bits of assessment information about the older adult. Physical construction of the genogram allows the nurse to observe the presence of functional hearing and/or visual problems, attention span, long- and short-term memory, expressive and receptive communication, fine motor skills, and behavior.

Genograms by their very nature stimulate reminiscence; they help older adults recognize the skills they have used to survive in the past that they can transfer to their current situation. Memories provide the older adult with an inner source of continuity and universality. As he or she reviews the lives of parents, grandparents, and distant ancestors, they recognize the significance of their own place in the process of birth, life, experience, and eventual death. Thus the genogram can boost self-esteem and a sense of well-being (Herth 1989).

Assisting Caregivers to Understand Their Roles

Nurses and other health care providers need to provide family caregivers with anticipatory guidance regarding the caregiver role. Family members who will serve in this capacity need to understand and weigh both the benefits and burdens (advantages and disadvantages) of accepting caregiver responsibilities. They need to identify the specific tasks and responsibilities they will have as caregiver and to identify whether these are realistic or whether a greater division of labor among family members will be required.

A job description should be written out in behavioral terms so that caregivers can articulate to

Table 19–5   Information Needed to Prepare a Genogram

Names

Age (or for deceased individuals, date and cause of death)

Location/residence

Major role/occupation/retirement status

Education

Health problems

Ethnic orientation

Religion

(Adapted from Herth 1989; Smoyak 1987; Ross and Cobb 1990)

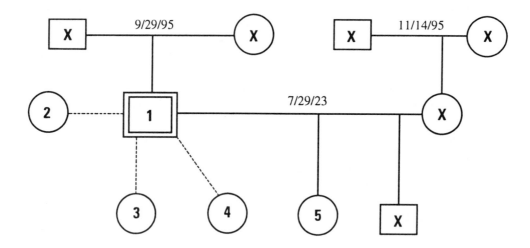

1. OLDER CLIENT
2. PAID CAREGIVER
3. NEIGHBOR CAREGIVERS
4. VOLUNTEER CAREGIVER WHO PROVIDES RESPITE CARE
5. DAUGHTER CAREGIVER

NOTE: ALTHOUGH THERE IS ONLY ONE FAMILY CAREGIVER, THERE ARE SEVERAL OTHER NONRELATIVE CAREGIVERS. THIS INFORMATION WILL BE HELPFUL TO THE NURSE.

Figure 19–1   Sample genogram

themselves and to others the expectations of caregiving (Green 1991). The job description also assists family caregivers in identifying the types of external support services (visiting nurses, homemakers, adult day care, and home health aides) that will be necessary to sustain the caregiving network.

Periodically, the job description needs to be rewritten and revised to reflect additional responsibilities and burdens acquired as a result of the client's changing physical and/or psychological status. Finally, the job description may be used by health care providers to assist caregivers in recognizing that they are performing a real job. The job description can be used to praise and evaluate successful performance and to identify areas of difficulty that will require supportive revision. For example, when asked what she does, the caregiver may respond, "I just take care of my husband." However, viewing the job descrip-

tion that lists thirty-five specific behavioral tasks will encourage her to redefine her role as organizing and coordinating complex nursing and social support services. She may also see the wisdom of building in respite and vacations from her responsibilities—a value held by all employed workers. If caregivers are unable to construct a job description, nurses may wish to construct and share sample behavioral task lists with the family to initiate discussion.

Caregivers should be warned from the outset of the burdens of long-term caregiving and the importance of the adherence to regular health maintenance activities. Specific strategies for maintaining health should be identified and commitments (such as the use of interpersonal contracts) should be obtained so that follow-through will occur. *The importance of rest and respite as essential activities should be presented to the caregiver.*

Managing Transition Periods

Changes in the health status of the care recipient may occur precipitously (as in the case of a stroke) or insidiously over time (as in the case of Alzheimer's disease). Precipitous events are marked by clear transition periods. Insidious progressions are marked by subtle turning points usually linked with changes in the performance of IADLs or ADLs. During transition periods families need help to group or regroup.

Following precipitous events, the initial period between client diagnosis and the commencement of family caregiving is often marked by shock, denial, grief, loss, and disorganization within the family system. Members of the system may vacillate daily from one set of emotions to another and flounder when making decisions. Initial decisions may prove wrong or impractical and the first family member to serve as principal caregiver may not ultimately be the most effective one.

Health care providers should recognize this period as one of intense disorganization and should not push family members to make permanent decisions for which they are not ready. Information should be provided regarding options open to the family and emphasis should be placed on the acceptability of making interim decisions that may be changed as the situation evolves. For example, caregivers may initially decide to take the client home and provide total care unassisted. The family should be helped to understand subsequent actions that they may wish to take without loss of face or stature as caregivers. Such actions may include help from the visiting nurse, placement in adult day care, or eventual nursing home placement.

Families should be cautioned to proceed slowly with decisions and warned against making too many major changes at once. Health care providers should assist the family to make decisions that are as compatible as possible with the current structure and operation of the family system until stability is achieved. Subsequently, well-researched and considered decisions may be made. Flexibility should be stressed as the key to sustained caregiving. No decision should be considered permanent. Change can, should, and will be required over time.

Attention should be given to the types of decisions that may need to be made over the course of caregiving. The principal caregiver should identify the family members who will need to be involved in these decisions. Family members who live in other cities or states should not be excluded from decision-making roles; they are often active participants in the family caregiving network. Their suggestions and feelings may be central to the decision-making process. These long-distance caregivers participate in the caregiving network by providing emotional and informational support by phone and instrumental support in the form of financial assistance to the principal caregiver or care recipient.

The family may also wish to select a principal spokesperson (may or may not be the primary caregiver). This person will deal with the physician or other health care providers and will issue bulletins to the remaining family members regarding changes in the care recipient's condition or treatment. This plan allows the family greater control over the flow of information and reduces garbled or conflicting information between the caregiving network and the health care system. This plan also helps health care providers who may become confused when confronted by demands for information from too many family members.

During the transition period, finances should be discussed. If the older adult will need to have health care costs subsidized by family members, the amount, distribution, and timing of such payments should be agreed to by contributors. If the care recipient desires to pay family members for services rendered, the exact nature of services expected should be delineated and agreed to in advance. The nature of such arrangements should be made clear to other members of the caregiving network so that jealousy and resentment do not inadvertently occur.

Learning Needs of Caregivers

Family caregivers usually have much to learn and need to understand that learning will take time. In the interval between ignorance and mastery of knowledge they will feel insecure and even panicky. They need to be warned about these feelings and assured that such feelings do not imply lack of current or eventual competence. Providers should create structure by clearly identifying what professional support systems will be available, what specific assistance they will provide, and how and when they can be accessed. Furthermore, types of emergencies and crises that may confront the family in the early caregiving period should be anticipated. The family should be given instructions for their management. For example, if a care recipient is discharged home with a new tracheostomy that family members must suction, the family may be offered the following plan for management of the situation:

1. The inpatient staff will teach caregiver(s) to perform suctioning techniques and observe at least ten return demonstrations from the caregiver(s) during the five-day period prior to discharge. The client will also be referred to the Visiting Nurse Association and a home visit will be requested for the afternoon of discharge.

2. The visiting nurse will visit on a daily basis for the first week after discharge to reinforce prior teaching and to provide additional instruction regarding management of the client's care. Following this first week the frequency of visits will be decreased, but the visiting nurse will remain involved with the family for a period of sixty days.

3. In case of an emergency (e.g., bleeding from the tracheostomy, difficulty breathing, or swelling and infection around the tracheostomy site or on client's neck and face), if unable to secure an immediate evaluation from the physician or visiting nurse, the client should be taken to the nearest hospital emergency room by ambulance.

In other words the family should be given a framework of support in which they can find safety. But they must also understand the benefits and limitations of the resources available to them.

During the learning interval, teaching of specific caregiving skills is a major role of the nurse in both inpatient and outpatient settings. Careful attention should be given to what the family identifies it wishes to learn. These learning requests should become the top priority of the nurse unless the need to teach some critical, lifesaving technique takes precedence over the family's desires. Nurses may supplement the family's priority list with additional skills or information that will be necessary to provide the desired level of care for both caregiver and care recipient.

It is helpful if the nurse collaborates with the family to create a time line for instruction. This plan helps family members establish realistic expectations regarding mastery attainment and reduces diminished self-esteem when tasks are not learned on the first try. As in the example great care should be taken to explain how tasks not yet mastered will be managed during the learning interval. Clients may be institutionalized by a family caregiving system that erroneously believes itself to be incompetent because unrealistic expectations were established for learning and no support was provided during the learning process. Trial-and-error learning is terrifying to families who perceive their loved one's life to be at risk if they make a mistake.

The family may also need help negotiating the health care system and need to be taught how to coordinate services delivered by many providers. For example, the client may have a primary care physician in addition to two or more specialists (e.g., an oncologist and a cardiologist), a visiting nurse, a home health aide, a physical therapist, a homemaker, a social worker, and a respiratory equipment vendor. The caregiver needs to acquire control over this group of health care providers and the associated appointment times that must be scheduled to accommodate their services without exhausting both the caregiver and care recipient. Initially, caregivers often become victims of the busy schedules of these providers. Caregivers need to be empowered to establish realistic and humane schedules compatible with the needs of the family.

Caregivers also need help in identifying the impact that caregiving will have on household arrangements and routines. For example, if the care recipient is bedfast, where is the bed to go and what are the implications of that decision? If the bed goes upstairs, will the caregiver have to run up and down all day? Will the care recipient be isolated from family activities such as communal dining, television viewing, or conversation? If the bed goes in the living room, will the children be able to bring guests home? Will the family be able to watch television? Will the care recipient be able to get adequate rest? Would a commode chair at the bedside render the living room unsuitable for family gatherings?

Scheduling of activities, including respite and vacations, needs to be reviewed. It is common for caregivers to become so consumed with caregiving that regular household activities such as cleaning, shopping, and attending religious services cannot be managed. Sometimes nurses can help caregivers step back and evaluate the schedule to see whether tasks can be grouped, delegated, reduced in frequency, or omitted altogether.

Caregivers need to develop strategies for managing visits to the physician or gerontological nurse practitioner. They need guidance in identifying information that should be maintained for provider review, such as blood sugar readings, weight and girth fluctuations, fluid intake and urinary output, dietary intake, timing and frequency of periods of disorientation, changes in size of and drainage from wounds, patterns of pain, and response to medications. Family caregivers need encouragement to identify and organize questions and requests to make of the physician or nurse provider. They need to develop confidence in their ability to actively collaborate in the creation and design of medical and nursing regimens. The members of the family caregiving network may need to discuss who should accompany the care recipient to appointments. Should it be the family member with the most health care training? The one with the best memory? The strongest to help with mobility? The one who learns the easiest? Should one, two, or three members of the caregiving network accompany the ill family member? In addition, criteria by which the family can evaluate the quality of care given to the care recipient need to be identified. Family members need to be taught the process for securing second opinions and/or changing primary care providers when care is deemed inadequate.

Caregivers from the younger generation may be unfamiliar with the Medicare program and may falsely believe that it covers all of the older adult's health-related expenses. The family will need clarification regarding covered versus uncovered Medicare expenses, participating providers, benefit periods and associated deductibles, copayments, and the distinction between a Medicare bill and a Medicare statement. They may need referral to a community resource that will aid them in filling out Medicare forms and analyzing the status of billing and payment. If the older adult's finances are limited, the caregiver may need instruction in how to apply for public assistance and Medicaid to cover expenses not covered by Medicare. Caregivers also need to be directed to other programs such as rent rebates, energy assistance, home repair and weatherization services, and medication subsidy programs. Family caregivers may also wish to explore the feasibility of enrolling frail older adults in community care option programs. These programs are selectively administered under Medicare and offer expanded benefits to targeted groups of recipients. If the care recipient is terminally ill, family members should be given information about the hospice benefit under Medicare and assisted to understand how the selection of that option will impact their standard Medicare services. They may also be taught the differences between palliative (hospice) and curative (standard Medicare) care and be willing to accept the benefit restrictions of the program chosen.

Finally, the caregiver may need information regarding community resources. When an older person becomes ill and begins to be more and more dependent, families might first think that nursing home placement is needed, probably because they are not aware of other alternatives and resources. However, the nursing home should be considered as a last resort in most instances rather than a first choice. There are an increasing number of various types of support services in most communities for older adults, see Table 19-6. Many of these services would help family caregivers continue to maintain older persons in their own home or the house of a relative for a longer period of time. (See chapters 20 and 21 for a more detailed discussion of these types of services.)

Support for Caregivers

The previous discussion centered around community services to help the caregiver provide care to an older family member. However, there is also a need to provide various kinds of specific support for the caregiver. Examples of support for caregivers are shown in Table 19-7.

The perceptive nurse—whether in the hospital, clinic, home, or nursing home—will recognize an adult caregiver who is experiencing personal problems and stress related to elder caregiving. The caregiver may appear tired, perhaps with little attention to personal grooming; anxious yet depressed, possibly with recent weight gain or loss; and overly concerned about the health status and perhaps nursing care being given to his or her parent. The nurse should recognize this need and provide specific written material about information and support groups in the community, see Figure 19-2. The caregiver may not want to admit that he or she needs

Table 19–6   Community Resources for Older Adults That Help to Relieve Family Caregivers

- Retirement centers (independent, but decreases need for house and yard upkeep)

- Congregate living (older persons living together)

- Foster home care (personal services and supervision)

- Share a home (prevents living alone)

- Live-in assistance (may be expensive)

- Senior centers (nutrition, recreation, counseling)

- Adult day care (social or medical)

- Home-delivered meals

- Transportation services (medical care and shopping)

- Lifeline or Careline (home emergency response systems)

- Errand and assurance (shopping assistance)

- Telephone reassurance (daily telephone contact)

- Home health care (intermittent care from nurses and allied health professionals)

- Carrier alert (postman reports on lack of mail pickup)

- Assisted living centers (personal care)

- Hospice care (help with the terminally ill)

- Homemaker service (help with household chores)

Table 19–7   Examples of Support for Caregivers

- Direct physical care of the care recipient (e.g., home health care by a licensed nurse or home health aide to help relieve fatigue)

- Homemaker services to relieve caregiver of household chores (e.g., assistance with cooking, cleaning)

- Information (e.g., about the aging process, communicating with older family members, and how to access community services)

- Individual and/or group psychological support and counseling (e.g., help with feelings of manipulation, anger, guilt, and depression)

- Respite care (e.g., volunteer relief for a couple of hours to go walking or shopping; nursing home care for one weekend or one week for a short vacation) help at the moment, but with written information in hand can decide at a later time to pursue such assistance. The nurse should provide other information about community resources, especially about respite care. Most of all if it is obvious that the person is very distressed, he or she should be referred for psychological and/or psychiatric counseling, preferably to a geropsychiatric nurse, gerontologist psychologist, or geriatric psychiatrist. The nurse should also help caregivers recognize that they have done everything possible for older family members and that they have no reason to feel guilty about their care.

Although the use of formal, external community services may be helpful and essential in many instances (e.g., skilled nursing care), Stoller and Pugliesi (1989, 236) found that the "use of formal support systems produces feeling of failure and guilt among caregivers." The caregiver may believe that "I should be able to do this for my mother." Nurses need to recognize this potential concern therefore in their care and support of the patient and the caregiver. The

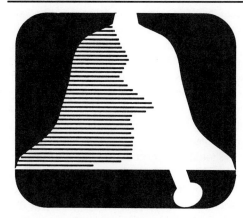

AS PARENTS GROW OLDER

A Series of Programs for Adults
With Aging Parents

IF YOU HAVE CONCERNS ABOUT

    *LIVING ARRANGEMENTS FOR YOUR AGING PARENT
    *PSYCHOLOGICAL AND EMOTIONAL ASPECTS OF AGING
    *CHRONIC ILLNESSES OF YOUR ELDERLY PARENT AND HOW TO MANAGE THEM
    *COMMUNITY SERVICES FOR THE ELDERLY
    *YOUR ABILITY TO MANAGE STRESSFUL TIMES WITH YOUR AGING FAMILY

THEN THESE PROGRAMS WILL BENEFIT YOU.

"As Parents Grow Older" is a series of six sessions designed to give information and support to adults caring for an aging family member. The sessions enable adult children to better understand the physical and psychological aspects of aging, identify their family needs, locate helpful community resources, and share feelings and coping strategies.

Sessions are held one night a week for six weeks. The following topics are discussed:

    WEEK 1 Understanding the Psychological Aspects of Aging
    WEEK 2 Chronic Illness and Behavioral Changes with Age
    WEEK 3 Sensory Loss and Improving Communication
    WEEK 4 Living Arrangements and Shared Decision Making
    WEEK 5 Availability and Use of Community Resources
    WEEK 6 Understanding Our Feelings

The series is offered on a continuing basis. For more information, call the Mental Health Association.

Figure 19–2 Example of caregiver information and support sessions

nurse should try to assure the caregiver that everything possible has been done for the family member.

Nurses should provide caregiver information (facts about normal aging and community resources) and support (listening and discussing alternatives). Nurses should not encourage either institutional or home care. Only the older person, caregiver(s), and other family members can make that decision based on their situation, resources, relationships, and a discussion of the advantages and disadvantages of all possible alternatives.

One of the major problems between caregiver and older person is often a lack of communication. Perhaps this problem occurs because of a lack of time or fatigue on the part of the caregiver or because the older person does not want to share his or her problems with the caregiver for fear of increasing the caregiver's burdens (Parsons, Cox, and Kimboko 1989). The nurse has a unique and important role in this situation, especially in the home, by sitting down and encouraging caregiver and older person to share individual and/or mutual problems and concerns. An objective facilitator can often help the other two persons share their concerns so that problems can be solved.

Caregivers may also need help in the management of unsatisfactory interpersonal relationships that evolve as a result of role conflict or role overload. One of the most common crises is marital discord resulting from a conflict between the attention needs of the spouse and the care recipient. Caregivers also need to develop assertiveness skills that can be used to manage and limit manipulative and demanding behavior of the care recipient and to defend himself or herself in intrafamily conflicts within the caregiving network. A critical need by the caregiver is the ability to distinguish which issues are his or her responsibility and which belong to another. For example, the caregiver may be struggling with guilt for not providing the care recipient with more contact time, but the care recipient may be having difficulty developing appropriate methods of dealing with loneliness (Green 1991).

Stress management techniques—e.g., diaphragmatic breathing, imagery and visualization, positive self-talk, meditation, humor, self-praise and self-reward, living one day at a time—are essential activities. These techniques are more easily mastered and reinforced with the aid of a support group. For caregivers who cannot participate in support groups, excellent audiotapes and videotapes are available for self-instruction. Respite care should be liberally used. Caregivers should be frequently reminded of the necessity of respite to prevent caregiver collapse and illness. If they will not readily accept respite for themselves, they should be encouraged to accept respite on behalf of the care recipient. Respite may be provided by substitute caregivers within the family caregiving network or by formal respite services within the community. Such services include domiciliary care, adult day care, paid companions and sitters, twenty-four-hour inpatient, and respite units (Baldwin 1990). Some caregivers are reluctant to leave home for fear that something will happen to the older adult. The use of an emergency call system, such as a pager or mobile cellular telephone, may give the caregiver freedom for a few hours and a sense of security that he or she can be reached at any time if really needed.

Nurses should remember that depression is a common concomitant in long-term caregiving. They should assess both caregiver and care recipient for the presence of clinical signs and symptoms of this disorder. A number of excellent depression screening inventories are available for this purpose, such as the Geriatric Depression Scale and the Beck Depression Inventory. Depression should be managed aggressively. Clients with abnormal scores on screening instruments should be promptly referred to a physician for diagnosis and treatment. Depressed caregivers may be unable to provide effective client care, participate in support groups, and use self-care techniques such as stress management.

Caregivers should be encouraged to actively seek and use support from others, whether provided by formal support groups (family caregiver support groups, caregiver skill workshops, family or caregiver therapy group); friendship networks (church groups, sororities, social clubs); or other members in the family caregiving network (siblings, aunts, uncles, and cousins). Caregivers must be taught the acceptability of asking for help and the graciousness of accepting help when it is offered. Care recipients also should be encouraged to provide support for caregivers by participating to the extent possible in their own care, through courteous treatment of caregivers, and by expressing periodic appreciation for services rendered. If behavior of the care recipient is a major issue, both parties of the relationship may need to learn behavior modification, using behavioral and cognitive therapy with the aid of a professional provider.

Riffle (1989) identified the role of support groups in relieving caregiver stress. She noted that support groups provide hope, a feeling of universality and the recognition that similar feelings and problems are experienced by others, interpersonal learning, catharsis, group cohesiveness, behavior modelling, information, and altruistic giving and receiving. She identified appropriate issues to be addressed in nurse-directed support groups. Among these are

- Values clarification

- Self valuing

- Physiological and psychological changes of aging

- Health, social, and emotional needs of older persons

- Home nursing strategies

- Stress management

- Assertiveness training

- Respite services

- Strategies for developing and strengthening social support systems

- Accessing community resources

- Goal setting

- Decision making

- Planning behavior change

- Implementing and maintaining lifestyle modifications

- Health-promoting behaviors

Riffle also recommended the use of telephone consultation with the nurse as a valuable source of social support.

The Power of Praise

Nurses should identify the significance of bringing praise and hope to family caregivers. The more isolated the caregiver, the more important these two gifts. Praise is especially important when caregivers are attempting to master new skills and are painfully aware of awkwardness. Nurses should find something to cite for special recognition or glowing praise during each contact with the caregiver. Even if every aspect of a procedure is performed incorrectly, praise can be given for the person's willingness to try. Caregivers need validation of their humanity and praise for their efforts. They need recognition for the job they are doing, positive reinforcement for successes, and gentle correction for errors. Sometimes they just need a listening ear. They need someone who can accept and validate the feelings of anger, guilt, pain, sorrow, jealousy, and resentment without being judgmental. At other times they may need a hug or may need to have tension relieved by humor. With laughter comes joy and with joy comes hope for the future as one is once again linked with all the emotions experienced by others not involved in the caregiving experience.

Promoting Changes in Eldercare Policy

Nurses have a responsibility to promote changes in the financing and delivery of health care for older adults. This can be done as individuals and through participation in professional organizations. Nurses can draft agendas and position papers. They can lobby legislators to support legislation that fosters the growth of family caregiving and protects the health and well-being of both members of the caregiving relationship. In addition nurses should actively support favorable changes that are occurring in the American workplace.

Currently the majority of married couples are both employed in the workplace, not only for financial reasons but also for the personal and professional rewards of an interesting occupation or career. Therefore when an older parent is no longer able to live independently safely, a decision should be made about where the older parent should live and receive needed care. A major problem occurs when the older person does not have adequate finances for an assistive living arrangement but does not qualify for Medicaid and really does not need to be in a nursing facility (home). All of the older parent's children probably are employed and unable or unwilling to quit work in order to care for the parent in the home. Live-in help is expensive, hard to find, and not always reliable. Therefore employees often experience problems in the workplace related to parent care, see Table 19-8.

A family medical leave bill was passed by Congress and signed by the President in 1993. This legislation requires employers to provide unpaid leave to employees during the acute illness of a dependent family member (including parents), with the employee's job assured upon return to work. In three western states—California, Oregon, and Hawaii—new laws took effect in 1992 that allowed relatives to take time off from work to care for ill relatives. California requires employers with fifty or more employees to allow employees "to take up to 16 weeks off without pay during a two-month period to care for. . .an ill spouse or parent" (*Fort Worth Star Telegram*, December 28, 1991). Oregon allows twelve weeks without pay every two years to care for sick relatives. A similar law in Hawaii applied to state and county workers in 1992 and private companies in 1994 (*Forth Worth Star Telegram*, December 28, 1991). Many countries, for example Norway and Sweden, have such laws that provide paid leave and contribute to quality family relationships and ultimately increase employee morale.

Employers are beginning to recognize the problem of eldercare and plan for it. "Recent surveys of major corporations show that one of every four employees *already* provide care to an elderly relative" (Duseel and Roman 1989). Executives and managers, more likely to be middle-aged and have older parents, are in a position to initiate and support programs that will help effective employees during a difficult time in their lives. Many large companies, corporations, and businesses have instituted an eldercare program as a fringe benefit to help their employees. Some of these benefits are listed in Table 19-9.

Ingersoll-Dayton, Chapman, and Neal (1990) studied a specific program for caregivers in the workplace. The program consisted of two phases: *(1)* a survey of employees for need and *(2)* services to employees consisting of a seven-week educational series in the workplace and a choice of three other services (case management by professionals, support group of peers led by professionals, or a caregiver buddy system). Twenty-three percent of more than nine thousand respondents said that they provided care to an older person. However, only 3 percent of the 23 percent attended the education sessions. The site where a small fee ($3.00 per session) was charged was better attended than the sites where the sessions were free. Still fewer employees participated in the case management (nineteen) and support group (thirty-two) options and no one chose the buddy system option. Only those employees who participated in the educational sessions knew about the service options and since many of them (36.7 per-

Table 19–8   Caregiver Problems in the Workplace

- Decreased productivity (because the older person telephones the employee many times during the day)

- Absenteeism (e.g., need to take a parent for medical appointments that can only be made during the day)

- Getting to work late (unexpected emergencies in the morning)

- Leaving work early (to run essential errands)

- Fatigue (because of caregiving responsibilities at night)

- Anxiety and stress (related to overall concern about a parent's condition and care)

cent) were "anticipatory caregivers" (127) rather than actual caregivers at the time, they may not have felt the need for the service options. On the other hand, caregivers who felt they did not need the education programs may have had a greater need for the service options but did not know about them. Participants evaluated the education sessions as very positive and their knowledge of services increased significantly. However, their absenteeism from work actually increased, possibly because their caregiving responsibilities increased, they had "affirmed the role of employees or caregivers," or they took time to investigate some of the services they had learned about in the educational sessions (128). The support groups were particularly helpful in learning "new ways of communicating with the older person and other family members" (129).

Some project staff members were afraid that education, and/or support sessions during the workday might depress employees. However, the employees stated that "having the opportunity to discuss these issues while on the job allowed them to work more effectively" (130).

Suggestions for revisions in future eldercare programs were

1. Offer the educational sessions at periodic regular intervals for a consortium of businesses.

2. Have videotapes of sessions for employees to view on their own time.

3. Have service options ongoing so that employees can use as needed.

4. Market and publicize the program to all employees whether or not they are current caregivers.

5. Change the name of the support group to something less threatening (e.g., "Technology of Caregiving").

6. Offer evening meetings.

7. Invite family members to educational sessions and support groups.

RESOURCES FOR CAREGIVERS

In addition to the resources cited in the text, many other valuable resources are available. The following are recommended for caregivers:

A Path for Caregivers. Washington, DC: American Association of Retired Persons [PF4013 (989) D-12957], 1987.

AARP; 1909 K St NW; Washington, DC 20049

Alzheimer's Disease and Related Disorders Association; telephone (800) 621-0379

Caregiving: Helping an Aged Loved One by Jo Horne. Scott, Foresman and Co.; 1865 Miner St; Des Plaines, IL 60016

Children of Aging Parents; 2761 Trenton Rd; Levittown, PA 19056

The 36-Hour Day by N.L. Mace and P.V. Rabins. Baltimore: The John Hopkins Press, 1991.

The Age Care Sourcebook by Jean Crichton. (Simon and Schuster; $9.95)

The Home Health Care Solution by Janet Zhun Nassif

Table 19–9   Eldercare Benefits in the Workplace

- Flexible-working schedules (flextime) (e.g., split schedules, later starts, part-time employment)

- Short-term personal leaves of absence without pay (during an acute illness of an older person)

- Information, meetings, support groups, and counseling in the workplace about caring for older parents (perhaps at lunch or in the evenings)

- Adult day-care units where an older parent who no longer is able to be alone during the day can stay while the adult child works

- Flexible vacation and sick time (often used for caregiving responsibilities)

SUMMARY

The majority of older persons eventually receive some type of care and support from other family members, most often a daughter, son, or spouse. Because more older persons are living into their 80s, 90s, and 100s, they often need some assistance. Adult children (usually in their 40s, 50s, and 60s) often have some responsibility for the care of parents and grandparents as well as children and grandchildren, which places them in the "sandwich generation."

Caregiving can be defined in many ways, but it usually involves physical, psychosocial, and/or financial support of some kind. There are both positive and negative aspects of caregiving. Caregiving can become very stressful, especially if there is a problem with relationships and communication between caregiver and care recipient.

There are an increasing number of community resources to aid caregivers and older persons. These include such services as home health care, adult day care, eldercare in the workplace, respite care, and information sessions and support groups for caregivers.

Nurses have a unique responsibility and the profession as a whole has an obligation to design services, programs, and patterns of service delivery that nurture and sustain family caregiving systems. Nurses are fortunate to be able to play a significant role in providing assistance to families experiencing stress as a result of caregiving. Their services as teacher, counselor, role model, mediator, and professional friend have the effect of fostering competence in the caregiving system. Their commitment to the well-being of both caregivers and care recipients enriches family life and supports older adults as they confront the developmental challenges of the eighth stage of family development (retirement and old age).

STUDY QUESTIONS

1. Why will there be more emphasis on family caregiving of older adults in the 1990s?

2. What are some ethnic differences in family caregiving?

3. Explain the developmental tasks of Stage VIII families.

4. Describe the major responsibilities of caregivers.

5. Who most often becomes the caregiver of older adults? How is this changing?

6. What are the primary problems and stresses of family caregivers?

7. What is the primary purpose of respite care?

8. How does caregiving affect the health of family caregivers?

9. What are the most important nursing interventions in assisting families with the care of older adults?

10. Why is there a need for eldercare programs in the workplace? Describe some examples.

REFERENCES

Baldwin, B. 1990. Family caregiving: Trends and forecasts. *Geriatric Nursing* 11(4):172–74.

Barer, B.B. and C.L. Johnson. 1990. A critique of caregiver literature. *The Gerontologist* 30(1):26–29.

Blazer, D. 1986. Depression: Paradoxically, a cause for hope. *Generations* 10(3):21–23.

Browning, M.A. 1991. Prevalence of depression in the Medicare home care client. Paper presented at the Phyllis J. Verhonick Nursing Research Conference—Quality of Care, Quality of Life—April 5, 1991 at the University of Virginia, Charlottesville, VA.

Connidis, I.A. and L. Davies. 1990. Confidants and companions in later life: The place of family and friends. *Journal of Gerontology* (4):S141–S149.

Dussel, C. and M. Roman. 1989. The elder care dilemma. *Generations* Summer:30–32.

Gaynor, S.E. 1989. When the caregiver becomes the patient. *Geriatric Nursing* 10(3):120–23.

Gaynor, S.E. 1990. The long haul: The effects of home care on caregivers. *Image* 22(4):208–12.

Gibeau, J.L. and J.W. Anastas. 1989. Breadwinners and caregivers: Interviews with working women. *Journal of Gerontological Social Work* 14(1/2):19–40.

Gold, D.T. 1990. Late-life sibling relationships: Does race affect typological distribution? *The Gerontologist* 30(6):741–48.

Green, C.P. 1991. Clinical considerations: Midlife daughters and their aging parents. *Journal of Gerontological Nursing* 17(11):6–12.

Herth, K.A. 1989. The root of it all: Genograms as a nursing assessment tool. *Journal of Gerontological Nursing* 15(12):32–37.

Ingersoll-Dayton, B., N. Chapman, and M. Neal. 1990. A program for caregivers in the workplace. *The Gerontologist* 30(1):126–30.

Johnson, C.L. and B.M. Barer. 1990. Families and networks among older inner-city Blacks. *The Gerontologist* 30(6):726–33.

Mercer, R. 1983. Assessing and counseling teenaged mothers during the perinatal period. *Nursing Clinics of North America* 18(2):293–301.

Meyers, B.S. and G.S. Alexopoulas. 1988. Geriatric depression. *Medical Clinics of North America* 72(4):847–63.

Morris, R.G., L.W. Morris, and P.G. Britton. 1988. Factors affecting the emotional wellbeing of the caregivers of dementia sufferers. *British Journal of Psychiatry* 153:147–56.

Naylor, M. 1990. Comprehensive discharge planning hospitalized elderly: A pilot study. *Nursing Research* 39(3):156–160.

Parmelee, P.A., I.R. Katz, and M.P. Lawton. 1989. Depression among institutionalized aged: Assessment and prevalence estimation. *Journal of Gerontology* 44(1):M22–M29.

Parsons, R.J., E.O. Cox, and P.J. Kimboko. 1989. Satisfaction, communication, and affection in caregiving: A view from the elder's perspective. *Journal of Gerontological Social Work* 13(3/4):9–20.

Pearlin, L.I., J.T. Mullan, S.J. Semple, and M.M. Skaff. 1990. Caregiving and the stress process: An overview of concepts and their measures. *The Gerontologist* 38(5):583–94.

Reed, B.R., A.A. Stone, and J.M. Neale. 1990. Effects of caring for a demented relative on elder's life events and appraisals. *The Gerontologist* 30(2):200–205.

Riffle, K.L. 1989. Stress: Nurses dealing with family members. *Journal of Gerontological Nursing* 15(7):18–25.

Ross, B. and K.L. Cobb. 1990. *Family Nursing: A Nursing Process Approach.* Redwood City, CA: Addison-Wesley Nursing.

St. Pierre, J., R. Craven, and P. Bruno. 1986. Late life depression: A guide for assessment. *Journal of Gerontological Nursing* 12(7):5–1.

Smoyak, S.A. 1987. Assessing aging families and their caretakers. In *Families and Chronic Illness*, edited by L.M. Wright and M. Leahey. Springhouse, PA: Springhouse Corporation.

Stoller, E.P. 1990. Males as helpers: The role of sons, relatives, and friends. *The Gerontologist* 30(2):229–35.

Stoller, E.P. and K.L. Pugliesi. 1989. Other roles of caregivers: Competing responsibilities or supportive resources. *Journal of Gerontology: Social Sciences* 44(6):231–38.

Talbott, M.M. 1990. The negative side of the relationship between older widows and their adult children: The mother's perspective. *The Gerontologist* 30(5):595–603.

White-Means, S.I. and M.C. Thornton. 1990a. Ethnic differences in the production of informal home health care. *The Gerontologist* 30(6):758–67.

White-Means, S.I. and M.C. Thornton. 1990b. Labor market choices and home health provision among employed ethnic caregivers. *The Gerontologist* 30(6):769–75.

20 Community Resources

Mary Flo Bruce

CHAPTER OUTLINE

FOCUS

Most communities have a variety of agencies, programs, and support systems whose primary purpose is to assist older persons and their families in some way. Often the problem is identifying those in greatest need and connecting them with the appropriate services available. The focus of this chapter is to describe the variety of community resources available to older adult clients and their families.

OBJECTIVES

1. Identify the role of the nurse in the community.

2. Discuss the role of the nurse in referring patients to needed community services.

3. Describe some of the services provided by home health care agencies.

4. Differentiate the two types of adult day-care services.

5. Discuss the value of senior centers.

6. Name three kinds of volunteer programs for older adults in the community.

7. Evaluate the value of nurse-directed wellness centers.

8. Relate how emergency help systems work in the home.

9. List six different general home services useful to older adults.

10. Evaluate the advantages and disadvantages of six different types of housing alternatives for older adults.

The maintenance of wellness is a vital concept that deals with the quality as well as the quantity of life. The biologic, sociologic, and metaphysical levels of assessment are encompassed. Wellness is an important goal for all age groups, but it is especially important during the last cycle of life. The notion that the life cycle is a curved line that *must* point down after the middle years is a misconception that leads many to the self-fulfilling prophecy of deteriorating mental and physical health and decline in intellectual capacity. But the nurse needs a comprehensive outlook to focus on high-level wellness for the older population. The definition of high-level wellness depends on many variables such as race, age, ethnic background, religion, and geographic origin.

OVERVIEW

To assess an older client in any given situation, the nurse needs to acquire some basic general knowledge about the aging process. This knowledge is essential for both the hospital-based nurse and the community-based nurse if there is to be continuity of care for the older population.

As the year 2000 approaches, bringing with it a new century, it will also bring an unprecedented number of people 65 years of age and older. Medical technology has produced a longer life expectancy, but there has been little concurrent increase in the quality of life for most older adults. The gain in life expectancy has brought changes that affect people of all ages in our society. Nurses can be initiators of social change for older people by learning about the various aspects and problems involved in the process of becoming "old."

REACHING NEEDY OLDER PEOPLE

Programs continue to be developed to meet the needs of older adults in the community. One of the challenges, however, is to get this information to those who are most in need of these programs. How can the nurse disseminate information about these programs to the older people who are most in need, those who are most isolated and most withdrawn?

Many frustrations confront those who work with older clients. There are frustrations over the slow change of attitudes toward aging, the lack of decent housing and adequate transportation, the grossly inadequate income of many older people, and the inability to reach many in need. Perhaps one of the major frustrations for a nurse is the inability to prevent or eliminate the multiple chronic diseases found in the older age group. In these cases the nursing goals must stress prevention of further disability

and acceptance of the chronic ailments that are present.

Yet there are tremendous rewards for those who are willing and take the time to work with the older population: the realization that the nurse has intervened to prevent a diagnosis of chronic organic mental disorder when all the while the client had been taking too much of the prescribed medicine, or the gratitude and appreciation that are expressed because someone has finally been willing to listen to the older client. The nurse needs to accept the person as he or she is and not as the nurse wishes the person to be. The greatest reward can come when the older client is accepted as an individual with specific strengths, needs, and problems, instead of as an "old man" or an "old lady."

Additional study is needed in this area. What are the attitudes of health care professionals in regard to aging? How does the belief in these myths and stereotypes affect the delivery of health care for this segment of the population? Studies could also be conducted to investigate the attitudes and beliefs that deter older people themselves from seeking health care.

ROLE OF THE NURSE IN THE COMMUNITY

The primary concern of the community health nurse is the population as a whole. At the same time, the nurse cannot lose sight of the client as an individual. Schwartz (1969) described five stages of health in which the nurse has specific responsibilities. The first two stages are completely preventive. Stage one deals with preserving the existing health status and stage two with recognition of high-risk individuals and populations. The third stage consists of early detection of any existing health problem. The last two stages consist of care of the acutely ill person and the rehabilitation of this individual.

The community health nurse is involved in all five stages. Prevention is the first and most important task of the nurse. Teaching good physical and mental health practices can preserve the existing health status. The older person should know about good nutrition and how to obtain it. Proper exercise is also essential. These needs require the nurse to be cognizant of the physical and emotional needs of each client. The second and third stages can be accomplished by thorough screening of this population. Screening must include all the components of physical, psychologic, and social status. When an older person must be hospitalized for acute illness, the community health nurse can assure continuity of health by checking on the progress of the client and by being involved in discharge planning along with the client, the hospital nurses, and the physicians. Such continuity will help ensure that the rehabilitation stage is not neglected and the client can return, as soon as possible, to the highest level of health possible.

In order to help older people maintain wellness and prevent illness, the nurse needs to be aware of all possible community resources that may be needed in providing holistic health care. Some of these resources are not specifically health related, but may be needed by older people to help maintain an active and healthy lifestyle in the community. Assessment of the client's specific needs—whether physical, psychological, social, or financial—is essential so that appropriate and timely references may be made.

Continuity of care is very contingent upon public policy. Therefore it is important that nurses develop political awareness. Public policy has a tremendous impact on what type of health care can be provided. Both the hospital-based nurse and the community health nurse have a vested interest in becoming politically astute in order to be able to offer clients the best health care possible. This political role is one nurses have too often ignored.

Teaching is a large and important component of nursing care for all nurses. They should be familiar with teaching/learning principles and strategies if they are to teach effectively. The community health nurse uses teaching in both preventive and rehabilitative stages. Thatcher (1988) contended that nurses should focus on those areas necessary to maintain, promote, or rehabilitate the health of the older client.

For learning to occur, the nurse must first develop a therapeutic relationship with the client. In so doing, two things occur: the nurse and the client learn to trust each other; and the nurse is able to assess how to approach the client. The nurse must identify the client's needs as the client feels them if any change is to occur. Then the nurse assesses the client's level of motivation and perception of the situation.

Health teaching is a need often voiced by groups of older people. An assessment of the personally identified needs of older adults in the Oklahoma City area was conducted by a group of baccalaureate students. The five most frequently identified areas of concern were hypertension, nutrition, arthritis, exercise, and the Heimlich maneuver.

SPECIFIC COMMUNITY RESOURCES FOR OLDER ADULTS

In order for nurses to assist older people to achieve a higher quality of life, it is necessary that both the hospital-based nurse and the community-based nurse be aware of the types of services available to older people. There has been a rapid proliferation of facilities and services for this age group, including programs that help meet social, recreational, economic, and health needs. Unless the programs are brought to the attention of those for whom they were created, however, they are worthless. One method of reaching older people in the community is an outreach program. Foley (1976) discussed a project funded by the California State Department of Aging. This project, "Outreach to Seniors," investigated means of reaching the older population. It was found that advertising is an effective method of reaching senior citizens. To make this approach most effective, different methods are needed to reach different people: television, radio, pamphlets, and newspapers should be used. The advertising must reach not only prospective clients but also friends, neighbors, relatives, and other professionals. "Hard-to-reach" people can be sought out by direct contact. Volunteers are used for this technique. Booth, one of the project participants, stated that ". . . to effectively reach out to the elderly, . . . we must stand close to the door" (Foley 1976, 10).

The increasing number of community resources available to older people covers a range of needs such as transportation, senior citizen activities, health care and home care facilities, housing, and income. Many larger communities have access to community resource books published by the United Way. Area Agencies on Aging are excellent referral centers. Some of these agencies publish directories of services specifically for older adults.

The nurse in many rural areas has an additional challenge in attempting to find community resources for the older client. While rural older people have the same need for continuity of care and its delivery, the nurse in the rural area may have a more difficult task in identifying available health care.

The Older Americans Act, 1978 Amendments, provides leverage for provision of health care for older people. If the services are not available locally, there may be provision for contractual agreement for resources in distant communities (Watkins and Watkins 1985). However, Krout (1987) conducted a study that demonstrated that senior centers in rural areas offer less activities and services. Other studies have shown that the older rural population is indeed interested in health care and health promotion. Bender and Hart (1987) developed a model for health promotion in rural Oklahoma. The number of older people to attend the meetings was "disproportionate to their numbers in the communities" (Bender and Hart 1987, 141). These findings emphasize the need for the rural community health nurse to become involved in developing innovative programs to provide activities and services to the older rural population.

Home Health Care

Belsky (1988, 263) stated that home health care is the "most widespread alternative to nursing home care." Also, the rising cost of hospitalization and other institutional care leads the way to a demand for increased home health care services. Home health care is believed to be less expensive than institutional care. However, Montgomery and Borgatta (1987) contended that it is not clear if home care is less expensive when families are not willing or not able to provide both much of the care and assume the cost of many of the community services. This belief received confirmation in regional public hearings conducted throughout the country in September and October of 1976, during which it was reported that home services were indeed cost-effective (*Report on Regional Public Hearings* 1976).

According to Ward (1983, 222), home health care "is the oldest formal mode of health care delivery in the United States." She traced its development to the mid-1700s, stating that "home health care was the only practical system" available to provide health care services for the acutely ill.

In the 1940s, Montefiore established the first hospital-based home health service. This program was established in the belief that the patient's hospital stay could be significantly shortened if home health care were provided to postacute patients. The pro-

gram required that the client have a support system at home that would provide homemaker care and unskilled services. The Visiting Nurse Association provided skilled nursing service, while the hospital provided home medical care, social service, and occupational and physical therapy. This was the first program to provide multiple professional services that considered the client more holistically (Ward 1983).

The role of home health service expanded in the late 1960s by the enactment of Title XVIII and Title XIX, which authorized federal payment for home care. These acts cast the federal government in the role of principal financier of home health service (*Report on Regional Public Hearings* 1976) and led to an increase in the types of services available.

Home health care agencies may be licensed, certified, or accredited. *Licensed* agencies have met basic legal requirements. They are not eligible for Medicare or Medicaid payment and employee training is not required. *Certified* agencies can accept Medicare or Medicaid payment. Government regulation requires a certain number of hours of staff training. *Accredited* agencies must meet requirements set up by a nonprofit organization that promotes high-quality home care. Accreditation is voluntary and requires the agencies to meet the most rigorous standards (Belsky 1988).

Home health care agencies offer a diverse number of services designed to meet specific medically related needs that do not require an intensive level of skilled care in institutions (*Report of Regional Public Hearings* 1976). This type of care, which must be authorized by a physician, includes medical, nursing, and homemaker services; home-delivered meals; physical therapy; crisis intervention; and counseling. These additional services add breadth to the much-needed care for older people and help achieve the aim of home health care, which is to prevent debilitation when possible and to allow clients to stay in their homes longer. The regional public hearings reported that these services were socially beneficial in fostering independence among older and handicapped people.

Adult Day-Care Services

Adult day-care centers were first established in England in the 1940s. They were established by psychiatric hospitals to provide ongoing care and decrease the number of hospital admissions. In the 1950s, England extended this care to the older population.

The first federally funded day-care center for older adults was established in 1972 in Hawaii. Since then, day-care centers for older people have been established throughout the United States. The purpose of these centers is to allow older people to reside in their homes as long as possible and yet provide them with therapeutic care during the day. This program allows disabled older people to live alone longer. It is also an important resource for working family members who do not want to leave older members alone (Dunkle 1988). Growth has been slow in the United States. However, the number has increased in the last ten years.

Adult day care can be divided into two types of services. One is the day-care social program for frail, moderately handicapped, or confused persons. This program is often confused with senior centers, but it is different. Most senior centers do not provide custodial care. The day-care facilities provide supervision, activities, rest periods, and at least one meal. The other type—the day-care hospital—provides additional services such as personal care services, skilled nursing care, and physical therapy. Both types serve as liaison with the client's family and home. Personnel of the centers are able to work with the families and provide them with advice and emotional support. At the present time, neither program is regulated by federal guidelines or requirements. Funds may be provided by the government through Title XIX or Title XX. Private sources of funds include businesses, grants, foundations, churches, and the United Way.

Adult day-care programs may be licensed and/or certified by the state. Type of *licensing* and licensing requirements vary from state to state. More stringent standards are usually required for health-related day-care programs. *Certification* is required to receive federal funding such as Medicare, Medicaid, and Older Americans Act funding. Centers may be certified for multiple funding (Weissert, Elson, Bolda, Zelman, Mutran, and Mangum 1990).

The necessity of working with family members cannot be overemphasized. Katz and Maginn (1989) urge that a thorough family assessment is essential. The nurse and/or intake worker assessment should include family expectations, ability to cope with the older person's aging changes, previous relationship with the client, and each family member's present situation. They emphasize that the family is a crucial part of the treatment team. They need to be included with the client in decision making. There also are informal services that the family can participate in when desired or able. Formal counseling services with individuals, families, or groups can provide emotional support for the caregivers, giving them an opportunity to express their feelings and concerns. Katz and Maginn (1989) stated that family members may be more comfortable in education and information-sharing groups than in counseling groups. They noted that other means of reaching families are peer support groups, newsletters, health-screening services, and an opportunity for family members to serve as auxiliaries. Necessity of involving families is demonstrated by Graham's (1989) study with families of dementia patients in adult day care. This study found that day care alone does not relieve family stress. These families reported feelings of guilt and defeat for not being able to manage and care successfully for the client. They also realized that nursing home placement would probably soon follow. Counseling was very important for the family.

Weissert et al. (1990) reported that a national survey of sixty day-care centers found that both clients and caregivers demonstrated high levels of satisfaction. They reported that adult day care is well received and appears to meet the needs of both caregivers and clients. Since women remain the primary caregivers and more women are working, day care is one method of resolving this dilemma.

Senior Centers

Senior centers are organizations designed to serve the needs of people 55 years of age and older. Funds are provided by United Way, donations, and government grants. The centers are usually scattered throughout the city to be easily accessible to older people and are often located in areas where there are large older populations.

In 1978 the Older Americans Act Amendments required that each Area Agency on Aging designate a site as a focal point for comprehensive service delivery to effect maximum colocation and coordination of services, thus giving impetus to the growth and development of senior centers. One of the purposes of these amendments was that the senior centers would serve as linkages in the community. Krout (1986) undertook a study to determine if the senior center did indeed colocate and coordinate activities with other community activities. His findings indicated that out of 755 senior centers, less than 10 percent reported colocation with other agencies and with county and local offices on aging; 10 percent with parks and recreation; 12 percent with other senior centers; and 25 percent with nutritional sites.

There is an increase in percentages for planning and coordinating services with the community. The largest linkage is with the Social Security office, 85 percent; 20–30 percent report linkage to health and related services; and less than 20 percent report linkage with agencies such as special disability groups, and like agencies. Receiving and sending referrals is the largest percentage. Some of the reasons listed for lack of colocation and coordination of services are lack of funds, time, personnel, and transportation (Krout 1986).

The purpose of these centers is to allow older people to remain independently involved in the community as long as possible. The centers are for the use of people who are able to be active and who do not require custodial or nursing care. The centers offer a wide variety of services such as recreational activities, shopping assistance, health education and screening, one or more nutritious meals, legal aid services, and transportation to and from the center. Many of the centers are also an excellent source of information about community resources for older people, besides providing participants fellowship with older persons the same age.

Ralston's (1987) review of research about senior citizen centers suggested that senior citizen centers are serving very diverse populations. As community-based organizations they need to reflect the diversity between and within communities. One of the challenges is to deal with this diversity especially when it is within one center. Also, government funding sources are decreasing, so these agencies are increasing the diversity of their services based on priority needs of older persons in the community. They are also actively seeking private funds to continue to expand their services.

Volunteer Programs

The federal government has four volunteer programs under ACTION specifically geared for people over 60 years of age. The Retired Senior Volunteer Program (RSVP) is a community-organized and community-operated program in which the older adult provides volunteer assistance to the community. The assignments of the volunteers are directed toward their talents and experiences (Gelfand 1988). The Service Corps of Retired Executives (SCORE) is sponsored by the Small Business Administration. Under this program, retired businessmen and executives provide advice to the small businessperson (Gelfand 1988).

Foster Grandparents is a program for low-income older adults. Foster grandparents work with children with disabilities for twenty hours a week and are paid for their services. Most foster grandparents work in institutions, providing children with companionship and guidance.

A relatively new service is the Senior Companion Program. This program hires low-income senior citizens to provide care and companionship for other older individuals.

Educational programs are also being expanded to meet the needs of the older population. Elderhostel is a summer program that provides educational courses for those over 60 years of age. Many diverse courses are offered for one week of concentrated study in colleges and universities. This program has been enthusiastically used by older adults who are in reasonably good health and have adequate financial resources.

Health-Screening Clinics

Since the early 1970s there has been a proliferation of multiphasic adult screening clinics. This important aspect of health maintenance is becoming available to more and more people. Clinics are conducted by city and county health departments, visiting nurse associations, medical schools, and private individuals. Many of the clinics are held in various sites throughout the city so that older people who have no transportation will have better access to these services. Many areas of the country do not have adult screening clinics, however.

Health-screening centers were established to offer

older people basic health screening services. All health screening is offered at no cost to the individual regardless of financial status, race, color, creed, or ethnic origin. The only requirement is that the individual be 60 years of age or older. The screening is performed by paid staff, volunteers, and supervised graduate and undergraduate students. Services range from blood pressure checks, medication counseling, and physician referrals to extended services such as physical assessments, glaucoma screening, hearing tests, dental screening and evaluation, nutritional assessment and counseling, diabetes screening, leisure-time counseling, foot care, and home visits.

Nurse-Directed Wellness Centers

The development of nurse-directed wellness centers is important in both urban and rural areas. These centers provide holistic, client-centered services to older clients and provide for the health maintenance and health promotion needs of the clients. Wilson, Patterson, and Alford (1989) described a wellness center that provides group health promotion programs, health screening, and individualized service through the clinic. In rural areas the nurse-directed clinic may be the primary health care resource in the community. The nurses in the center need to gain support of the community, decrease barriers to health care and make services more widely available. The centers must be able to be reimbursed in some way (Fenton, Rouk, and Kha 1988).

Transportation

Transportation is frequently a problem for older clients, especially for those who are physically or visually disabled or fragile. In the 1970s the federal government attempted to encourage the use of mass transportation by older adults. Programs that provided reduced fares during nonpeak hours were instituted. The number of older people using mass transit has increased since the programs began. However, mass transit is not usually direct to one's destination, and it is considerably slower than a private car or taxi. It is not a feasible solution for some of the fragile or disabled older people.

The Urban Mass Transit Act (1975) provided financial assistance for transportation programs to non-profit organizations. By 1977 more than 1,400 organizations had utilized these funds to purchase specialized vehicles. Over 75 percent was used to purchase passenger vans for older persons. One of the major stumbling blocks in this program has been the difficulties encountered by agencies in obtaining adequate insurance. However, this has been somewhat resolved by new insurance ratings (Gelfand 1988).

Transportation problems are one of the major problems for older people. A person's lifestyle is greatly hampered if the person is unable to make plans somewhat at his/her own convenience. The family is often willing to transport older people to appointments and the bank, for example. However, it is often difficult to arrange schedules where neither the older individual nor the family feels burdened. The nurse needs to investigate what transportation is available in the community. Often, a local unit of the American Red Cross, churches, the Salvation Army, and other charitable organizations provide transportation for older persons or those with disabilities. The transportation may be for limited reasons, such as physician or dentist appointments, or may be used for any reason. There may be a charge or the service may be free. Also, some senior centers and day-care centers offer free transportation to and from the center. Most of the centers accept but do not require donations. Many communities have developed minibus or van service for those in wheelchairs for a minimal fee, especially for the disabled and for older people. The vans often transport several clients at a time so the nurse needs to assess the client to determine if the client can withstand a prolonged ride.

Emergency Help Systems

Careline-Lifeline Systems. The Careline-Lifeline systems are home-based electronic emergency systems available for homebound individuals. These systems provide a telephone link to a base station in case of an emergency. The individual signs up for the service and is given a medallion that is worn around the neck. The individual provides information such as health history, name of physician, medications, and telephone number of three responders. When an emergency arises, the individual pushes a button on the medallion and a signal is received at the base station. The base station operator calls the individual. If there is no answer, the first responder is called. If the first responder does not answer, the second responder is called and then the third. If no responder is available, the police are called to investigate. When one of the responders answers, he or she goes to the home to check on the older person. The responder calls the base station and informs them about the situation and appropriate measures are instituted.

These systems are an excellent method of monitoring a homebound individual and are utilized widely by older people, especially those in their 90s. However, there are a number of problems with the system. One is that the user must reset the medallion each day. Even though it provides a measure of safety, some users resent the device and feel it is an intrusion on their privacy. Some are afraid of the electronic device. False signals are frequent; that is, some individuals forget to reset it or to inform the home base that they are away from home.

Another type of electronic monitoring is the monitoring of cardiac clients. The individual is monitored around the clock. Any arrhythmias activate a signal that rings a telephone at the local hospital. The client is called immediately. Appropriate emergency assistance can be sent at once.

There are many case studies of individuals whose life has been saved or injury has been minimized because of electronic monitoring systems. The following is just one example.

Case Study 1. During July a 76-year-old woman who lives in North Texas was in her garden working when she fell. It was about noon, the temperature was already more than 100°F, and she was lying in the sun. Unable to get up, she pushed the button activating the system. The first responder was available and went to the home, finding the woman in the garden. An ambulance was called. The woman had a broken hip. A potentially life-threatening situation was averted. Instead of lying hours in the sun becoming dehydrated, she received immediate attention. Within three hours she was in surgery. In a short time she was back home.

General Home Services

Home Security Programs. Many older adults live in fear of being robbed or violently injured in their own home. Frequently, older people are a target for crime. For this reason, a number of home security programs have been developed to help older homeowners make their homes more safe. There are numerous types of programs. Basically they offer a free home check of windows and doors. Identified security breaks are repaired or installed free. For example, substandard doors are repaired or replaced and supplemental window security and dead-bolt locks installed. The requirements are usually that the client live in the community, be buying or own his/her own home, and be 60 years of age or older. Some programs require that the individual have a limited income. The nurse should be knowledgeable about these programs and be instrumental in bringing the program to the attention of the client if needed. These measures can make older individuals feel more secure in their own homes.

H.E.A.T. Program. This is a federally funded program that offers financial assistance to help pay fuel bills during the winter. Eligibility is determined by one's income.

Home Care Programs. There are various types of home care programs. These programs consist of services such as housecleaning, lawn care, snow shoveling, painting, general house repairs, and winterizing and insulating of home. Some of the programs are established and funded by governmental or private organizations. Other programs are conducted by churches, fraternities, sororities, and organizations such as the Scouts. These programs may provide a one-time-only service or an annual service. The work is done by other older persons, high school and college students, and church members. The nurse can be aware of the latter programs by reading the newspaper or watching television.

Errand Services. Errand services are being developed to aid the homebound older individual with tasks the individual cannot do. One such program— Errand Service, Inc., developed in Austin, Texas—is nonprofit. The individual can apply for the service by telephone. There is a fee, based on the individual's income (Gillis 1985).

Telephone Services. Telephone service may be socializing for the isolated individual or for reassurance. Telephone reassurance services began in Michigan in the 1960s (Gelfand 1988). These programs are privately or publicly funded. The reassurance service is offered to individuals who are able to maintain an independent living style but whose daily well-being is questionable. Usually the telephone reassurance service calls the individual twice a day. If there is no answer, someone is dispatched to the home to investigate the person's well-being. Individuals must inform the service when they will not be at home. The telephoning is usually done by volunteers.

Telephone visiting service frequently is available through senior centers, churches, and other voluntary organizations. This service is offered to the homebound, isolated individual. The individual may be called daily, weekly, or as needed. Often the telephone visitor is the main contact for the homebound, isolated person.

Senior Companions. There is a federally funded senior companion program that provides aid to homebound older adults. Companions are paid a nontaxable stipend, and their transportation is reimbursed. The senior companion must be at least 60 years of age and have a low monthly income. The companion assists the client with household duties and provides support and friendship to the homebound individual. The nurse should be alert not only for older individuals who need this service but also for individuals who might provide the service.

The Consolidated Neighborhood Services, Incorporated in St. Louis developed a program called the System to Assure Elderly Services (STAES), which trained volunteers to maintain regular contact with assigned neighbors, to refer them to needed service agencies, and to provide various supports such as telephone reassurance, shopping, and transportation. The purpose was to develop a network of older volunteers at a minimal cost (Morrow-Howell and Ozawa 1987). They caution, however, that for a program of this type to be successful, the staff must be committed and energetic.

Family and Friends Support

The benefits of social networks are demonstrated in research. Mor-Borak, Miller, and Leonard (1991) conducted a longitudinal study with 3559 older subjects that demonstrated that social relationships have significant effect on the health of poor and/or frail older adults. When one's social network is improved, one's health status is often improved. Lubben (1988) modified a Social Network Index and found that social networks were a positive influence on mental health, individual health practices, and days in the hospital. Antonucci and Akiyama (1991) contend

that relationships that assist one in meeting challenges reinforce a sense of worth and competency. They noted that this was a reciprocal relationship and not a rescue relationship.

The majority of long-term care provided older adults is by family, friends, and neighbors. Most individuals receiving formal care also get informal assistance. A study by Chappel (1991) found that older adults named friend and spouse and children as both primary caregiver and givers of emotional support. Friends were named more than siblings or neighbors. Armstrong (1991) believes that support of friends is underestimated. It is not secondary to or a substitute for the family. Friendship is an optional, personal choice while family may not be.

HOUSING ALTERNATIVES

Kart et al. (1988) stated that about one in four older adults lives alone and that this number is increasing because of the increase in the number of widows and the change in economic status of older people. Almost half of the older adults live with their spouses, and approximately 20 percent live with some other older person. Approximately 71 percent of these older people live in single-family homes that they own. The remainder of the older adults live in diverse types of housing described below. Older people must take many things into consideration when they plan to move. The nurse can help the older person by discussing the types of housing available as well as the advantages and disadvantages of each. Among the factors that determine where the person should live are *(1)* financial status, *(2)* the amount of social contact preferred, *(3)* the preference for either age-segregated or age-integrated housing, and *(4)* the importance of a quiet and safe environment.

Age-Segregated Housing

Many older adults live in age-segregated housing, which includes retirement villages, high-rise complexes, mobile home parks, retirement hotels, congregate living facilities, and nursing homes. The number and types of age-segregated housing are on the increase. Age-segregated housing affords older people security and a chance to meet their peers. At the same time, it isolates them from other age groups.

Retirement Communities. Retirement communities are found mostly in the warmer climates, such as California, Arizona, and Florida. The cost of living in these areas is high, but for the person who can afford it, these communities offer protection, privacy, recreation and social opportunities. Before investing in a retirement community, the buyer should conduct a thorough investigation of all related factors. Most retirement communities offer an excellent alternative for those who want that type of living. However, some of the companies that sell such housing are frauds.

High-Rise Apartments. Age-segregated high-rise apartments are another type of housing for older adults. These apartment complexes may be privately or government funded. Older people qualifying for low-income housing apply through the local housing authority under the Department of Housing and Urban Development. Rental fees are based on income. There is a wide array of services offered at these apartment complexes. Many of them have a senior center within the complex. Recreational and social activities are offered. Many have health screening, social services, and legal services. The apartments afford each resident the amount of privacy they want while they may also have as much social contact as they wish. Some of the complexes offer one meal a day. Most are equipped with an emergency alarm bell that rings in the main office.

Single-Room Occupancy Hotels. Single-room occupancy hotels may or may not be age segregated. These hotels are usually situated in the downtown areas of larger cities. They offer their residents low rent and nearby facilities. However, they are frequently located in noisy, high-crime areas. More men than women live in these hotels. Lally and coworkers (1979) found that these residents were very suspicious of social service agencies and did not use the services available to them. Gelfand (1988) stated that they avoided government programs and had an unstable work history. These residents are some of the hard-to-reach older people who present a challenge to the nurse. They value independence and privacy and often pride themselves on being nonconformists. Nurses working in these areas need to make a concerted effort to identify these people and establish a relationship with them. Lally and coworkers suggested that the nurse should develop a relationship with the hotel staff and inform them about the services available for their residents.

Congregate Housing. Congregate housing was authorized in 1970 by the Housing and Urban Development Act. Gelfand (1988) stated that in 1985, three thousand older persons were housed in sixty-eight federally funded congregate housing projects. Congregate housing provides shelter and can also provide housekeeping services, food services, emergency health services, and recreation. However, residents are responsible for their own care and congregate housing serves as an intermediate housing option. Congregate housing may be age segregated or age integrated. This commune type of housing allows the residents to share costs and responsibilities. It can provide emotional and social ties similar to a traditional family.

Foster Home Care. Foster home care for adults is another alterative for older adults who cannot be entirely independent but who do not want to be institutionalized. The foster home care programs aim to provide a protected home situation and some personal supervision (Sherman and Newman 1977). This type of housing allows more freedom than an institution. These programs emphasize family care and offer the client a chance to participate in family activities. The majority of homes provide room for four to six residents. Many states are presently investigating the establishment of foster home care for adults. This is an area devoid of research and there is a need to explore the effects of foster home care on older adults.

Gelfand (1988) reported that three-fourths of foster home caregivers state that they include the resident in family activities, three-fourths interacted in the neighborhood, and two-thirds participated in community activities. A large number of foster home caregivers are females over age 55 and living alone. However, the sense of family is still present. He also reported that a study was conducted in Massachusetts and Maryland to determine the social functions and cost-effectiveness of the program compared to nursing homes. It was found that the cost of foster home care was 20 percent less than that of nursing homes. However, the social functioning was not assessed.

Board and Care Homes. Board and care homes are very similar to foster care homes except there is little supervision of many boarding homes. If federal or state agencies refer to boarding homes, they can require the home follow certain regulations. The Select Committee on Aging in 1979 reported that one million older and/or disabled adults lived in 68,850 licensed and unlicensed boarding facilities. McCoy and Conley (1990) stated that these facilities provide room and board, provide some degree of protective services and protective oversight, and may provide nonmedical personal care. They question if foster care does not fall under board and care homes.

Shared Housing. Another option that is being used more is shared housing. Gelfand (1988) claims this approach of matching individuals with similar housing needs is creating excitement in many areas. Shared housing may be devised of very diverse individuals who share the home, rent, and food. Some shared homes have very clear cut roles and expectations while others are more vague. Local social agencies frequently provide the locating services.

Life-Care Communities. Continuing care retirement centers or life-care communities are another source of housing for older adults. These communities provide a wide range of housing, dependent on the individual's physical and/or mental abilities. The retirement centers may be established as private nonprofit, private for-profit, or religious denomination centers. Residents may have a private home or apartment on the premises. As they become unable to stay in the home, they can move to a high-rise housing apartment and then to a nursing home, also on the premises. These retirement communities integrate people, housing, health, and social services. Fox and Abraham (1991) stated that continuing care retirement centers promote quality of life, relative independence, and continuity of care. The nurse needs to alert clients that these centers have several plans available. The most comprehensive includes all care until death. Other plans provide partial care or must pay additional costs. Some older adults sell their homes and then invest the money in a continuing care retirement center. If they are financially able to purchase the most comprehensive plan, they are then relatively secure for life.

NEEDS OF RURAL OLDER PEOPLE

Rural older adults face an even greater degree of isolation than their urban counterparts. Health care resources and services in rural areas are frequently deficient or not available. Social services are few. The older people who live alone often must travel long distances to visit friends or family at an age when they find driving difficult and dangerous. Even the belief that rural older people have better housing than their urban counterparts has been shown to be false. Rural older adults occupy 15 percent of the substandard housing in the United States. Although the majority of rural older people own their own homes, over half the homes do not have running water (Coward 1979). Obtaining adequate and safe heat, so important for older people in winter, is also a major problem.

The physical and mental health problems of older people who live in rural areas are compounded by the lack of an available health care delivery system. Nowhere is the inadequate distribution of health care more apparent. There are no clinics and few, if any, physicians in many rural areas. An administrator of the Texas Facilities Commission believes that public education and public involvement would help. He has advised the people of Texas to get involved and to write local, state, and federal agencies in an attempt to improve the situation (Johnson 1979).

Nurses should become involved in issues affecting older people in their local areas. Nurses in rural regions should assess what resources for older adults are available in their areas. By working with agencies that already exist and using the community support system, nurses can help make health and social service care available to rural older adults. Day-care centers could be started in rural areas by neighbors with large homes. Although the facilities would accommodate only a few and the services would probably be minimal, such services would be a great improvement over the existing situation and would help meet some of the health needs of older people in the community.

Taetz and Milton (1979) conducted a research study in which the differences between rural and urban services for older adults in upper state New York were discussed. They found that services that allow the rural older population to remain noninstitutionalized have greatly increased since a study completed in 1967.

In many regions in the country, however, the health problems of rural older adults are compounded by the lack of auxiliary services. Homebound clients cannot receive Meals-on-Wheels because they live outside the city limits. There is no transportation to take these people to clinics or physicians' offices. These problems increase their dependence on their families. The community health nurse who works with rural clients quickly learns the frustration of the situation.

Harbert and Wilkinson (1979) suggested that health professionals who wish to work in rural areas should use the positive strengths and values of these older people, who exhibit such traits as self-reliance, independence, and a strong sense of responsibility. The nurse who wishes to institute change for these people must recognize these values and not work against them.

More research is needed to explore the role of the nurse in meeting the health needs of the rural resident. Comparative studies of rural and urban older people would help determine what facilities and services are needed. This type of research could also identify the effects of the services on the two populations.

Caring for the older rural client provides additional challenges for the nurse. If the nurse is not from the rural area, it is necessary for the nurse to become aware of the ethnic and cultural traditions of the particular community. Overall, rural residents are more conservative and hold more traditional values than their urban counterparts. Johnson (1991) found

that the main concern of the older rural residents was to remain independent and in their own homes. Johnson (1991) also urged that the programs for rural residents be based on their needs and not copy urban programs. Each community should be assessed to identify the beliefs, norms, and traditions of that community. Programs should be set up to meet the perceived needs of that population of older clients.

Rural clients have identified the same needs for health promotion programs as the older urban client, i.e., blood pressure screening, nutrition classes, exercise classes, and other health teaching (Davis et al. 1991; Johnson 1991). However, Johnson (1991) found that the older rural resident was not using positive health practices on a regular basis, while Davis et al. (1991) found that her subjects reported adhering to balanced diet, exercise, and other positive health practices.

Rural areas are not only underserved in health promotion programs but also have less resources to provide other types of programs that promote overall well-being. Johnson (1991) found that older adults in the rural areas felt that their intimacy needs were not met and that they felt that they had no one to share their concerns and problems. Social programs can help meet these needs to some degree. Money has been allocated for local Area Agencies on Aging for programs to serve these needs. An example of a program instituted from these monies was one for rural and isolated older adults in rural central Oklahoma. The program was an art appreciation program that involved both active older residents as well as cognitively and physically impaired individuals (Belzer and Rugh 1991). The goal of the program was to add meaning, purpose, and enjoyment to the lives of these individuals. It involved underachieving junior high school students, professional artists, and college art students. The program was received enthusiastically and the older adults reported that it was a success.

SUMMARY

Both hospital-based and community-based nurses must be cognizant of the many community services

available for older adults, since members of this age group are often unaware of such services. The resources available in each community can be found in community resource books and telephone books, and from the local Area Agency on Aging. Many of these services are geared for older people who have various types of health needs.

Some of these community resources are home health care; adult day-care services; senior centers; various volunteer programs such as foster grandparents, RSVP, and SCORE; health-screening clinics; nurse-directed wellness centers; special transportation services; house emergency help systems; home security programs; assistance with fuel expenses; home care programs; errand services; telephone as-

surance; and senior companions. Family and friends are also an important part of the older adult's support system.

The nurse should share his or her knowledge of housing alternatives with the client, so that together they may arrive at the most suitable arrangement.

The needs of rural adults are also a problem. There has been a great increase in the type of services available in some rural areas, but many areas have few or none. However, the nurse can find ways of being an effective force in implementing services for rural older adults.

STUDY QUESTIONS

1. Identify two of your negative beliefs concerning older adults and defend your viewpoint.

2. Name at least three community services that provide some form of health care for older people.

3. Describe the services provided by one of the community health agencies.

4. Identify four governmental volunteer programs especially geared for individuals 60 years of age or older.

5. Discuss the services provided by each of these volunteer programs.

6. Name four general home services that are available for older people and discuss the purpose of each of them.

7. Compare and contrast urban and rural community health care services for the older population.

8. Develop one creative way to improve home health care for older people in rural areas.

9. Why is transportation a major problem for many older adults?

REFERENCES

Antonucci, T. and H. Akiyama. 1991. Social relationships and aging well. *Generations* 15(1):42–43.

Armstrong, R. 1991. Friends as a source of informal support for older women with physical disabilities. *Journal of Women and Aging* 3(2):63–84.

Belsky, J. 1988. *Here Tomorrow*. Baltimore: The Johns Hopkins University Press.

Belzer, A. and M. Rugh. 1991. Making your own mark. *Generations* 15(2):49–51.

Bender, G. and P. Hart. 1987. A model for health promotion for the rural elderly. *The Gerontologist* 27(2):1339–42.

Chappell, N. 1991. Living arrangements and sources of caregiving. *Journal of Gerontology* 46(1):51–58.

Coward, R. 1979. Planning community services for the rural elderly: Implications from research. *The Gerontologist* 19(3):275–82.

Davis, D.C., M.C. Henderson, A. Boothe, M. Douglass, S. Faria, D. Kennedy, E. Kitchens, and M. Weaver. 1991. An interactive perspective on the health beliefs and practices of rural elders. *Journal of Gerontological Nursing* 17(5):11–17.

Dunkle, R. 1988. Alternatives to institutionalization. In *Aging, Health and Society*. 2d ed., edited by C. Kart, E. Metress, and S. Metress. Boston: Jones and Bartlett Publishers.

Fenton, M., L. Rouk, and S. Iha. 1988. The nursing center in a rural community: The promotion of family and community health. *Family and Community Health* 11(2):14–24.

Foley, L., ed. 1976. *Stand Close to the Door*. Sacramento, CA: School of Social Work, California State University.

Fox, J. and I. Abraham. 1991. Designing continuing care retirement centers: Toward a partnership of formal and informal care providers. *Family and Community Health* 14(2):68–80.

Gelfand, D. 1988. *The Aging Network: Programs and Services*. 3d ed. New York: Springer.

Gillis, J. 1985. *A Guide to Compassionate Care of Aging*. New York: Thomas Nelson.

Graham, R. 1989. Adult day care: How families of dementia patients respond. *Journal of Gerontological Nursing* 15(3):27–31.

Harbert, A. and C. Wilkinson. 1979. Growing old in rural America. *Aging* 291(292):36–40.

Johnson, J. 1991. Health care practices of rural aged. *Journal of Gerontological Nursing* 178:15–19.

Johnson, K. 1979. Rural health woes. *Erath County Electric News* December 6–8.

Kart, C.S., E.S. Metress, and J.F. Metress. 1978. *Aging and Health: Biologic and Social Perspectives*. Menlo Park, CA: Addison-Wesley.

Katz, K. and P. Maginn. 1989. Family services in adult day care. In *Planning and Managing Adult Day Care*, edited by L. Webb. Owings Mill, MD: National Health Publishing.

Krout, J. 1986. Linkages in the community. *The Gerontologist* 26(5):510–15.

Krout, J. 1987. Rural-urban differences in senior center activities and services. *The Gerontologist* 27(1):92–97.

Lally, M., E. Black, Thornock et al. 1979. Older women in single room occupant (SRO) hotels: A Seattle profile. *The Gerontologist* 19(1):67–74.

McCoy, J. and R. Conley. 1990. Surveying board and care homes: Issues and data collecting problems. *The Gerontologist* 30(2):147–53.

Montgomery, J. and E. Borgatta. 1987. Values, cost and health care policy. In *Critical Issues in Aging Policy*, edited by E. Borgatta and R. Montgomery. Newbury Park: Sage Publications.

Mor-Borak, M., L. Miller, and S. Leonard. 1991. Social networks, life events, and health of poor, frail elderly: A longitudinal study of buffering versus direct effect. *Family and Community Health* 14(2):1–13.

Morrow-Howell, N. and M. Ozawa. 1987. Helping networks: Seniors to seniors. *The Gerontologist* 27(1):17–20.

Ralston, A. 1987. Senior center research: Policy from knowledge. In *Critical Issues in Aging Policy*, edited by E. Borgatta and R. Montgomery. Newbury Park: Sage Publications.

Report on Regional Public Hearings. 1976. (Publication 76-135). Washington, DC: Home Health Care, United States Department of Health, Education, and Welfare.

Schwartz, D. 1969. Aging and the field of nursing. In *Aging and Society*, edited by M. Riley, A. Funer, M. Moore, et al. New York: Russell Sage Foundation.

Sherman, S. and E. Newman. 1977. Foster-family care for the elderly in New York state. *The Gerontologist* 17(6):513–20.

Taetz, P. and S. Milton. 1979. Rural-urban differences in the structure of services for the elderly in upper New York counties. *J Gerontol* 34(3):429–37.

Thatcher, R. 1988. Health promotion in older adults. In *Nursing and the Aged: A Self Care Approach*. 3d ed., edited by I. Burnside. New York: McGraw-Hill Book Co.

Ward, S. 1983. Home health care. In *The Aged Patient*, edited by N. Ernst and H. Glazer-Waldman. Chicago: Year Book Medical Publishers.

Watkins, D.A. and J. M. Watkins. 1985. Policy responses to the needs of rural elderly. In *The Elderly in Rural Society*, edited by G.R. Lee. New York: Springer.

Weissert, W., J. Elston, E. Bolda, W. Zelman, E. Mutran, A. Mangum, R. Wilson, M. Patterson, and D. Alford. 1989. Services for maintaining independence. *Journal of Gerontological Nursing* 15(6):31–37.

21   Governmental Resources

Patricia F. Cheong

CHAPTER OUTLINE

FOCUS

This chapter describes governmental programs that assist older adults and that have increased gradually since the Older Americans Act was passed in 1965. These programs include those related to income, health care, housing, nutrition, transportation, and in-home services. Many of these programs help older adults maintain their independence in the community.

OBJECTIVES

1. Evaluate the value of universal governmental programs for older adults.

2. Describe the major governmental income programs that benefit older Americans.

3. List the major benefits of Medicare and Medicaid.

4. Evaluate the effectiveness of Medicare and Medicaid.

5. Explain the sources of Medicare and Medicaid funding.

6. Describe housing needs and alternatives for the indigent poor.

7. Describe the components of the aging network.

8. List several in-home services for older adults.

9. Evaluate the use of the food stamp program for older adults.

10. Discuss the major purpose of the National Institute on Aging.

In the course of a health crisis older patients or their families may turn to their primary care provider (often a nurse) for help with a variety of other problems that may have arisen as a result of or have been intensified during the health crisis. A number of governmental resources are available to address such problems as lack of insurance, lack of adequate income, need for home care, need for alternative housing, nursing home care, and need for social contact or social services.

However, the number of programs administered and funded through federal agencies has reached monumental proportions. In its 1986 annual report, the United States Senate Special Committee on Aging included reports on aging programs from thirty-one separate departments and agencies. The level of involvement varies greatly. Governmental programs may be funded by the federal government, by state governments, by local governments, or by a combination of all three. The eligibility of these programs may vary, depending on state or local guidelines. This fragmented array of services is administered through a complex maze of regulations that is challenging for a professional but especially daunting for a lay person to negotiate. As a result older persons may be underserved even by programs to which they are entitled.

GOVERNMENTAL PROGRAMS

Governmental programs can generally be divided into two kinds: *universal* programs, for which all or most of the population at risk is eligible, and *categorical* programs, for which only those individuals within a specifically defined subgroup may be eligible (e.g., only those people over age 65). However, when discussing programs for older people, differentiating between the two types of programs based on the level of funding and participation is useful. Those programs that reach most older people may be referred to as *universal* programs while those that reach significantly fewer may be viewed as *categorical*. However, this distinction is difficult to apply.

Impact of Universal Programs

Four programs reach the majority of older persons: Social Security, Supplemental Security Income, Medicare, and Medicaid. Two primary programs, both funded by the federal government, reach most older adults in the United States: Old Age Survivors and Disability Insurance (OASDI)—commonly referred to as Social Security—and Medicare. Social Security ensures a minimum level of income for retired workers, while Medicare provides a minimum level of health insurance for most persons age 65 and over. In 1985 about 94 percent of all Americans age 65 or over were drawing or were eligible to draw Social Security benefits. All older people are or should be covered by Medicare, Medicaid, or both.

Two secondary programs that enhance Social Security and Medicare benefits for special and low-income populations are Supplemental Security Income (SSI) and Medicaid. SSI provides additional income support for persons eligible for Social Security who have very low incomes. Medicaid is a federal/state funded program that covers the cost of Medicare deductibles and premiums for Medicare-eligible persons living on low incomes if they qualify.

Funding for these four programs accounts for over 80 percent of all federal dollars earmarked for programs for older adults, thus providing the broad base of financial support and health care for the entire population of older people in the United States (U.S. Senate Special Committee on Aging 1986).

Impact of Other Programs

On the other hand, less than 1 percent of all federal funds for older adult programs is allocated to community-based programs operated under the Older Americans Act of 1965, as amended. Although the services are available to all persons over age 60 without regard to income (therefore technically *universal* services), fewer individuals participate in these programs. However, for those who do, the services may greatly enhance their quality of life.

Older Americans Act funds are allocated to states based on each state's population over age 60. Within states the funds are allocated to regions, based on a statewide formula that may take into consideration the number of people over age 60 who are minority, who are poor, or who live in rural areas. The act calls for the development of locally coordinated systems of services to carry out its intent, which is to ensure that older people have adequate health, housing, income, transportation, and other services to enable them to continue to live independently.

The act requires that state funds and local funds match the federal funds in varying percentages. Therefore the level of services available will vary from state to state and from one community to another. It will depend on the level of federal funds allocated by population to a specific state, the level of additional state funds allocated over and above the required match, and the level of local support generated. Therefore to receive services, an older person must be fortunate enough to live in a community where these programs exist and are well-coordinated.

Increasingly, with the federal administration's concern for balancing the federal deficit, responsibility for care of older people has been pushed from the federal level to the state and local levels. Older Americans Act service providers have been under increasing pressure to respond to the needs of a growing population. These kinds of government-supported community-based services are essential to enhance the quality of life for older residents. The range of services available may include information and referral, case management, home-delivered meals, home health care, senior centers, meals in centers, transportation, wellness programs, legal services, and advocacy services for nursing home residents. Pushing state and local elected officials as well as federal legislators to recognize the growing demand in the face of diminishing dollars has been a focus of advocates for the aging population during the late 1980s and continues into the 1990s.

UNIVERSAL FEDERAL PROGRAMS

Income Programs

It has been said that if the income of the older people were adequate, all their other problems would disappear. This obviously overstates the case, but there is no question that an adequate income makes a significant difference in most other areas of life. The federal government in general and the Senate Special Committee on Aging in particular have sought to eliminate poverty among older Americans. The major portion of federal funds supporting programs for older people is devoted to the two income programs, Social Security (OASDI) and Supplemental Security Income (SSI). The reduction in the percentage of older people living in poverty to less than 15 percent is attributable to the fact that the number of people age 65 and older receiving OASDI increased from two out of ten in 1950 (U.S. Department of Health, Education and Welfare, Social Security Administration 1973) to nine out of ten in 1984 (U.S. Senate 1986), in addition to the introduction of SSI in the early 1970s. However, in 1989, although only

11.4 percent of people age 65 and over lived on income at the poverty line, another 8 percent had income between the poverty level and 125 percent of the poverty guideline, making a total of 19 percent, nearly one-fifth of the older population, being poor or near-poor (American Association of Retired Persons and Administration on Aging 1990).

The Social Security Act was passed in 1935 after many years of study and struggle. Many observers say it passed Congress only because of the impact of the Great Depression in the 1930s. Since that time there has been a gradual shift from a program that was intended to provide a minimal supplement to retirees' other sources of income (which were found to be extremely limited) to one that is the primary source of retirement income for most American retirees. Other provisions of this act that are significant for people under 65 are the disability and survivors' insurance provisions. But for the purposes of this discussion, attention will be directed to the provision that provides income in retirement based on prior earnings and contributions from those earnings and the SSI program.

Social Security (OASDI). The Social Security check that more than 39 million people receive each month represents, in reality, a transfer of funds from the working population to the nonworking population. It is a commonly held notion that the amount people receive each month comes from the payments that they and their employers personally have deposited into the Social Security Trust Fund during their working lives. That this (erroneous) notion is held is not surprising, since for years it has been the basis on which the program has been "sold" to the American public. A number of factors have brought the "Social Security issue" to the forefront of the public's attention. Among these are the following:

- The number of recipients 65 and older has dramatically increased in a relatively short period of time (from approximately 5 million in 1950 to more than 38.9 million in 1989).

- The average monthly payment to retirees has increased more than twelvefold. For example, in 1940 the average payment to an aged couple was $36.40 (U.S. Department of Health, Education and Welfare, Social Security Administration 1973), whereas in October 1985 it was $464 (U.S. Senate 1986).

- The contribution deducted from workers' pay has increased dramatically (lower-income workers now face the fact that they pay more in Social Security taxes than in income tax).

For 15 percent of the population age 65 and over, Social Security is their only source of income; for more than one-fourth of older people (26 percent), Social Security accounts for almost all their income (90 percent or more); and for almost two-thirds (62 percent) of older Americans 65 years and older, Social Security is the major source of income (50 percent or more).

In general, workers with average earnings can expect Social Security benefits to replace just over 40 percent of their earnings (U.S. Department of Health and Human Services, September 1990). Benefit increases are made annually based on the change in the Consumer Price Index (CPI) from the third quarter of one year to the third quarter of the next (U.S. Department of Health and Human Services, January 1990).

If a client is entitled to Social Security benefits or the nurse believes the client may be so entitled, the person should be encouraged to gather certain documents. The person should take his/her Social Security card or number, proof of age, record of citizenship or legal status, proof of income, and proof of resources to the nearest Social Security office or call the Social Security Administration's toll-free 800 telephone number. Each person's entitlement must be calculated by the Social Security Administration. The Social Security worker can check the person's earnings record, age, and contributions record to determine eligibility and the amount the person should receive.

The services of the Social Security Administration are free of charge. Older people should be wary of advertisers offering to help them obtain Social Security benefits for a fee or those charging a fee for books on how to obtain benefits. The recipient can request that Social Security checks be deposited directly in the bank. This method is safe, convenient, and reliable and it prevents theft, special trips to the bank, and incorrect accounting.

In the case of an individual who is deemed by the Social Security Administration to be unable to manage the benefit check, a representative payee may be appointed. A representative payee is an individual or group—relative or nonrelative—who volunteers to oversee the financial management of the monthly payments. Approved payees promise to act in the beneficiary's best interest and must provide to the Administration an accounting of how the benefits were used. The Social Security Administration requires medical evidence and other documentation before appointing a representative payee.

Because benefits vary, choosing the best retirement date is advisable. Several factors to consider are the individual's age, expected earnings for the year, estimated benefits, and whether family members will also receive benefits. Notifying the Social Security Administration some months before impending retirement will ensure that the applicant receives helpful information on which to base the retirement date decision.

The Social Security Administration publishes a pamphlet entitled *Personal Earnings & Benefits Estimate Statement* (PEBES). This pamphlet includes instructions for estimating monthly benefits depending on whether the individual retires at age 62, 65, or 70. The major types of coverage are listed here.

- A retired worker who starts drawing benefits at age 65 may draw full benefits.

- A retired worker who wishes to begin drawing benefits as early as age 62 will receive reduced benefits, due to the longer drawing period.

- A worker who waits to retire until after age 65 will see benefits increase.

- If both the wife and the husband are covered workers, each may elect to receive the Social Security benefits to which he/she is separately entitled, if it would be to their advantage to do so.

- A retiree's spouse receives one-half of the amount of the retired worker's monthly amount.

Although taking a job will affect Social Security benefits, it may not necessarily mean losing benefits if the individual is blind or disabled.

Supplemental Security Income (SSI). Supplemental Security Income (SSI) pays monthly checks to certain people with limited income and resources. SSI is designed to provide a minimum income for persons age 65 or older or blind or disabled who have limited income and resources. In 1987, approximately 70 percent of SSI recipients also received Social Security benefits.

The SSI program is funded from general tax revenues—not from Social Security taxes—but it is administered by the Social Security Administration. SSI benefits are not based on prior work. In 1987 about 65 percent of SSI recipients were disabled, about 33 percent were older adults, and 2 percent were blind. About 11 percent were both older and disabled (American Association of Retired Persons and Rio Grande Council of Governments Area Agency on Aging 1988).

The economic status of older adults is far more varied than that of any other age group. Although some older persons have substantial resources, a surprising number have practically none. Comparing average income statistics conceals the simple fact that an unusually high proportion of older adults has income and other economic resources below or slightly above the poverty level. Each person should contact the local Social Security office to determine whether income and resource levels would meet SSI eligibility requirements.

In 1987, 75 percent of those entitled to SSI on the basis of age were women, while more than 50 percent of those entitled on the basis of disability were women. Among SSI recipients entitled on the basis of age, over 40 percent were age 80 or more, compared with the fact that only 21 percent of the older population is over age 80. The application for determination of SSI eligibility is important for reasons other than income alone. In many states, eligibility for Medicaid benefits as well as other welfare services provided by states, such as food stamps, is based on SSI eligibility. Some states provide financial benefits for SSI recipients in addition to those from federal resources, a fact that the staff of the local Social Security office will share. A determination of SSI eligibility might produce a monthly check of only $1.80 but also provide free prescription drugs, transportation to and from medical services, and home health services, for example. These added benefits would make an appreciable net impact on spendable income.

If a claim for SSI is denied, the applicant has the right to appeal the decision. In the majority of cases, SSI appeals are successful. Therefore it is important that the applicant not become dissuaded by those who might suggest that the individual has too much income or resources. He/she should complete the full application process and receives notification of either eligibility or ineligibility. Notification of ineligibility becomes the basis for the appeal.

Occasionally a person may have been disqualified from SSI because of higher than allowable income or resources. If subsequently the income or resources have been depleted, the individual should be encouraged to reapply. The most common changes that affect one's eligibility for SSI are a decrease in income or resources, the death of a spouse, the move of a spouse into a nursing home, a move to another state, a medical condition that worsens, or a disabled child who reaches age 18 (U.S. Department of Health and Human Services, Social Security Administration 1990). Since every case is determined individually, the importance of contacting the Social Security Administration directly cannot be overemphasized.

Health Programs

Some facts relating to the health status of older people are worth noting at this point. Only 5 percent of those age 65 and older are institutionalized, mostly in nursing homes. However, the likelihood of nursing home care being needed increases with age; women are at greater risk of institutionalization than are men (U.S. Senate Special Committee on Aging 1990). So, approximately 95 percent of our nation's older adults live in the community. Although almost 80 percent may have some chronic condition, the majority claim that they are not mobility impaired.

Because of declining physical health, the demand on health care services is higher by older people than by younger people. In 1989, people age 65 and over averaged almost twice as many contacts with physicians (nine contacts) as those under age 65 (five contacts). This age group also experienced hospital stays averaging about two-thirds longer than those under age 65 (8.9 days compared with 5.3 days) (American Association of Retired Persons and Administration on Aging 1991).

Therefore the cost of health care is of major importance to the older population overall and of crisis proportions to certain individual older people. The total per-capita medical cost for people age 65 or older had risen from $419 in 1963—before the advent of Medicare—to $5360 in 1987; while for younger people, the total per-capita cost was still only $1290 (AARP 1990). Although public funds covered about three-quarters of these costs for older persons in 1987 (compared to only 26 percent of health care costs for younger persons), the smaller percentage of out-of-pocket expenses represented a much higher dollar amount ($1500) for older people than the average of $967, which represented 75 percent of the much lower total cost of $1290 for younger people (American Association of Retired Persons and Administration on Aging 1991). The majority of out-of-pocket expenses for older people are for physician visits and services, health care services, and nursing home care not covered by Medicare, Medicaid, or private insurance (American Association of Retired Persons and Administration on Aging 1991).

In 1986 the Catastrophic Health Care Act was passed by Congress and then repealed after pressure was brought to bear by advocacy groups and older people. Older citizens objected to the fact that much of the coverage was available through coverage they already had. They also objected to the fact that older people would be taxed for benefits to younger or disabled beneficiaries. The move for a national health insurance program has gained momentum in the 1990s.

Medicare. Medicare, the nation's only federal health insurance program and the principal federal program to help older people meet the costs of health care, was enacted as part of the Social Security amendments of 1965. This program was the result of decades of congressional and special-interest-group attempts to create some form of national health insurance. The program is financed by a portion of the payroll taxes paid by employers and employees. Despite the deficiencies of the program, Medicare has provided some cushion for the rapidly escalating health costs that often decimate the savings of many older people.

Medicare provides health insurance for people age 65 or older, certain disabled people under 65, and people of any age who have permanent kidney failure. It provides basic protection for the cost of health care but it does not cover all expenses (U.S. Department of Health and Human Services, Social Security Administration 1991).

Among the kinds of health care not covered by Medicare that many older people will need but will end up paying for out of their own pocket or going without are:

- home health care that does not require skilled personnel

- nursing home care (except for a limited time)

- routine medical checkups and related tests

- prescription drugs

- testing for and the cost of eyeglasses and hearing aids

- routine dental care and dentures

The Health Care Financing Administration (HCFA) is the federal agency in charge of administering the Medicare program. The Social Security Administration handles enrollment and provides information to the public about the program.

There are two parts to Medicare: hospital insurance (also called Part A Medicare) and medical insurance (also called Part B Medicare), which covers costs related to physicians' charges and certain other medical expenses. The hospital insurance is financed by a portion of payroll taxes that also fund Social Security. Eligibility for hospital coverage is based on Social Security eligibility. The medical insurance is provided through monthly premiums paid by people who choose to enroll. In order to be eligible for Part A Medicare hospital insurance, a 65-year-old person must be getting or be eligible for Social Security or railroad retirement benefits, be a retired government employee, or be the spouse of an individual 62 or older who is entitled to Social Security benefits. Most older people are eligible for the Part A hospital coverage. However, individuals who are 65 but do not qualify under these conditions can buy the coverage for a premium (which was $221 per month in May 1993) with the stipulation that they must also enroll in and pay a monthly premium for Part B medical coverage as well ($36.60/month in 1993).

Almost anyone who is 65 or older can enroll in Part B Medicare medical insurance. Those who are getting Social Security or railroad retirement benefits will be automatically enrolled in both parts of Medicare but have the option of turning down the Part B coverage for which they must pay the premium. The Part A hospital coverage is subject to certain annual deductibles and benefit periods. A benefit period is defined as beginning the day an individual enters the hospital and ending when the patient has been out of the hospital for sixty days in a row. Medicare covers a portion of hospital costs for up to ninety days within a benefit period. For hospitalization within the first sixty days an individual must pay a deductible, which in 1993 was $676, but Medicare pays all covered services. For the last thirty days of a ninety-day stay, the individual must pay $169/day for covered services, with Medicare paying the remainder. The same benefits are renewed in the next benefit period. If a patient needs to be hospitalized for more than ninety days, some of the sixty lifetime reserve days may be used. If reserve days are used, the individual must pay $338 per day for covered services.

One of the flaws in the Medicare system is that a seriously ill patient may run out of Medicare coverage. Once a seriously ill older patient has been in the hospital, it may not be possible for a family to keep the patient out of the hospital for the sixty days required to start a new benefit period with renewed coverage. Once all of the sixty lifetime reserve days are used, a patient who has not been out of the hospital sixty days has no more Medicare coverage.

Medicare hospital insurance helps cover the cost of such services as semiprivate room and meals, regular nursing care, anesthesia, operating room costs, recovery room costs, intensive care costs, and coronary care costs. While in the hospital, medications, lab tests and Xrays, medical supplies and appliances, and rehabilitation services such as physical therapy are covered. Hospital insurance also will cover some of the costs related to skilled nursing home or rehabilitation services, skilled nursing care at home or therapy services at home (but not custodial care), and hospice care.

Part B Medicare medical insurance helps pay for physicians' services and many other medical services and supplies that are not covered by Medicare hospital insurance. In 1993 a beneficiary had to pay a $100 annual deductible for medical insurance before Medicare would start paying. He/she also had to pay 20 percent of the approved charges for covered services for the rest of the year. Medicare generally pays for 80 percent of the *approved charges* after the deductible has been met. Examples of physicians' services covered by Part B Medicare medical insurance are medical and surgical services, including anesthesia, diagnostic tests that are part of treatment, Xrays, inpatient or outpatient radiologists' and pathologists' services, services provided by the physician's office nurse,

medications that cannot be self-administered, blood transfusions, and medical supplies. Other services covered by medical insurance include outpatient clinic or emergency room, ambulance transportation, home dialysis equipment and support services, outpatient physical therapy and speech pathology services, radiation treatments, and in certain cases, home health care (U.S. Department of Health and Human Services, Social Security Administration 1991).

Since Medicare has out-of-pocket expenses such as deductibles, premiums, and co-insurance, many older people opt to purchase private insurance. Types of private insurance include major medical, employer group insurance, association group insurance, or Medicare Supplement policies. Medicare Supplement or Medigap policies are the most common and provide useful coverage. Medicare Supplement policies are specially designed to interface with Medicare and to pay all or part of Medicare deductibles and coinsurance amounts. Some also pay for health services that Medicare does not cover (U.S. Department of Health and Human Services, Social Security Administration 1991). Medigap policies have been increasingly regulated by state departments of insurance to ensure that coverage meets certain standards and that coverage is clearly spelled out (see Chapter 18 for more details).

Some insurance policies are designed to offer a particular kind of coverage, such as nursing home coverage, specific disease coverage (such as cancer policies), or hospital indemnity policies, which pay a fixed amount per day for hospital stays. Individuals are warned to read such policies very carefully to avoid pitfalls such as escalating hospital costs that in the future will far exceed the daily rate covered when the indemnity policy was purchased; stipulations in nursing home policies that cover only skilled nursing home care when an individual may require custodial care in such an institution; waiting periods before benefits begin; or lack of coverage for pre-existing conditions by disease-related policies.

As was the case with Social Security benefits Medicare is explained here in general terms. Each person's particular case must be examined with regard to eligibility and payment for services to which he or she is entitled.

Medicaid. The Medicaid program is designed to provide payments for medical services for the poor, including the older poor. Federally funded through Title XIX of the Social Security Act, Medicaid is administered by the states. Before the enactment of the legislation, some states paid a portion of medical and health care costs for the poor. States' policies varied widely as to what costs were covered, who was eligible, and even whether there was any coverage at all. With Medicaid (or its counterpart under other names in some states), a universal program for the poor was established. States were required to provide at least as much coverage as was provided before the legislation took effect. In some instances, but not all, the states increased the coverage with the addition of federal funds.

Eligibility also varies among the states, since each state is allowed to establish its own criteria for determining eligibility. The Medicaid program is related to poverty level, but the income eligibility criteria are not consistent from state to state.

Another variable with which applicants and recipients must contend is the fact that each individual medical service provider may decide whether or not to participate in the Medicaid program. For example, some nursing homes accept Medicaid patients; others do not. It is not uncommon to hear older people complain that a certain doctor would not see them because the doctor does not accept Medicaid patients. The provider's right to decline to accept Medicaid reimbursement severely limits the availability of services to Medicaid patients. Many providers do not wish to adhere to the state-determined fee structures. Providers also complain about the amount of paperwork required and the delay in reimbursement by the paying agency.

Although Medicaid is administered through the state welfare departments (e.g., in Texas, the Texas Department of Human Services), eligibility for Medicaid usually rests upon determination of entitlement for SSI payments, which is made at the local Social Security office. Every case is determined on its merits, requiring close coordination with the Social Security office and the local office of the state welfare department.

Housing Programs

In 1989, more than 20 percent of all households in the United States were occupied by persons age 65 and older. Of those households, 75 percent were owned and occupied by older persons; 83 percent were owned free and clear (U.S. Senate Special Committee on Aging 1990, p. 117). Most older people tend to remain in their homes and over the years develop special housing needs because of age-related changes including health, income, and household size. About 12 percent of older homeowners have disabilities or health problems that dictate the need to modify the home and obtain supportive services in the home (American Association of Retired Persons 1987).

With increasing age, people tend to rent rather than own. This is due in part to increasing dissatisfaction with their housing situation and an inability to maintain the home because of physical deficiencies or spiraling costs. It is not uncommon for homes purchased by couples who grew old along with the neighborhood to be located in neighborhoods now classified as run-down and crime ridden. Older people find themselves saddled with property of low value and low incomes, increased maintenance costs, and need to escape from an unhealthy environment. Rapidly rising property taxes, home insurance, utility bills, and maintenance costs are forcing some older homemakers to sell their homes and seek other living arrangements. In 1985 the percentage of income spent on housing (excluding maintenance) was higher for older households than for younger households, including those owners with and without a mortgage and among renters.

Recognizing that housing for older citizens is a problem of national scope, Congress has passed a number of legislative acts designed to help alleviate the situation. One of the key programs is rental assistance for lower-income families, the elderly, and the disabled, established under Section 8 of the Housing Act of 1937 as amended. This program is designed to pay part of the cost for low-income families or older/disabled persons to live in rental housing. It provides for paying part of the rent and utility costs in existing rental units (houses or multiple dwellings), for building new units for use by eligible families or persons, or for rehabilitation of existing units owned by the Department of Housing and Urban Development (HUD) for occupancy by eligible families or individuals.

People age 62 and over who meet the income and asset eligibility requirements may participate in the Section 8 rental assistance program. After computing the applicant's total income, the administrative agency guarantees to the landlord the monthly payment of that portion of the rent and utilities cost that exceeds 30 percent of the applicant's income. To investigate the availability of housing under this program, the person should contact the local housing authority or the nearest HUD area office.

Another major program provides housing for older people and the disabled under Section 202 of the Housing Act of 1959. Section 202 allows private nonprofit organizations to obtain funds for the construction or rehabilitation of housing for rental units for older adults and the disabled. Direct loans at a low interest rate from the federal government support this program. These loans are provided to enable sponsors who would not otherwise be able to secure loans to develop housing that can be rented at a lower-than-market value due to the reduced level of interest at which the principal is loaned. For example, a church that sees the need for a more protective living environment for older citizens in its community could obtain a Section 202 loan to construct a facility that it would manage, repaying the loan from the rents charged to the residents. It is not uncommon for Section 202 housing to include a site manager, congregate meals, and social services, all of which provide an environment conducive to enhancing the lives of the residents.

A third program is aimed at housing for low- and middle-income families under Section 236 of the National Housing Act, as added by the Housing and Urban Development Act of 1968. Under this program, private corporations can construct housing with federal guarantees and payment of a portion of the interest to private lending institutions. Because of the reduced costs to the builder, the units can be rented at rates below the existing market level.

The federal government also makes provisions among its housing programs to support the construction and rehabilitation of nursing home facilities (Section 232, National Housing Act 1952). This program provides government guarantees and insurance for loans to private, nonprofit, or profit-making groups to construct or rehabilitate nursing home facilities for patients requiring skilled nursing or intermediate care.

The programs just discussed here constitute only a small part of the federal housing programs developed by the federal government. They are, however, among the most important in their impact on housing for older people. The practitioner with a client in need of housing is encouraged to contact the local public housing authority, the nearest HUD area office, or, in the case of rural clients, the county Farmers Home Administration Office.

THE AGING NETWORK

The Older Americans Act (OAA) of 1965, as amended, has guided and governed many of the nation's efforts to respond to the problems and enhance the opportunities of a rapidly growing population of older Americans. The Act, through the Federal Administration on Aging and a network of state, area, and local agencies, fosters economic and personal independence for older persons.

Although many people point to the first White House Conference on Aging in 1961 as the catalyst that brought together the necessary congressional forces to enact the OAA, the struggle predates the 1961 White House conference. For a number of years before 1961, educators, social scientists, human service providers, and special interest groups representing the older population had been stressing with increasing intensity the need for a focal point for older adults' concerns at the national level. This national concern, plus the favorable climate for social legislative action during the Great Society years of Lyndon B. Johnson's presidency, led to the first White House Conference on Aging in 1961 and to the passage into law of the Older Americans Act of 1965.

The Older Americans Act made major strides towards organizing and establishing programs and services for many older people across the country. It designated a special office—the Administration on Aging (AoA), within what is now the federal Department of Health and Human Services—to be the agency through which concerns of older Americans were to be addressed.

Some older people had problems that could not be solved solely by increases in Social Security benefits and payments for health care. Some of them needed safe, reliable transportation to the grocery store or medical facilities; some needed more nutritious diets; some had lost their friends and family and needed companions and advisors; and some older people needed information and motivation to maintain active healthy lifestyles. Through the aging network, gerontologists, social service providers, and

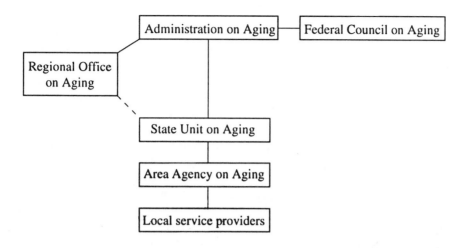

Figure 21–1   The aging network

planners as well as others interested in older people are taking steps to alleviate these and similar problems. The OAA programs are not as pervasive as the income and health programs discussed earlier, but they do offer services that can be of specific use to a nurse's patients.

Older Americans Act programs are not based on income and therefore are not welfare programs. Under Title III of the Older Americans Act, programs are available to persons age 60 or older without regard to income. Individuals cannot be refused service based on their inability or unwillingness to pay a fee, but are encouraged to contribute toward the cost of services. Depending on the service, some services, such as fitness classes, may request voluntary contributions, while others, such as home-health care services, may rely on a sliding contribution scale to encourage appropriate levels of participant cost-sharing.

The Older Americans Act is reauthorized every four years. With each amendment come new areas of emphasis. The act was due to be amended in 1991, but Congress did not develop an amendment that could pass both the House and the Senate. Therefore, it was 1992 before the amendment was finalized. Reauthorization issues that continue to be debated include the need for additional levels of funding, cost sharing, outreach efforts to minority and frail older

persons, the need for more local flexibility to address local needs, more appropriate funding formulas, elevation of the Commissioner on Aging position to a higher level position within the federal Department of Health and Human Services, and the role of the area agencies on aging in providing direct services such as information and referral. The uniqueness of the aging network is that it provides for a nationwide network of locally administered and coordinated aging services. Although the specific services may vary, the generic services—information and referral, case management, senior centers, nutrition services including congregate and home-delivered meals, home health care services, legal services, nursing home ombudsmen programs—should be available in most regions throughout the country. To nurses and social workers one value of this network is in being able to refer families and those caring for older relatives to similar services in other areas of the country.

Structure

The Administration on Aging, Fig. 21-1, is the heart of the federal government's attempt to formulate policy and influence and coordinate the delivery of services to older people across the country. The early programs of services to the older citizens of each state were organized with technical assistance and funding through the state units on aging. In 1973, amendments to the Older Americans Act called for the organization of subagencies on aging; that is, the individual states were divided into regions and each region (frequently a multicounty area) had an Area Agency on Aging. Operating with funds allocated through the state units, the Area Agencies on Aging (AAAs) are responsible for providing leadership in the coordination and development of services for older adults throughout their geographic areas of responsibility. The Area Agencies on Aging dispense federal and state funds allocated to the region by the state units to local service providers to finance a wide variety of services for older people.

Local service providers have traditionally been the point of contact between the aging network and older adults. Most local service providers operate with a combination of federal (sometimes state) and local funds. Municipal and county governments, charitable organizations and individuals, volunteers, and churches have all joined forces to ensure the continued availability of services that have been shown to be essential to a number of people in their communities. Amendments to the act, made by Congress every four years, have required the aging network periodically to refocus its service delivery efforts to increase accessibility or to address changing needs. In some states the AAAs have been encouraged to address emerging service needs by providing services directly rather than subcontracting to local providers, if appropriate, for initiating demonstration projects or to increase the visibility of the AAA as a pivotal access point in the aging network. This strategy has been implemented in order to obtain increased visibility and funding from state governments and local foundations. Some of the more significant aging network programs and services carried out in communities throughout the country are discussed next in this chapter.

The 1987 amendments to the Older Americans Act called for services to be targeted to at-risk groups of older people. They also called for AAAs to budget an "adequate proportion" of funds for "access" services (which in 1992 include information and referral, outreach, case management, and transportation), for "in-home" services (as described further in the chapter), and for legal services (as defined in the following section). However, the following discussion of services pays some attention to the historical development of the programs.

Senior Centers

Senior centers existed in some parts of the country before the OAA was enacted. However, as a result of the act, the number of centers established increased substantially to meet the need for a central place for older people to congregate and, in many cases, develop new interests (or expand existing interests) and meet new friends. The 1978 amendments to the OAA strengthened the senior center as not only a gathering place but also the focal point of aging programs and services, such as information and referral, meals, and transportation. As they are discussed below, the relationship of these programs and services to the senior center concept will be apparent.

Senior centers enjoyed a period of growth in the 1980s. However, amendments to the Older Americans Act in the late 1980s shifted the focus to target existing services to those in greatest social and economic need, including low-income minority older persons, and to require the AAAs to budget an "adequate proportion" of funds on in-home services.

Nutrition Program

The nutrition program was started with the 1972 amendments to the Older Americans Act. It had become evident that a positive step had to be taken to provide for nutritious meals for older people. At the same time, it was felt that ancillary programs and services should accompany the meals. Therefore the nutrition program was designed to provide meals in a setting that would afford the opportunity for other meaningful activities for the participants. Recreational, educational, and health activities are a regular part of nutrition programs. The nutrition program lends itself to inclusion in a senior center if the community has a center.

The nutrition program guidelines recognize that some older people are not able to leave home for their meals. Therefore funding provisions allowed the development of home-delivered meals service. In most cases, home-delivered meals are delivered from the kitchen that services the nutrition site. With Medicare regulations now limiting the length of hospital stays, many older Americans depend on home-delivered meals during their convalescence at home. The demand for home-delivered meals has increased dramatically. Most home-delivered meal programs depend heavily on donations from local churches and foundations to meet the need that has outstripped federal funding increases.

The needs of those older people requiring special diets have not been overlooked. Nutrition sites are required to provide low-cholesterol meals, low-salt or salt-free meals, soft diets, and the like, both at the congregate site and in the home-delivered meals service. From the inception of the nutrition program, participants have been given the opportunity to contribute to the cost of the meals. Funds from participants must go back into the program to provide for additional meals.

Transportation

Numerous federal, state, and local programs have been developed to meet the transportation needs of older people. As the funding that flowed through the Area Agencies on Aging for services gained momentum from 1973 to 1975, small buses and vans were purchased by service providers to provide transportation for older people in their communities. Additional funds available through the Urban Mass Transit Act of 1975 provided for purchase of small buses equipped with wheelchair lifts for transportation of older people and the disabled. Transportation in a community with these vehicles is usually available by contacting a central dispatching office. Other communities establish special fares for older adults on existing transit routes, sell low-cost coupons for taxi fares, or use volunteers in personal automobiles. Transportation designed to take older people both to senior centers and to medical or social service appointments received increased attention in the 1987 amendments to the Older Americans Act. This was done to improve access to services by an increasing number of older adults.

Information and Assistance

The 1992 amendments to the OAA changed the service title "information and referral" to "information and assistance." An aging information and assistance (I&A) service is designed to collect and disseminate information relating to services that will meet the needs of the older population. The I&A office refers the older person to the appropriate agency or agencies that have been established to provide the ser-

vices meeting his/her needs. In addition to these referrals the I&A office has access to or information about transportation available to help the older person take advantage of the services. The more sophisticated I&A offices have workers who are trained to determine whether the callers have needs other than the ones expressed. They may also have outreach workers to visit a person if a call indicates that such a visit is warranted. Escort personnel may be available for assisting the disabled in visiting offices, filling out forms, carrying groceries, and so on.

After a referral is made, the worker places a follow-up call to both the older person and the agency to which referral was made to ensure that the older person's need was met. If the need was not met, the worker determines whether another agency or agencies could be called on to provide that service.

Many I&A services publish directories of services that list local social service agencies and other providers of services to older adults and their families. These directories are an invaluable resource not only to nurses and social workers but also to assist individuals and families to begin accessing needed services.

Another important function of the I&A service is to compile data regarding the demographics of its callers, the types of problems older callers or their families are experiencing when they call, the frequency of such problems, the nature of the referrals made, and the outcome of the referrals. An annual or periodic report of such information by the aging I&A service provides valuable information to Area Agencies on Aging to enable them to track trends and to plan and fund services to meet emerging needs.

Case Management

With Medicare patients being released from hospitals "quicker and sicker" as a result of regulations linking approved and reimbursed care to their diagnosed condition, many AAAs have initiated community case management services to enhance their ability to assess the need for in-home services. The 1992 amendments to the OAA formally mandate AAAs to provide case management. Case management usually involves a home visit and a comprehensive physical, social, and mental assessment, followed by the development of a coordinated care plan. The AAA may administer case management services directly or subcontract with a local provider.

In-Home Services

In-home services were defined by the 1987 amendments to the Older Americans Act as "homemaker and home health aide, visiting and telephone reassurance, and chore maintenance." In-home services often fill the homemaking gap that functional disability has created, enabling older people to remain in their own homes rather than being forced into an institutional living arrangement. In 1987, a new section to the act, Title III-D, provided for specially targeted in-home services to frail older people, including low-income minorities and persons with Alzheimer's disease.

Homemaker services provide personnel who make periodic visits to the homes of older persons to perform the household tasks that are difficult or impossible for older people to do for themselves. Such services as washing clothes, house cleaning, changing linen, bathing, food preparation, and obtaining adequate supplies of prescribed medicines are provided. Home health aides are certified to provide assistance with personal care such as bathing, feeding, or assisting with toileting the older person.

Visiting and telephone reassurance are designed primarily for the older person who lives alone and whose physical condition prevents most social interaction. Usually provided by volunteers these services are rendered through periodic home visits or telephone calls (usually daily) to assure the older person that he or she is not alone in the world and to provide the person with a regular contact with the network of services available in the community. Telephone reassurance has been credited with saving lives. A regular feature of the service includes an emergency plan that goes into effect if an older person does not answer a call. A sudden onset of illness or a fall that prevents the older person from reaching the telephone can be discovered by those designated to investigate the older person's residence. However, as the number of available volunteers has decreased with the entry of many women into the work force, electronic emergency response systems (ERS) have increasingly been used to meet an older person's need for safety and security. (See chapter 20 for more details on these systems.)

Chore maintenance services provide personnel to do heavy maintenance tasks for older people, such as small plumbing chores, cleaning windows, putting up storm windows, moving heavy objects into basements or attics, and lawn and yard care.

Some agencies provide the homemaker, home health aide, and chore maintenance service for a fee; some charge fees on a sliding scale; and some services have been furnished exclusively by volunteers. The nurse who has a patient with such needs should get in touch with the nearest I&A office for information about in-home services in the particular community.

Legal Services

The 1987 amendments to the OAA required that an "adequate proportion" of Title III funding be used to provide legal services for older people. Legal services may include not only assistance with basic wills, estate issues, and benefits counseling but also guardianship services. Guardianship services assist those deemed by the court to be unable to manage their own affairs. "Benefits counseling" is also available to assist clients to apply for financial, health, or social service benefits to which they may be entitled, such as SSI, Medicaid, or food stamps. Legal services may be provided by attorneys, paralegals, or qualified social service personnel. Services may be available in senior centers, county hospitals, or through other local providers.

Nursing Home Ombudsman Program

The Ombudsman (commissioner or official) program was mandated nationwide to bring community volunteers and representatives into nursing homes to function as a liaison between nursing home residents and the nursing home administration and to act as advocates for nursing home residents. The state ombudsmen, based in the state agencies on aging, give leadership by directing program activities and providing training and certification for volunteers and staff recruited at the local level. Usually a regional ombudsman for the AAA region recruits volunteer ombudsmen who are matched with local nursing homes and commit to visit on a regular basis. Local ombudsmen may also accompany health department officials on inspection visits.

The ombudsmen play an integral role not just in visiting residents or acting as a "community watchdog" in institutions housing our most vulnerable residents, but also in effectively working with the nursing home industry to maintain and enhance the standards of care for residents.

Other *Older Americans Act* Services

The 1987 amendments to the Older Americans Act authorized two new programs for which Congress was not to appropriate funding until funding levels for existing programs had reached certain levels. The two new program areas authorized were Title III-G, "Prevention of Elder Abuse, Neglect and Exploitation" and Title III-F, "Preventive Health Services." In the area of abuse, neglect, and exploitation, the role of the AAAs was prescribed as being supportive to the state agencies legally responsible for investigating reports of such cases. The small initial level of funding provided in the early 1990s was intended primarily to include public awareness campaigns or other preventive activities. Preventive health services, not funded until 1993, include a spectrum of counseling and health assessment srvices. The 1992 amendments moved the elder abuse agenda to a new Title VII and Title III-G focused on services to caregivers. By focusing on prevention, both of these new areas of emphasis add to the continuum of services maintained by the Older Americans Act.

OTHER FEDERAL PROGRAMS RELATING TO OLDER ADULTS

Although the Administration on Aging is the only federal agency and the AAAs are the only local agencies mandated by Congress to develop and promote programs solely for older adults, there are programs relating to older adults in many other agencies. Some governmental agencies (e.g., the National Institutes of Health) have a division exclusively concerned with programs or research related to aging. Many of the programs are primarily funding mechanisms that are not specifically for older persons but rather allow older persons to be considered eligible for the program. The allocations decisions for many of these programs are made at the local level. This is characteristic of Title XX of the Social Security Act, General Revenue Sharing, and the Community Development

Block Grants of the Department of Housing and Urban Development (Gelfand and Olsen 1980).

Title XX of the Social Security Act

Title XX of the Social Security Act provides federal monies for a variety of social programs, many of which are available to older people. They are determined by the state, frequently by the state public welfare department. Often these entitlement services are provided through contracts or purchase-of-service arrangements with community service providers such as the Visiting Nurse Association. Among the services available to those who qualify for assistance on the basis of income, usually SSI entitlements, are

- *Homemaker service*—nonmedical personal care of the client in the home, with limited support services such as some household tasks and transportation

- *Chore services*—performance of such essential household tasks as shopping, meal preparation, simple home repairs

- *Congregate and home-delivered meals*

- *Health assessment service*

- *Day activity services*—both personal and social care in a protected environment and rehabilitative day care with a full range of rehabilitative services. Support services, such as transportation, may be included.

- *Alternative living plans*—includes such placements as foster homes

- *Protective services*—social and legal services for those who are abused, neglected, or exploited and have no one willing or able to act on their behalf

As has been noted repeatedly, not all these Title XX services are available in every community. Each nurse must talk with the local representative of the agency that implements Title XX to determine availability of services.

Food Stamp Program

The food stamp program is a nationwide program that helps low-income people obtain more nutritious diets.

Food stamps can be redeemed for foodstuffs at authorized grocery stores and other outlets. Older persons may also use their food stamps to obtain meals at congregate nutrition programs and home-delivered meals programs. The program is administered by the Department of Agriculture at the federal level and by state or county social service departments at the state and local levels. These social service departments determine the eligibility of low-income persons and set the benefit levels. Special provisions address the needs of persons age 60 or over. For example, households with older persons are able to deduct more expenses from their income to establish eligibility and may be subject to a more lenient financial resources standard. Older persons may apply for food stamps at Social Security offices, may apply through an authorized representative, or have the office interview waived if they cannot come to the office. Sometimes other services, such as reduced telephone rates, are available based on an individual's receipt of certain benefits such as food stamps. Therefore, the nurse should encourage the older person not to decline a seemingly small food stamps benefit for which he/she may be eligible.

National Institute on Aging

The National Institute on Aging was established in 1974. It conducts research on the biologic population and sociologic aspects of aging at its Gerontology Research Center in Baltimore, Maryland. It also supports research by others at universities and laboratories across the United States. It has a limited publications program but does not engage in support of service delivery.

Veterans Administration

The Veterans Administration (VA) has the responsibility for meeting the health, human services, and income maintenance needs of eligible veterans. The VA's health care system includes acute medical, surgical, and psychiatric inpatient and outpatient care; extended hospital, nursing home, and domiciliary care; noninstitutional extended care; and a range of special programs and professional services for older veterans in both inpatient and outpatient settings (U.S. Senate 1988). Disability and survivor benefits, such as pension, compensation, and dependency and indemnity compensation, administered by the Department of Veterans Benefits provide all or part of the income for certain persons age 65 or older. For information or assistance in applying for veterans benefits, interested persons should contact any of the VA offices throughout the United States and territories.

SUMMARY

The growing impact of older Americans on the national economy and political scene is evidenced in the tremendous increase in public and private programs placing new emphasis on the older population. Although a wide variety of social, medical, and income-support programs are available to older people in the United States, they still are uncoordinated, fragmented, and poorly distributed geographically. For example, at least four federal agencies or programs support home health care for older people in some fashion, yet home health care is available only to a minority of the older Americans who need it. Such basic needs as legal services are only just beginning to be recognized as a component of social services. Information and referral services, the basic "glue" necessary to hold together a system as fragmented as the one that now exists, are frequently not available, not known to service providers, or woefully inadequate. However, shifts are taking place that affect the scope of services and clarify the responsibility of the major organizations providing services. Most observers believe that the next few years will be a time of consolidation and coordination, with the emphasis on determining service priorities and making currently established programs more widely available. The nurse can be an important catalyst in ensuring this goal for the community.

STUDY QUESTIONS

1. Name four programs that reach most older adults in the United States.

2. In what year was the Social Security Act passed?

3. What are the major benefits of the Social Security Act?

4. Explain the differences between Social Security and SSI (Supplementary Security Income).

5. In what year was Medicare enacted into law?

6. List the major benefits of Medicare hospital insurance and Medicare medical insurance.

7. What is the difference between Medicare and Medicaid eligibility and benefits?

8. What were the major provisions of the Older Americans Act (OAA) of 1965?

9. Describe several programs that were instituted as a result of the Older Americans Act.

10. Evaluate services for older adults provided for in Title XX of the Social Security Act.

REFERENCES

American Association of Retired Persons (AARP) and Administration on Aging (AoA). 1991. *A Profile of Older Americans*, Brochure PF3049 (1291)-D996.

American Association of Retired Persons (AARP). 1987. *Understanding Senior Housing*. Washington, DC: American Association of Retired Persons.

American Association of Retired Persons and Rio Grande Council of Governments Area Agency on Aging. 1988. *SSI Training Materials*. Produced for SSI Outreach Project. Washington, DC: American Association of Retired Persons.

Gelfand, D. and J. Olsen. 1980. *The Aging Network, Programs and Services*. New York: Springer.

U.S. Department of Health and Human Services. *Social Security Information Items*. January 1990.

U.S. Department of Health and Human Services. *Social Security News*. September 1990.

U.S. Department of Health and Human Services, Social Security Administration. *Medicare*. SSA Publication No. 05-10053. May 1991.

U.S. Department of Health and Human Services, Social Security Administration. *Press Release #5*. May 1990.

U.S. Department of Health, Education and Welfare, Social Security Administration. 1973. *Social Security Programs in the United States*. Washington, DC: United States Government Printing Office.

U.S. Senate Special Committee on Aging. 1986, 1990. *Aging in America, Trends and Projections*. Washington, DC: United States Department of Health and Human Services.

U.S. Senate Special Committee on Aging. 1988. *Developments in Aging: 1987*. Vols. 1, 2, 3. Washington, DC: United States Government Printing Office.

Part 6

SPECIAL CONCERNS

22 Maltreatment of Older Adults

Linda Cox Curry
Joy Graham Stone

CHAPTER OUTLINE

FOCUS

The phenomenon of maltreatment of older adults is hidden and largely unreported. This chapter describes types of maltreatment, profiles of victims and perpetrators, assessment criteria, prevention and intervention strategies, and current legislation.

OBJECTIVES

1. Identify the incidence of maltreatment of older adults in domestic and institutional settings.

2. Analyze problems in defining the categories of maltreatment of older adults.

3. Define the categories of maltreatment of older adults.

4. Compare and contrast the early (1980s) profiles of the victims and perpetrators of maltreatment

of older adults with those from current comparative research.

5. Explain why it is difficult to apply existing theories to the problem of maltreatment of older adults in view of current research findings.

6. List assessment indicators used to identify maltreatment of older adults.

7. Discuss appropriate intervention strategies for maltreatment of older adults.

8. Identify current legislation related to maltreatment of older adults and how it influences prevention, reporting, and intervention.

9. State ways to aid in the prevention and intervention of maltreatment of older adults.

DEFINITIONS

Even though the problem of maltreatment of older adults is not a new social concern, definitions are not clear. Baker has been given credit for the earliest reference to maltreatment of older adults dating back to 1975 (Homer and Gilleard 1990). He used the term "granny battering" to describe and draw attention to maltreatment of older adults in Great Britain. The study of maltreatment of older adults remained somewhat dormant for almost ten years while the focus of abuse literature and research centered on child abuse and spouse abuse (Douglass 1983). However, in the 1980s maltreatment of older adults began receiving heightened attention by researchers and publishers.

Despite the massive volume of literature and research on maltreatment of older adults in recent years, definitions remain varied, conflicting, and unique to the author. A review of the literature indicated an absence of a common frame of reference regarding maltreatment of older adults. Authors, researchers, and even state legislatures differ in their operational definitions. Variance persists among the descriptive definitions used to label, conceptualize, categorize, and describe maltreatment of older adults. What constitutes abuse in one study may constitute neglect in another. To further complicate matters, each state in the United States may have its own unique statutory definition with differing requirements for reporting and varying statutes regarding prosecution. Therefore legally, what is considered abuse of older adults in one state may not be considered abuse of older adults in another (Wolf 1988). The lack of uniform definitions for the terms associated with maltreatment of older adults has complicated the identification, description, and conceptualization of the phenomenon.

Although the literature exhibits no uniformity in the definitions, common terms have emerged (Hirst and Miller 1986; Valentine and Cash 1986; Wolf 1988; Callahan 1988; Pillemer and Finkelhor 1988; Brewer and Jones 1989; Hall 1989). However, the terms differ in defining characteristics and organizational groupings. Furthermore, the terms lack a standardized operational definition and are not mutually exclusive when compared between different authors and researchers. For instance, neglect may be separated into physical neglect, psychological neglect, and material neglect (McDonald and Abrahams 1990). Conversely, all forms of neglect might be joined together into a single descriptive category. Physical abuse and physical neglect may be divided into two categories or coupled together into a single category. Likewise, psychological abuse and psychological neglect may be categorized into a single grouping or separated into two distinct groups. Interestingly, the literature on maltreatment of older adults does seem to maintain a relatively exclusive and distinct category for material abuse. Different labels (i.e., exploitation, financial abuse) may be applied to the category of material abuse by differing researchers and authors, but the definition seems to remain the same (American Medical Association 1990).

Definitions of common terms used in literature and research on maltreatment of older adults are listed in Table 22-1. Readers are cautioned again that maltreatment definitions are unique and individual to each author. Therefore readers must understand each author's definition when reviewing the phenomenon of maltreatment of older adults. Otherwise they may find themselves in the dilemma of trying to understand and compare "apples to oranges." The descriptions used in this chapter were derived from examples and definitions commonly used in the research and literature on maltreatment of older adults. These definitions may be identical, similar, or dissimilar to definitions used in other literature, depending on the author.

Table 22–1 Terms Used Regarding Maltreatment of Older Adults

Term	Definition	Examples
Physical Abuse	Direct, nonaccidental physical or sexual assaults that result in harm to an older person's body. Physical abuse involves the active attempt of the perpetrator to inflict pain, injury and/or restraint on the victim	Beatings, slappings, shakings, sexual molestations, burns, cuts, threats with a weapon, harsh physical restraints, intentional rough handling, unnecessary physical confinements (Hirst and Miller 1986)
Physical Neglect	Failure to provide for physical safety and failure to prevent physical harm (Foelker, Holland, Marsh, and Simmons 1990)	Failure to provide the essential necessities of daily life (i.e., shelter, food, clothing, exercise and mobility, cleanliness, responsiveness to calls for help, appropriate temperature, hygiene); inappropriate restraints due to lack of knowledge; rough handling due to improper technique; withholding or depriving assistance with activities of daily living (ADL); failure to provide assistance with meal preparation or feeding when needed; delayed or denied medical treatment (Hirst and Miller 1986; Pillemer and Finkelhor 1988)
Psychological Abuse	Direct infliction of emotional pain or manipulative coercion on an older person	Intimidation, ridicule, verbal threats, yelling/screaming, name calling, insults, humiliations, harsh tones, harsh orders, withholding of affection, social isolation, abandonment

Category	Definition	Examples
Psychological Neglect	Failure to provide for the emotional needs and security of an older person; has been commonly labeled benign neglect, even though the emotional consequences to older persons may not be so benign	Leaving the older person alone or isolated for prolonged periods of time; withholding visitation from others; failure to listen and communicate effectively; failure to provide psychological stimulation; failure to provide a supportive, nurturing environment; unpleasant physical surroundings (i.e., no television, few personal belongings, a lack of color and luster to surroundings, no calendars or clocks large enough for the person to see); unpleasant odors (i.e., urine smells, vomitus, body odors); unpleasant sounds (i.e., the cries or screams of others, noise during a rest period)
Material Abuse	Direct, nonaccidental, infliction of financial, property, or material loss to older persons through exploitation and improper or illegal use or misuse of their funds, valuables, and material resources	Theft; mismanagement of an older person's material resources for one's own gain; use of an older person's material resources for one's own gain; use of an older person's money for payment of perpetrator's own bills and valuables; embezzlement; various schemes/scams/cons
Material Neglect	Failure to provide for the proper management, protection, and security of an older person's finances, property, and valuables, resulting in material loss to the older person	Poor investments of an older person's money; improper financial advice; coercion to the older person regarding financial materials; failure to assist the older person with paying bills in a timely manner; failure to maintain the upkeep of an older person's property when the responsibility is given to perpetrator (i.e., car maintenance, yard care, home repairs, dusting furniture, failure to prevent children or pets from damaging or destroying valuables and property)

(continued)

Term	Definition	Examples
Active Maltreatment	An intentional act of omission or commission that results in physical or psychological pain or injury, or material loss to an older person. The perpetrator directly refuses to fulfill his/her responsibilities and obligation to the older person. The act is considered to be consciously derived with active knowledge, foresight, awareness, and/or planning by the perpetrator. The focus of this descriptive term is on the motivational characteristics underlying the maltreatment of the older adult. Therefore this term may be used in conjunction with the other terms that focus primarily on the manner in which harm is manifested on the older person.	(See physical, psychological, and material examples.)
Passive Maltreatment	An unintentional act of omission or commission that results in physical or psychological pain or injury, or material loss to an older person. The perpetrator indirectly or unintentionally fails to fulfill his/her responsibilities and obligation to the older person. The act is believed to occur unconsciously, unknowingly, or without the active foresight, thought, knowledge, or awareness of the perpetrator. The focus of this descriptive term is on the motivational characteristics underlying the maltreatment of the older adult. Therefore this term may be used in conjunction with the other terms that focus primarily on the manner in which harm is manifested on the older person.	(See physical, psychological, and material examples.)

Violation of Personal Rights	Denial or deprivation of the personal rights of an older person	Loss of privacy; lack of confidentiality to medical records; decision making without the active involvement of the older person; disregard for the older person's values; forcing the older person to change place of residence without his/her expressed or direct consent; interference with the transmission of mail; involuntary discharge from a care facility; forced or prevented will alterations, divorces, or marriages (Sengstock, McFarland, and Hwalek 1990)
Self-Abuse	Direct and willful self-infliction of pain, anguish, or loss	Cutting oneself with razors; burning oneself with cigarettes or matches; hitting oneself with objects; willful noncompliance to medical treatment for the purpose of harm to oneself
Self-Neglect	Failure to provide for the personal care and needs of oneself	Refusal to request or receive assistance when necessary; wearing clothing inappropriate for the weather, resulting in hypothermia or hyperthermia; forgetting to take medications as prescribed; forgetting to eat or drink fluids
Domestic Maltreatment	Maltreatment occurring in the domestic setting or the personal home in which the older person resides	House, apartment, duplex, etc.
Institutional Maltreatment	Maltreatment occurring in an institutional setting	Nursing homes, retirement centers, community centers, hospitals, jails, prisons

THEORIES OF MALTREATMENT OF OLDER ADULTS

Many theories have been proposed in an attempt to understand and explain what would compel one human being to hurt another, particularly when the victim is perceived to be weak and vulnerable. Explanations concerning abuse of older adults have included theoretical suppositions that highlight *(1)* the stress of the older adult's dependency and disability exhausting a caregiver; *(2)* enhanced external stresses; *(3)* the intergenerational transmission of violence; *(4)* familial retaliation on the older parent by caregiving adult children for physical and/or psychological abuse or neglect during their childhoods; *(5)* the negative attitudes toward older adults and the entire aging process that encourage dehumanization and victimization of older persons; *(6)* the social exchange theory; *(7)* the theory of psychopathology of the perpetrator. Many of the proposed theoretical explanations overlap and conceptually blend together, while lacking conceptual exclusivity.

Kosberg (1988) underscored the importance of understanding the unique and individual characteristics of each case of maltreatment of an older adult. While each theoretical explanation may hold some validity, singularly they may only partially explain maltreatment of older adults. Perpetrators may be victimizing older persons due to multiple theoretical causations.

Theoretical assumptions should undergo the rigors of validation through testing with stringent research methodology before they are accepted as theoretical truths. However, some concepts and beliefs regarding maltreatment of older adults, which are now being disputed by findings from comparative research, quickly achieved acceptance. Research is still underway testing out the proposed theories regarding maltreatment of older adults. Hence the final word is not in regarding "why" maltreatment occurs in this population.

SCOPE OF THE PROBLEM

Domestic Abuse

The prevalence of abuse of older adults is difficult to estimate. Legal and research definitions of abuse or neglect vary widely as do state laws, local police practices, social service assistance levels, and pro-

secutorial or court-related activities. The problem is viewed differently by mental health, medical, law enforcement, and other professionals (Douglass 1987). The U.S. Bureau of Justice Statistics (1982) on victimization indicate that people over age 65 have the lowest victimization rate for crimes of violence. However, the most recent report by the House Select Committee on Aging estimates that over 1 million older Americans are physically, financially, and emotionally abused by their relatives or loved ones annually (Douglass 1987). Estimates cited by Pedrick-Cornell and Gelles (1982) run as high as 2.5 million per year, affecting perhaps one in ten older adults who live with a family. Steinmetz (1981) estimates the incidence of abuse of older adults as one in ten families when a frail older person is part of the family—a statistic comparable to that for child abuse.

Wolf (1988) summarized a study by Gioglio and Blakemore conducted in 1983, in which a random sample of older adults in New Jersey were interviewed. A structured questionnaire was used that included vignettes of physical abuse, psychological abuse, financial abuse, and neglect. Only 5 of 342 (or 15/1000), people interviewed reported experiencing abuse. Both Wolfe (1988) and Haviland and O'Brien (1989) concluded that methodologic flaws made the results of this study questionable.

The first large-scale random sample survey of abuse in community-dwelling older Americans was conducted by Pillemer and Finkelhor (1988). They interviewed 2020 persons age 65 and over to assess their experience of physical violence, verbal aggression, and neglect. The prevalence rate of overall mistreatment was 32/1000, with physical violence being the most widespread form of abuse at a rate of 20/1000. This study represents a rigorous methodology and more accurate data than many previous reports (Haviland and O'Brien 1989; Wolf 1988).

Block suggested that approximately 66 percent of maltreated older adults are victims of neglect. Deprivation of adequate food, medication, clothing, or shelter, as well as essential corrective or remedial devices such as eyeglasses, hearing aids, dentures, canes, walkers, and wheelchairs, were reported (Valentine and Cash 1986).

In 1985 the House Select Committee on Aging estimated that only 20 percent of all cases of maltreatment of older adults are reported; other studies suggest that 95 percent of those reported are repeat offenses (Douglass 1987). As the population ages, the proportion of those vulnerable to maltreatment will increase. As life expectancy increases, the incidence of chronic illness and debilitation rises with more older persons needing caregiving. Yet the decreasing birth rate results in fewer people to share in adult caregiving (Delunas 1990).

There are elder abuse laws in all fifty states and the District of Columbia, with forty-seven states and the District of Columbia possessing mandatory reporting or investigation laws (Brewer and Jones 1989). Still, cases of abuse of older adults continue to be underreported (Gelles and Strauss 1988; Douglass 1987). With society's reluctance to intervene in family problems and the limited resources allocated for investigation and intervention, only the most offensive occurrences may be receiving attention (Hall 1989).

Factors believed to contribute to the underreporting of abuse of older adults were identified by Kosberg (1988). Those factors included: family secrecy, acts occurring out of sight within family dwellings, reluctance of older persons to report abuse by relatives, professional lack of awareness of the problem, and failure of responsible persons to report. Other contributing factors to underreporting identified by Brewer and Jones (1989) and Callahan (1988) included the lack of a federal policy for abuse of older adults, the lack of a universal definition of abuse of older adults, vague and broad state statutes, and lack of funding for meaningful interventions. Callahan (1988) pointed out weak political support, which may be due to the relatively small number of citizens actually experiencing serious physical abuse.

Institutional Abuse

Most of the literature addresses domestic abuse, as 90 percent of older adults live at home (McDonald and Abrahams 1990). Most reported cases of maltreatment of older adults occur in the home (Douglass 1983); the abusers are usually a relative or loved one (Myers and Shelton 1987). However, it is estimated that one of four people who reach age 65 will spend some portion of their life in a nursing home (Gerety and Winograd 1988). Evidence of some form of abuse in institutional settings is growing.

This is of concern because institutionalized older persons are a particularly vulnerable group who often do not even complain when abuse has occurred (Sengstock, McFarland, and Hwalek 1990). Kimsey, Tarbox, and Bragg (1981) speculated that fear of retaliation by caretakers, threat of discharge, being unaware of their rights and legal remedies, and apathy may be factors contributing to older adults' acceptance of an abusive situation. A sense of the inevitability of impending wrath may enhance their feelings of helplessness and depression.

The American Medical Association (1990) "White Paper on Elderly Health" reviewed numerous studies documenting the high incidence of treatable medical conditions among nursing home residents, including malnutrition, low serum albumin levels, dehydration, hyponatremia, and depression. Myers and Shelton (1987) reported that 25 percent of medications are given in error and that overmedication is also a problem. Reynolds and Nelson gave indirect evidence of abuse from Studies of Selective Mortality (Myers and Shelton 1987). They found that depressed and self-destructive older persons in nursing homes are more likely to die than those with higher life satisfaction.

Pillemer and Moore (1989) surveyed 577 nursing home staff from 31 nursing homes to determine the extent of physical and psychological abuse. They concluded that abuse may be a common part of institutional life. Substantial portions of staff reported observing abusive behaviors toward patients—36 percent were incidents of physical abuse and 81 percent were considered psychological abuse. In addition, 10 percent reported personal acts of physical abuse toward patients and 40 percent reported psychological abusive acts. Kimsey et al. (1981) reported that theft of personal belongings was one of the most common complaints by residents. They also identified misuse of funds as a problem in nursing homes. Material abuse included embezzlement of trust funds, improper charges for services, failure to notify the state of death or departure, artificial upgrading of Medicaid recipients' classifications, and improper handling of drugs.

No studies have addressed the prevalence of abuse in hospitalized older adults or those seen in ambulatory care settings (Haviland and O'Brien 1989). Cassell (1989) stated that maltreatment might arise during the course of medical treatment that is, in itself, apparently proper. Such instances arise when the older person lacks the capacity to give consent for treatment and has a chronic, irreversible mental incapacity. Because life-sustaining treatment is given despite previously expressed wishes to the contrary, or contrary to the wishes of the older person's surrogate(s), this constitutes maltreatment through violation of rights. Cassell (1989) believed that the maltreatment from rights violation occurs as a result of the failure of physicians to allow older persons the responsibility and obligation to determine the extent of technologic power used in their treatment. The question must be asked, "Is keeping the person alive proper treatment or maltreatment?"

Cassell (1989) believed medical maltreatment occurred for three reasons. First, the sick person is not being treated. Rather, the events that happen to the person are being treated, such as treating related episodes of illness separately instead of as part of a person's ongoing history as a sick individual. Second, treatment reflects what the technology of medicine and the fiscal allocations from insurance agencies allow a physician to do, rather than what a person requires. Third, though physicians have good intentions, they may express their obligations and responsibilities to the sick body instead of to the sick person. What is good for the person may be uncertain, difficult to determine, and ambiguous. Needs of the body are more apparent.

Material Abuse

Material exploitation is a form of crime. The older American is a prime target. While people over age 65 constitute only 12 percent of the population, they are estimated to make up 30 percent of scam victims (Bekey 1991). Scam artists play on fears of older people about maintaining a comfortable lifestyle on a fixed income, surviving inflation, preparing for recession, affording medical care, and providing for their families. Since many own their own homes or have considerable equity, they are eligible for loans secured by their homes. This attracts swindlers. In addition they are vulnerable, frequently seeking investments for their savings, and they are more likely to be home when the con artist calls (Bekey 1991).

Violation of Personal Rights

There is almost no discussion in the literature of violation of personal rights as a dimension of maltreatment (Sengstock et al. 1990). This problem usually occurs in conjunction with other types of maltreatment. Yet control over major and routine matters should remain the right of every person regardless of age.

Sengstock and Hwalek (1986) included in this category incidents in which older persons had been forced to marry, change a will or deed, or take actions against their will, or had been prevented from doing things they wished. Being forced to move, not having one's privacy respected, and not being allowed to participate in discussions regarding one's own welfare are also areas of concern (Sengstock et al. 1990).

Sengstock et al. (1990) noted that personal rights of residents were included in the policies and procedures required of long-term care facilities by Titles XVIII and XIX of the United States Department of Health and Human Services. A copy of these policies and procedures should be made available to residents. Such rights include that each person admitted to a long-term care institution be: *(1)* fully informed of his/her rights; *(2)* free from mental and physical abuse; *(3)* allowed to handle personal affairs; *(4)* assured of confidentiality of medical needs; *(5)* accorded the opportunity to associate privately with persons of his/her choice; *(6)* allowed to retain and wear personal clothing; *(7)* allowed to receive and send mail; *(8)* assured privacy for visits by his/her spouse (Sengstock et al. 1990). In 1986, McFarland conducted personal interviews with nursing home clients and found that violations of personal rights caused great concern, even more than concerns about the physical environment. Areas of concern voiced by the clients included: *(1)* absence of a lockable closet or drawer to keep personal items; *(2)* inability to wear and enjoy their personal clothing without fear it would be lost or stolen; *(3)* lack of privacy for visitors or for themselves (Sengstock et al. 1990).

LEGISLATION

State Statutes

States have been passing legislation on abuse of older adults since 1973. Laws within each state may define the rights of older persons, resources available to aid the victims, as well as the responsibilities and liabilities of health care practitioners. Yet, there is no federal policy for maltreatment of older adults, so each state has established its own definitions, criteria, and reporting system (Brewer and Jones 1989).

Many laws were passed quickly—frequently using child protective service legislation as a model—without adequate knowledge of the causes of abuse of older adults or the effectiveness of programs (Wolf 1988). Laws are continually changing. Though all fifty states and the District of Columbia have elder abuse laws, only forty-seven and the District of Columbia have mandatory reporting or investigation laws, most passed since 1986. Three states—Colorado, New York, and Wisconsin—have voluntary reporting laws (Brewer and Jones 1989).

Brewer and Jones (1989) reviewed state legislation addressing abuse of older adults. They found that seventeen states had enacted specific abuse laws, thirty-four covered abuse through protective service statutes, and eleven had domestic violence laws with provisions for older adults. In some instances there were different laws for those residing in nursing homes or other health care facilities and for those residing in the community.

Statute Models

Palinscar, in 1982, categorized elder abuse laws within three models: child abuse statutes, domestic violence statutes, or advocacy statutes (Brewer and Jones 1989). Each one of these posed problems for working with cases of abuse of older adults. Brewer and Jones (1989) support use of the 1982 model and identified the problems of each model. When the child abuse model was used, there was a threat to human dignity and the right to due process. The older person's right to free choice was affected. An investigation might be carried out without the victim's consent because the law portrayed the person as helpless, dependent, and unable to make competent decisions. Institutionalization was a frequent outcome that could attribute to an earlier death.

Domestic violence statues were designed to provide short-term solutions to crisis situations and did not deal with neglect. Older persons must be assertive and appear in court to obtain a protective order against their perpetrator (Brewer and Jones 1989).

Advocacy statutes were designed to protect devel-

opmentally disabled adults 18 years and older and were designed to allow the individual maximum independence. If the person decided to remain in an abusive environment, protective intervention could only occur if the situation became life-threatening (Brewer and Jones 1989).

Statute Dilemmas

As stated earlier maltreatment definitions vary from state to state. Legally, many of the definitions are broad; some do not even use the word abuse. Few of the definitions clearly delineate between neglect and abuse (Thobaben and Anderson 1985; Brewer and Jones 1989). In some states, neglect laws focus on the condition, while others focus on the intentionality of the perpetrating caregiver to deprive the older person (Brewer and Jones 1989). In most states, abuse includes physical injury not caused by accident. Some laws cover neglect separately or as part of the definition of abuse. Others do not cover neglect at all (Rosado 1991).

Texas passed new legislation in 1989 to address neglect. In Texas anyone who accepts responsibility for a person over 64, a child, or an invalid—regardless of relationship—must provide care. The first case to test this law is currently being pursued (Rosado 1991). A young couple, ages 19 and 22, have been charged with criminal abuse of the young wife's grandmother. If convicted, they face not only a $10,000 fine, but from five years to life in prison. The case involved a 70-year-old grandmother who was treated in the emergency room in Houston in June 1990. She was covered with pressure ulcers and maggot-infested wounds that went through the bone. The woman weighed only ninety-five pounds at 5'7". She had suffered a loss of forty pounds in six months. Not surprisingly, she suffered from dehydration and malnutrition.

California clearly delineates between physical abuse and neglect definitions. Additionally, California defines fiduciary abuse (stealing money/property) and abandonment. Yet, Delaware law only covers exploitation (Thobaben and Anderson 1985). Material maltreatment means different things in different states and is not even covered in the laws of one-third of the states (Brewer and Jones 1989).

Mandatory Reporting

Mandatory reporting of abuse varies from state to state. In Alabama, if a visiting nurse assessed signs that an older person had been abused and the nurse did not report it, the nurse could be found guilty of a misdemeanor and fined up to $500 or jailed. In California the nurse could still be guilty of a misdemeanor, but could be fined up to $1,000. In Maine the nurse may have licensing penalties. In other states there are no provisions for any penalty (Thobaben and Anderson 1985).

To determine one's legal responsibilities, state laws must be understood. In every state the nurse and physician are named as reporters, being required to immediately report cases to protective service departments responsible for investigation. Some state statutes have no penalty for failure to report. Brewer and Jones (1989) found thirty states outlined penalties for failure to report, with fines up to $1,000 with no imprisonment. The District of Columbia and Maine additionally assessed licensing sanctions. Arkansas and Minnesota laws make one liable for damages incurred by the victim.

State laws have increased the number of cases reported (Salend et al. 1984), but underreporting still remains a major problem. Many medical professionals are either unaware of state laws or disregard them. O'Brien reported that 70 percent of responding physicians in 1986 in Michigan and North Carolina were unaware of their states' laws, yet 25 percent had encountered abuse of older adults in their practices (Clark-Daniels 1990). In another study in Alabama (Daniels, Baumhover, and Clark-Daniels 1989) licensed physicians were surveyed. One-half of those responding were unsure if Alabama had standard procedures for working with abuse, three-fourths were unsure how to report cases, and one-half did not know the state agency responsible for receiving abuse reports.

Physicians report other barriers to reporting abuse of older persons. Reasons include: *(1)* doubt in confidentiality; *(2)* concern about angering the abuser; *(3)* need for subsequent court appearances; *(4)* damage to their professional relationship with the patient; *(5)* skepticism regarding prompt follow-up investigation (Daniels et al. 1989).

In a similar study of emergency department personnel in Alabama (Clark-Daniels 1990) most personnel did not understand the requirements of the state laws, were unaware that anonymity would be guaranteed if a person reported a case of abuse, and were concerned about being required to make lengthy court appearances. While most personnel had seen cases of abuse of older persons and felt reporting was a responsibility of care providers, differences existed in their satisfaction with the disposition of cases reported to state authorities. They did not believe sufficient support services existed, were unsure how to report cases, and doubted their abilities to identify and diagnose abuse. Interestingly, personnel reported seeing an average of 41–48 patients over 65 years old per day, with an average of 1.8–2.6 cases of abuse seen in the last year. However, they had only reported an average of 0.1–3.0 cases in their entire career.

Clark-Daniels and Daniels (1990) surveyed both licensed and practical nurses who currently were practicing in Alabama in home health care. They identified reasons for not reporting abuse of older adults. Two main categories were defined: obstacles to intervention and obstacles to reporting. The most common obstacle to intervention included a lack of government response or resources (25 percent) and a lack of evidence that abuse had occurred (23 percent). Another identified obstacle to intervention was the lack of cooperation by the family or the patient. The most common obstacle to reporting related to the nurse's involvement with the patient. Fear of involvement with and responsibility for the patient was the main reason nurses underreported maltreatment of older persons. Twenty-five percent of the nurses cited this obstacle. Other reasons given for underreporting were: someone else reported the abuse; reporting would only make life worse for the patient; not understanding the requirements of reporting or the outcomes following the report. Only 5 percent reported never have seen abuse of older adults.

Some professionals believe mandatory reporting prevents older persons from seeking medical care or other types of assistance (Brewer and Jones 1989). Lack of awareness, combined with an unquestioning acceptance of explanations for symptoms suggestive of abuse, interferes with reporting (Kosberg 1988).

Meaningful intervention following a report can be a problem because states do not provide adequate funding (Brewer and Jones 1989). The Council on Scientific Affairs (1987) noted that the 1985 U.S.

House of Representatives report on abuse of older adults indicated that states spent an average of $22.00 per child for protective services, while only $2.90 was spent for each older person. This converted to only 4.7 percent of the average state's budget (a drop of 2 percent since 1980), despite the fact that 40 percent of all reported cases of abuse involved adults or older persons. Such lack of funding may cause potential reporters of abuse to question the advantage of their report, especially if the situation might be worsened.

In addition mandatory reporting laws conflict with statutes providing privileged communication for physicians, lawyers, and other practitioners (Brewer and Jones 1989). The person must consider and deal with the advantages and disadvantages of reported suspected maltreatment of older adults, such as losing a client's/patient's trust or jeopardizing the therapeutic relationship. Violating the law is not a consideration.

Underreporting is a serious problem. Despite obstacles perceived by health care providers, the responsibility for reporting remains. If more reports were filed when abuse was suspected, the issue would come to the forefront as a major social problem, gain more political support, and lead to laws—particularly federal laws—that more clearly protect the older person and provide adequate support services when abuse occurs (Clark-Daniels and Daniels 1990).

Limited Investigation

Mandatory reporting is inadequate without provision of support services. Responsibilities for investigation and services may be assigned to as many as fifteen different types of agencies by different state laws. Brewer and Jones (1989) found that thirty-three states assigned responsibility to the state social service agency, three states identified a law enforcement agency, and in twenty-one states more than one agency was specified. Most states did not have supportive services to intervene constructively. Without adequate investigation and support, the family may experience a traumatic intervention without satisfactory resolution (Ambrogi and London 1985). In addition, time frames for investigation differ. While some states specify seventy-two, twenty-four, or even one hour in life-threatening situations, others use terms

such as "promptly," "immediately, or "as soon as practical" (Brewer and Jones 1989).

Another problem facing the investigator is interviewing the abused family members. Family members may deny access within the home, where most cases occur. An agency can gain access but only after a judicial proceeding and a showing of probable cause (Brewer and Jones 1989).

The lack of support services can create an expectation that cannot be met. If constructive intervention cannot be offered to resolve family problems, the older person is frequently institutionalized (Ambrogi and London 1985). The older person may prefer to remain in an abusive situation rather than be placed in a strange nursing home. Older adults' refusal to accept help may be construed as proof of impairment warranting involuntary assistance, yet many older adults do refuse help. In Ohio, 700 of 4900 older persons requiring protective services refused help in 1987 (Carlson 1989). Possible reasons for older adults refusing help may include: reluctance to have family privacy invaded, fear of reprisal, embarrassment and shame, reluctance to bring litigation against a relative, beliefs that they themselves are responsible for the problem due to their dependency or their own earlier abusive behaviors toward another, and fear of institutionalization (Kosberg 1988). Those in institutions may also fear being discharged, be unaware of their rights and legal recourse, lack social supports, and be apathetic (Sengstock and Hwalek 1986).

Well-funded adult protective services laws are needed as an integral part of public policy on violence (Cash and Valentine 1987). In some states the caseload is so high for each adult protective services specialist that only limited time can be spent on each case. In Texas there is a mandatory law to report abuse of an older adult to Adult Protective Services (APS). However, there is less than one APS specialist for every two counties (Theiss and Anderson 1987). Even when cases are followed, many states do not have laws establishing penalties for perpetrators. When laws exist, there may be no discrimination for varying degrees of maltreatment (Brewer and Jones 1989).

Lack of Police Involvement

A problem affecting intervention and resolution is that police are unlikely to become involved in cases of abuse, neglect, or exploitation of older persons (Sengstock and Hwalek 1986). The police usually become involved when the police department is contacted by social agencies to help with difficult cases. These are usually not classic cases of maltreatment of older adults.

Typical police referrals deal with landlord-tenant problems, people with mental problems, or general domestic violence cases. Agencies are unlikely to contact police and do not believe the police will be of much assistance to the abused older client. When police referrals are made, they usually deal with very dangerous cases, forced entry into a home, or the need to acquire court orders for a commitment. Sengstock and Hwalek (1986) identified several reasons police are reluctant to help with cases of abuse of older adults. The researchers defined police distaste for domestic relations cases, police observations that victims are unlikely to follow through with prosecution, the frequent lack of hard evidence, eyewitnesses who are less than effective, and victims who do not desire police involvement as obstacles for police involvement in maltreatment of older adults.

Problems within the criminal justice system, such as prosecutorial resistance and frequent reversals in higher courts, add to the difficulty in successfully bringing cases to court. Cases must be very serious for court intervention. Legal remedies are seen as a last resort and few prosecutions are successful (Salend et al. 1984). Yet, there are cases of physical abuse that clearly break criminal law and should be prosecuted. A better working relationship between social agencies and the police clearly is needed.

PROFILES OF PERPETRATORS

The research and literature on maltreatment of older adults show many discrepancies in the area of profile descriptions. As interest in the phenomenon of maltreatment of older adults has increased over the past fifteen years, writings and research have flourished. This has brought additional pieces of data to the picture of abuse of older persons, resulting in a new look at the phenomenon.

Analytic comparison of the research on abuse of older persons has been slowed by the differing definitional categories and classifications the researchers use when sampling their populations, analyzing their data, and presenting their findings. Some researchers clump all forms of maltreatment of older persons together. Others distinguish abuse from neglect. Others differentiate physical, psychological, and material abuse from active and passive neglect. Understandably, differing research presents differing profiles of victims and their perpetrators. Hence, the victim and perpetrator profiles remain conflicting and unclear. Nonetheless, varying research profiles have been presented in an attempt to highlight the profile findings on maltreatment of older persons. Space limits an exhaustive presentation of the research on profile descriptions, but major contributors have been included. Tables 22-2–22-5 give summaries of recent profile findings from literature and research on maltreatment of older persons.

Table 22–2   Older Victim Profile for Abuse

GENERAL ABUSE DATA

- *Female*: middle class; presently with poor income; physically disabled or mentally impaired; dependent on the caregiver (Hamilton 1989)
- *Females*: because females outnumber males in general older population; older; physically disabled or mentally impaired; physically dependent on caregiver; alcohol or substance abuser; passive (i.e., less likely to resist abusive behavior or sexual molestation); self-blaming; self-deprecating; excessively loyal to perpetrator; history of past abuse; stoicism; tolerance; resignation to life's events; socially isolated; demanding; belligerent (Kosberg 1988)
- Lower cognitive functioning; poor mental health; low self-esteem; recent decline in mental status prior to abuse or neglect; recent decline in physical health; did not have more numbers of physical disabilities; difficulties with activities of daily living; not more financially dependent; socially isolated; poor relationship with perpetrator (Godkin, Wolf, and Pillemer 1989)
- Natural mother to perpetrator; older; physical disabilities or mental impairments (Anetzberger 1989)
- *Female*: age not a significant factor (Miller and Dodder 1989)
- Alone at time of offense; Black and Caucasians are victims most often of Black perpetrators; more likely to report victimization from stranger than relative (Fattah and Sacco 1989)
- *Female*: 75 years of age or older; widowed; cared for by perpetrator for 9.5 years; one or more physical or mental impairments; dependent physically, emotionally, or financially on the caregiver; socially isolated; alcohol abuse; aggressive and combative at times; history of family violence; poverty (McDonald and Abrahams 1990)
- Physically disabled; dependent physically on perpetrator (Delunas 1990)
- Few admitted to abuse; previous abuse over many years; no difference in physical dependency between abused and nonabused older persons; no significant difference in physical or mental disabilities of abused and nonabused groups; not significantly more socially isolated (Homer and Gilleard 1990)

OTHER DATA

PHYSICAL	PSYCHOLOGICAL	MATERIAL	INSTITUTIONAL
• Less affluent older persons (Douglass 1987)	• Less affluent older persons (Douglass 1987)	• Affluent older persons (Douglass 1987)	• Frail older persons (Myers and Shelton 1987)
• Men at almost twice the risk of abuse than women; spouse of perpetrator (Pillemer and Finkelhor 1988)	• More independent in activities of daily living; poor emotional health; but no recent decline in mental status; social network available on emergency basis only (Wolf and Pillemer 1989)	• Not married; financial difficulties; transportation difficulties; recent loss of support network (Wolf and Pillemer 1989)	
• *Female or male*: Caucasian; over age 75; physically disabled or mentally impaired; dependent on the caregiver; has problematic management behaviors; living with a relative; minimal social supports (Haviland and O'Brien 1989)		• Impaired judgment or cognitive functioning; emotional dependency; passivity, especially in financial matters; socially isolated (Weiler 1989)	

(continued)

Table 22–3 Older Victim Profile for Neglect and Passive and Active Maltreatment

PHYSICAL	PSYCHOLOGICAL	MATERIAL	INSTITUTIONAL
• Males are more likely to have physical assaults from nonrelatives or strangers (Fattah and Sacco 1989)		• Has financial or material resources; desire economic gain from perpetrator; may not realize exploitation has occurred (Fattah and Sacco 1989) • 65 years of age and older (older persons comprise 12 percent of the population and 30 percent of scam victims); greed exceeds caution; willingness to believe what told; intelligence and normal cognitive functioning not an adequate safeguard against professional perpetrators; have been "scammed" before; no one is immune; eager for easy opportunities to save or make money (Bekey 1991)	
GENERAL DATA ON OLDER VICTIMS OF NEGLECT AND MALTREATMENT			
• Female or male; Caucasian; over age 75; physically disabled or mentally impaired; dependent on the caregiver; have problematic management behaviors; living with a relative; minimal social supports (Haviland and O'Brien 1989)	• Lower cognitive functioning; poor mental health; low self-esteem; recent decline in mental status prior to abuse or neglect; recent decline in physical health; did not have more numbers of physical disabilities; difficulties with activities of daily living; not more financially dependent; socially isolated; poor relationship with perpetrator (Godkin, Wolf and Pillemer 1989)		
SPECIFIC DATA ON OLDER VICTIMS OF NEGLECT AND MALTREATMENT			
INSTITUTIONAL NEGLECT		ACTIVE MALTREATMENT	
• Institutionalized, frail older persons (Myers and Shelton 1987)		• Physically dependent for activities of daily living; emotionally dependent; socially isolated (Wolf and Pillemer 1989)	

Table 22-4 Perpetrator Profile for Abuse of Older Persons

GENERAL DATA ON PERPETRATORS OF ABUSE OLDER PERSONS

- *Female*: Caucasian; adult daughter or daughter-in-law; middle-age (45 years or older); increased external stresses (Hamilton 1989)
- *Nonrelative*: male; acting singularly or in pair; less likely to be group or gang offense; Black and Caucasian are victims most often of Black perpetrators; less likely to use a weapon when victimizing older persons; more likely to complete offense to older persons when in daytime (Fattah and Sacco 1989)
- *Men*: history of mental illness; recent decline in mental status; dependent on the victim financially and socially; recent external stress (e.g., death of another family member, unemployment); poor relationship with victim; unrealistic expectations of older victim; caregiving stress; external stresses (Godkin, Wolf, and Pillemer 1989)
- *Psychopathology of the perpetrator*: psychiatric illness; alcohol or substance abuse; external stresses ("the straw that breaks the camel's back"); some gain for the perpetrator (Fulmer 1989)
- *Relative*: spouse, child, grandchild; dependent on the victim; lives with victim; negative attitudes toward older persons; anger with caregiving role; mentally ill; psychologically disturbed; impaired judgment; alcohol or drug abuse; cared for older person(s) 9.5 years; caregiver stresses (e.g., time, emotional, physical, and financial burdens of caring for older person); external stresses (e.g., unemployment, major illness, death of loved one); formerly abused by victim or others (McDonald and Abrahams 1990)
- Violence in childhood (Delunas 1990)
- *In institutions*: relative; staff; visitor; another resident or patient of the institution (Sengstock, McFarland, and Hwalek 1990)
- *Spouses*: longstanding mutually abusive relationships; 45 percent admitted openly to maltreatment of older spouse; alcohol use was most significant risk factor; disturbed, disorganized personalities; poor communication; poor relationship with victim; previous abuse over many years; stopped working to care for older victim; open to discussing abuse (Homer and Gilleard 1990)

SPECIFIC DATA ON PERPETRATORS OF ABUSE OLDER PERSONS

PHYSICAL	PSYCHOLOGICAL	MATERIAL	INSTITUTIONAL
<ul><li>*Relative of the victim*: 40 percent spouses; 50 percent adult children and grandchildren</li><li>*If adult child*: most often middle-class female; 40–50 years old; sons tend to be more physically abusive than daughters; socially isolated and poorly integrated into society</li><li>*If grandchildren*: not married; unemployed</li><li>*If other relative*: frequently polite; well dressed; pillars of community (Kallman 1987)</li></ul>	<ul><li>Unemployed; alcohol abuse; poor relationship with the victim; dependent on the victim (Douglass 1987)</li><li>Lives with older victim; mentally ill; recent decline in mental status; poor communication skills; poor relationship with victim (Homer and Gilleard 1990)</li></ul>	<ul><li>*Younger*: does not live with victim; alcohol abuse; no recent decline in mental status; no recent medical illness or complaints; financially troubled and dependent; external financial stresses (e.g., unemployment, change in job status, financial problems), no family support (Wolf and Pillemer 1989)</li><li>*Stranger*: brief, fleeting contact with older victim; polite; seem knowledgeable (Fattah and Sacco 1989)</li></ul>	<ul><li>*Facility characteristics*: custodial orientation; lack of supervision; understaffed; high turnover; at times, small facilities; smaller number of beds; lower rates for care; for-profit institutions</li><li>*Staff characteristics*: young; nurse's aide position; negative attitude toward older adults; lower levels of education; inexperience with geriatric population; burnout; willing to discuss abuse or neglect; external stresses contributed to more psychological abuse (Pillemer 1988) *(continued)*</li></ul>

Table 22–5 Representive Profiles for Neglect and Active and Passive Maltreatment of Older Persons

GENERAL DATA ON PERPETRATORS OF NEGLECT AND MALTREATMENT OF OLDER PERSONS

PHYSICAL	PSYCHOLOGICAL	MATERIAL	INSTITUTIONAL
• Dependent adult sons; spouses; most often husbands; alcohol and drug abuse; unemployment; postretirement; depressed; low self-esteem; history of child abuse (Douglass 1987)	• Relative: spouse—most likely; adult children—second most likely; may be mentally ill; poor communication and coping skills; history of family violence; may be "pushed over the edge" by stresses of caregiving; substance abuser; poor relationship with the victim; dependent on the victim for residence and finances (Haviland and O'Brien 1989) • Females commit more neglect: combined neglect and abuse; self-neglect (60 percent), family member (19 percent) (Miller and Dodder 1989) • History of mental illness; recent decline in mental status; dependent on the victim financially and socially; recent external stress (e.g., death of an-	other family member, unemployment); poor relationship with victim; unrealistic expectations of older victim; caregiving stress; external stresses (Godkin, Wolf, and Pillemer 1989) • Poor communication skills; poor relationship with victim; socially dysfunctional (Homer and Gilleard 1990)	• *In institutional settings:* young; inexperienced; low educational level; low staff wages; high patient-to-staff ratio; high staff turnover; staff burnout (McDonald and Abrahams 1990)

SPECIFIC DATA ON PERPETRATORS OF NEGLECT AND MALTREATMENT OF OLDER PERSONS

PSYCHOLOGICAL	ACTIVE MALTREATMENT	PASSIVE MALTREATMENT	INSTITUTIONAL
• Mentally ill; demented; may not know they have committed offense (Quinn and Tomita 1986)	• Older; female; no history of mental illness; stressed by caregiving to victim (Wolf and Pillemer 1989)	• Realistic expectations of older victims; recent medical complaint; no financial dependency; stressed by caregiving to victim; loss of social supports (Wolf and Pillemer 1989)	• *Facility characteristics:* custodial orientation; lack of supervision; understaffed; high turnover; at times, small facilities; smaller numbers of beds; lower rates for care; for-profit institutions • *Staff characteristics:* young; nurse's aide position; negative attitude toward older persons; lower levels of education; inexperience with geriatric population; burnout; willing to discuss abuse or neglect (Pillemer 1988)

Initially research focused primarily on older persons who were victims of domestic abuse. Some studies obtained their sample population exclusively from cases reported to protective service agencies (e.g., Cash and Valentine 1987; Hall 1989). Others obtained their sample population from surveys (Wolf 1988; Pillemer and Finkelhor 1988; and Pillemer and Moore 1989). The findings from these differing studies have produced differing profiles of older victims and their perpetrators.

Initially, older victims were profiled to be frail, dependent, disabled females who lived with the perpetrator of their abuse. Perpetrators were typically identified as the adult children of the older victim. Additionally, perpetrators were viewed as overburdened caregivers, exhausted from the stresses of their caregiving role. Daughters were more frequently identified as perpetrators. Yet, when sons were labeled as potential perpetrators of maltreatment, older persons were considered to be at greater risk.

Concerns had been identified (Pillemer and Finkelhor 1988) that these profiles focused more on the characteristics of the victim than on the characteristics of the perpetrator. These concerns highlighted the "victim-blaming" overtones of earlier profile descriptions. In the last two to three years, researchers have expanded their view on domestically abused older persons and have begun comparing sample populations of abused older persons to nonabused older persons. This more recent research appears to present findings that contradict the initial profiles (see Tables 22-2–22.5). Furthermore, recent profile presentations have shifted from a heightened focus on victim characteristics to a focus on the defining characteristics of the perpetrator.

Callahan (1988) was probably the most accurate of profile researchers, noting that there was no typical victim. However, the new profile data that have been emerging are worth noting as they have begun challenging the older profiles of maltreatment of older adults. Most surprisingly, the recent comparative research on domestically abused and nonabused older persons did not validate the profile descriptions of older victims of maltreatment from earlier research. This newer comparative research did not corroborate the profile of the older victim in which frailty, disability, and dependency on the caregiver were high-risk factors for maltreatment. Rather, some of the more recent research profiled older victims as younger older persons, who were no less disabled, frail, or dependent than their nonabused counterparts. In fact, Wolf and Pillemer (1989) noted that older victims of domestic abuse tended to be somewhat more independent in activities of daily living than the nonabused. Further, this more recent research profiled victims of maltreatment as affluent older adults who shared a residence with the perpetrator for nine or more years. In unprecedented accounts, spouse abuse emerged as a foremost factor in domestic maltreatment of older persons.

Along with this finding, older males have begun to surface as an underreported population of victims of maltreatment. In fact, Pillemer and Finkelhor (1988) found in their research of over two thousand older persons from the metropolitan area of Boston that the risk of abuse for older men was more than twice the risk for older women. Furthermore, their calculations utilized raw numbers and did not factor in the differential risk percentage considering the fewer numbers of men than women in the older population. Thus older women may present in higher numbers to health care and protective services and may have larger raw numbers of those who are abused; but proportionately, men seem at higher risk.

The identification of a spouse perpetrator conflicts with the previous identification of an exhausted adult child as the typical caregiving perpetrator. The adult child still is listed as a potential abusive caregiver. But spouses are being identified in increasing research studies as the more common perpetrator of maltreatment in domestic settings. The focus is beginning to shift away from the characteristics of the older victim onto the characteristics of the perpetrator.

In direct inversion to early studies a heightened degree of dependency of the perpetrator on the older victim (rather than the degree of dependency of the older victim on the perpetrator) has been identified as a risk factor for domestic maltreatment of older adults. The maltreatment perpetrators have been profiled to have heightened dependency on the older victim for financial support, lodging, transportation, and socialization.

Multiple factors that point to the psychopathology of the perpetrator consistently have been highlighted in perpetrator profiles. These profile characteristics of maltreatment perpetrators include: psychiatric illness, substance abuse, aggressive tendencies, history of antisocial behavior, dependency on the older victim (i.e., financially, socially, emotionally), unemployment and/or employment problems, unrealistic expectations of the elder, and overall poor coping skills. Recent external stresses in a preceding year, such as job loss, illness, interpersonal conflicts, and death of a loved one, also have been identified as potential drains on the limited coping capacity of an impaired caregiver. Hence external stresses may become the final catalyst that causes impaired caregivers to lose what limited control they possess and mistreat elders. In summary, recent accounts of domestic maltreatment of older adults have been profiled to occur within settings in which older people who are financially stable share their home with a dependent, emotionally unstable person who has undergone external stresses in the past twelve months. Spouse abuse and male victims should not be overlooked when profiling domestic maltreatment of older persons.

In an attempt to understand how the apparently incongruous earlier research reports on domestic maltreatment fit together with more recent findings, Fulmer (1989) compared seemingly conflicting research findings on abuse of older persons. Fulmer believed that the seemingly incongruous findings resulted from different phenomenological perspectives of the same date. Some researchers were comparing abused to nonabused older persons, while other researchers were comparing independent to dependent older persons. Fulmer reported that both sets of research were valid and reliable, despite their disagreement regarding the role of dependency in the profiles of abused older victims.

In addition to older adults who have been domestically mistreated, older adults who have been institutionally abused, materially exploited, and whose rights have been violated recently have been the subject of research and literature on maltreatment of older adults. It is common for multiple types of maltreatment to occur simultaneously to older victims.

Second to domestic maltreatment, institutional maltreatment and material exploitation of older persons have received leading attention in research literature on maltreatment of older persons. As with the data on domestic maltreatment of older persons, research findings conflict regarding the profile descriptions of victims and their perpetrators. However, some commonalities do persist. In contrast to older victims in domestic settings, older victims in institutional settings have been profiled to be aged, frail, disabled, and dependent. These victims have limited capabilities to protest the maltreatment, to defend and to protect themselves. Neglect is believed to be far more common than abuse in these settings.

Some researchers have profiled perpetrators in institutional settings as young, inexperienced staff with low educational levels. Pillemer and Moore (1989) rebutted these perpetrator profile characteristics, and found correlation with age, level of education, and level of experience in their research on institutional maltreatment. However, research findings were consistent in profiling perpetrators of maltreatment of older persons in institutional settings as persons who had frequent conflicts with older persons, additional personal stresses, a childlike view of the older victim, and an impaired capacity for coping and communication. Consequently, control battles and power struggles between the older victim and the perpetrator were common in institutional settings. Perpetrators of institutional maltreatment were profiled as depressed, substance abusers, callous toward older persons, personally stressed, and vocationally burned out.

Some studies also highlighted characteristics of institutions in which maltreatment of older adults occurred. Often, the institutions were profiled to have difficult working conditions with high patient-to-staff ratios, high staff turnover, low staff wages, long working hours, and minimal staff supervision. Facilities that operate on a for-profit status have been profiled by some researchers as institutions that possess higher risk for maltreatment of older adults. However, Pillemer and Moore (1989) found no correlation with this characteristic.

The research on material exploitation of older persons has identified affluent, socially isolated, and emotionally dependent older persons as high-risk profiles for victimization. Older victims of material exploitation possess impaired judgment. This impairment may be due to a cognitive disability, a general passivity in financial matters, or a desire for quick and easy economic gain. Bekey (1991) reports, however, that no older adult is totally immune to material exploitation. In fact, victims may not even realize that exploitation has occurred (Fattah and Sacco 1989).

Perpetrators of material exploitation are more likely to be strangers to the older victim. These individuals are smooth talkers with an uncanny ability at presenting themselves as trustworthy and reliable. While portraying a friendly and concerned demeanor, perpetrators prey on typical fears of elders, such as safety concerns, financial security, and health. Often these material-exploiting perpetrators only engage in brief and fleeting encounters with the older people they victimize. Phone solicitation, mail fraud, and person-to-person encounters have been used to victimize older adults. These perpetrators often have fragmented business operations, if any at all. They may have an office in one city, a mailing address in another, and a warehouse in a third locality. Also, they relocate frequently. In an interesting note, Bekey (1991) found that perpetrators who materially exploit older adults typically operate out of warmer states (e.g., Southern California, Florida, Texas, Arizona, and Nevada).

The final definitional category of maltreatment of older persons to appear in the literature of maltreatment is one that is most lacking in clarity and testing through research. This category has been labeled the violation of rights. The definition of violation of rights has shown up in maltreatment literature as a distinct and separate category since 1984 (Giordano and Giordano 1984). But no distinctions have been made regarding profile characteristics for either older victims or the perpetrators of this type of maltreatment of older adults. Instead, this category maintains only a descriptive quality. Violation of rights and the denial of an older person's personal rights seem to occur in conjunction with the other types of maltreatment. This assumption has yet to undergo the rigors of research testing. Therefore this specific type of maltreatment of older persons lacks profile descriptions for victims and perpetrators.

As is apparent from this discussion, all of the pieces of data concerning descriptive profile characteristics on the different types of maltreatment of older persons have yet to be defined. Furthermore, the more recent profile data from comparative research has offered a different view of victim and perpetrator profiles. As research continues on the phenomenon of maltreatment of older adults, there will be a continuation of the changing perspective on the profile's characteristics.

THE PROGRESSION OF VIOLENCE

There is a progression of violence that is frequently discussed in the family violence literature. Figure 22-1 shows a graphic representation of the progression of violence. Stages have been identified that describe and clarify the progression of violence in abusive relationships.

In the beginning all is calm. Then, over time, individuals will begin to have an increased sensitivity and irritability to interpersonal situations, external stresses, and internal intrapsychic demands. Certain words, discussions, interactions, and external pressures can serve to trigger increasingly intense emotional responses from an abuser. In the initial stages, triggers begin to set off the abuser and tension mounts. As time continues, sensitivity to triggers increases. Subsequently, irritability, tension, and aggression build.

When the tension can no longer be contained in the abuser, an explosion occurs. Depending on the characteristics of the abuser and the situation this explosion could be limited to brief psychological abuse (e.g., name calling) or it could encompass physical abuse that culminates in the death of the older victim. After the explosion there is a gradual decline in the state of tension in the abuser. However, an abuser may readily recycle into the tension-building stage and a second explosion if the aggression does not thoroughly defuse. If recycling does not occur, an abusive individual will eventually defuse.

The progression of violence ends when the abuser moves into the "hearts and flowers" phase of guilt and remorse. This is the best time to begin intervention and to attempt to talk about the incident of violence. Unfortunately, gradually the tension will again build and the cycle may repeat itself over and over again.

Perpetrators progress through the cycle of violence at their own rates and will express their individualized manifestations for release of aggression. Some abusers require months to progress through a cycle; others recycle in days or even hours. The degree of explosion and acting out will vary with each abuser, as will the duration and extent of the guilt and remorse phase.

ASSESSMENT

Assessing maltreatment of older persons requires a multifaceted approach. The complexity of the clinical

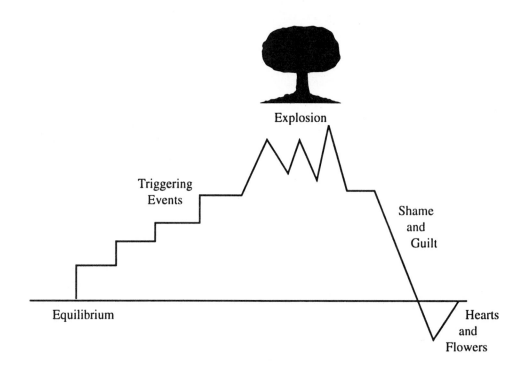

Figure 22–1   Graphic representation of the progression of violence

assessment, in and of itself, can seem overwhelming. Evaluation of maltreatment of older persons requires a comprehensive diagnostic workup in physical, psychological, and social areas. The older person, the caregiver, and the living environment need to be assessed.

Professionals are challenged to differentiate aging processes, accidents, and illness from abuse, neglect, and exploitation. O'Malley et al. (1983) noted that maltreatment of older adults often is misdiagnosed as dementia, paranoia, frequent falls, noncompliance of the elder person, failure to thrive, accidental medication errors, or a decline due to aging.

The process of aging along with the complexities of intrapersonal and interpersonal dynamics complicates assessment of maltreatment of older adults. For example, older persons are at high risk for falls and fractures. In a report of the Council on Scientific Affairs by the American Medical Association (1990)

falls were identified as the leading cause of nonfatal injury to the elderly. Furthermore, the report stated that falls accounted for 87 percent of all fractures among older adults. Determining the extent to which an older person's falls were accidental, due to neglect, or the result of an intentional push by a perpetrating caregiver requires a thorough investigation along with a comprehensive multidimensional assessment.

Bruising of the skin occurs quite easily. If professionals do not extend their assessments beyond symptom and disease identification, maltreatment of older adults may be erroneously attributed to aging and thereby continue to be unrecognized and underreported. Extensive bruising on an older person's arms could easily be dismissed as a common part of the aging process complicated by medication. Still, investigation as to how the bruises occurred might reveal maltreatment. Not all older persons with falls and bruising are victims of maltreatment. However, assessing the geriatric population requires specialized training and comprehensive workups.

McDonald and Abrahams (1990) noted that emergency medical personnel may have a complex challenge in distinguishing abuse-related trauma from nonabuse-related trauma. Older victims often present for evaluation with a medical problem and deny abuse. Kallman (1987) noted that older victims of abuse may passively fail to bring up the issue of abuse when questioned regarding their most serious problems, actively deny abuse accounts, and even refuse further evaluation if questioned too intensely.

The lack of universally accepted profile characteristics for victims and perpetrators inhibits the process of identification of high-risk persons of maltreatment. With the initial profile data, professionals could heighten their observations for maltreatment on frail and disabled older persons. However, the more recent findings from competing comparative research profiled less disabled older adults as abuse victims in domestic settings. Therefore professionals must keep an ever watchful eye on all older persons for indications of maltreatment and exploitation.

Guidelines for assessing potential maltreatment of older persons are presented in this section. Indicators of maltreatment have been identified. However, the presence of indicators, even a clustering of indicators, is not an indictment of maltreatment of an older adult. Rather the indicators have been presented to serve as a guide in the interviewing and assessment process. Typically a multidimensional and interdisciplinary assessment process is required prior to diagnosing maltreatment. This assessment process can vary from a seemingly quick and easy procedure, to one that is complex, confusing, and shrouded in mystery. For example, if an older person presents to the emergency room with repeated old fractures of the radius and ulna, hand and wrist glovelike burns from scalding water, and both the victim and the perpetrator possess the cognitive and emotional capacities to reveal the abuse, professionals may quickly obtain an accurate diagnosis of maltreatment of the older adult. However, if an abused and neglected older person presents to the emergency room with confusion, paranoia, malnourishment, and a history of frequent falls, and both the victim and perpetrator are heavily entrenched in a complex denial process, discovery of maltreatment of the older adult may be delayed or averted.

Professionals' Attitudes

The professional's attitude can set the tone for the interview and assessment process. This tone can facilitate or inhibit information gathering. Table 22-6 lists guidelines for the assessment and interview process. Maintaining therapeutic neutrality is essential in establishing the type of rapport that encourages disclosure of emotionally laden content like maltreatment.

Denial of maltreatment by both the older victim and the perpetrator presents a challenging problem for maltreatment identification, especially in the domestic setting. McDonald and Abrahams (1990) identified that older persons value independence and that more than 90 percent want to remain living in their own homes. Therefore older clients may refrain from disclosing the familial, emotional, or financial difficulties that occur in their homes. Likewise, Homer and Gilleard (1990) found in their research that few of the abused older clients would complain of the abuse.

West, Bondy, and Hutchinson (1991) discussed the difficulties in interviewing older persons in institutional settings. They proposed strategies to strengthen the validity when interviewing impaired institutionalized older clients. Suggestions included: *(1)* interviewing the older person as soon after an event in question as possible, *(2)* waiting patiently (even for several minutes) for the response, *(3)* listening for themes, *(4)* translating and interpreting communications from the elder by restating the communication in the form of a question back to him/her (e.g., "Do you think that. . . ?" "So you think/feel/believe. . . ?"), *(5)* making frequent contacts to build rapport with the older person and overcome problems of disorientation and memory deficits, *(6)* allowing long blocks of time because older persons may fall asleep, become disoriented, or have to break away from the interview temporarily. These suggestions may well be applicable in interviewing older adults and perpetrators of all types.

Interestingly, Homer and Gilleard (1990) found the caregiving perpetrators more willing to admit to and discuss the incidents of domestic abuse than were their victims. These researchers reported that the perpetrators were willing to disclose events of

Table 22–6   Guidelines for Assessment and Interviewing

- Use nonjudgmental approach with neutral tones.

- Avoid sounding surprised, excited, or angry.

- Avoid disapproval; it may only serve to increase feelings of shame and anger.

- Perform interviews in private.

- Interviewing suspected perpetrators in their home environment may facilitate trust and eventual self-disclosure.

- Remember that close proximity of the perpetrator may alter responses of the victim. For instance, the victim's responses may be more guarded if they were brought for evaluation by their perpetrator or if the perpetrator is waiting in the next room.

- Interview suspected victim and perpetrator(s) separately, as well as together. Pace questions, beginning with less threatening questions to establish rapport. Ask each to describe their typical day. Listen for conflicting and changing stories.

- Assess the suspected perpetrator for characteristic profile concordance. Especially note perpetrator dependency on the older person and any psychopathology. Assess social lifestyle of the suspected perpetrator and the older person for dependency and isolation.

- Open-ended questions may be helpful initially (e.g., "What is your life like at home?" "How are things at your home?" "What can you tell me about yourself?")

- Direct questions regarding maltreatment must be included (e.g., "Have you ever felt that you had been neglected, abused, or taken advantage of?" "Have you ever been hit, pushed, or shoved?" "Have you ever been tied to a chair or bed or restrained in some way?" "Have you ever had medication or food withheld?" "Are you afraid of [*suspected perpetrator*]?").

- Documentation of specifics is essential.

---

maltreatment when the interviewer maintained a nonjudgmental attitude and performed the interview in private, preferably in the home setting. Homer and Gilleard (1990) even noted that the perpetrators expressed relief at having the opportunity to share their problems with others. The proper professional attitude can enhance self-disclosure and establish rapport that may facilitate change during the intervention stage of maltreatment management.

After setting the stage for eliciting assessment data, professionals must keep in mind the need for clear, precise documentation. Photographs, videotapes, audiotapes, direct quotes, and the use of psychological screening instruments have been used in the documentation of maltreatment of older adults (Haviland and O'Brien 1989). Findings from the physical examinations should be systematic and exact. Measurements and outlined descriptions on body charts may facilitate the documentation process of physical findings. Documentation of the nursing process (i.e., assessment, diagnosis, plan, intervention, and evaluation) is an important part of the legal medical record, but it can also be an essential part of a legal investigation.

Suspicious Indicators

Suspicious indicators alert professionals to potential victims of maltreatment. Typically the profile characteristics of victims and perpetrators are used to red flag high-risk persons and situations. The present state of the body of knowledge on profile characteristics limits professional reliance on clearly identified high-risk individuals for maltreatment. Professionals are challenged to continue their review of research data and professional literature. Current data are still valuable to alert professionals of high-risk situations.

Table 22-7 lists suspicious indicators of maltreatment of older adults. These indicators function to alert professionals to potential maltreatment situations. However, an apparent absence of these indicators does not exclude the possibility of maltreatment of older persons.

Physical Abuse and Neglect Indicators

The indicators of physical abuse and neglect are essential in the assessment of possible maltreatment of older adults. These indicators include observable physiological conditions and emotional reactions to abuse and neglect. It is difficult to imagine any individual enduring physical abuse and/or neglect without psychological suffering. In fact, researchers (Fulmer and Cahill 1984; Pillemer 1988; Homer and Gilleard 1990) have noted that victimized older persons commonly sustain more than one type of maltreatment.

Tables 22-8 and 22-9 outline common indicators of physical abuse and neglect. Chen et al. (1981) noted that victims of physical maltreatment often evidenced signs of bruising, cuts, injuries, sexual molestation, malnutrition, and poor hygiene. The extensive research from child abuse studies on the unique signs and symptoms of physical abuse can be useful in assessing atypical injuries in older victims. Kelley (1988) differentiated that bruising from accidental injuries typically was found on the lower arms, knees, shins, iliac crests, forehead, and under the chin. Whereas, bruising on the buttocks, genitalia, thighs, ears, side of face, trunk, and upper arms were suspicious and warranted further investigation.

Kelley (1988) further noted that warning signs of physical abuse included bruising at various stages of healing. Estimates as to the age of bruises can be determined to some extent by their color. Table 22-10 outlines the common age-related color characteristics of bruises (Kelley 1988; Haviland and O'Brien 1989). Thin, loose, and fragile skin, such as the skin around the eye, genitalia, and on some older persons' arms, bruises quickly and easily. Tissue that has greater muscular support, such as the

Table 22–7 Suspicious Indicators of Maltreatment of Older Persons

- Matching of profile characteristics for situation, victim, or perpetrator
- Physician or hospital "hopping"
- Frequent visits to the emergency room
- Delays in treatment
- Missed appointments
- Noncompliance with treatment recommendations
- Unexplained prior injuries
- Inconsistent explanations for injuries
- Injury explanations inconsistent with medical findings
- Recurrent injuries of a similar nature
- Past history of maltreatment

Table 22–8   Physical Abuse Indicators

1. Welts

2. Bruising

   a) multiple bruising, in various stages of healing, in the configuration of loop-marks indicate inflicted injuries from being struck with doubled cords, ropes, chains, etc. The pattern of the bruise may indicate the method or object used to cause the injury (Besharov 1990).

   b) on wrists, ankles, or around the abdomen, indicating manual or physical restraint

   c) on upper arms, indicating holding or shaking

   d) of unusual shape (similar to an object)

   e) multiple bruises with different levels of healing, indicating old and new bruising

   f) inside thighs and inner arms

   g) small bruising over fatty, soft-tissue areas, indicating pinching

   h) genital bruising

   i) bruising on the pinna, from pinching the ears and injury to the ears from "boxing the ears" (Kelley 1988)

   j) bruising on the corner of the mouth from gagging

3. Sexual molestation

   a) sexually transmitted diseases

   b) genital or breast bruising or trauma

   c) pain, itching, or bleeding in the genital-rectal area

   d) painful, unusual gait on ambulation

4. Fractures, dislocations and recurrent sprains

5. Abrasions or lacerations with various stages of healing

6. Head and face injuries (particularly orbital fractures, black eyes, broken teeth)

7. Scalp injuries, hemorrhage beneath the scalp

   a) erratic alopecia (hair loss) from hair pulling

8. Burns

   a) unusual shape or in unusual places

   b) burns resembling hot implements such as cigarettes, curling irons, hot plates, stove burners, radiators

   c) atypical hot-liquid burns (e.g., glovelike, socklike)

   d) rope burns and chain burns

   e) carpet burns from being dragged or restrained on carpet

   f) chemical burns (Rathbone-McCuan and Goodstein 1985)

9. Human bite marks, which usually are circular or crescent shaped lesions. Denoting specific characteristics in the bite mark and measuring the size of the bite's arch may assist in determining the perpetrator.

10. Scratches (older persons might scratch themselves).

(continued)

11. Emotional indicators (Rathbone-McCuan and Goodstein 1985):

    a) high level of fear (huddled in corner) or nervousness

    b) confusion in the presence of the abuser

    c) depression

    d) anger

    e) severe emotional liability

    f) passivity and withdrawal

Table 22–9   Physical Neglect Indicators

- Malnourishment and dehydration (wasting away of subcutaneous tissue).

- Hypernatremic dehydration.

- Poor hygiene, pressure ulcers, oral thrush.

- Clothing inappropriate for weather and/or unclean.

- Frequent falls.

- Incontinence.

- Fecal impaction.

- Decayed teeth.

- Broken or missing glasses.

- Noncompliance with medical recommendations.

- Hyperthermia, hypothermia.

- Unexplained delay in seeking treatment.

- Signs of overmedication or undermedication.

- Long-standing diarrhea, dehydration, malnutrition.

- Lack of eyeglasses, hearing aids, false teeth, walkers, crutches, or other supportive/assistive devices.

- Contractures may be due to a lack of adequate range-of-motion exercise and activities.

- Neglect may also be evident by not preventing the older person from self-injury and self-harm.

buttock and thigh areas, may not evidence bruising until several days after the injury (Kelley 1988).

Besharov (1990) differentiated between accidental and nonaccidental hot-liquid burns. He described burns such as those in which the perpetrator immerses the victim in hot or scalding water to have clearly demarcated and symmetrical boundaries. In contrast, accidental hot-liquid burns tend to have irregular, asymmetrical boundaries with identifiable splash marks. However, all splash burns are not accidental. Splash burns on the back or face may be indicative of hot liquid thrown on the victim by the abuser. Socklike or glovelike burns and round, doughnutlike burns on the buttocks and genitals are examples of the burns most noted from perpetrator-inflicted physical abuse.

A similar differentiation can be made with cigarette burns. Accidental cigarette burns typically result in first or second degree burns. However, perpetrator-inflicted cigarette burns can leave deep, penetrating, third-degree burns.

Kelley (1988) discussed a particularly dangerous form of physical abuse to children identified in the last 1970s as "Munchausen's syndrome by proxy." In this unusual disorder associated with child abuse, the adult caregiver/parent presents the child with a fabricated illness or disease to a health care practitioner for treatment. Unknowingly the health care professionals assist in the abuse to a child through unwarranted tests and the erroneous prescription of treatments (i.e., medications, enemas, intravenous fluids). Although mothers of children less than 8 years old typically have been identified as perpetrators, research may be warranted to assess the possible prevalence in association with physical abuse to older adults by caregivers in domestic and institutional settings.

Individuals should not assume that the consequences of physical neglect are less serious than the consequences of physical abuse. Himmelstein, Jones, and Woolhandler (1983) researched fifty-six patients with hypernatremic dehydration, twenty-nine of whom developed the condition while at nursing homes. This common electrolyte imbalance can be induced from free water loss due to hyperglycemia, diabetes insipidus, acute renal failure, vomiting, or diarrhea. It also can evolve because of severe fluid deprivation, as when older persons are dependent on others for ambulation to fluid resources and/or assistance with fluid intake. Twenty-six of the fifty-six patients in the study died. Fifteen of those deaths were patients who had been admitted from nursing homes. Himmelstein, Jones, and Woolhandler (1983) reported that hypernatremic dehydration should be considered a dangerous but preventable indicator of neglect.

Indicators of Psychological Abuse and Neglect

Emotional maltreatment can easily be seen to occur in conjunction with the other forms of maltreatment. The process of victimization affects the emotional well-being of older persons. Tables 22-11

Table 22–10   Estimating the Age of Bruising

Time	Color of Bruise
first few hours	red, inflamed, tender
24–40 hours	reddish blue
2–4 days	brownish purple
5–7 days	yellow-green
7–10 days	yellowish brown
10–14 days	brown
2–4 weeks	clear

and 22-12 list indicators of psychological abuse and neglect.

Chen et al. (1981) identified withdrawal, fear, anxiety, depression, insecurity, powerlessness, confusion, passivity, and dependency as common indicators of maltreatment of older adults. Fear, and even disorientation, can become intense and generalized. When an older person has been maltreated by a caregiver, as is commonly the case, the older person can become highly suspicious of any individual who assumes a helping role. A premature diagnosis might conclude that the older person is simply paranoid or cognitively impaired. A more thorough assessment would attempt to ascertain the reasons behind the fears. Rathbone-McCuan and Goodstein (1985) noted that even disoriented older persons generally are calm in the familiar surroundings of their own homes. Therefore they encouraged professionals to assess fearful older adults in their own surroundings. As is evident, this necessitates home visits.

Frieze, Greenberg, and Hymer (1987) identified immediate, short-term, and long-term reactions to victimization. Table 22-13 lists these reactions and their respective time frames. Immediate reactions of shock and disbelief enhance disorientation in the victim. Sleep disturbances with nightmares are common. Autonomic nervous system arousal in response to the stress is typical. Hence, rapid heart rates, hypertension, diaphoresis, and various somatic complaints such as headaches, stomach aches, and diarrhea are common. These responses may occur separate from physiological reactions directly associated with physical injuries from physical abuse or neglect. Visceral stress responses normally subside with time. However, they may become long-term reactions if the victim remains in an abusive, neglectful, or exploitative situation and if the victim does not receive supportive interventions.

As the immediate shock begins to wear off, feelings begin to surface in the victim. The temporary

Table 22–11   Indicators of Psychological Abuse

- Extreme guardedness or clinging to abuser

- Paranoia

- Wariness of strangers

- Expression of extreme ambivalence toward family/caregivers

- Fear in the presumed safety of the older adult's own surroundings

- Frequently may deny the abuse due to fear of retaliation; may feel that aggression was appropriate; fear of the unknown and potential fear of being removed from present residence (Anderson and Thobaben 1984)

- Erratic and changing explanations of injuries

- Depression

- Confusion and disorientation

- Conflicting accounts with caregiver

- Anger, rage

- Imposed social or physical isolation

- Conflictual interactions (e.g., hostile overtones; overt, heated arguments between the older person and the perpetrator)

- Threats used by the perpetrator to control/coerce the older person

Table 22–12   Indicators of Psychological Neglect

* Hunger for attention and socialization; clinging responses to the professional
* Impoverished socialization history
* Depression
* Withdrawal
* Confusion and disorientation
* Anger
* Low self-esteem
* Minimal verbal interactions between the older person and the perpetrator
* Attitude of indifference toward the older person by the perpetrator
* Perpetrator speaks for the older person
* Perpetrator denies the older person an opportunity to interact with others
* The older person is not included in the decision-making process regarding personal well-being and care

numbness of the immediate disorientation fades and a wide multitude of feelings may emerge. Fear is one of the primary feeling states that becomes evident. Major fears include: recurrence of the event, fear of death, safety fears, fear of being alone and fear of being abandoned. Rage is another common feeling state during this stage. The anger can include fantasies of revenge and retaliation, self-blame, blaming others unassociated with the event, and blaming fate.

Victims' symptoms typically diminish within six months. However, some individuals will evidence a delayed reaction. This syndrome has been identified as the Delayed Posttraumatic Stress Response by the American Psychiatric Association's Diagnostic and Statistic Manual (DSM-III-R 1987). Individuals with delayed posttraumatic stress disorder experience a complex myriad of symptomatology that includes: recurring, intrusive recollections or dreams of their victimization; flashbacks; emotional distress at "triggers" (i.e., symbolic or related stimuli such as: objects, dates, events that resemble or are associated to the event of victimization); numbness; avoidance of triggers; amnesia or memory blocking to parts of the victimizing event; detachment; anhedonia (without pleasure); decreased range of affect; reduced future

orientation and view; and persistent symptoms of arousal.

Indicators of Material Abuse and Neglect

Material exploitation by strangers is one area in which older victims do tend to report abuse and neglect. Perpetrators of material exploitation who are strangers to their older victims are typically con artists and swindlers. The challenge with material exploitation by strangers is that the scam may be so "slick" that the older persons do not even realize that they have been had.

Material abuse and neglect also can be caused by caregivers in domestic and institutional settings. When the older person has experienced material exploitation at the hands of a caregiver, the disclosure is more complicated than when the older person has been scammed by a stranger. The psychological components of victimization play a larger role when the perpetrator is someone who is known to the older person and who may continue to play a vital role in his or her life (e.g., institutional staff, spouse, relative/caregiver). Thus older victims may withhold information of material exploitation from fact-seeking professionals. The material price they pay may seem

Table 22–13   Reactions to Victimization

CATEGORY	TIME	REACTION
IMMEDIATE	few minutes to hours	disorientation shock numbness disbelief weak helpless
	hours to days	frozen fright detachment regressive behaviors vulnerability
	days	anger anxiety sleep disturbances psychosomatic reactions
SHORT-TERM	first weeks	masked affect or expressive affect (fear, crying, rage)
	two to three weeks after incident	attempts at coping phobias nightmares seeking support
	first three to eight months	mood swings: fear and anger, self-pity and guilt fears of future attacks anger and revenge
LONG-TERM	can be more than six years	less pleasure in daily living continued fear trust issues impaired sexuality flashbacks physical pain depression low esteem relationship difficulties

small in comparison to their suspected fears of being placed out of their current living setting, abandonment, or retaliation by the perpetrator (Fulmer and Cahill 1984; Sengstock, McFarland, and Hwalek 1990).

Questioning anyone regarding their financial matters is a delicate matter. Yet questions regarding financial arrangements, thefts, loss of income or property, poor investments, and financial status are essential parts of the assessment for material exploitation. These data also may be useful in identifying caregivers in domestic settings who are financially dependent on the older person and who therefore may be potential perpetrators of domestic physical abuse. Table 22-14 lists indicators for material abuse and neglect.

Research data and literature on assessment tools for material abuse and exploitation are lacking in the professional arena. One might speculate that perpetrators would not be willing to reveal material exploitation of older persons due to the criminality of such confessions and the direct loss of resources to the perpetrator. This is known to be true when the perpetrator is a stranger, since few con artists confess and turn themselves over to authorities. In fact these perpetrators are quite adept at slipping away from the rigorous pursuits of legal authorities. However, the prevalence and disclosure rate of the material exploitation of older adults by their caregivers in domestic

and institutional settings have yet to receive thorough research exploration.

Perpetrator Assessment

Rathbone-McCuan and Goodstein (1985) judiciously warned professionals to assess suspected perpetrators cautiously, even though many caregiving relatives who perpetrate in domestic settings confess their deeds of maltreatment. Perpetrators come in all sizes, shapes, and personality clustering. Hence their responses to assessment and intervention vary widely. Professionals should be on guard for signs of impulsiveness and destructive or aggressive behaviors. Safety is crucial for all involved. Although probing questions may not be avoidable, the interviewer continually should monitor and titrate the emotional tension during the interview process. Assessing verbal tone, content, physical movements, and gestures gives clues to the emotional level of the interaction. Aggressive or highly seductive syntax, verbal threats, threatening gestures, or the displaying of weapons should be taken seriously by the interviewer. Ultimately it may be better to terminate an interview session and continue the assessment at another time than to overstimulate an aggressive individual who is close to losing control.

The assessment of the suspected perpetrator will give information that is essential in determining the

---

Table 22–14   Indicators of Material Abuse and Neglect

- Victim is the best source of information.

- Victim is constantly out of money.

- Recurrent thefts of significant items from the victim's home.

- Older victim is unaware of monthly income or financial status.

- Suspected financial status is considerably less than actual financial status.

- Financial affairs are turned over to others.

- Inconsistent, unexplained draining away of older person's material possessions or financial resources.

- History of financial losses due to repeated unwise investments.

- Reluctance of financial manager for older person to allow review of financial affairs by outside services.

---

dangerousness of the situation and appropriate interventions. For example, deep-rooted psychopathology, such as with severe antisocial or sadistic personality disorders, may warrant separation between the perpetrator and the older victim. Table 22-15 outlines important indicators frequently assessed in perpetrators. These indicators can serve to guide the assessing process. Still, a comprehensive knowledge base in mental health and psychopathology is indispensable in assessing suspected and known perpetrators.

Marin and Morycz (1990) underscored the importance of creating a trusting atmosphere during the interview process with suspected perpetrators to

Table 22–15   Common Indicators Noted in Perpetrators

- Reacts with indifference or hostility to questions that seek to assess potential for abuse (Anderson and Thobaben 1984; Rathbone-McCuan and Goodstein 1985)

- Ease in answering questions regarding abuse, especially with domestic maltreatment by a victim's relative

- Poor interpersonal skills with the interviewer: poor listening, self-centered, defensive

- Unpredictable responses (Rathbone-McCuan and Goodstein 1985)

- History of mental illness, psychiatric hospitalizations, substance abuse/use, major illness, recent death or loss of significant other or friend, job loss, financial dependency on the older person, resides within the older person's home

- History of aggressive episodes

- Feelings of powerlessness, vulnerability, and dependency

- May perceive aggression as a normative coping strategy, but also may have regrets

- Poor social skills

- Poor skills in power control; pushes through versus backing off (Rathbone-McCuan and Goodstein 1985)

- Erratic and changing explanations (e.g., of injuries to the older person; explanations of care, personal history, or history of the older person)

- Resistance to the older person being privately interviewed

- Encouraged isolation by the caregiver showing reluctance for the older person to be allowed to become involved with outside social contacts; resistance to "watchdogging" by outsiders (Fulmer 1989)

- Refusal to permit repeated interviews (O'Malley et al. 1983)

- History of being abused as a child (Rathbone-McCuan and Goodstein 1985)

- Discrepancies in perpetrator's account of injuries and physical findings

- Financial dependency on older victim

- Access and/or control over older victim's material or financial resources

- Increased marital conflict, especially in spousal maltreatment

facilitate candor and prevent impulsive acting out. They recommended that questions be framed in a manner that elicits responses from the suspected perpetrator to cooperate in problem solving for the well-being of the victim and himself/herself. Soft tones and supportive words by the interviewer can imply support to sensitive areas of questioning. For example, phrases like: "Can you help me understand how. . . ," "I'm wondering if you could shed some light on this for me; when did. . . ," "You must have some times when you feel _____ , how do you manage that?", or "Have you ever wished/feared that. . . " can be useful in establishing rapport with suspected perpetrators.

The attitudinal frameworks are quite similar for the interview process for both the suspected victim and the perpetrator. Yet many professionals struggle to maintain supportive tones when dealing with known or suspected perpetrators. The psychoanalytic field labeled these struggles of professionals countertransference. Professionals may benefit from supervision or additional training if they have difficulty maintaining a professional attitude and therapeutic stance with suspected and known perpetrators.

Evaluating Incidents of Maltreatment of Older Persons

One of the crucial elements in evaluating incidents of maltreatment of older persons is determining the dangerousness of the situation and the element of risk to the older person. Death can be a realistic outcome of maltreatment.

Table 22-16 offers guidelines to questions that evaluate potential risk factors to the older person. High-risk situations include the following: severe psychopathology of the perpetrator, refusal of outside intervention, and repetition of maltreatment incidents with increasing severity (Quinn and Tomita 1986).

Valentine and Cash (1986) distinguished between acute and chronic abuse of older persons. In situa-

---

Table 22–16 Assessing the Extent of Maltreatment

- Is this an isolated event? Has this happened before?

- How long has this been happening?

- Has the perpetrator/victim received help for this problem before? If so, what type of intervention?

- What are the functional and coping capacities of the perpetrator and the older victim?

- Are family members, friends, or resource persons available to monitor the situation (play watchdog)? (It has been proposed that watching prevents acting out.)

- Is the older victim in immediate danger of abuse and/or neglect?

- What are the consequences of the abuse/neglect on the victim and how severe are these consequences?

- What is the will of the victim? Is the older client willing to carry out the recommended treatment interventions?

- Sengstock and Hwalek (1985) and Quinn and Tomita (1986) emphasize the importance of assessing the deliberateness of the mistreatment and assessing true remorse from expressed remorse due to being "caught."

- It may be necessary to verify information through additional relatives, friends, neighbors, and other collateral resources who may have had contact with the suspected perpetrator and the victim.

- Does the older victim have the capacity to report subsequent maltreatment and elicit help if needed?

---

tions of acute abuse, the perpetrator frequently is reacting to a recent stress or crisis. These incidents are typically isolated occurrences and the perpetrator is generally responsive and receptive to supportive intervention. Conversely, incidents of chronic abuse represent persistent patterns of maltreatment and are more resistant to change. Perpetrator psychopathology is greater when protracted chronic abuse occurs, rather than isolated, stress-related incidents of maltreatment.

Assessment of the Residence

One of the final aspects in assessing maltreatment of older persons includes the evaluation of the living situation of the older victim. Table 22-17 lists items for assessment of the older person's residence. With the continuing expansion of health care services into home health care, home evaluations are becoming more prevalent.

The old saying that a picture is worth a thousand words is a true metaphor for the value of home visits. People tend to relax and show more of their true selves in the home surroundings. Information concerning numerous safety variables are assessable visually when visiting a person's home. Comprehensive home assessments in situations of maltreatment of older persons, particularly those in which the victim and/or the perpetrator are mistrusting of outside resources, may require prolonged or multiple visits.

If the perpetrator or victim is resistant to interventions from outside sources, gaining access into the residence may be challenging. Multiple phone calls may be required to begin establishing rapport prior to the first visit. Unfortunately, many agencies and reimbursement companies do not compensate health care professionals for telephone contacts or prolonged or multiple client visits for assessment.

INTERVENTIONS

Intervening in health care problems such as maltreatment of older persons takes a three-faceted approach: *primary* intervention, *secondary* intervention, and *tertiary* intervention (Anderson, McFarlane, and Helton 1986; Pender 1987). *Primary* interventions

---

Table 22–17 Criteria for Assessment of the Home

- Safety from physical hazards
- Cleanliness and sanitary conditions
- Safe access and mobility for the older person
- Adequate heating and cooling
- Adequate food supply
- Locks on doors and closets, possibly indicating restriction of the older person in certain areas
- Damage to furniture, indicating restraint (such as rope marks on chairs or bedposts)
- Cramped quarters for the older person
- Adequate space and privacy versus overcrowding (especially in shared residences and institutions)
- Adequate supply of personal items (soap, shampoo, toiletries, towels)
- Adequate assistive devices and/or personnel for assisting with activities of daily living (ADL)
- Presence of substances (e.g., alcohol, marijuana, cocaine, amphetamines)
- Access and availability to support persons and/or intervening resources
- Safety and support provided by local community

---

focus strategies on the prevention of maltreatment of older persons. *Secondary* interventions focus on identifying and treating the immediate effects of the maltreatment in an attempt to minimize the degree of trauma from the victimization. *Tertiary* interventions, utilized after maltreatment has occurred, facilitate long-term recovery and rehabilitation from the trauma of the victimization. Interventions for maltreatment have been separated in the following discussion as either primary, secondary, or tertiary interventions. Often, strategies for intervening in maltreatment of older persons, like other health care problems, incorporate a combination of primary, secondary, and tertiary components. Therefore some of the interventions of the sections may seem to overlap with other intervention modalities.

Table 22–18   Primary Interventions for Maltreatment of Older Persons

1. Education:
   a) educational seminars
   b) public service announcements
   c) newspaper articles/advertisements
   e) movies addressing issues of elder persons, such as normal changes of aging, developmental issues, emotional and social needs of older persons, relationship issues with older couples, and abuse and exploitation of older persons

2. Legislation:
   a) regulations regarding the care given to older persons
   b) tax laws
   c) Medicare regulations
   d) institutional regulations (e.g., nursing home regulations, health department codes)
   e) stiffer penalties for maltreatment of older persons

3. Frequent visits to older persons

4. Strengthening support networks of potential older victims

5. Counseling/psychotherapy to potential perpetrators

6. Marital counseling for older couples

7. Attitudinal changes in society:
   a) value of older persons
   b) dignity versus greed
   c) hard work versus quick riches
   d) empathy versus exploitation
   e) enhanced social or familial networks to replace lost family ties

8. Alternatives for placement of older persons

9. Research on:
   a) profiles
   b) treatment strategies for perpetrators
   c) theoretical assumptions
   d) primary interventions

Primary Interventions

Primary interventions focus on preventing the occurrence of maltreatment of older persons. For years, little attention was directed to prevention strategies against maltreatment of older adults. Rather, the first line of defense for maltreatment was secondary interventions, such as the assessment and treatment of injuries of older victims. As professionals and the public have turned their attention to the phenomenon of maltreatment of older adults, strategies for primary intervention have been expanding. Table 22-18 offers examples of primary interventions for maltreatment of older persons.

Education is a major strategy for primary intervention. As professional literature has increased on maltreatment of older persons, education has been expanded in the professional arena. However, newspapers, magazines, and the television media have begun to report problems associated with maltreatment of older adults. The media have been a very powerful tool for increasing public awareness of the problems of maltreatment of older persons.

Sometimes informing the public about health care problems can occur in the form of advertisements for services or programs that provide secondary or tertiary care to victims or perpetrators of maltreatment. For example, hospitals, community agencies, or even legal and financial institutions may advertise to help older victims of physical or psychological abuse or neglect or material exploitation; they also offer help for perpetrators. These advertisements may appear as public service announcements. The added plug usually applied at the end of the announcement can assist individuals in distinguishing between true public service announcements and paid advertisements.

Pillemer and Finkelhor (1988) believe that education needs to focus on informing older persons about spouse abuse. Their research noted that older persons were more likely to be abused by their spouses than by any other person. Many of today's older adults grew up in an era when women were more tolerant of wife abuse and when men certainly did not report being abused by their wives. Education that identifies spousal abuse as a problem, reduces the shame and denial associated with such abuse, and identifies resources that assist in the treatment of spouse abuse is a major component to preventing the recurrence of spousal abuse among older persons.

Education through the use of the television and newspaper media has been helpful in keeping older populations, and the public at large, aware of the current scams that perpetrators of material abuse are performing. Although these perpetrators of material exploitation are extremely difficult to catch and prosecute, public awareness decreases the number of potential unsuspecting victims available for their scams and con jobs. The public is informed which agencies and resources to utilize when reporting attempts at material exploitation and victimization.

Legislative efforts that focus on the protection of older persons from maltreatment also can be viewed as a form of preventive primary intervention. Lobbying for regulations on individuals and institutions that provide care for older persons, establishing programs that assist older persons to maintain their independence in healthy environments of their choice, and creating structures that protect the financial autonomy of older persons are important prevention strategies. It has even been argued that stiffer penalties for perpetrators of maltreatment of older adults might serve as preventive deterrents (Mathias 1986; Homer and Gilleard 1990).

Several national actions may help in the identification of abuse of older adults in the future. Clark-Daniels (1990) reported that The Elder Treatment Act (HR 1674) is an attempt to clarify the definition of abuse. In 1965 the United States Congress passed the Older Americans Act (Public Law 89-73). It was amended in 1987 (PL100-175) to add services and to make the prevention of abuse of older Americans a priority for government funding. In addition state offices on aging were expected to become more involved (Foelker, Holland, Marsh, and Simmons 1990). Carlson (1989) reported the creation of a six-member advisory committee of the National Aging Resource Center on Elder Abuse by the Administration on Aging. The committee will function to provide information and suggestions regarding the recognition and treatment of abuse.

Counseling individuals who are at high risk of perpetration on older persons is a primary intervention that many hope will prevent potential perpetrators from offending. The goal of this strategy is to try to emotionally heal, correct the pathology, or provide social and vocational support to potential perpetrators before they offend. There are many challenges to accomplishing this strategy of intervention. First, identifying potential perpetrators is difficult with the present flux in profile descriptions. Second, interventions require access to potential perpetrators. Rarely do nonoffending potential perpetrators volunteer for psychological treatment. Legally mandated access typically requires an offense to have occurred. Potential perpetrators, like other participants of health care services, have a right to refuse treatment. Third, the scientific knowledge regarding which treatment approaches more successfully correct the issues underlying perpetration of maltreatment is lacking. Fourth, the agencies and financial resources that provide and pay for these types of services for potential perpetrators are severely limited.

Community and societal changes are warranted to prevent the continuation of maltreatment of older persons. Society's attitudes toward older persons must be changed. The normal process of aging and the unique and specific needs of older persons must become known. Value and empathetic understanding for persons of increased age must occur if maltreatment is to be prevented. A return to the work ethic replacing the current desire for quick and easy riches is judicious. The desire for easy riches makes older persons easy prey for scams and material exploitation and encourages perpetrators to steal and exploit older victims. The strengthening of community and family supportive networks provides an important protective watchdog effect against crime and victimization. Strong supportive networks also expand the options older adults have for residential placement outside of institutions.

Hirst and Miller (1986) noted that a final primary intervention strategy was research. As research clarifies profile descriptions, screening tools, treatment approaches for perpetrators, and theoretical causations for maltreatment of older persons, preventive strategies can more effectively intervene that may be helpful in dealing with maltreatment. The list is by no means exhaustive but is provided to serve as a stimulus to preventive strategies against maltreatment of older persons.

Prevention of Material Abuse. The types of crimes perpetrated against the public are endless. Though older Americans experience the lowest crime rates for ordinary crimes, such as rape, theft, murder, burglary, and robbery, they are still victims of crime. Police observations have indicated a definite increase in purse snatchings on the days Social Security checks

are received in the mail. There is also a continuing problem of Social Security checks being stolen from mailboxes and residences. Most crimes occur in the evenings, in public places, and by young male offenders. The fact that the older American tends to stay home more and tends to associate more with other persons of their own age decreases their exposure to crime (Yin 1985).

Police records have been unreliable in assessing the prevalence of crime due to nonreporting, deliberate manipulation of records, and irregularities in the ways complaints are reported. Victims frequently do not report crimes. Reasons for this include reporting procedures that are too troublesome, beliefs that the police cannot do much, fear of revenge from the criminal, or fear that exposing the crime may incriminate them (Yin 1985). Fear can also be based on reality. Sundeen (1977) reported high levels of fear among older adults who perceived themselves in ill health and who had been prior victims. If neighbors had been hesitant to call police after witnessing a crime, this factor increased fear in the older people living nearby.

Older Americans probably make up 30 percent of scam victims. Such scams include, but are not limited to

1. Medical, health, nutrition schemes

2. Real estate schemes

3. Investment schemes

4. Fraud by mail

5. Telemarketing fraud

6. Home repair schemes

7. Death vulturism

8. "Medigap" insurance schemes

9. Confidence games

There are many varieties of consumer fraud. The more common devices have been described in an effort to alert professionals in the detection of fraud schemes being used on older populations.

Older people are considered frequent targets for fraud for several reasons. They are more likely than other age groups to be at home. Many have fears about maintaining a comfortable lifestyle on a fixed income, surviving inflation, preparing for a recession, having adequate medical care, and providing for family. Many have considerable home equity, which can secure bank loans. Many want higher returns than they are making on savings accounts and are vulnerable to promises of high yield and quick returns. Unfortunately once a person has been the victim of a scam, he/she is a prime candidate for con artists to hit again (Bekey 1991).

Prevention of Medical Fraud. Consumer frauds may be committed by small companies as well as by individuals. Medical fraud is common. Drugs or medical equipment may be offered with false claims of their powers. Common medical problems for which cures are offered include arthritis, hearing loss, denture problems, cancer, and epilepsy. People suffering such problems are eager to try anything to reduce their chronic suffering. Health and nutrition fraud is also common, claiming to meet special needs of older people (Yin 1985).

Hearing Aid Fraud. Older adults make up the largest proportion of people who need hearing aids. Most hearing aid dealers are reputable, but a few are unqualified and dishonest. Some disreputable dealers pose as audiologists, offering free hearing testing and one-day-only specials on hearing aids. The main loophole in the legitimacy of the hearing aid industry is the fact that hearing aids can be sold without a prescription. Nerve deafness, the most common deafness in the older population, cannot be helped by hearing aids. Nurses should inform their clients that:

- Reputable audiologists do not go door-to-door looking for business.

- There is no degree known as a hearing-aid audiologist.

- They should check questionable hearing aid dealers with the local Better Business Bureau.

- The hearing aid, by law, must have stamped on it the manufacturer's name, name of model, serial number, year of production, and a + symbol to indicate positive battery connection.

- An instruction booklet should accompany the hearing aid.

- They should avoid one-day-only specials.

Health Quackery. Arthritis sufferers are popular targets for illegitimate health professionals. Everything from moon dust to free electrons has been proposed as cures for this painful disease. Other conditions that attract quacks are hernias, psoriasis, anemia, hair loss, cancer, obesity, and alcoholism.

Nurses should know about such quackery in their communities and be alert to cues that their clients are seeking this type of care. In their teaching, nurses should emphasize that their clients

- select reputable health care practitioners and practices

- avoid people who make magical or inflated claims of a cure for an incurable disease

- obtain a second opinion when they are suspicious of a prescribed treatment or regimen

Prevention of Real Estate Fraud. Real estate fraud is common, preying on people's strong desire to own land and possibly on the older person planning to move to a warmer climate (Yin 1985). Falsely presenting real estate is not difficult when the buyer lives too far to visit the land. Real estate schemes aimed at the retiree's savings are all-too-common news items. Some swindlers have bilked millions of dollars from many older people before being exposed. The loss of their entire savings has a devastating effect on the physical and mental health of older adults.

The free lot (for which a buyer pays only a deed transfer fee of $149) is another scheme. The sales pitch is: "All you have to do to get this beautiful half-acre in this garden spot development is pay the deed transfer fee." The salesman does not explain that the developer paid $1000 an acre and the zoning law requires homes to be built on one-acre lots. The half-acre attached to the free half-acre will cost $2000.

The pressure on the buyer to buy now is difficult to resist. The land salesman carries a walkie-talkie over which an accomplice indicates lots are going like hot cakes. This device is designed to make the prospective buyer fearful that no lots will be left to buy. Older clients should be taught to

- investigate before investing

- resist buying under pressure

- base the decision to buy on fact, not promise

- explore hidden costs such as assessments, insurance costs for the area, and municipal improvements (sidewalks, streets, and water utility access)

Prevention of Investments Fraud. Investment fraud can cheat people out of millions of dollars, with the heaviest losses in the area of commodity futures. This type of fraud capitalizes on selling stocks and bonds that are financially unsound. The pyramid game is another scheme used by fraudulent investors. With this scheme, investors are promised returns that are unrealistic and impossible to keep. A third scheme involves work at home. Working at home to make extra money appeals to older people who do not drive and are living on fixed incomes. Some work-at-home schemes are devious and require that a person buy something before starting employment. For example, the job may entail assembling a product, buying reading materials, or customer lists. This scheme requires the victim to purchase the parts or products at wholesale cost, and the supplier promises to buy back the finished products. The older worker finds, however, that the product is never up to specifications, and the employment does not bring in the financial rewards promised.

The work-at-home schemes are many and varied. Everything from frog feeders to testing laxatives has been used fraudulently. Professionals who suspect problems with work-at-home schemes can advise their clients to follow certain guidelines:

- If contemplating a home business, obtain information from the Better Business Bureau.

- Be suspicious of work-at-home schemes that offer great rewards for no experience. These plans are probably get-rich-quick schemes for the schemer.

Prevention of Mail Fraud. Most mail-order companies are reputable and represent products fairly. But of the $183 billion in annual sales, 1 percent ($1.8 billion) may be spent on fraudulent schemes. Mail order con artists state opinions and stretch the truth. The scheme may fail to deliver prepaid merchandise, late deliver products, send unsolicited merchandise, or overcharge on credit cards (Yin 1985). Some mail-order frauds have included the following:

1. A "universal coat hanger" for $3.99 that was a $.10 nail

2. A "solid-state compact food server" for $39.95 that was a spoon

3. A "solar clothes dryer" for $39.99 that was a clothesline and clothespins

4. A "hide-a-swat" to kill flies at $9.95 that was a rolled-up newspaper (Bates 1991)

How can one avoid falling for such scams? Some of the more typical sales pitches to avoid are listed here. The American Association of Retired Persons (AARP) recommends that individuals beware if they hear these lines in a sales pitch (Bates 1991):

1. A "secret" plan for success.

2. An offer available only to a few select people.

3. You must respond immediately.

4. A chance for high pay in a short time for little effort.

5. A guarantee for a refund if you follow instructions.

6. Testimonials by people identified by initials.

7. Ads showing money trees and fistfuls of dollars.

Prevention of Telemarketing Fraud. Telemarketing fraud accounts for $10 billion in investor losses a year according to the North American Securities Administrators Association in Washington, DC. Since telephoning is easy and cheap, it is a vehicle of choice—900 numbers are frequently used. Individuals may lose $300,000 or more on such schemes, though inexpensive items may be sold as well. Telemarketing may be used to sell any product from vitamins to vacations to high-dollar investments. It may be used to fraudulently represent you as a contest winner in order to sell products, or to obtain credit card numbers to make unauthorized purchases later (Bekey 1991).

Telephone scams seem to be increasing, as indicated by a rise in complaints. But it is hard to estimate because these operations change addresses, telephone numbers, and names frequently. Southern California is reported to have as many as three hundred telemarketing scams working at any one time. They are hard to stop because by the time victims complain, the setup has moved. Too many people are embarrassed to even report the loss. In addition the operations are fragmented with an office in one city, telemarketers in another, and the mailing address in another (Bekey 1991).

AARP (Bekey 1991) recommends the following ways to avoid a telemarketing scam:

1. If you suspect a problem, hang up.

2. If you converse with a telemarketing person, ask the following questions:

   Where did you get my name?

   Explain all the risks involved in this investment.

   Can you send me a brochure or other written material to back up your claims?

   Could you explain your proposal to my attorney, accountant, or banker?

   What governmental or other regulatory agencies supervise your activity?

   How long has your company been in business?

   How much of my money will go for fees and commissions?

   Where will my money be held, exactly? In what form?

   What type of written statements do you provide and how often will I receive them?

   Who are your firm's principals? Can you provide references for them?

Legitimate callers will answer questions, provide written materials supporting their claims, and not rush your decisions. Con artists typically follow prepared scripts designed to persuade or bully. Rarely are they thorough enough to cover unanticipated consumer responses and persuasive comebacks (Bekey 1991).

Protection from Home Repair Schemes. Clients should be warned to beware of the person who "happened to be working in the neighborhood." This is the type of swindler who claims to be in the neighborhood sealing driveways and has some compound left over from a job a block away. He can let you have it cheap because he does not want to haul it back. The sealer might be crankcase oil or chemical waste. The older person who has been cheated will be unable to pursue complaints because the name, address, and phone number of the company are false.

The city furnace inspector may be a salesman in inspector's clothing. Clients should ask for identification from any public official who comes to the door. They should suspect that someone who wants to use a home as a model for siding or roofing is usually selling the product and service at an inflated price.

Some swindlers of home repair services peddle fear. Older people living alone are particularly vulnerable. One older lady, after receiving newspaper clippings about older people being beaten, robbed, and raped in their homes, was then approached by a burglar alarm system salesman. The alarming clippings had been sent to her by the burglar alarm company. The fire and police departments should be asked for recommendations regarding this type of equipment.

Protection from Death Vultures. The death vulture is the most unsavory kind of swindler. He or she capitalizes on the grief of older people. The newly widowed person is sent false bills for merchandise supposedly ordered and not paid for by the deceased. Frequently, the swindler claims the deceased person ordered the overpriced merchandise before death as a surprise for the bereaved. The names of newly widowed people typically are selected from the obituary columns of local newspapers.

A similar scheme involves funeral vultures. These people use a casket showroom, a rented hall, or a limousine as a base of operation. They talk mourners into purchasing caskets at outrageous prices. Costly funerals are paid for by the deceased's estate, death benefits, or relatives. Nurses can encourage their clients and their families to consider the five suggestions listed here to prevent excessive expenses and anxiety when a death occurs.

1. Select a reputable funeral director in advance.

2. Leave written instructions for funeral arrangements.

3. When making decisions on funeral arrangements, take an uninvolved person with you.

4. Check the license of the funeral home if the state requires such a license.

5. Do not accept products in your spouse's name unless you are aware of it being ordered and wish to accept it.

Protection from Confidence Games. Confidence games are theft by trickery and devices. The person does not mean to relinquish title to his or her property, only possession, handing it over to the con artist for a specific purpose (Yin 1985). Popular games are the bank examiners or embezzler game, and the pack game or the pigeon drop.

Bank Examiner Fraud/Embezzler Game. Older people

are becoming victims of this game with increasing regularity. The game is played with many variations. In one such variation the confidence person picks an old-sounding name out of the phone book, e.g., Hattie. He or she then calls Hattie and claims to be employed in the security department of the bank. He or she "has reason to believe" that one of the tellers is dishonest and has taken money out of her account. He needs Hattie's help in exposing the culprit. Hattie is then instructed to withdraw all of the money from her account, so the embezzler will need to steal from another account to cover the withdrawal. After the withdrawal the con person instructs Hattie to turn over the money as evidence of the dishonesty of the crooked teller. She is assured her money will be redeposited in her account. The results of this scheme are obvious. Frequently the victim's entire life's savings are taken. When police are aware that a confidence team is operating locally, they sometimes publish a security bulletin. A person who answers "yes" to the following questions is likely to be an intended victim of a confidence game.

- Have you received a call from a person who represented himself or herself as a bank examiner?

- Have you been asked to help in apprehending a dishonest teller?

- Were you instructed to withdraw a large amount of money from your account?

- Were you told to turn the money over to a special agent at a given location?

- Were you told that the money would be returned to your account?

- Were you instructed not to tell anyone about this plan?

The nurse should watch for these cues. If a client were to answer "yes" to any of these questions, the nurse should warn the client that he or she may be an intended victim.

Pack Game Fraud/Pigeon Game Fraud. The pack game, so called because it involves a pack of money, begins when a stranger asks a victim directions to Pea Green Street or the Star Motel. During the conversation a second stranger excitedly approaches the victim and stranger and tells him he/she "just found" an envelope with a "lot of money." This second con artist displays the envelope with a genuine $100 bill showing. The victim and the first con artist are invited to share the money if they promise not to tell anyone about it. Good faith money is then requested of the victim and the first con artist. The victim is accompanied to the bank by the first con artist. The money is withdrawn and the two (victim and first con artist) go to a designated place to divide the money. While the stranger or first con artist goes to find the second con artist to hand over the money, the victim is encouraged to ask the motel clerk if an envelope has been left for him or her. By the time the victim opens the envelope to find it full of worthless paper, the con artists are gone. Frequently the victim is so embarrassed because of his or her involvement in the dishonesty, the crime is not reported to the police. A "yes" answer to these questions indicates a person is the intended victim of the pack game

- Have you been approached by a stranger?

- Were you joined by a second stranger who claimed to have found an envelope or package that contained a large amount of money?

- Have you been offered a share of this money? Have you been asked to put up some of your money to show good faith?

- Has anyone accompanied you to the bank?

There are many other forms of fraud, such as scams involving magazine subscriptions, the lottery, carpet cleaning, and solicitations for groups, agencies, individuals. These appear in Table 22-19, "The Ripoff Repertoire," which shows twenty of the most common fraudulent operations (AARP 1991).

Secondary Interventions

Secondary interventions emphasize accurate assessment and diagnosis of maltreatment of older persons with timely treatment. Secondary interventions seek to limit the extent of physical, psychological, social, and/or material injury, loss, or damage that older victims experience as a result of maltreatment. The hope of prompt and effective secondary interventions is to allow older victims to retain or regain their normal functioning or material assets as soon as possible. Table 22-20 outlines suggestions for secondary interventions for maltreatment of older adults. Appendix E lists helpful resources.

Secondary interventions begin with assessment and screening efforts that identify victims of maltreatment. Accurate and early assessments might minimize or prevent more severe forms of maltreatment. For instance, early diagnosis might be able to prevent psychological abuse from escalating into physical abuse.

Once maltreatment has occurred, the secondary interventions of nursing and medical professionals are concerned with the diagnosis and treatment of the older victim. Emergency nursing and medical care may be necessary in certain instances of physical abuse or neglect. Psychological abuse or neglect also could facilitate a need for emergency health care intervention. If the older victim became profoundly suicidal in his or her depression, emergency hospitalization for psychological reactions might even be necessary.

The attitude and responsiveness of health care professionals throughout the assessment and intervention phase of treatment of older victims are essential in preventing what Gottfredson, Reiser, and Tsegaye-Spates (1987) termed a "second injury." They reported a study in which victims had to wait up to five hours for medical treatment that then was delivered with an impersonal and harsh approach. Gottfredson and his associates discussed the importance of victims receiving emotionally tender and responsive care from health care professionals. Victims are quite vulnerable in the early stages following an incident of abuse or maltreatment.

Secondary interventions also include a thorough assessment of the safety factors surrounding the maltreatment incident(s). Determining the safety of older persons returning to their previous environment must be evaluated. However, family members and even professionals can become perpetrators of maltreatment themselves if they violate the older person's rights by determining placement plans without allowing them to participate in the plans for their own care.

The desire to protect the mistreated can stimulate strong rescuing impulses in many individuals. These impulses can be so overwhelming that older victims become excluded in their own treatment planning. Some older victims of maltreatment have even had decisions made that change their place of residence without the older victim's knowledge. This constitutes maltreatment by violation of rights, even when

motivated by care and concern of loving family members and helping professionals. This desire to rescue the older person at all costs is a common pitfall of secondary interventions. It occurs so frequently that it has received slang monikers such as "the rescuing syndrome" and "the savior syndrome."

The goal of secondary interventions is to benefit the older victim. Still, older adults maintain the right to consent to the treatment approaches of their choice. O'Malley and associates (1983) noted that older adults possess a "right to be abused." They defined health care professional's obligations as twofold: ensuring decision making without coercion and ensuring informed and competent decision making. Still, many states have legal structures that direct professionals when older persons are exhibiting self-harm behaviors and making choices that may endanger themselves. Table 22-21 provides a questioning guideline for assessing the safety of older victims returning to their place of residence, especially if that was the site of their maltreatment.

Regular visits to the older person's residence, whether that place of residence is a home, retirement center, or institution, offer ample opportunity for assessing multiple parameters of safety and care when older victims return to their home environment. Hamilton (1989) noted that subtle changes between caregivers and care receivers may be difficult to notice. That difficulty is reduced if ongoing assessments occur through recurrent visits. Further, early indicators of increasing tension or aggression may be noticed by outside resources if frequent, recurring visits are made. Early assessment of rising tension and aggression may allow for successful intervention prior to an act of violence or exploitation against the older person. These interventions might include directing a cooling off period between the potential perpetrator and victim, reinterpreting or relabeling behaviors for potential perpetrators and victims, accessing potential perpetrators to counseling resources, or providing financial management resources or consultants to potential older victims.

Typically maltreatment intervention programs have focused on the theoretical assumption that older victims are mistreated because their caregiver is exhausted from the care of a severely disabled and frail older individual. These programs generally provide in-home assistance with the care of the older victim, respite care, and caregiver support

Table 22-19   The Ripoff Repertoire

The ripoff repertoire

The 20 most insidious cons operating

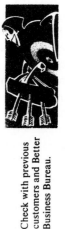

THE CON	THE CONSEQUENCE	THE PARRY
Bank examiner: Bank "official" asks you to take out money for him/her to hold to lure embezzler.	Person takes your money and disappears.	Call bank to verify legitimacy of "official."
Carpet cleaner: Ad offers very low price to clean carpeting in one or more rooms of your house.	Regardless of carpet's condition, cleaner says it's too worn/soiled for this offer and charges more.	Report operation to consumer authorities and Better Business Bureau.
Charity/religious group: You're solicited by an organization you know nothing about.	No such group exists, or only fraction of money donated is used for charitable/religious purposes.	Ask for verified financial statement to see where money goes, or only contribute to known groups.
City inspector: "Inspector" says he needs to check plumbing, furnace, heater, wiring, trees or whatever.	Person finds "serious" defect and must disconnect some critical service immediately. Offers to call friend who can do repair fast and cheap. Work is shoddy or unnecessary, charge exorbitant.	Call city department the "inspector" claims to represent to verify credentials before okaying job (get number from phone book, not his business card).
Contest winner: You're told you've won vacation, auto or other prize, but must send $5 for postage or registration, or call 800 number for details.	You get nothing or something worthless, or you're sent catalog of overpriced or nonexistent products.	Steer clear.
Credit/phone card: Person asks for your credit- or phone-card number to send you a product, check unauthorized charges, verify insurance, etc.	Product never arrives or is of inferior quality; or unauthorized purchases or calls are charged to your card number.	Never give credit- or phone-card number to anyone.
Government service: Official-sounding firm (e.g., with "Social Security" in name) offers Social Security service that is "required" (plastic-coated ID cards), "critically needed" (to help keep agency solvent), or useful (earnings form).	Services aren't from government, aren't required, aren't needed, or can be obtained free from Social Security itself.	Ask Social Security Administration about any such organization.
Home repair/inspection: "Contractor" offers to repair, inspect or remodel your home, exterminate pests, check for radon, etc.; or offers work with leftover materials from another job in area.	Person does nothing, does it wrong, or does unnecessary work.	Check with previous customers and Better Business Bureau.
Land sale: You're promised cheap land or complete retirement and recreational facilities in sunny, gorgeous site.	Promise is never fulfilled after site is purchased.	Visit site, investigate area before considering any land purchase; deal only with reputable firms.

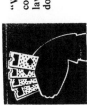

Lottery: Person offers to sell you winning lottery ticket he/she can't cash because "I'm an illegal immigrant," or "I'm behind in my child-care payments"; or "law firm" says anonymous donor has bequeathed a winning lottery ticket to you, but first you must send $20 for a computer search to verify your identity.

"Winning" ticket is counterfeit; law firm and donor don't exist.

Don't buy ticket from individual or send "search" fee. Be suspicious of any stranger offering to share money with you.

Magazine subscriptions: Young person is selling "subscriptions" to earn money for school/camp/team.

Money never goes beyond young person's pocket.

Buy subscriptions only through people or groups you know, or directly from magazines.

Mail-order health care/lab tests: You're promised medical care by mail, or lab screening for AIDS, cholesterol, cancer, etc.

You're stuck with expensive long-term and useless treatments, no tests are performed, or results are phony.

See your doctor for all tests and treatments.

Medical products: You buy health, beauty-care or "cure" product by mail, or you're sent newspaper clipping extolling magic diet with note scribbled across it: "It works—try it!" Signed "J."

Product is never sent or is overpriced, useless or harmful.

Ask your doctor about product first.

Need help: Man says his wife is sick, his car's been impounded, he's run out of gas, or some such; he needs just $10–$20, promises to pay it back, and shows extensive identification.

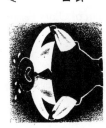

There's no emergency and his IDs are fake or stolen.

Don't loan money (or anything else) to anyone you don't know.

900 number: Products are offered via special 900 number. (Such numbers are common and legitimate.)

Call costs more than advertised, you're put on hold to pad your bill, and products are worthless.

Know cost before you call; avoid credit card, credit repair and contest-confirmation calls.

Obituary: You're recently widowed; C.O.D. box arrives for product "your husband/wife ordered."

"Messenger" is imposter and package contains cheap item at substantial price.

Tell person your spouse is deceased and you cannot accept product.

Pigeon drop: Person offers to share "found" money with you if you'll put up some of your own money "to show good faith."

You're asked to put your money in envelope. Diversion distracts you, envelope containing your money is switched with one containing paper.

Ignore come-on in the first place.

Product demonstration: Agent offers to describe only (not sell) new product if you'll sign paper "for my boss" proving he/she did it.

Paper you sign is actually contract ordering product.

Read every form before you sign.

Travel club: Firm offers bargain airfare/hotel package in glamorous foreign locale.

It's for only one person, price for others is sky-high, fees add more, hidden conditions could cancel trip, and if you ever go, it's fleabag city.

Ask travel agent if package sounds feasible; if you decide to go, read all paperwork carefully.

Unknown callers: Woman with child knocks on door and asks for some favor requiring entrance.

You're distracted by one while other steals cash or jewelry.

Give location of nearest public restroom/phone or whatever they need—but don't let them in.

Legitimate firms are injured too when cons imitate their sales methods. Learn to sort the bad apples from the good.

groups (Myers and Shelton 1987; Pillemer and Finkelhor 1988). However, most of the programs overlook the information provided by comparative research that highlights spousal abuse and perpetrator pathology as high-risk profile characteristics for domestic maltreatment of older persons. In such cases, interventions that focus on marital counseling, psychotherapy for perpetrators, and financial assistance and vocational training for perpetrators is warranted.

Legislative efforts that focus on penalties for maltreatment offenses, provide adequate shelter programs, provide psychological treatment for perpetrators, and provide for payment for treatment of physical and psychological injuries of older victims are examples of secondary intervention. Ambrogi and London (1985) recommended legislative changes to assist in the treatment, follow-up, and discharge options for older victims of maltreatment. They specifically recommended that the reduction in Social Security income benefits be eliminated when older adults share a residence with others. Additionally, legislative changes that provide for psychological and social services and protective follow-up for older victims and their perpetrators would enhance treatment options during secondary interventions.

There is controversy regarding secondary interventions for perpetrators of maltreatment of older persons. Some support criminal prosecution, while others believe legal action is an inappropriate form of punishment. Those opposing legal interventions for

Table 22–20 Secondary Interventions for Maltreatment of Older Persons

- Utilizing hotlines for maltreatment of older persons
- Reporting maltreatment of older persons to appropriate protective agencies and abuse registries
- Utilization of assessment tools for identification of victims and perpetrators
- Clear and precise documentation
- Crisis intervention strategies
- Emergency medical treatment, as needed
- Shelters for older victims
- Temporary shelters/placement facilities for perpetrators
- Legal penalties for perpetrators
- Frequent visits to older victims and perpetrators
- Effective treatment techniques for perpetrators
- Substance abuse treatment
- Effective treatment techniques for perpetrators
- Financial assistance/counseling for victims and perpetrators
- Protective services for older persons
- Home health care
- Public guardianship
- Marital counseling for older couples
- Vocational training for perpetrators

Table 22–21   Questioning Guideline for Determining Placement for Elder Victims

- Do older victims want to return to their place of residence?
- Do older victims want to continue to share their residence with the perpetrator?
- Are other resources or persons available to assist the older person with home care?
- Is the older victim agreeable to outside resources?
- Can the perpetrator's behavior be modified?
- Is the perpetrator agreeable to treatment and intervention?
- Are watchful or protective resources available to the older victim?
- Is the older victim capable of making a competent and informed decision regarding his or her care?
- Are legal statutes for adult protection being followed, while allowing older victims and perpetrators appropriate treatment choice?

perpetrators recommend that perpetrators receive psychotherapy interventions and support services (Ambrogi and London 1985). Valentine and Cash (1986) reported chronic abuse by perpetrators to be less amenable to change. They further supported court involvement when perpetrators were uncooperative or resistant to intervention. Homer and Gilleard (1990) were pessimistic regarding prevention strategies, available services, and the effectiveness of intervention strategies on perpetrators. They proposed that criminal prosecution may be more successful with perpetrators of physical and material abuse.

Mathias (1986) addressed the difficulty in treating perpetrators of domestic violence. She reported that these types of perpetrators tend to minimize the seriousness of their behavior, blame others, and maintain strong denial systems that are highly resistant to counseling. In her article she discussed an experiment conducted by the Minneapolis Police Department. Officers were divided into groups with different intervention strategies. One group of officers provided mediation for domestic abuse. The other group arrested perpetrators. Among the arrested abusers 19 percent repeated their abuse in the following six-month period. The recurrence of domestic violence among the perpetrators who received mediation as an intervention strategy was 35 percent. Mathias declared that jail may not be therapy, but it

gets the attention of the perpetrator and stops the abuse.

Researchers have noted that legal actions against perpetrators were seldom completed, even when restraining orders and criminal charges were available options to older victims (Myers and Shelton 1987; Homer and Gilleard 1990). Many studies have reported that older victims were reluctant to press charges due to embarrassment, a desire to protect a perpetrator who is a member of their own family, fear of reprisal from the perpetrator, and fear of loss of their current place of residence.

The controversy on treatment for the offending perpetrators of maltreatment continues. Quantitative experimental research is severely lacking in this area. Until treatment strategies can be tested for validity, reliability, and effectiveness, treatment interventions are likely to remain varied with conflicting accounts of success and failure.

Tertiary Interventions

Tertiary interventions are appropriate once victimization has occurred and the immediate treatment has been delivered. Tertiary intervention of maltreatment of older persons focuses on the rehabilitation and recovery of older victims. Rehabilitative services may begin during the treatment phase of

Table 22–22   Tertiary Interventions for Maltreatment of Older Persons

---

1   Occupational therapy

2. Physical therapy

3. Speech therapy

4. Assistive devices (e.g., wheelchairs, walkers, transfer boards, electric hospital beds)

5. Structural changes in the home residence (e.g., widening doorways for wheelchairs, lowering sinks for use from a sitting position in a wheelchair)

6. Assistance with meals (e.g., home-delivered meals)

7. Assistance with activities of daily living (e.g., home health aides, family/friend assistance)

8. Socializing activities:

   a) day programs

   b) community center activities and programs

   c) church activities

9. Counseling and psychotherapy:

   a) individual counseling for the victim and perpetrator

   b) marital counseling

   c) family counseling

   d) survivor groups

10. Alternative living arrangements

11. Vocational retraining and education

---

secondary interventions, but typically begin after secondary interventions have been completed. For example, an older victim of physical abuse might begin to receive secondary intervention for injuries in a hospital emergency room. The secondary interventions might continue throughout a period of inpatient hospitalization for the older victim. Some tertiary interventions may occur if the patient is referred for rehabilitative services while still being hospitalized for the injuries. However, most aggressive rehabilitation programs wait to begin their interventions until after the patient has achieved acute recovery from his or her injuries.

Assisting older victims of maltreatment to recover can encompass a wide variety of resources. If the maltreatment caused physical disabilities, occupational, physical, speech, and even vocational therapies may be authorized. Psychological intervention is crucial for dealing with the short-term and long-

term effects of all types of victimization. Overt manifestations of psychological trauma from the experience of victimization may remain dormant for years, even though the effects are being felt and experienced by the victim (Gottfredson, Reiser, and Tsegaye-Spates 1987).

Lobbying efforts that provide for programs and funding for the long-term rehabilitative process of older victims of maltreatment and that outline criminal penalties and rehabilitative structures for perpetrators expand tertiary intervention strategies. Legislative regulations that provide funds for the treatment of victims can provide needed financial assistance for the long-term recovery process. Further, programs that offer psychological treatment for the rehabilitation of perpetrators offer options other than incarceration. Even if incarcerated, most perpetrators of maltreatment will eventually be released. Therefore strategies that focus on preventing reoffending by perpetrators are crucial for tertiary intervention. Identifying which strategies provide the best rehabilitation for perpetrators of maltreatment has yet to be determined.

Table 22-22 lists tertiary interventions that may be helpful for victims and perpetrators of maltreatment. Professionals are challenged to assess the needs and choices of individuals involved in maltreatment of older persons and assist them in maintaining access to the appropriate treatment and assistive resources that facilitate their recovery. Victims who have recovered from trauma such as maltreatment have been called "survivors." These survivors at times have reported emotional growth from the experience of recovering from victimization. Although comprehensive and prolonged use of resources often are needed to assist older victims to simply return to their previous level of functioning, the ultimate hope of tertiary interventions would be that all victims could rise above their experiences of victimization to an even higher level of functioning.

SUMMARY

Maltreatment of older persons only now seems to be moving into the spotlight of professional and public attention. Society has maintained stubbornly resistant and blasé attitudes regarding the care of older persons. Many older individuals became a part of a forgotten society when they advance in age. History accounts report devaluement, negative attitudes, and prejudice against older persons more often than value, respect, and appreciation. For years, older individuals have endured abuse, neglect, and exploitation. But only in the past few years have news reports begun to focus on the maltreatment of older persons.

Maltreatment of older persons received professional examination only after abuse research thoroughly concentrated itself on child abuse and spouse abuse. The topic of maltreatment of older persons remained relatively dormant in professional literature until the past ten years.

The data base now is growing immensely. Research is hampered by definitional clarity and commonality. Precise determinations of the scope of the problem of maltreatment of older persons may never be achieved until terms have universally accepted definitional categorization. More research also is needed to clarify the conflicts in profile characteristics of victims and perpetrators. Nonetheless, assessments can be made and three-staged interventions (i.e., primary, secondary, and tertiary) can be utilized to intercede in the phenomenon of maltreatment of older persons.

The last years in a person's life should be reflective time in which the person is able to relive the joys and heartaches of a lifetime. For an older person to be constantly fearful of becoming a victim of abuse, neglect, or exploitation in these last years is appalling. Health care professionals can make a difference by educating older persons on how to protect themselves from maltreatment, lobbying for legislative changes that protect older persons, identifying high-risk individuals and situations, intervening with potential and offending perpetrators, and utilizing primary, secondary, and tertiary intervention strategies.

STUDY QUESTIONS

1. What are three types of maltreatment of older persons?

2. Differentiate between abuse and neglect of older persons.

3. What new profile characteristics of older victims and their perpetrators have been identified in recent research that compares domestically abused to nonabused older persons?

4. Identify three theories of maltreatment of older persons.

5. Define five indicators of physical abuse.

6. Describe three indicators of physical neglect.

7. Identify three indicators of psychological abuse; of psychological neglect.

8. List three indicators of material abuse or neglect.

9. Name five types of material abuse to which older persons are particularly vulnerable.

10. Discuss primary, secondary, and tertiary interventions for maltreatment of older persons.

REFERENCES

Ambrogi, D. and C. London. 1985. Elder abuse laws: Their implications for caregivers. *Generations* Fall:37–39.

American Medical Association. 1990. White paper on elderly health: Report of the council on scientific affairs. *Archives of Internal Medicine* 150(12):2459–72.

American Psychiatric Association. 1987. *Diagnostic and Statistical Manual of Mental Disorders.* 3d Edition Revised. Washington, DC: American Psychiatric Association.

Anderson, E., J. McFarlane, and A. Helton. 1986. Community-as-client: A model for practice. *Nursing Outlook* 34(5):220–24.

Anetzberger, G.J. 1989. Implications of research on elder abuse perpetrators: Rethinking current social policy and programming. In *Elder Abuse: Practice and Policy*, edited by R. Filinson and S.R. Ingman. New York: Human Sciences Press.

Bates, D.G. 1991. Fraud by mail. *Modern Maturity* 34(2):33.

Bekey, M. 1991. Dial s-w-i-n-d-l-e. *Modern Maturity* 34(2):31–32, 36–37, 40, 44, 88.

Besharov, D.J. 1990. *Recognizing Child Abuse: A Guide for the Concerned.* New York: The Free Press, A Division of Macmillan.

Brewer, R.K. and J. Jones. 1989. Reporting elder abuse: Limitations of statutes. *Annals of Emergency Medicine* 18(11):1217–21.

Callahan, J.J. 1988. Elder abuse: Some questions for policy makers. *The Gerontologist* 28(4):453–58.

Carlson, M.J. 1989. Evidence of elderly abuse growing. *Ohio Medi-Scene* 85(5):346–49.

Cash, T. and D. Valentine. 1987. A decade of adult protective services: Case characteristics. *Journal of Gerontological Social Work* 10(3/4):47–60.

Cassel, E.J. 1989. Abuse of the elderly: Misuses of power. *New York State Journal of Medicine* 89(3):159–62.

Chen, P.N., S.L. Bell, D.L. Dolinsky, J. Doyle, and M. Dunn. 1982. Elderly abuse in domestic settings: A pilot study. *Journal of Gerontological Social Work* 4(1):3–17.

Clark-Daniels, C.L. 1990. Abuse and neglect of the elderly: Are emergency department personnel aware of mandatory reporting laws? *Annals of Emergency Medicine* 19(9):970–77.

Clark-Daniels, C. and S. Daniels. 1990. The dilemma of elder abuse. *Home Health Care Nurse* 8(6):7–12.

Council on Scientific Affairs. 1987. Elder abuse and neglect. *JAMA* 257(7):966–71.

Daniels, S., L. Baumhover, and C. Clark-Daniels. 1989. Physicians' mandatory reporting of elder abuse. *The Gerontologist* 29(3):321–27.

Delunas, L.R. 1990. Prevention of elder abuse: Betty Neuman health care systems approach. *Clinical Nurse Specialist* 4(1):54–58.

Douglass, R.L. 1983. Domestic neglect and abuse of the elderly: Implications for research and service. *Family Relations* 32(July):395–402.

Douglass, R.L. 1987. Domestic mistreatment of the elderly: Towards prevention. *Criminal Justice Services Program Department, AARP (American Association of Retired Persons)*. Washington, DC.

Fattah, E.A. and V.F. Sacco. 1989. *Crime and Victimization of the Elderly.* New York: Springer-Verlag.

Foelker, G.A., J. Holland, M. Marsh, and B.A. Simmons. 1990. A community response to elder abuse. *The Gerontologist* 30(4):560–62.

Frieze, I.H., M.S. Greenberg, and S. Hymer. 1987. Describing the crime victims: Psychological reactions to victimization. *Professional Psychology, Research, and Practice* 18(4):299–315.

Fulmer, T.T. 1989. Mistreatment of elders: Assessment, diagnosis, and intervention. *Nursing Clinics of North America* 24(3):707–16.

Fulmer, T.T. and M.V. Cahill. 1984. Assessing elder abuse: A study. *Journal of Gerontological Nursing* 10(12):16–20.

Gelles, R.J. and M.A. Strauss. 1988. *Intimate Violence: The Causes and Consequences of Abuse in the American Family.* New York: Simon and Schuster.

Gerety, M.B. and C.H. Winograd. 1988. Public financing of Medicare. *Journal of the American Geriatrics Society* 36:1061–66.

Giordano, N.H. and J.A. Giordano. 1984. Elder abuse: A review of the literature. *Social Work* May/June:232–36.

Godkin, M.A., R.S. Wolf, and K.A. Pillemer. 1989. A case-comparison analysis of elder abuse and neglect. *International Journal of Aging and Human Development* 28(3):207–25.

Gottfredson, G., M. Reiser, and R. Tsegaye-Spates. 1987. Psychological help for victims of crime. *Professional Psychology: Research and Practice* 18(4):316–25.

Hall, P.A. 1989. Elder maltreatment items, subgroups, and types: Policy and practice limitations. *International Journal of Aging and Human Development* 28(3):191–205.

Hamilton, G.P. 1989. Using a prevent elder abuse family systems approach. *Journal of Gerontological Nursing* 15(3):21–26.

Haviland, S. and J. O'Brien. 1989. Physical abuse and neglect of the elderly: Assessment and intervention. *Orthopaedic Nursing* 8(4):11–19.

Himmelstein, D.U., A.A. Jones, and S. Woolhandler. 1983. Hypernatremic dehydration in nursing home patients: An indication of neglect. *Journal of the American Geriatrics Society* 31(8):466–71.

Hirst, S.P. and J. Miller. 1986. The abused elderly. *Journal of Psychosocial Nursing and Mental Health Services* 24(10):28–34.

Homer, A.C. and C. Gilleard. 1990. Abuse of elderly people by their carers. *Br Med Journal* 301(December):1359–62.

Kallman, H. 1987. Detecting abuse in the elderly. *Medical Aspects of Human Sexuality* 21(3):89–99.

Kelley, S.J. 1988. Physical abuse of children: Recognition and reporting. *Journal of Emergency Medicine* 14(3), 82-90.

Kimsey, L.R., A.R. Tarbox, and D.F. Bragg. 1981. Abuse of the elderly: The hidden agenda. *Journal of the American Geriatrics Society* XXIX:465–72.

Kosberg, J. 1988. Preventing elder abuse: Identification of high-risk factors prior to placement decisions. *The Gerontologist* 28(1):43–50.

Marin, R.S. and R.K. Morycz. 1990. Victims of elder abuse. In *Treatment of Family Violence*, edited by R.T. Ammerman and M. Hersen. New York: Wiley and Sons.

Mathias, B. 1986. Lifting the shade on family violence. *Networker* (May/June), 20–29.

McDonald, A.J. and S. Abrahams. 1990. Social emergencies in the elderly. *Emergency Medical Clinics of North America* 8(2):443–59.

Miller, R.B. and R.A. Dodder. 1989. The abused: Abuser dyad: Elder abuse in the state of Florida. In *Elder Abuse: Practice and Policy*, edited by R.

Filinson and S.R. Ingman. New York: Human Science Press.

Myers, J.E. and B. Shelton. 1987. Abuse and older persons: Issues and implications for counselors. *Journal of Counseling and Development* 65(7):376–80.

O'Malley, T.A., D.E. Everitt, H.C. O'Malley, and E.W. Campion. 1983. Identifying and preventing family mediated abuse and neglect of elderly persons. *Annals of Internal Medicine* 98(6):99–1005.

Pedrick-Cornell, C. and R. Gelles. 1982. Elder abuse: The stakes of current knowledge. *Family Relations* 31:457–65.

Pender, N.J. 1987. *Health Promotion in Nursing Practice.* 2d ed. Connecticut: Appleton and Lange.

Pillemer, K. 1988. Maltreatment of patients in nursing homes: Overview and research agenda. *Journal of Health and Social Behavior* 29(3):227–38.

Pillemer, K. and D. Finkelhor. 1988. The prevalence of elder abuse: A random sample survey. *The Gerontologist* 28(1):51–57.

Pillemer, K. and D.W. Moore. 1989. Abuse of patients in nursing homes: Findings from a survey. *The Gerontologist* 29(3), 314-320.

Quinn, M.J. and S.K. Tomita. 1986. *Elder Abuse and Neglect: Causes, Diagnosis and Intervention Strategies.* New York: Springer.

Rathbone-McCuan, E. and R.K. Goodstein. 1985. Elder abuse: Clinical considerations. *Psychiatric Annals* 15(5):331–39.

Rosado, L. 1991. Who's caring for grandma? *Newsweek* (July 29):47.

Salend, E., R.A. Kane, M. Satz, and J. Pynoos. 1984. Elder abuse reporting: Limitations of statutes. *Gerontologist* 24(1):61–69.

Sengstock, M.C. and M. Hwalek. 1986. Domestic abuse of the elderly: Which cases involve the police? *Journal of Interpersonal Violence* 1(3):335–49.

Sengstock, M.C., M.R. McFarland, and M. Hwalek. 1990. Identification of elder abuse in institutional settings: Required changes in existing protocols. *Journal of Elder Abuse and Neglect* 2(1/2):31–50.

Steinmetz, S.K. 1981. Elder abuse. *Aging.* (January/February):6–10.

Sundeen, R.J. 1977. Fear of crime and urban elderly. In *Justice and Older Americans*, edited by M.A. Rafai. Lexington, MA: D.C. Health.

Theiss, J.T. and J.M. Anderson. 1987. Services to prevent abuse needed. In *Gerontology Newsletter*, edited by I. Iscoe. 5(June). Austin, TX: Institute of Human Development and Family Studies.

Thobaben, M. and T. Anderson. 1985. Reporting elder abuse: It's the law. *American Journal of Nursing* 85(4):371–74.

United States Bureau of Justice Statistics. 1982. *Criminal Victimization in the United States* (NCJ 84015). Washington, DC: United States Government Printing Office.

Valentine, D. and T. Cash. 1986. A definitional discussion of elder maltreatment. *Journal of Gerontological Social Work* 9(3):17–28.

Weiler, K. 1989. Financial abuse of the elderly: Recognizing and acting on it. *Journal of Gerontological Nursing* 15(8):10–15.

West, M., E. Bondy, and S. Hutchinson. 1991. Interviewing institutionalized elders: Threats to validity. *Image: Journal of Nursing Scholarship* 23(3):171–76.

Wolf, R.S. 1988. Elder abuse: Ten years later. *Journal of the American Geriatrics Society* 36(8):758–62.

Wolf, R.S. and K.A. Pillemer. 1989. *Helping Elderly Victims: The Reality of Elder Abuse*. New York: Columbia University Press.

Wood, J. 1991. Ripoff repertoire. *Modern Maturity* 34(2):46–47.

Yin, P. 1985. *Victimization and the Aged*. Springfield, IL: Thomas.

23

Legal Concerns

M. Kathryn Nichols

CHAPTER OUTLINE

FOCUS

This chapter will focus on some of the legal concerns that arise as people become older. The role of health care providers in assisting older patients to utilize available resources will be considered.

OBJECTIVES

1. Describe some of the more common legal problems of the older adult.

2. Emphasize the need for planning while older people are still in control of their mental and physical faculties.

3. Provide information on legal resources available for both health care providers and older adults.

4. Emphasize the need for competent legal advice to assure that the person's desires are fully understood and executed.

5. Assist health care providers in determining their own responsibilities in assisting clients.

Older people often need legal assistance; they are sometimes unaware of this need. Many older citizens have led lives uncomplicated by legal entanglements and are not acquainted with legal needs and services. Often they have not given much thought to the need for a will or any other form of estate planning. It may not have occurred to them that they might become unable to care for themselves or their families. The emphasis on youth and independence in our present social structure discourages thoughts of old age, dependency, and death. It is as though we think we are immortal and therefore refuse to accept reality and prepare for events such as illness, disability, or death. Many families find themselves having to go through unpleasant and sometimes expensive legal procedures to remedy these situations.

Older people are victimized by unscrupulous outsiders, greedy family, or both, because they did not plan ahead and/or did not know where to go for assistance. Those who are on limited incomes may find it difficult to obtain competent legal assistance unless they are able to get help from community or government agencies. Limited income, increasingly impaired mobility because of physical or mental problems, inadequate knowledge of available resources, and limited or nonexisting resources all contribute to the problem. However, the Older Americans Act of 1965 has caused most states to focus efforts and funds on remedying many of these deficiencies. An example of increased availability of legal services is the Texas Community Services Advisor (CSA) program, funded by the Governor's Committee on Aging and created to train legal advisors. The need for the services was confirmed in the Texoma Region when, in one county (Grayson) alone, 236 requests for legal services were processed in one year. The advisors trained in the CSA program responded to the need for help with advice and assistance about various problems such as income maintenance (through Social Security and Supplemental Security Income), health maintenance (through Medicare and Medicaid), and establishing the need and eligibility for other public assistance such as food stamps. The advisor would usually have older people get in touch with local lawyers' referral services or legal aid agencies for help with strictly legal issues such as protective services, guardianship, commitment, power of attorney, or consumer problems (Governor's Committee on Aging 1978). More recently, the federal government included a provision in the Omnibus Reconciliation Act of 1990, called the Patient Self-Determination Act. It requires certain Medicare-participating agencies to provide written information to patients regarding their rights under state laws to accept or refuse medical treatment. This new law is discussed in more detail later in this chapter.

Health care personnel, especially nurses who work with older people, should be aware of the role they can play in dealing with the specific legal problems of the older population. It must be emphasized that there is no substitute for competent legal help from qualified lawyers. The health professional should be informed enough to know when to refer and where to find help for those who need it. Just as the medical profession has become highly specialized, the legal profession has many branches. Not every lawyer is skilled at writing wills or trusts. Not every lawyer is interested in the problems of senior citizens, especially those with limited financial resources. There are many national and local groups, such as the Gray Panthers and the American Association of Retired Persons, who will refer people to agencies where legal help is available free or for reasonable charges. There are Legal Aid Societies, Legal Services for the Aging, senior citizens groups, and other agencies that provide such services. Health care workers should become aware of all such resources in their area.

As adults grow older, there is a tendency for others to begin to treat them as if they were less and less capable of making life decisions with the competency readily granted them a few years before. Older children of aging adults frequently begin to assert their influence on many issues, especially those involving property, financial decisions, and health care. Physicians also frequently talk to the children rather than the older parents about what is "best" for them. It would therefore be ideal if all people could keep their legal affairs in proper order, write wills, and complete other estate planning while in full control of their faculties and affairs. Such is not always the situation, of course, and health care personnel frequently find themselves involved in situations where they need to be knowledgeable about legal affairs.

As has been well documented in several chapters of this book, there is an increased number of citizens who are in their 80s and 90s, most of whom continue to function independently both physically and mentally. However, as the total numbers increase, the numbers of those who are not able to handle their own affairs and make decisions for themselves increase. There is an increased effort by many groups to make information and assistance available to both citizens and caregivers. All efforts should be made to encourage people to take the necessary steps to ensure that they are the ones who make the decisions, before they are unable to make them or to convey their wishes to a person they trust to carry out their plans.

WILLS AND ESTATE PLANNING

People usually want to decide for themselves who will receive their property, whether they have large, involved estates or simply a few sentimental items.

Dispersal of resources may be a source of great anxiety to the older person. If the nurse can help the person to relieve that anxiety, it is worth the personal involvement and effort necessary. The nurse who has taken the trouble to gain some basic knowledge of the legalities involved will feel less apprehensive about advising the older person. Too many nurses shy away from witnessing legal documents when they might be of great service to the people involved by their willingness to testify to facts as they have observed them. Nurses have learned to make objective observations and assessments accurately and have little hesitation in recording this information on charts. The same type of observations and assessments are crucial in determining whether older people are competent to execute valid wills or manage their own affairs. There is no need for the nurse to give opinions about the decisions being made; all that is needed is an accurate account of the circumstances and facts as observed. It is wise for the nurse to keep notes about facts being attested to if there is a chance those facts will be challenged later. The nurse should also be informed about any policy of the particular institution where employed regarding the witnessing of legal documents before becoming involved. Legally, anyone over 18 years of age can witness the signing of a will. There are some types of documents for which a family member or health provider cannot be the witness signing, such as the advance directives form.

The nurse is actually testifying that the testator, to the best of the witness's knowledge, is of sound mind, is lucid, and understands what is being done. The nurse might be questioned later on these points and may also be asked whether there was any indication of coercion. Almost anyone can execute a will, even people who have been committed involuntarily to mental institutions, but it is possible for heirs to challenge such wills, charging that the testator was not competent at the time. The nurse should confine testimony in such challenges to facts surrounding the testator's mental competence, memory, and ability to make decisions and should not give opinions as to intent or feelings.

Inheritance Patterns

Before examining the basic structure of wills, it should be of interest to review some studies concerning trends in our society that have influenced and may continue to influence inheritance patterns. Rosenfeld (1979) studied inheritance and disinheritance in a social perspective and suggested that retirement communities and increased institutionalization of older adults have a marked influence on the transmission of family wealth. As children feel less obligated to be actively involved in the care of aging parents, the parents feel less obligated to leave their estates to children and may choose instead to leave their estates to people or organizations with which they have had more recent involvement. When older citizens consider moving to retirement communities such as apartment complexes, planned communities for older adults, and condominiums, there is frequently a concerted pressure by the community developers for the total commitment of the person's assets, which then become property of the community developers upon the death of the individual.

Rosenfeld (1979, 37) compared retirement communities to "greedy institutions," which expect the commitment of total resources to the institution in return for lifetime care. The pressure may be more subtle—e.g., the use of sophisticated advertising techniques, such as testimonials from celebrities, directed at a vulnerable segment of the population who are anxious to exercise their last hold on freedom of choice concerning their lives. The retirement community programs are frequently designed to isolate and encompass the lives of the older residents, replacing family interactions and loyalties with community activities. These newly developed loyalties will possibly encourage the resident to redirect any remaining assets to the most current ties (i.e., the community developers). Rosenfeld (1979) pointed out that his study was not conclusive but that it had important implications for future studies. He also pointed to trends in recent legislation that have changed inheritance laws to permit greater portions of estates to go untaxed. However, any taxable portion is now assessed at higher rates on large estates. He quoted other writers who speculated that these changes in inheritance laws may encourage older people to spend more of their assets while they are alive to reduce their estate to the tax-free limits. Other factors such as inflation and increased costs of living for the retired person probably have had similar effects on what might have been considered large estates in earlier times. The recessional years of the late 1980s and 1990s, with decreased interest rates on savings and increased bankruptcies of many banks, savings and loans, and supposedly stable companies, have had a marked influence on the independent status of many older adults who depended on these sources of income.

Trusts

Estate planning may involve a simple will or complicated trusts. A will is the basic document of most estate plans. It usually contains only three simple primary provisions: *(1)* signature of testator (the one who executes the will), *(2)* the name and powers of an executor who will carry out the provisions of the will, and *(3)* specific instructions about who is to receive the testator's property after all debts, final expenses, taxes, and cost of administration of the will are paid. If the will is handwritten, it is called a holographic will.

To carry out the intentions of most testators effectively, a qualified attorney should be consulted. The attorney will advise the testator concerning the laws of the state where the will is to be executed, aid the testator in avoiding excessive taxes for the heirs or beneficiaries, and assure the distribution of property as desired. Competent advice would cover the selection of an executor who is prepared to fulfill the role, as well as successor executors should the first one named be unable to serve. The experienced lawyer can help determine in which situations a trust is beneficial and can explain such terms as *wife trusts*, *family trusts*, *living trusts* (also called *inter vivos trusts*), and Medicaid Trusts. It may be more stressful to some clients than the benefits are worth and families in these cases may choose to simply drop the subject. In many cases, however, if people understand how a will or trust can simplify financial matters if they become incapacitated, most would choose to take these simple steps.

An important part of preparing a will is the provision that empowers an executor or trustee to carry out the testator's directions. For instance, a testator who owns a business should stipulate that the executor has the authority to carry on the business. There have been instances where this power was not given and a family business has been forced into liquidation before the court could give its permission to the executor to take charge. Husbands and wives should discuss how to proceed if the husband should die first. If the wife is not involved in the business and is not capable of making sound decisions regarding the business, the husband should leave instructions in his will to provide for such eventualities. Many widows have probably wished their husbands had done just that, especially if they have never been involved in the family business or finances. There should also be provisions for such possibilities as the death of husband and wife in a common disaster. Such provisions are especially important if minor children are involved, but they may also ensure that the estate is distributed among the testator's intended beneficiaries. If no provision is made, the entire estate may go to the husband's heirs only, depending on the laws of the particular state. Any major change in a person's life situation indicates the need to re-examine a will or trust. A remarriage, death of one child, divorce of a child, or additional children and grandchildren born after a will has been executed are all examples of common changes that could affect the will.

When There Is No Will

Health care personnel do not give advice on the construction of a will, but they may be in a position to point out to a patient the need for the services of a competent attorney. A person who has no written will should be aware that, upon his or her death, the state will determine how the estate is to be distributed. Most states have a formula for the distribution of the property of a person who dies intestate (without a will). In most states this type of formula gives a wife only one half of the estate if there are children. Such provisions often are inadequate for the needs of the wife, especially if the estate is small. This problem can also cause an estate to be tied up in probate for a prolonged period, leaving the heirs with unnecessary financial burdens.

A surprising number of previously unknown relatives appear when even a small estate is to be distributed without a will. Consider the case of a middle-aged couple who raised a young, homeless girl as their own daughter. While the girl was in college, the "parents" became seriously ill and consequently very dependent on the girl for physical help and management of their business affairs. The girl was never adopted officially but was as devoted as any natural child could have been. The parents had also neglected to make a will. The wife became confused and increasingly disoriented. She was diagnosed by a physician as having an organic mental disorder. She had not been willing to discuss the preparation of a will before she became grossly confused, even though her husband had suggested that a will was needed. He had not been willing to push the issue. He became critically ill with circulatory problems, which made the amputation of his legs necessary. The wife could not cope with the stress and became incoherent, and she had to be hospitalized. The young woman was faced with a major legal problem when the surgeon required a signature for permission to amputate. The husband was unable to sign his own permission and the wife was not only incoherent, she was seriously, even critically, ill. It is not surprising that about this time several cousins who had not visited in years appeared and exhibited concern. The young woman was distraught over her "parents'" conditions, and she was harassed by the relatives because they felt they should inherit the "parents'" property. This unpleasant, unjust situation might have been avoided by simple legal advice before the couple became virtually incapacitated and unable to care for their own business affairs. The "daughter" they loved and who loved them could have continued to care for them without legal entanglements and without the problem of greedy, uncaring cousins who were interested only in the property and money that might be involved. It is likely that the little that was left after both parents died was lost in court costs and thus did not benefit the beloved "daughter." Without any legal authority the "daughter" could not pay bills or authorize care until the court so ruled.

POWER OF ATTORNEY

The case discussed in the previous section points out another legal procedure that is frequently needed for older adults. Investing *power of attorney* is a relatively simple procedure that provides for someone to carry on the affairs of another person when that person cannot continue to do so. If the couple mentioned earlier had executed a power of attorney legally authorizing the "daughter" to act for them, she could have carried on business affairs while they were ill. A power of attorney is a written document in which a person appoints someone as an "attorney in fact" to act as that person's agent. The provisions of the document can be broad, allowing the agent to do almost anything on the person's behalf; or they can be specific, permitting the agent to undertake only certain functions. The person may designate the particular time or circumstances under which the person given power of attorney may act. Such a document is essential if the person should become ill or physically impaired or should be out of the country for an extended period of time, during which certain functions must be performed on the person's behalf.

The activities that the agent is empowered to carry out may be as simple as paying monthly bills or filing an income tax return while the person is away or incapacitated. A power of attorney should state the length of time it is to be in effect, up to the time of death if that is the intent. Power of attorney terminates with death. In some states if a person is ruled incompetent, this fact may also invalidate any power of attorney previously delegated. If this is the law in a specific state, the person may choose to create a revocable living trust before becoming incapacitated.

Power of Attorney for Health Care

There has been increasing emphasis on the need for a Power of Attorney for Health Care. This may also be called Medical Power of Attorney or Health Care Proxy. This is a different document than the Living Will. The Living Will (more accurately, Directive to Physician) is a document prepared to give directions or instructions regarding the decisions about life-sustaining procedures in the event of a terminal illness or major injuries that incapacitate the person. Many states now recognize these as valid when the instructions are followed. The rules may differ in different states. The document generally must be signed and witnessed by someone other than family members or health care providers. Copies of the properly executed document should be filed with the client's physician and with the family or the person given power of attorney for health care. The document should be reviewed, dated, and initialed by the client periodically. It can be revoked at any time verbally or in writing. The execution of this document does not alter the ability to make decisions as long as the person is able to do so (*Implementation of the Patient Self-Determination Act* 1991).

Power of Attorney for Health Care is a document

that designates and authorizes someone selected by the person to make health care decisions for that person if he or she becomes unable to make those decisions. It may also include more specific directions or guidelines if the person so desires. Some suggest that in addition to placing copies of this document in the medical files of the person's physician and other places, a card should be carried in the person's wallet that gives instructions on how to reach the person designated.

There are specific guidelines related to the preparation and execution of this document. The agent designated may be anyone 18 years of age or older (or a younger person who has had the disabilities of minority removed). For practical reasons this person should be someone trusted and who is geographically near and able to carry out the responsibilities. It is wise to designate alternates, should the first person named be unable to serve in this position. Individuals executing these documents should discuss their religious and moral beliefs concerning health care and should make their expectations clear before the document is signed. Many agencies, such as a local health care agency (e.g., hospital), local bar association, or the American Association of Retired Persons, provide copies of documents that can be used.

The Power of Attorney must be signed in the presence of two or more witnesses. These witnesses *may not* be the designated agent; a health care or residential care provider of the client or an employee of these providers; a spouse; any lawful heirs or beneficiaries of the client's estate; or creditors or persons who have claims against the estate.

All people should strongly consider executing such a document, regardless of age, but especially those in high-risk groups, such as the older adult or anyone with a chronic illness who has the potential for partial or total incapacity.

The Patient Self-Determination Act (Public Law 10 1-508) became effective December 1, 1991. This act was passed to assure patients' rights to participate in the decisions surrounding their care in Medicare-participating hospitals or other Medicare provider agencies. The law requires that the Medicare-participating agency provide, in writing, to every patient admitted, information that outlines the personal right to freedom of individual choice under state law. The agency must document on the patient's record that the individual has been given the information and has signed a form that states that he or she does understand the content. *It does not require the patient to execute any kind of document.* The staff also should explain to the patient any policy or philosophy the agency has about whether or not they will honor or carry out directives that might be contrary to the directive. The staff should make every effort to assist the patient to transfer to another agency if the patient so desires (*Implementation of the Patient Self-Determination Act* 1991).

Abuses of Power of Attorney

Powers of attorney should not be used indiscriminately, however. There is always the risk of abuse. Those who work with older people are aware of many instances in which a maid or "companion" employed to assist the person at home may be "trusted" to sign checks so they can buy groceries or shop for the person or household. When family members do not fulfill these needs, the person may turn to the maid or companion for help in an attempt to avoid institutionalization. Such employees may abuse this responsibility and cheat the older person out of substantial sums, thereby limiting the older person's future alternatives in maintaining independence. Administrators of nursing homes and other health care facilities may be given power of attorney so that they can write checks and carry on business for incapacitated residents who do not have a family or guardian. Care must be taken to prevent abuse by unscrupulous people in any position.

Most directors of health care facilities prefer the courts to appoint a guardian or conservator for older patients to avoid suspicion and the responsibility involved. In one case, a 78-year-old woman who lived alone and had no close relatives became more and more dependent on several friends to help with her shopping and other activities. When she became unable to do so, they even helped her pay bills. Eventually they became concerned that it was unsafe for her to live alone and helped her to be admitted to a nursing home. When some distant relatives appeared and attempted to take charge of the older woman's affairs, the nursing home administrator advised the friends to petition the court to appoint a guardian. The judge determined that it was not advisable to appoint either the family or friends and instead appointed an attorney as guardian. The attorney was a neutral party and did not represent either group.

APPLICATION FOR SOCIAL SECURITY BENEFITS

Many older people need assistance in applying for benefits for which they are eligible. The forms may not appear complicated to the nurse, but they may be confusing to someone not accustomed to filling out such documents. Benefits under the Old Age Survivors and Disability Insurance (OASDI)—Social Security—are available to most older Americans. These benefits are not automatic; they must be applied for by the eligible worker. Applications are available from Social Security Administration (SSA) offices throughout the country. The person must fill out the application and furnish proof of eligibility with such information as requested. If needed, a person can receive assistance from the SSA in filling out an application form but must sign the form unless physically or mentally incapable of doing so. An indication of intent to file for benefits by any means other than an official application blank, such as a telephone call or a letter, may sometimes be considered an application but must be followed by official application within six months. The older person should investigate the advantages and disadvantages of applying for Social Security benefits as early as age 62. Social Security Administration workers can supply the person with facts so that the best decision can be made. An application should be filed about three months before the time the applicant expects to receive the benefits, whether at age 62 or 65. If the application is not filed promptly, some benefits could be lost. Benefits, whether they are for retirement, survivors' pension, or disability payments, will not be paid retroactively for more than twelve months.

Establishing Eligibility

Establishing eligibility for Social Security benefits is the responsibility of the applicant. Social Security Administration workers must have the necessary evidence available and will inform the applicant of the kind of evidence required. Pamphlets containing this information are available at SSA offices. The nurse can be helpful by reminding the client to locate birth certificates, marriage licenses, or death certificates to take along to the SSA office. Even if these documents are not readily available, the application should not be delayed, although the lack of these documents often complicates the establishment of eligibility and legal aid may be needed. Usually, however, other types of documents will be acceptable, if available. Some of the more acceptable substitutes are church records of birth or baptism, if made before the fifth birthday, or a certified copy of these records. School or census records, church records of religious confirmations or baptisms, military records, labor union records, insurance policies, passports, and other authentic documents may be used to aid in establishing eligibility for benefits. In some cases the testimony of friends or relatives may be accepted. Usually older documents are given more consideration than more recent ones. When evidence of a marriage is needed, common law marriage is accepted as valid if the state where the agreement existed considers it legal. An affidavit from both parties may be needed stating that the agreement existed. If one spouse is deceased, two affidavits from friends or, preferably, blood relatives who know of the agreement should be submitted with the application (Brown 1979).

Need for Legal Assistance

Many different problems may arise for which a claimant needs expert legal assistance. The SSA office can provide much help, but if the claimant has great difficulty or unique problems, legal aid societies or other similar agencies will provide needed assistance.

A California agency established for legal assistance to senior citizens reported that the most common problem for which they are asked for assistance is to help older people prove eligibility for disability claims that have been denied. If the nurse believes that a client is eligible for benefits that have been denied, referral to a legal aid group is indicated. Older people who have private pensions, veterans' benefits, or railroad retirement benefits are usually able to get assistance from those agencies, but the nurse may need to help the patient locate the agency and follow through with instructions (Brown et al. 1979).

There are many sources of information about legal assistance. The telephone directory lists addresses and phone numbers of groups such as the

Grey Panthers, American Association of Retired Persons, the Alzheimer's Association, the local Bar Association, Mental Health Association, and many official state or federal agencies. Many agencies furnish free publications, e.g., *Health Care Powers of Attorney*, published by the Commission on Legal Problems of the Elderly and the American Bar Association, and *Legal Considerations for Alzheimer's Disease*, published by the Alzheimer's Association.

GUARDIANSHIP AND CIVIL COMMITMENT TO INSTITUTIONS

Because many legislators and judges believe that one of the inevitable aspects of old age is deterioration, either physical or mental, the courts frequently intervene in the lives of older people through a process known as guardianship. The intent of this process is usually to protect older adults from injury to themselves or from others. The courts, family, or friends may also be trying to prevent older people from squandering their resources or from being victimized by unscrupulous, designing people.

Most deterioration is not inevitable. As pointed out in several other chapters of this book, the confusion and memory loss experienced by many older people may be the result of factors that are treatable and thus reversible. It is incumbent upon nurses and other health professionals involved in the care of the older person to be aware of the laws governing the declaration of incompetence, the appointment of guardians, and commitment to institutions. In many instances nurses can assist older people in exercising their rights and avoiding unnecessary and undesirable institutionalization, which may lead to increased problems or early death. The serious implications of removing a person's basic decision-making power regarding his or her own life should be kept in mind during all proceedings. Frequently, health professionals are in a position to be involved with either the person or the family or both. A basic knowledge of the law may help all concerned reach a more reasonable and satisfactory solution to the problem.

Powers of the State

Thee are two general principles or justifications for legal action in the areas of guardianship and civil commitment. It is important to distinguish between

them. The state has the authority and responsibility to intervene when a person's actions threaten or harm another's property or person. This authority involves the states' police powers and is based on laws designed to protect society. People who are convicted of violations of these laws can be removed from society, thus losing their freedom. Involuntary commitment to a mental institution can be based on this authority if a person is ruled as being dangerous to society. It is generally agreed that such action is justifiable and necessary in many, perhaps even most, cases. But one role of the nurse or other health professional is to help prevent abuse or misuse of this authority by those who may not hold the client's rights as a high priority. This attitude may be the result of inadequate knowledge or, in some cases, simply unscrupulous or unethical motives.

The second power of the state that may be more involved with incompetence or guardianship decisions is the doctrine of *parens patriae* or "parentage of the state." This power involves the states' right to protect people who cannot protect or care for themselves, their dependents, or their property because of incapacitation as a result of disease or other causes. This power is exercised to protect the individual rather than society. The laws of each state that govern the process of declaring a person incompetent and the appointment of a guardian to be responsible for that person are based on this concept.

Many people are concerned about abuses of governmental authority. Because of this concern, groups such as state mental health associations have been active in monitoring and investigating practices in their own states in an attempt to change laws to include safeguards in the procedures set forth by the law. Some states have been more successful than others in accomplishing reforms. Each state will of course differ somewhat in the procedures and definitions included in the law. Even more crucial sometimes are the interpretations of the statutes as they are enforced.

Procedures for Commitment and Incompetency Determinations

Quite often health care workers and others assume that medical decisions and opinions are the basis for commitment and incompetency determinations. This assumption is not the case. Commitment is a legal procedure based on the two principles of state power described above. The final decisions are made by official representatives of the law, e.g., a probate court judge. These officials may rely heavily on medical information, sometimes perhaps to the disadvantage of the client if the medical personnel are not familiar with the law and the process of aging and are not concerned about the client's interests and rights.

Role of Health Care Personnel

Health care personnel can be most helpful by their careful observation, accurate assessment, and appropriate detailed reporting of the behavior of the people in question in regard to their ability to participate in decisions about their own care. The avoidance of vague diagnostic terms is essential. Instead the emphasis must be on the patient's communication skills, memory, and judgment. These are the functions that are most in question when an incompetence ruling is sought and should be described in simple, descriptive terms that will help those responsible to make a fair and sound judgment regarding the person's ability to handle his or her own affairs. *Incompetence* is a legal term that means that a person is not capable of managing or caring for his or her own affairs properly because of disease or other conditions. It is not necessarily related to mental disease, although it frequently carries this connotation. Different states have varying requirements or procedures that must be satisfied before a person is determined to be incompetent, thereby allowing the appointment of a guardian. However, most states require that someone, usually a relative, file a petition with a court specifically requesting that court to declare a person incompetent. Then there must be a hearing to allow both sides adequate opportunity to convince the court of the true facts regarding the person's capabilities.

Competency and the Need for a Guardian

The determination of the need for a guardian is not a criminal proceeding, and the client is not referred to as a defendant. One similarity to a criminal proceeding exists, however, in that a person is assumed to be competent until proven otherwise. The burden of proof rests with the party requesting the ruling of incompetence. Most states require a stated time period for notification of the person about the time, place,

and purpose of the hearing. It is usually required that the person be informed that he or she may have a lawyer present to safeguard his or her rights. In some areas a lawyer (guardian *ad litem*) is automatically appointed to represent the person whose competency is under question, unless that person chooses to retain his or her own lawyer. The person must be told that he or she has a right to be present at the hearing. The person who wishes to contest the proceedings should invite to the hearing friends, business associates, or anyone who has direct knowledge of his or her ability to function effectively in decision making and financial management. The court will hear all testimony and see all evidence submitted before reaching a decision.

If there are insufficient safeguards regarding guardianship in the statutes of a particular state, nurses in that state should become active in gaining the attention of various groups and legislators who can facilitate reforms and work for necessary changes until they are accomplished. Although the competency ruling and the appointment of a guardian are two separate court actions, they may be done at the same time. The nurse should be clear that the two are not at all the same. A person may be deemed to need help with financial affairs or an estate, while being judged competent to make other decisions about his or her life. However, the procedures for both court actions are similar.

Effects of Incompetency Determinations

Brown (1979) declared that the determination of incompetency reduces the person to the status of a child because so many commonly accepted functions and rights are removed. He pointed out that each state imposes its own specific limitations. In general a person who is declared legally incompetent can no longer vote or hold office; negotiate contracts; manage property by selling, buying, leasing, or mortgaging; determine where he or she will live independently; divorce or marry; babysit or otherwise care for children; travel; drive an automobile; and appoint representatives. Certain other legal functions are also curtailed, such as practicing certain professions, serving on juries, operating a business, witnesses legal documents, and initiating lawsuits or defending against one.

The nurse should be aware that the determination

of incompetency also limits a person's ability to refuse treatment and, in many instances, to give permission for treatment. Nurses caring for a person who has impaired competency should investigate the legal status of that person to avoid liability for their own actions and possibly for the institution or agency where they are employed. If a patient has a legally appointed guardian, only the guardian can sign for the patient for any reason. There are instances in which family members disagree among themselves about what is best for the patient. An institution such as a bank, a nursing home, or a hospital may have been designated as guardian. A friend, relative, or even the person may object to decisions about treatment, confinement, or any other invasion of the person's life activities. It is important, therefore, to determine who can legally give permission before initiating procedures that require consent.

Types and Responsibilities of Guardians

There are different types of guardians with different types of authority that are determined by the statutes of the particular state. Most guardians have total power and control of all aspects of the person's, or *ward's* (the term frequently used), life. There is also the position of partial or limited guardian, usually called a conservator or curator. This title usually implies narrower powers than those of guardian, limited mostly to the ward's property and finances and may be for a specific time period.

The courts may designate anyone deemed capable who is not clearly antagonistic to the ward's best interest to be guardian or conservator. It may be a friend, relative, lawyer, or public agency such as a bank. The Veterans Administration and Social Security Administration each has its own system of limited authority of guardianship that is separate from court-appointed guardianship. Unfortunately the person is not necessarily consulted to determine if the guardian appointed is acceptable. There may also be limited supervision of the parties appointed as guardians by the courts. Many states have poorly written guidelines for the removal of the incompetency designation and the return of the person's powers to manage his or her own affairs again. *It should not be assumed that incompetency is permanent.* Proper treatment may restore capabilities and the patient or ward may need an active advocate. It is usually the

responsibility of the ward to sue for return of his or her legal status and to prove that whatever condition existed before has been overcome. The older person may not know his or her rights and may need help in obtaining effective assistance. The nurse should be aware that neither the appointment of a guardian nor a ruling of legal incompetence is necessarily permanent.

Brown (1979) pointed out that the control a guardian has over a ward is very similar to that of a parent over a child. Therefore it is rare that a court will overturn an action taken by a guardian even if the guardian has exceeded his or her authority, provided the court has determined that in its judgment the guardian acted in good faith for the ward's best interest. Every state requires that a guardian post a bond and make a periodic accounting and report. Usually the amount of the bond is a percentage of the estate to be managed. By negligently wasting the ward's assets or failing to report, the guardian may forfeit all or part of the bond or be removed as guardian.

The intent of the appointment of a guardian for persons unable to care for themselves is protection of the individual. However, when plenary or total guardianship has been granted or assigned by the judge, in some states the "guardians assume the incapacitated person's right to make all health care decisions, including commitment to a psychiatric facility and consent to participate in experimental medical research" (Stevenson and Capezuti 1991, 11). Unfortunately, too frequently the rights of the client are not sufficiently protected. The client may not understand the full implications of the procedure and might not even attend the hearing. The client may be temporarily confused or impaired because of reversible physical conditions. Nurses should take responsibility and initiative when needed to assure that clients are informed of the process and, if indicated, are properly and fully assessed. As Stevenson et al. pointed out, nurses provide the bulk of care to vulnerable clients. They can exert a crucial influence over care and participate in gaining reforms in laws and rules that will safeguard the civil rights of clients.

A guardian who is negligent or exceeds the authority specifically assigned may be sued by the ward. The courts may appoint a temporary guardian, called a guardian *ad litem*, who can represent the ward at trial.

Usually the ward is expected to pay a guardian a percentage of the estate to manage the estate. The court must grant approval each year for the payment. For wards with limited assets it may prove difficult to find someone willing to assume the responsibility of a guardian. Therefore some states have created the position of public guardian. Public guardians receive salaries for their services from the state government.

Volunteer Guardians

Some counties or areas have programs such as Volunteer Guardians. This is a program that recruits, trains, supports, and provides supervision for volunteers who serve as court-appointed guardians for older citizens who have no family or friends able to assist them in managing personal and business affairs. This agency gives priority to those cases where health and safety are factors and where the appointment of a guardian will enable a client to avoid institutionalization. The court defines the responsibilities of the guardian. In addition to managing the client's financial affairs by such activities as receiving payments, paying bills, and keeping records, the guardian may advocate for needed social services and monitor the quality of care provided. The guardian also may arrange for any authorized medical treatment, if needed, and will usually visit the client regularly. Similar programs are available in most areas and older citizens frequently need help in finding the agency that can best serve their needs. In addition to making it possible for the client to maintain some independence and dignity longer, the cost savings of avoiding institutionalization are considerable to both the client and the taxpayers.

The following is an example of a typical client situation regarding the need for a volunteer guardian.

Volunteer Guardians. . .
More Than Just a Volunteer

My first week as an employee at Volunteer Guardians was an experience that I will never forget. I was so excited to tackle my first case that I blindly committed to handle a "difficult" case and to serve as the guardian for a lady named "Sarah." Sarah was referred to Volunteer Guardians from Adult Protective Services (APS). Many of our clients are referred from

APS and are sometimes victims of abuse, neglect, and/or exploitation.

My first visit to see Sarah was shocking. She came to the door and reluctantly stepped out of her small house to talk to me. I had to stand four feet away from her in order to bear the terrible smell of a lady who had not bathed in several years. She was apologetic for her appearance and the condition of her home. She told me that she did not trust anyone because she had been robbed so many times. Only after repeated assurances was I allowed to enter her house and assess the situation.

Nothing in my life could have prepared me for what I saw when I entered her home. The interior of the house was filled from floor to ceiling with garbage, newspapers, broken furniture and soiled clothing. A tiny pathway through the living room to a hall and bedroom was the only area through which a human being could pass. In the bedroom, I found a cocoon hollowed out of the debris that served as Sarah's only place to sit or lie down. The closet light nearby was her only source of light in a house darkened by piles of paper and garbage that blocked all windows. This lady had lived for years in a house without running water, without heat, without a refrigerator or stove, and with only one bedroom closet light. Sarah had been abandoned by her family and had been exploited by a home repairman who took all her savings. She was confused and paranoid about everything. She was malnourished and dirty. My heart went out to her because she was a survivor, and she desperately needed help to live a better life.

I was appointed in Tarrant County Probate Court as guardian of Sarah's person and estate until her situation was improved and a volunteer could be found to take over her case. I have never felt so needed and appreciated as I have in helping this wonderful lady for the past five months.

The clean up of the house was the first milestone we passed. The initial garbage pick up included 250 large bags of trash and two dumpsters of newspaper to be recycled. With the house cleaning progressing, Sarah went for a four day "vacation" to a personal care facility to be bathed, fed and pampered with air conditioning and TV. Her clothes were cleaned and she was taken to the beauty shop. The beautician had to cut the rock-hard bun from the back of her head because her gray hair had not been washed or combed in years. Sarah came back to her house looking beautiful and most of all clean.

Through all of this, Sarah and I became friends. I will never forget the day when she first returned my hug, or the day when she responded to my "I love you" with "I love you too." This lovely lady had not known love or attention from anyone in so long that it was very difficult for her to respond. The words did not come easily for her. I was so proud when she began to hug me and trust me and even love me in her own way.

During this time, my concern was increasing that Sarah would not be safe in her own home. At least twice, the police were called about robberies at her home. The repairman came to her house again and forced her to go with him to her bank and withdraw her Social Security funds. This incident confirmed my decision that it was unsafe for Sarah to live alone. While she did not need to be in a nursing home, I decided that she should be moved to a supervised living facility where someone would provide meals, cleaning, and assistance with personal grooming.

Now I visit a safe, healthy and content Sarah every week in a local supervised living facility. No longer afraid and distrustful of others, she talks and laughs with other residents who have become her friends. She enjoys such "luxuries" as a working bathroom with hot water, having her hair shampooed and set, eating three meals a day in a cafeteria, laundry service and clean clothes, and of course, a devoted guardian.*

LEGAL CONCERNS OF NURSING HOME RESIDENTS

When older persons become unable to live alone because of physical or mental incapacitation and have no family able or willing to take them into the family's home or who will move in with the older person, a nursing home is often the only solution to the problem. Most families explore all other possibilities first: home care services, visiting nurse associations, day-care centers for older adults, and home-delivered meal programs. The negative publicity about nursing homes in recent years has increased the reluctance of many families to place their older members in such homes, and many older people view this alternative with fear, anger, and resentment. Unfortunately, some of the publicity was earned and the fears are well grounded in many institutions. Only the concern and education of the consumer and the health care provider can correct the problems that exist and improve the care given to nursing home residents.

Planning for entry to a nursing home can help avoid many legal problems. The family or the prospective resident or both would probably benefit from seeking the counsel of an attorney to assist the family with an evaluation of the prospective resident's legal status. An attorney could advise them on any needed changes, such as writing a will, updating an existing will, appointing a trustee, executing a power of attorney, listing assets, arranging for a transfer of property, or planning for a method of handling bills. It is important to emphasize the value of such action before the admission. Legal advice need not be a terribly expensive procedure in most cases, and it may save needless expense and avoid many problems later. When such decisions are difficult for a family, they may not act rationally. The nurse can be helpful by suggesting legal consultation. The family frequently respects the nurse's judgment and experience and accepts such suggestions readily,

---

Source: Ann Hill, Supervisor of Volunteer Guardians of Tarrant County, Senior Citizen Services of Greater Tarrant County, Inc., Fort Worth, TX, December 1991. Reprinted with permission.

whereas the same suggestions from relatives might be viewed with suspicion.

Resident's Income and Property

One of the principal problems encountered by a guardian or conservator is that of managing and preserving the resident's income and property. Imprudent decisions, such as joint bank accounts or giving power of attorney to acquaintances or institutions, can result in problems that may be costly and not easily remedied. Any contracts signed with institutions should be reviewed carefully, especially the "life care" agreements. If the obligations of the facility are not clear to the resident in written form, the resident or family should request a letter stating clear, detailed information about the obligation of the facility, its charges, and the resident's obligations. Family members should realize that by signing any kind of papers, they may be incurring financial responsibilities along with the resident. Having the contract reviewed by an attorney before admission to the facility may be the best investment the family or resident can make. A contract means exactly what it states. The failure to understand its contents does not invalidate a contract that has been signed. A contract for "life care," for instance, may provide for a probationary period of six months or longer to allow both parties to evaluate the specific provisions before it becomes effective. Such a plan is desirable, because if the person or family is not pleased with the care, either may cancel the agreement and choose a home that will more nearly match the expectations of the resident and family.

Standards of Nursing Home Care

Standards of care in nursing homes are defined in specific regulations that are part of the Federal Medicare Health Insurance Programs for the Aged under the Social Security Act. An institution that expects to participate in this program and receive funds must meet these standards. The regulations define standards for different levels of care and are specific concerning the physical plant, space per resident, programs offered, and qualifications and numbers of personnel per resident. It is easy to become confused by the different levels of care because the regulations are sometimes unclear, but these regulations also define the rights of the resident and prohibit discrimination for any reason. The institution is inspected periodically, but residents or families may report violations to the state department that licenses the facility. The Department of Health and Human Services requires that agencies receiving federal funds must open their records, and inspection reports must be available to the public. It is wise for families to examine these reports before admitting the family member to a particular institution.

Nurses working in nursing homes or involved in any way in the care of residents in nursing homes should keep in mind that these older residents are entitled to the same rights as any patient/client. The same principles of care apply, except that the nurse may be held to a higher standard of responsibility because older people usually are high-risk patients. If these people have any physical or mental impairment that limits their capacity to participate fully in their care or the decisions regarding their care, the nurse is more liable for any injuries that may occur.

The resident does not give up any rights because of admission to a nursing home and is not incompetent unless a legal ruling has been made. Nursing home residents may therefore refuse treatments, medications, and participation in activities and leave at any time. The resident cannot be restrained unless the physician has specifically ordered the restraint in writing for a specific medical reason. The practice of tying residents to beds or chairs or medicating them heavily is subject to both state and federal regulations. When restraints are employed, the resident must be checked frequently. Proper documentation of the reasons for the restraints and the precautions taken are highly advisable to avoid assault and battery charges if a resident or family should feel that their use was not necessary.

The resident's right to privacy is as important in the nursing home as in the hospital. The nurse should see that all employees respect the resident's dignity and rights when giving care and discussing the resident's condition. No information should be given to any unauthorized party. In short, *residents of a nursing home are considered to be competent citizens with full control of their lives unless and until they are ruled otherwise.* If a ruling of incompetency has been made, the legal guardian must give permission for all treatments, including medications, transfers, and inclusion in programs of the institution.

Employees may not seclude a resident, censor mail, restrict visitors or communications, or treat the resident without specific orders from the physician for that resident for specific periods. The plan of care must be reviewed periodically, and the physician must see the resident periodically if the resident is receiving Medicare or Medicaid benefits. Private institutions are generally held to similar regulations by the state agency that licenses them.

Death Certificates and Autopsies

Nurses employed in nursing homes encounter problems with the legalities surrounding the death of residents more often perhaps than other nurses. The meaning of the term *death* may itself be a problem. Many state medical associations and state legislatures are examining this issue. It has received so much attention because of transplants, organ donations, and the increased availability of life support systems that are expensive and sometimes of questionable value in terms of "quality of life." Even though these issues may not be the primary factor in the death of nursing home residents, problems may arise because of the hesitancy of medical associations and legal bodies to define *death* and to determine under what circumstances a "dead" person's body may be released to a funeral home or for autopsy. Quite often when an older resident who has been in a nursing home for a long period of time or has been in a comatose state for some time expires, some physicians do not see the need to make an appearance to pronounce the resident dead or sign the death certificate immediately. Some local statutes prohibit removal of the body without the physician's signature on the death certificate. Nurses in some states have sought the assistance of their state nurses' associations, state joint-practice committee, and licensing boards to resolve this problem, but with limited success. It is an area that is still in much need of further study and attention. If there is any reason to suspect any unusual circumstances surrounding the death, the coroner's offices should be notified even though nursing home residents' deaths are generally not viewed as "unattended" deaths, since the residents are under the care of a physician. The nurse should be informed about specific state or local regulations but should be aware that only a physician may "diagnose" death and sign a death

certificate. If the nurse encounters problems in this area, a review of the home's policies by the administration should be requested. Nurses should not allow themselves to be intimidated but should be fully informed of the legalities involved and exercise their right to refuse to participate in questionable practices.

INFORMED CONSENT, RIGHT TO TREATMENT, AND LIVING WILLS

The patient who is mentally competent and who willingly signs a contract for admission to a care facility is obviously asking for and consenting to a certain implied, if not defined, measure of care. When treatment or care involves more complicated procedures and thus greater risk, the patient has a right to expect that these procedures will be explained sufficiently for an informed decision to be properly made. Older patients sometimes are not given full credit for their capabilities, and health caregivers, families, and friends may usurp this authority and make decisions for the patients. Such actions by health care personnel can result in technical charges of assault and battery. Hemelt and Mackert (1978, 91) stated that the necessary elements constituting valid written consent include "the patient's signature attesting that the procedure to be performed was the one to which he consented and evidence that the person consenting understood the risks involved, and the probable consequences." Most nurses understand this principle; but when an older patient is involved, they often have difficulty determining whether the patient can fully understand the explanation given and reach a reasonable decision. The nurse should be careful to remember that informed consent involving medical treatments is legally the fiduciary responsibility of the physician.

The nurse who wishes to conduct research involving older patients will also be concerned with consent forms. Frequently, older adults hesitate to sign forms for research, perhaps because they do not understand the purpose of the consent form (Kelley and McClelland 1979). They usually are pleased to participate and eager for the contact and attention, but signing consent forms can be frightening. Older patients can be encouraged to sign if the nurse shows patience in explaining the forms and their purpose clearly and carefully. It is important to determine the patient's legal status and the need for a guardian's permission if the patient has had one appointed.

Patients have the right, as long as they remain competent, to refuse treatment and to execute a living will. The living will instructs those giving care what to do when there is no reasonable expectation of recovery from mental or physical disability, so that patients may be allowed to die and will not be kept alive by artificial or *heroic* measures. Not all states recognize the legality of the living will, but the document may help to persuade those involved to honor the wishes of the patient. Some states have enacted legislation in this area. The living will has been studied and legislation has been passed in many states, twenty-two in 1985 ("The Living Will—Where It Stands," *Geriatric Nursing* 1985). This action represents concern for the rights and dignity of the dying as well as protection of the caregivers who are faced with the dilemma of such awesome decisions. The laws in each state vary, but most laws require certain types of declaration forms to be executed and filed in the patient's record with two witnessed signatures. Those witnessing may not be relatives, heirs, physicians or their employees, or the patient's health facility's employees ("The Living Will—Where It Stands," *Geriatric Nursing* 1985). However, these restrictions vary from state to state. The Texas Natural Death Act became law in 1977. It was passed after careful scrutiny of other states' laws, e.g., those of California and Oregon. Farabee (1977, 92) reported on the Texas law, which was designed to protect those patients who do not want life-sustaining procedures to be used for them but who also want to leave the physician free to make all necessary medical decisions concerning the patient's condition, and "in the alternative, to allow the doctor to make the traditional decision to terminate life-sustaining procedures when warranted by the patient's condition without interference from the law." The Texas law has specific requirements that may differ from other states. It provides that living wills are valid only for five years and that they are binding only "if the patient is qualified and has signed or reexecuted the will at least 14 days after being notified of his or her terminal condition" (Farabee 1977, 1992). The physician who is not willing to honor the directive must transfer the patient's care to a physician who is willing to do so. Refusal to transfer a patient is considered unprofessional conduct. The Texas law has the other usual provisions regarding the right to revoke the will at any time. Unfortunately it also has specific provisions that make enforcement difficult. The Texas law requires a specific form to be used and stipulates that the will must be notarized. It states that concealment or destruction of the will is a class A misdemeanor.

If older people are concerned about this problem and wish to avoid having their lives prolonged by heroic measures, the nurse should help them do whatever they choose and should assist them in finding legal assistance to carry out their wishes.

THE ROLE OF THE NURSE IN LEGAL ISSUES

The 1980s will be remembered for many changes in the health care field. The increase in malpractice insurance rates—because of the numbers of lawsuits filed and the huge awards granted in those cases where the courts found the institutions or caregivers or both guilty—is perhaps one of the more significant changes. As a result Congress has begun to introduce comprehensive legislation intended to bring about reforms in the quality of services delivered in nursing homes and by other agencies that provide care for older citizens. The support for this action was greatly strengthened by the National Academy of Sciences, Institute of Medicine (IOM) report on "Improving the Quality of Care in Nursing Homes." The American Nurses' Association (ANA), the National League for Nursing (NLN), and other nursing organizations have strengthened their previous efforts to support and influence the content of health care legislation. They particularly have addressed the qualifications of nursing staff in nursing homes. There have been many organizations, such as the American Association of Retired Persons, that have worked to form coalitions such as the National Citizens' Coalition for Nursing Home Reform. These coalitions have produced consensus papers and have testified before congressional committees. The Omnibus Budget Reconciliation Act of 1987 and additions in 1990 have helped to improve the care of residents in nursing homes (see chapter 18).

The role of nurses in the care of older patients is not only changing but also is in the forefront of other changes. Gerontological nursing content was often not identifiable in nursing curricula before the 1980s.

Both the ANA and the NLN are working to require all accredited schools to include specifically identified content in gerontological nursing in their curricula. Those nurses who are already working in this specialty must become more aware of their expanded responsibilities for the quality of care. These responsibilities include more than just technical advances and an expanded scientific knowledge base. The legal and ethical components of this type of nursing practice are sometimes overwhelming.

There has been much discussion regarding the patient's role, the health care provider's role, and the family's or significant other's role in the decision-making process about whether or not to institute or discontinue life-sustaining measures. Cushing (1984) cited precedent-setting cases in California and New Jersey involving the withdrawal of nutritional support and respiratory support measures. She also discussed the need for adequate documentation of assessment measures taken to determine prognosis, especially whether a patient's condition is irreversible or not. This assessment is important because it is the major deciding factor in many instances. While the outcome of the case in California is uncertain, "What is certain is that this case will encourage nurses and other care providers to define how 'care and comfort for the dying, supportive care, and keep the patient comfortable' translate into nursing action" (Cushing 1984, 191).

Decisions by legal authorities related to discontinuing life-sustaining measures have differed. The factors considered in reaching those decisions also differ. For example, the definition of invasive or non-invasive measures sometimes is considered important. Other factors to be considered may be requests by patient and family to discontinue treatment, evidence of patient's intent, economic considerations, benefits and burdens of continued treatment, and quality of life. (A complete discussion of this issue can be found in *Patient Care Law*, edited by John Horty in the April/May 1986 issue.)

It is essential that nurses recognize the importance of knowing the policies of the agency or institution, the laws in their own state, and the current guidelines for professional standards of practice (e.g., the American Nurses' Association). Ethical issues are difficult, and increased litigation in our society produces an even more complicated situation. It is generally agreed that the patient, or the proxy decision maker

for the patient, and the physician are the most appropriate decision makers regarding life-sustaining measures. Nurses may, however, find that questions regarding the continuation of treatment may be directed toward them because of their close relationships with patients and their families. The courtroom is not the most appropriate place for decisions regarding continuation or termination of treatment. However, when family and caregivers have different opinions, the courtroom frequently is the place where decisions will be made. (Ethical considerations are discussed in more detail in chapter 24.)

Older patients are more vulnerable to abuse because of their reduced capacity to maintain independent functioning. Therefore nurses—especially charge nurses—must be alert to potential and actual abuse. The person responsible for prevention and detection of abuse is most frequently the charge nurse. Careful selection, in-service education, and supervision of all employees are essential. Sometimes supervisory nurses respond to administrative pressure to "not make waves" and retain employees to cover patient care. Therefore they might not terminate employees who are believed to neglect or abuse patients. This situation may happen more frequently when salaries are low and unqualified personnel are employed. It may be viewed that "somebody" is preferable to "nobody." This attitude may place the nurse supervisor in legal jeopardy because the supervisor is responsible for the actions of his or her nursing staff. Such actions also cause discomfort because of the violation of personal moral and ethical standards.

Awareness of legal rights and responsibilities should guide all nursing decisions and actions. The concepts of patients' right to refuse treatment, informed consent, and assault and battery are important for the nurse to review. The mental confusion experienced by some older patients is frequently considered ample justification for treating or medicating the patient. It should be remembered that these actions are justified only in emergencies to protect the patient and others. Jakacki and Payson (1985) pointed out that *expressed* or *implied* consent derived from the general consent form signed on admission to an institution is applicable only to routine procedures. The doctrine of informed consent is applicable to more complex and unfamiliar procedures. They list three factors in the doctrine of informed consent: "competency to decide, voluntary choice, and knowledge of the pros and cons affecting the decision" (Jakacki and Payson 1985, 1335). Mental illness no longer automatically conveys incompetence. Jakacki and Payson (1985, 1335) cited a general guideline of informed consent to be "whether the patient understands the circumstances and appreciates the consequences of his decision." Unless one of the emergency criteria is present, incompetency to make the decision does not give nurses the right to force treatments or procedures on a patient. This permission must be granted by the appropriate substitute legally appointed to give permission.

When nurses ignore this consent doctrine, they may be found guilty of *assault* or *battery* charges made by either the patient or the designated responsible parties. The term *assault* means the perceived or actual threat of force or harm. *Battery* is the actual touching of the patient without consent. The application of patient control devices (restraints) may fall into this category. The nurse must weigh carefully the patient's consent against the possibility of harm that may result from failure to take action. This harm may be either to the patient or to others. All possible factors must be considered, and agency policy must be followed. The doctrine of the least restrictive measure necessary to handle the situation must also be remembered, even when the decision is to act. Complete documentation of factors in the decision, as well as documentation of the decision and action, is essential. It must be remembered that any decision in situations of this type is potential for future litigation. While protection of the patient's rights and safety is the most important factor, the nurse and other health caregivers need to have adequate data available if an injury to the patient or others should occur. Clear, accurate, legible documentation on the patient's record is the only reliable defense when any situation results in charges of neglect, abuse, assault and battery, or malpractice.

Documentation is perhaps one of the most important roles of the nurse. Some nurses are resentful of the amount of time they must spend on paperwork in their positions. However, there are ways to minimize the time without jeopardizing the completeness of the records. Many hospitals are employing computer methodology. Computers may be more expensive than some institutions can afford, but the savings may quickly offset initial costs. Checklists and properly designed forms also can be great time-savers. In-service education for staff in proper documentation can be cost-effective. The often repeated statement that "what isn't charted wasn't done" is a good principle to remember when staff tend to become too brief or too ritualistic in documentation.

The nurse's role in assuring quality care involves not only the nurse's action but the performance of all those who come under the nurse's supervision. It is essential that the charge nurse observe, firsthand, nursing care by all employees. Frequent rounds, which include contact with patients and families to observe and hear what occurs daily, are one way to guarantee that the nurse will be aware of the quality of care being given. Contact with patients may ultimately save time if potential problems are detected early before they require more time or outside consultation or evaluation. A good manager will find ways to supervise adequately. The nurse who exemplifies professional behavior will not hesitate to "make waves" if the situation demands it and will do everything possible to ensure every patient quality care.

Knowing employees is essential. Frequent contact can help the nurse identify not only the skill level of employees in delivering care but also attitudes that enhance or endanger quality care. Some personnel may have prejudices that interfere with their work. These may be racial, ethnic, religious, or age-related or involve resentment against behaviors such as alcohol or drug abuse. If such behaviors are undetected, the result could be neglect or blatant abuse. (Abuse is discussed in chapter 22.) The nurse's responsibility for preventing, detecting, and reporting abuse in an institutional setting is important to consider in the nurse's legal role. Reporting may be required by law in many states. The nurse must take action, whether or not it is required by law.

The reader is urged to refer to more comprehensive sources for detailed information on legal issues. It is important to stress the importance of adequate policies in every institution and a thorough knowledge of individual state laws governing practice in that state. All nurses also should have their own professional malpractice insurance and not rely on the insurance of the employing institution.

SUMMARY

Many older citizens remain active, well, independent, and able to carry on their activities effectively until death. Others fail to plan ahead and find themselves unable to handle their own affairs; they are often victimized by opportunists or greedy relatives. Health care workers are frequently in a position to help the older person obtain the needed assistance and they should feel obligated to become involved. Health care workers should keep informed of basic legal rights and available legal resources. They should never attempt to practice law but should rec-ognize that competent legal assistance is as important as competent health care. Health care personnel who work with older adults have a greater degree of responsibility to assist with legal affairs because of the vulnerability and decreased ability of older clients to participate actively in their own decision making and planning.

New federal and state laws have been the result of increasing awareness and interest in helping people exercise their rights to make their own health-care and life-or-death decisions.

STUDY QUESTIONS

1. Discuss the need for nurses to develop an awareness of legal issues facing older patients.

2. Cite the importance of estate planning before reaching an age or state of being in which decisions are not possible.

3. Discuss wills and trusts as alternatives in estate planning.

4. What happens to an estate when there is no will?

5. Show how investing power of attorney in a reliable, trusted person can benefit an older person.

6. Cite possible abuses of the power of attorney.

7. What does power of attorney mean?

8. Describe the power of attorney for health care.

9. Describe the role of nurses in assisting patients with obtaining Social Security benefits.

10. Compare and contrast the benefits of guardianship versus declaration of incompetency.

11. Identify the state's role in guardianship and civil commitment.

12. Who are volunteer guardians?

13. Discuss problems the nurse may encounter in helping families when a patient dies in a nursing home.

14. Analyze the problems surrounding informed consent for older adults.

15. Describe the patient's right to competent and caring treatment and right to refuse treatment.

16. Analyze the Patient Self-Determination Act.

17. Identify legal problems surrounding the nurse's role in decisions to withhold (discontinue) life-sustaining measures for older patients.

REFERENCES

Brown, R.N., C.D. Allo, A.D. Freeman, and G.W. Nelzarg. 1979. *The Rights of Older Persons, An American Civil Liberties Union Handbook.* New York: Avon Books.

Cushing, M. 1984. The implications of withdrawing nutritional devices. *Am J Nurs* 84(2):191–94.

Farabee, R. 1977. The Texas natural death act. *Texas Medicine* 73:91–95.

Governor's Committee on Aging. 1987. *Biennial Report.* Austin: Office of the Governor, State of Texas.

Hemlet, M.D. and M.E. Mackert. 1978. *Dynamics of Law in Nursing and Health Care.* Reston, VA: Reston Publishing Co.

Horty, Springer, and Mattern Law Firm. 1986. The controversy will continue. In *Patient Care Law* (April/May), edited by J. Horty.

Implementation of the Patient Self-Determination Act. October 1991. An action kit for the new federal law. Texas Hospital Association—Texas Medical Association.

Jakacki, M. and A.L. Payson. 1985. Legal side: Out of control. *Am J Nurs* 85(12):1335–36.

Kelly, K. and E. McClelland. 1979. Signed consent: Protection or constraint? *Nursing Outlook* 27(1):40–42.

Rosenfeld, J.P. 1979. *The Legacy of Aging*. Norwood, NJ: Ablex.

Stevenson, C. and E. Capezuti. 1991. Guardianship: Protection versus peril. *Geriatric Nursing* 12(1):10–13.

The living will–Where it stands. 1985. *Geriatric Nursing* 6(1):18–20.

24 Ethical Issues

Sister Rose Therese Bahr

CHAPTER OUTLINE

FOCUS

Ethical decision making is especially important in the health care of older adults. This chapter focuses on the many ethical issues facing older adults and their families. The nurse needs to understand these issues in order to provide information, support, and assistance as needed.

OBJECTIVES

1. Review the purpose of the American Nurses' Association Code for Nurses.

2. Discuss the concept of ethical decision making.

3. List major ethical decisions facing older adults and their families.

4. Evaluate the issue of quality versus quantity of life.

5. Relate Maslow's hierarchy of needs to older adults.

6. Evaluate availability of health care to older adults.

7. Analyze the issue of age as related to distribution of scarce health care resources.

8. Discuss the use of older adults as research subjects.

9. Relate the issue of resuscitation to the care of older adults.

10. Differentiate between active and passive euthanasia.

How sacred is human life? This question faces society today (Bernardin 1986; Gress and Bahr 1984). The founding fathers of America stated in the document upon which this country was established that the pursuit of life, liberty, and happiness was a right of every person. Yet today a growing portion of older adults are faced with difficulties in attaining these goals and in experiencing lifestyles that should rightfully be theirs. In this regard, Tobin, Ellor, and Anderson-Ray (1986) noted that the lifestyle they strive to preserve is slowly being eroded by conflicts in the application of moral principles. Principles are legislated through rules and regulations that stipulate eligibility criteria for services to be rendered by agencies whether an older person's needs are to be met in an institution of his or her choice, home health care for older adults, or retirement village. Values are the foundation for principles regulating actions to promote the welfare of each person and have been passed on from one generation to the next. The United States was founded on the Judeo-Christian value system which should, if implemented, promote the well-being of all citizens. A value system must be viable. It should provide the organizational framework for living. Thus a basic respect for human life is reflected in a value system that regards the older members of society with esteem (Bernardin 1986).

WHAT CONSTITUTES THE FIELD OF ETHICS?

The field of ethics is concerned with moral conduct based on principles of behavior that promote the goodness of the human being. For those who base their principles on the Christian tradition, ethical or moral behavior is patterned after the life of Jesus Christ as He lived it on earth and in His teachings as recorded in the Scriptures (National Conference of Catholic Bishops 1979). Ethics, a branch of philosophy, is concerned with what is good and evil and with moral obligation. To be ethical is to be true to one's basic nature. The natural law transcribed into ethical conduct projects guidelines that promote the welfare of all human beings regardless of age, creed, or color. This welfare includes attention to all aspects of the human condition. The needs of the human being become paramount in providing an environment conducive to growth and development along the entire continuum of life. Each person is responsible for sharing in the growth of the human being. To stunt this growth is to act unethically.

The human dignity of each person forms the basis for the ethical behavior called forth from other people. Human beings must have the respect of their fellow humans throughout their lifetimes. This respect enables each person to realize his or her own personal worth so that the person can, in turn, respect himself or herself sufficiently to motivate his or her own growth toward self-actualization. Ethics therefore projects guidelines useful to people in resolving

situations where the welfare of people is the main focus (Bernardin 1986; Husted and Husted, 1991).

COMMON ERRORS IN ETHICAL THINKING

Weber (1976) noted that several common errors in thinking may occur when ethical or moral situations are confronted. These errors are usually a result of societal attitudes toward a given population or particular situation. These common mistakes in thinking include the following:

1. "Morality and practicality" are synonymous (Weber 1976, 6). In this type of thinking, what is sought is the greatest good for the greatest number. In this light, whatever steps are deemed necessary to resolve an ethical dilemma, regardless of the consequences to the individual or to society as a whole, are considered practical and therefore good from an ethical standpoint. This type of thinking is called situational ethics. The tenets upon which situational ethics is based hold that what is good for a particular situation and resolves the ethical situation or problem in this instance is acceptable as a rightful, moral decision. A major proponent of this cognitive approach is the prominent ethicist Joseph Fletcher.

   The resolution of the ethical dilemma, using the practical approach, may be observed in discussions concerning the so-called worldwide food shortage. A proponent of the practical ethics would resolve the problem of worldwide food shortage by ensuring an adequate supply to those nations that already have a bountiful food supply, so they will continue to survive in the future. A lesser concern of the proponent would be those unfortunate countries where an inadequate food supply exists. This practical approach is futuristic in that a future is ensured for one segment of the world population but not another. In actuality the rights of some human beings are ignored; it is a case of the haves and have-nots.

2. "Morality and opinion" are considered under the same guise (Weber 1976, 7). This approach is a direct result of the emphasis on the scientific orientation to society; that is, that unless a fact is verifiable through objective quantification, it

remains pure opinion. The moral questions and problems faced by society are matters of values. The way the hierarchy of values is implemented promotes the welfare of the citizens. Morality as opinion emerges as the prominent idea when it is clear that no scientific verification can be placed on a value. Morality therefore becomes merely an opinion. The rightness or wrongness of an action by its very nature cannot be considered. Personal preference becomes the norm for dealing with ethical issues through this ethical orientation.

This type of thinking is deemed tolerance of another's actions—one person should not express to another what action should be taken. It is merely a case of opinion and no one opinion dominates another for the resolving of an ethical situation.

3. "Subjectivity and morality" (Weber 1976, 9): (*a third approach to ethical thinking that can cloud the meaning of the situation*). Subjectivity deals with the attitudes and the motives of the individual who achieves the completion of the action. Here again it becomes impossible to judge the action objectively because of the very private nature of the action. It is so personal to the individual that it is impossible to judge the rightness and wrongness of the action from a moral perspective. There is no attempt to analyze the moral principles involved rationally.

Any of these three ethical perspectives can therefore be applied in an individual ethical situation. The various approaches and the resulting outcomes are entirely different from each other, depending on the approach used in analyzing the social event or medical-moral condition.

In reviewing these approaches it should be noted that there are two ethical viewpoints that determine the manner in which the situation is resolved from a moral perspective. These ethical viewpoints are *(1)* contemporary nature and *(2)* the ancient, or as Weber (1976) stated, the "classical" nature. In the contemporary viewpoint the individual human being is at the center of the world or the universe and is consequently in control of the world through this dominant position. Using this approach, the morality of the situation is seen in terms of what is good for the person from a subjective, pragmatic, and individual orientation. The individual person becomes the all-pervasive presence in determining

the goodness and badness of actions. On the other hand, in the more ancient or "classical" viewpoint, the individual person is perceived in another light. Here the human being is not the center of the world, although the individual person is an important part of that world. The universe in and of itself has a meaning and a value apart from that of the individual. Each human being has a moral obligation to respect, accept, and live life according to the meaning and purpose of that life and that of the universe. Each species has its own purpose for existence. The human person must follow the dictates of his/her nature so that he/she truly is a fully potentiated human. This fulfillment, of course, comes with application of knowledge to his/her particular orientation to life. Weber (1976) further noted that in the classical viewpoint the person comes to a deep appreciation of the inherent value of each human being and consequently holds each life as worthy of dignity and respect. In addition many other pervading viewpoints are prevalent that allow an individual to personally derive a philosophic attitude toward life and its purpose without embracing either of the viewpoints as noted by Weber (1976).

Differences lie, therefore, in the two opposing viewpoints in relation to ethics. In the modern or contemporary viewpoint the decision of what is right or wrong resides within the individual; whereas in the ancient tradition the person feels that he or she can discover what the purpose of the world is and that should impose moral obligation for action. Thus the action itself becomes an important component of the person's total behavior. Each action has a consequence that must be taken into consideration when performing the act. The action can be destructive of the good for human beings, even if the purposes for which it was intended were perceived as good and doing no harm. Freedom of action is afforded to a person only when the action does not infringe on another person's rights as a human being worthy of respect and dignity. Thus the value of the human being takes on dimensions of worth that outweigh the good of the universe or the good of the person who perpetrates the action. Values, then, become the all-pervasive guideposts that gently lead a person toward moral conduct that enhances rather than destroys life.

A third viewpoint revolves around the concept of morality and historical consciousness (Rigali 1979).

In this view, morality or the moral law is seen, not as an imposition from the past, but as an evolutionary process, as one discovers how life is lived in contemporary society. Historical consciousness is the transformation or the transcendence of cultures of the past to focus on the present as the point of departure for the morality to be experienced and lived. History is "the realm of contingency and singularity, just as essence bespeaks necessity and universality; and human life is history. For persons, to live is—for better or worse—to create history, indeed ultimately the encompassing history of humankind. Historical consciousness views each human life in terms of creating history rather than in terms of a universal code of behavior, preordained in a time-transcending human nature" (Rigali 1979, 165).

When moral law is viewed within this frame of reference, living becomes creative, rather than a passive acceptance of laws projected into the twentieth century from previous centuries. Its design molds the substance of life lived in the now rather than in the past. The hope is that the way life is lived now, based on solid moral principles meaningful to the times, will aid in building a better future for coming generations. In other words, the precedents and foundations laid today will have consequences for either the betterment or the detriment of future generations of society. The implications of this approach are indeed grave, arising out of the responsibilities laid upon the human beings comprising the present generations (Rigali 1979).

The question is raised: How do the philosophic stances of ethics and values affect the professional nurse?

THE VALUE SYSTEM
OF THE PROFESSIONAL NURSE

To value someone or something is to attach a degree of goodness that elevates that object or person to a place of prominence in one's thinking. Values may be positive or negative in their basic composition. Positive values are measures directing one's conduct toward cherished people and elements. Negative values lead a person away from those items or human beings that are not treasured. A value system becomes entrenched in each person through childhood, adolescence, and adulthood. Values continue to change as a person grows in knowledge of human nature and the world. Purposeful living should reveal what is of value in one's life.

The professional nurse enters the world of health care with a set of values formed on the basis of parental example and guidance, home environment, experience, and educational preparation. With this value system in operation, the nurse encounters a world of life-and-death decision making that may or may not coincide with the nurse's ethical viewpoint. One reason for choosing the profession of nursing is the value placed on helping people with health care problems and providing the information, care, and concern that the nurse feels will contribute to a purposeful and meaningful existence and the strength and health needed to carry out life goals. The nurse is in a key position to evaluate situations from a moral perspective as they are experienced (Ketefian 1987). Many factors come into play that may cloud the situation in terms of expediency, conflict of interest, and the good of the many versus the good of the individual. Issues raised because of decisions made by others rather than by the person who is principally involved must be resolved; that is, medical treatment plans imposed on an individual (once entered into the health care system) without proper knowledge of consequences by the person involved, elective surgery intervention performed without proper documentation of need, and wrong surgical interventions such as amputation of nondiseased limbs. With the passage and implementation of the Patient Self-Determination Act (PSDA) (see chapter 23), informed consent to treatments is required. Information must be made available to all patients regarding their right to make their preferences and wishes known about the treatment of acute illnesses in case they become cognitively incapable or incompetent to make such decisions. These directives are meant to provide that these wishes will be respected and that the rights of the ill person will be executed in the event that he or she cannot speak for himself or herself.

Code of Ethics

One important document nurses use to guide ethical conduct is the Code for Nurses (American Nurses' Association 1985). This document emphasizes the need for the nurse to look for the good in all people and to treat each person with dignity and respect. These directives may sometimes create a conflict within the nurse who, while functioning in a professional capacity, observes clinical situations involving clients and other health professionals that are contrary to the code. Nurses must not allow themselves to be coerced into executing an action that will be contrary to their preferred behavior and conscience. Nursing students are encouraged to study the Code For Nurses as part of their educational preparation before they enter the world of professional nursing. Once practicing as licensed professionals, they are committed to implementing this guide daily in the ethical situations they encounter. Some state boards of nursing have incorporated the code into the legal definition of nursing in their nurse practice acts. The code then has legality and nurses are required by law to implement its provisions (Yeaworth 1985; Bahr 1987; Kileen 1986).

Code for Nurses

1. The nurse provides services with respect for human dignity and the uniqueness of the client, unrestricted by considerations of social or economic status, personal attributes, or the nature of health problems.

2. The nurse safeguards the client's right to privacy by judiciously protecting information of a confidential nature.

3. The nurse acts to safeguard the client and the public when health care and safety are affected by the incompetent, unethical, or illegal practice of any person.

4. The nurse assumes the responsibility and accountability for individual nursing judgments and actions.

5. The nurse maintains competence in nursing.

6. The nurse exercises informed judgment and uses individual competence and qualifications as criteria in seeking consultation, accepting responsibilities, and delegating nursing activities to others.

7. The nurse participates in activities that contrib-

ute to the ongoing development of the profession's body of knowledge.

8. The nurse participates in the profession's efforts to implement and improve standards of nursing.

9. The nurse participates in the profession's efforts to establish and maintain conditions of employment conducive to high quality nursing care.

10. The nurse participates in the profession's efforts to protect the public from misinformation and misrepresentation and to maintain the integrity of nursing.

11. The nurse collaborates with members of the health professions and other citizens in promoting community and national efforts to meet the health needs of the public.

American Nurses' Association, 1985*

These directives, to be implemented by the nurse, imply that a process for ethical decision making is put into motion.

There are important factors to be considered in ethical decision making. These factors must be understood by the nurse specializing in gerontological nursing so that intelligent guidance may be offered to older clientele seeking assistance in the health care system.

ETHICAL DECISION MAKING: THE PROCESS

The process of ethical decision making is necessary whenever a person faces a moral question. Each person's conscience dictates the particular process of moving from a dilemma through the use of a problem-solving approach to answering the question. Weber (1976) identified several steps to be followed in the implementation of the decision-making process.

The first point is the determination of general principles based on one's perspective of the human being's relationship to the universe. How is the human being viewed? Is the person seen as being good only for society and its welfare or for the inher-

---

*From *Code for Nurses with Interpretive Statements,* © 1985, American Nurses Association, Washington, DC. Reprinted with permission.

ent goodness of being human? If in general the human being is perceived as possessing inherent goodness, that is, the essence of the person is good in itself, then that person's life is worthy of respect and dignity and has certain rights. These principles suggest two closely related statements.

- That human life is sacred by the very fact of its existence; its value does not depend upon a certain condition or perfection of that life.

- That, therefore, all human lives are of equal value.

Weber 1976, 18*

The second step is to identify guidelines that provide more specific direction. As a logical sequel to the idea that people are intrinsically good, the guideline would be that one would not harm oneself and would avoid endangering one's life.

Third, moral decision making rests on the analysis of a specific human act to discover if it is permitted or not permitted by the specific guidelines.

Finally, the situation and its ramifications have implications for the moral decision that must be considered. Thus, in ethical decision making, the focus moves from the general to the specific. A person must be attuned to many factors in judging actions to determine if the morality of the action is in accordance with the basic humanitarian tenets of society (Weber 1976).

These basic principles, then, should provide the general framework for gerontological nurses in assessing ethical decision-making situations involving older people and their families. From this general stance the nurse, as moral agent of the older adult (Husted and Husted 1991), moves into a specific approach to the decision-making process and interacts intimately with the older client and family in analyzing all factors impinging on the situation (Bahr 1987). This analysis should result in a decision that is acceptable to all parties involved in the process.

Wheelock (1976) noted that professional nurses are in a key position to assist the clients in their care in coming to terms with ethical decisions that must be made regarding matters pertaining to their health care. Husted and Husted (1991) stated that the con-

temporary ethical standards useful to the nurse are autonomy, veracity, fidelity, beneficence, freedom, and privacy. Outlined here are the major points Wheelock (1976) makes about the process that nurses should follow.

1. Get as many facts as possible. Listen for hints of problems other than the one being presented. Often, the first thing mentioned is not that which is truly bothering the patient. It would not be out of place to probe a bit here, as long as one is sensitive to the patient and goes only so far as the patient is ready to go.

2. Identify options: *(a)* What is the present situation? *(b)* What is the patient doing about it? *(c)* What other things can be done? There are usually more than two choices. The more options that can be presented to the patient, the better, although some may obviously be unacceptable. It is important to show patients that there are many options and that they are not boxed in.

3. Separate those aspects of the patient's situation that can be changed from those that cannot. What is beyond his/her control, and what can be controlled? Encourage the patient to believe in the ability to change that which can be changed. Sometimes the most important thing a nurse can do is to show the patient that he or she believes in the patient's ability to change. Many people have already given up on the patient or told him/her that he/she cannot change the situation. It will be a tremendous help to the patient to know that someone at last believes in him/her.

4. Help the patient sort out the underlying issues of the situation, especially the value issues. Every option involves a value of some kind, and the nurse should discuss it. Ask the patient to identify the positive and negative consequences of his/her actions or contemplated actions. Encourage the patient to think through his/her value commitments. Ask questions, such as, "What do you stand for?" "What do you treasure or really believe in?" "How intensely do you believe in these things for yourself and for others?" Help the patient see that there is no easy or ideal choice. All

---

*Reprinted with permission from The Catholic Health Association of the United States.

solutions involve risks and the renunciation of other choices.

5. Help the patient make decisions in the light of his/her personal value system. At times the nurse may disagree with the choice and may tell the patient so, but it still must be the patient's choice. The nurse should emphasize reality, especially if the patient's choice is obviously unrealistic. The nurse must convince the patient that one cannot base one's life on an illusion.

Wheelock 1976, 50, 51*

Every nurse, to be effective in the process of ethical decision making, must focus on the welfare of the client as the nurse/patient contractual agreement connotes (Husted and Husted 1991).

Payton (1979) has schematically diagrammed the decision-making process for ethical situations, providing helpful and practical approaches for the professional nurse in clinical situations, see Figure 24-1. These guidelines, if used consistently by professional nurses, should prove beneficial to clients who need assistance in moral decision making. Nurses who are caring people should assume this responsibility in order to protect the dignity of people coming under their jurisdiction in the health care world. Moral decision making is not easy, but it is an essential part of the fabric of daily living and cannot be ignored (Ketefian 1987; Husted and Husted 1991). To consider the rightness or wrongness of an action in light of what is best according to a person's conscience fosters growth in the person and gives dignity to his or her actions. Such a goal is a truly sublime mission for the professional nurse.

This overview of ethics, ethical principles, and the decision-making process lays the foundation for consideration of the ethical questions and issues faced by older adults and the nurses providing their care. Many older people, because of varying circumstances, have been considered nonentities rather than human beings to be afforded dignity and respect based solely on their humanity. Professional nurses must take the risk of countering this societal attitude and take a stand on their moral beliefs and principles about aiding older people to preserve their human-

ness. Nurses should become involved in the resolution of the ethical issues facing the older population so that society will implement a model of morality where human life is indeed considered valuable and worthy of efforts to preserve it.

ETHICAL ISSUES FACING OLDER ADULTS, THEIR FAMILIES, AND SOCIETY

Older Americans—who should be considered wise and venerable and who should be sought out for guidance, counsel, and general information because of their wide experiences and understanding—are today some of the most forgotten people on the face of the earth. We read of them in the newspapers every day. Some have been in the back wards of state mental institutions for years, isolated from reality and humanity simply because they are old. Some have no place to lay their heads except on a piece of cardboard under a bridge or a hole in the dirt alongside a river or creek bank (Health Care for the Homeless 1986). Some have no food except that obtained by rummaging through garbage cans or the city dump as they seek something that appears edible. Some have little or no money and cannot afford health care, housing, or the other necessities of a lifestyle in conformity with human dignity.

To appreciate the ethical dilemmas faced by older people, their families, and society, six aspects must be considered.

1. Quality of life versus quantity of life

2. Age: its effect on decisions in ethical situations

3. Availability of health care to older adults

4. Health care decisions for the disoriented older adult: whose responsibility?

5. Resuscitation decisions

6. Euthanasia: active and passive

Quality of Life versus Quantity of Life

Quality of life versus quantity of life raises serious questions in contemporary society. Numerous view-

---

*Reprinted with permission from The Catholic Health Association of the United States.

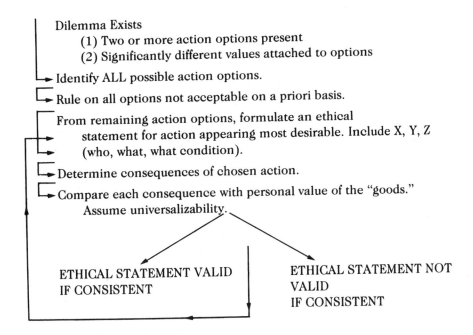

Dilemma Exists
    (1) Two or more action options present
    (2) Significantly different values attached to options
Identify ALL possible action options.
Rule on all options not acceptable on a priori basis.
From remaining action options, formulate an ethical
    statement for action appearing most desirable. Include X, Y, Z
    (who, what, what condition).
Determine consequences of chosen action.
Compare each consequence with personal value of the "goods."
    Assume universalizability.

ETHICAL STATEMENT VALID
IF CONSISTENT

ETHICAL STATEMENT NOT
VALID
IF CONSISTENT

One cycle return in case of invalid results:
    (1) Ethical Statement may be reformulated modifying the conditions.
    (2) Alternate action option (still available after the rule in) may be explored
       going through all remaining steps.

REMEMBER—the decision to take no action is in itself action.

Figure 24–1 Pluralistic ethical decision-making model. Reprinted with permission from "Pluralistic Ethical Decision-Making" by Rita Payton, in *Clinical and Scientific Sessions,* 1979 © 1979, American Nurses Association, Washington, DC.

points are being formulated to grapple with these terms and the ramifications of each line of ethical thinking. There are "prolife" and "respect life" groups of citizens and groups such as "prochoice" who oppose the first two viewpoints. Many "battles" are waged each day—in and out of courtrooms, on television and radio, and in the newspapers—in the attempt to convince the general public of the ethical meaning of quality versus quantity of life. This issue becomes more prominent as the attitude grows in the United States that life has little inherent value. Doing violence to life through injury and destruction appears to be the order of the day.

Where does the initiation of the concept *quality of life* begin in the life of a person? Logically, it begins in a family unit, the basic unit in society (National Conference of Catholic Bishops, 1991). Life in a family should provide the important foundation of this value system leading to ethical decisions based on solid principles engendering respect for each person's life and the human dignity to be afforded each member of the family. The quality of a person's life is based on certain rights given primarily because the person is a human being with needs. If these needs are met, the person can live according to the moral principles of justice, love, and peace.

Some of the rights of people appear to be threatened in today's society.

- *The right to life*: This right is basic and inalienable.

- *The right to eat*: This right is directly linked to the right to life. Millions today face starvation.

- *Socio-economic rights*: Reconciliation is rooted in justice. Massive disparities of power and wealth in the world, and often within nations, are a grave obstacle to reconciliation. Concentration of economic power in the hands of a few nations and multinational groups, structural imbalances in trade relations and commodity prices, failure to balance economic growth with adequate distribution (both nationally and internationally), widespread unemployment and discriminatory employment practices, as well as patterns of global consumption of resources, all require reform if reconciliation is to be possible.

- *Politico-cultural rights*: Reconciliation in society and the rights of the person require that individuals have an effective role in shaping their own destinies. They have a right to participate in the political process freely and responsibly. They have a right to free access of information, freedom of speech and press, as well as freedom of dissent.

- *The right of religious liberty*: This right uniquely reflects the dignity of the person as this is known from reason itself. Today it is denied or restricted by diverse political systems in ways that impede worship, religious education, and social ministry.

Synod of Bishops 1974, 2–3

In 1976, the bicentennial year of the United States, the Commissioner of Aging, Dr. Arthur Fleming, officially promulgated a Statement of Rights for Older Americans. These rights address the quality of life that all Americans should support for this segment of the population. This statement is reprinted here.

BICENTENNIAL CHARTER FOR OLDER AMERICANS

STATEMENT OF RIGHTS AND RESPONSIBILITIES OF CITIZENS

I. The right to freedom, independence, and the free exercise of individual initiative.

II. The right to an income in retirement which would provide an adequate standard of living.

III. The right to an opportunity for employment free from discriminatory practices because of age.

IV. The right to an opportunity to participate in the widest range of meaningful civic, educational, recreational, and cultural activities.

V. The right to suitable housing.

VI. The right to the best level of physical and mental health services needed.

VII. The right to ready access to effective social services.

VIII. The right to appropriate institutional care when required.

IX. The right to life and death with dignity.

Federal Council on Aging 1976

The needs of older people and their relation to the idea of quality versus quantity should be examined with these rights in mind (Harper 1990; Aroskar 1987; Bahr 1991).

Needs and Rights of Older Adults. What are the specific needs of older people in the United States? How can these needs be met and violations of rights be rectified to ensure a high quality of life for older people?

Hierarchy of Needs. Maslow (1970) theorized a hierarchy of needs ranging from the lowest level of a pyramidal base to its highest point. In this hierarchy the needs of the person include: physiological, safety, love, esteem, and self-actualization. For many older people, fixation at the first level of need on Maslow's hierarchy seems to be the rule rather than the exception. At this level, physical needs constitute the essence of quality of life. Older people must provide themselves with the bare necessities for the maintenance of life itself. The level at which physical needs are met is that of survival, a far cry from the level at which the potential for self-actualization is fully achieved. The economic problems stemming from the inadequate retirement income of so many older Americans are pressing issues as inflation and recession take their toll.

Housing. Housing is another need for the older American (Selby and Schechter 1982). Many own their own homes, but the house is often too large for their needs or is in disrepair and perhaps too costly to maintain. Additional senior citizen housing must be developed to assist those older people who no longer can live in their own homes because of architectural barriers or the hazards of living in certain neighborhoods. These housing units should be located near houses of worship, shopping centers, and recreational facilities so that older people may interact with others and not be isolated by their living arrangements.

Food Costs. The cost of food is a serious problem for older adults. Many are on restricted diets or, because of financial restrictions, are unable to plan meals that are nutritious and wholesome. More assistance through food stamps, home-delivered meals, and nutrition sites that are open seven days a week would alleviate this condition tremendously.

Thus it can be seen that many older people have difficulty meeting the basic physical needs for life maintenance and therefore do not enjoy a better quality of life. Life for older adults becomes a daily endurance test in maintaining themselves against great odds. This situation raises many ethical dilemmas for older people, such as whether to use money from fixed incomes to pay for utilities or to obtain necessary medications or food (Selby and Schecter 1982).

Safety. Safety is also a major problem for older people (Ebersole and Hess 1985; Ebersole and Hess 1990). Violent crime is on the increase in the United States and a great portion are attacks against older adults. Muggings, robbery, rape, and beatings are being endured by older people in ever-increasing numbers. Because they feel neither safe nor secure in their own homes and neighborhoods and because they are unable to enjoy a walk or just being on the streets in the daylight hours, older adults suffer greatly from tension and anxiety. This psychologic stress eventually takes its toll on the older person's frail physique.

Belongingness. Belongingness—a sense of being wanted, loved, and cared for—creates a major problem for older people as their own family members (sons and daughters) find it more and more difficult to be with their older parents, to care for them in their own homes, and to provide for them other than by placing them in institutions. Many older people are isolated from their friends and neighbors because of physical or psychologic distance. Depression is often

the consequence of such treatment. The feeling that "no one cares" can have devastating results for the older American. Humanness is denied in terms of self-respect and dignity. Newspaper articles contain stories of old persons who are especially depressed at Christmastime as well as other special holidays and want the gift of a visitor—a son, daughter, nephew, neighbor, or friend—who can offer an opportunity to share warmth, affection, and friendship.

Self-Esteem and Self-Actualization. Self-esteem and—the ultimate in quality of life—self-actualization cannot be achieved and maintained if the developmental characteristics of a personal life venture mentioned above are unachievable for the older American (Maslow 1970; Ebersole and Hess 1985; Ebersole and Hess 1990).

The philosophical dilemma inherent in the concept of quantity of life versus quality of life cannot be resolved easily. The quality of life depends on several elements: continued growth of the personality; control of environmental factors; and continued appreciation of cultural values and beliefs. These traits, if freely chosen, encourage the older person to live fully and reach full potential. In American society older people fortunate enough to have had jobs that afforded them enough money to support themselves comfortably in their retirement years and the capability of enjoying a high standard of living pose no ethical dilemma for the nation. For millions of other older people, however, the main concern is mere existence and survival. For them the question becomes one of quantity of life: how to survive from one year to the next on the minimal monetary compensation of the monthly Social Security or pension checks they receive.

Professional nurses who specialize in gerontological nursing must become political activists on behalf of the older adults in our society. There are practical ways for nurses who work with older people to alleviate the current conditions that are so demeaning to the quality of life for the older population. Nurses should

1. Become members of such organizations as the Gray Panthers to resolve problems through legislative lobbying and writing congressmen;

2. Speak out on issues relating to older adults to raise public consciousness and initiate social justice action on local, state, and regional levels;

3. Request the ANA to lobby for increases in Social Security payments and the availability of housing for older adults so health and the quality of their lives are improved.

Aging, Illness, Death, and Quality of Life. When an older person becomes seriously ill and is hospitalized, an ethical question arises. Does the quality of life consist in mere existence, without sufficient health to carry on one's daily responsibilities? Or is the prolongation of life, that is, the quantity of life, to be the basic consideration for the professional nurse, the family, the physician, and older patients themselves? This crucial question is not easily resolved. The ethical decision-making process should be used to gather as many facts as possible about the patient's potential. When the question is one of prolongation of life through extraordinary measures, that is, those measures deemed "experimental or exceptionally difficult procedures" (Kosnik 1976, 25) in medical standards of practice in a given community or region, this issue of the quality of life must be considered. Kosnik (1976) noted that, because of the readily available newer medical procedures that in most instances can prolong life, consideration is now being given to the "hope that a given procedure offers the patient." The person, not the procedure, becomes the focus for ethical decision making. This shift in emphasis within recent years has changed the issue from the emphasis on ordinary and extraordinary measures for the prolongation of life to a focus on the person and judgments regarding the quality of life (Kosnik, 1976).

The quality of life for a person may be described in terms of the ability to love, which "requires consciousness and rationality. Thus, the ability to love (humanly) becomes the critical value which gives life its meaning and ultimate purpose" (Kosnik 1976, 29). Since life is more than physical existence, it becomes important in ethical decisions to consider the spiritual, psychologic, and emotional well-being of the person. It becomes clear then that the totality of the personality must be considered in evaluating the quality of a patient's life. Where relationships and the expression of love are no longer a possibility, it can be concluded that the purpose for which that person was given life has been completed and does not call for medical or health measures to preserve physical existence. This conclusion, of course, must be reached only after serious consultation among the family, clergy, physician, and health care members, primarily the professional nurses.

Professional nurses should take an active part in the decisions to be made regarding the welfare of the older clients in their care. By so doing, they enter the world of reality where many ethical dilemmas exist for the health professional. Two prominent belief systems or viewpoints with which the professional nurse must deal when caring for older people and that may evoke value conflict are *(1)* the view of the *vitalist*, who believes that the quantity of life is all that matters regardless of its quality; and *(2)* the view of the *pluralist*, who believes that the quality of life is most important. Each of these viewpoints gives certain moral directives to professional conduct in relation to the older person (Mosely 1989; Office of Technology Assessment 1987; Bahr 1991).

The nurse plays an important role in preserving the welfare of the patient through an intimate knowledge of the person in all aspects of his or her humanness. Consequently the nurse must continue to assess the data regarding the older client and alert the physician and family of subtle changes in the physical, psychosocial, and spiritual domains exhibited by the older person. In caring for the older patient who no longer has the capacity to relate to others, the nurse must continue to treat the patient with dignity and respect until such time as death occurs. The quality of life becomes a key issue in the ethical decisions regarding the value system to be involved when caring for older clients (Benjamin and Curtis 1981; Bahr 1991; Hunter 1992).

The Executive Committee of the American Nurses' Association, the Council of Gerontological Nursing (1989-1992) is drafting a proposed *Position Statement on Quality of Life* (February 1992). It presents a framework for addressing approaches gerontological nurses may use in caring for terminally ill older adults. This statement is currently under review by official committees of the ANA.

Age: Its Effect on Decisions in Ethical Situations

In ethical decision-making situations, all aspects of life, including age, become important. If a society is truly civilized, then human life is given a higher value of worth than any other form of life. When life becomes a thing to be manipulated, discarded, or destroyed without considering that the ramifications of such an attitude may lead to the breakdown of the fabric of society itself, the path is open to unpredictably destructive attitudes and customs, e.g., promulgation of life destruction measures by Hemlock Society "assisted suicide" machines and suicide pacts by older couples. The right to life, the fundamental principle that applies to each human being, is the foundation on which American society is built. Any interference with this principle brings with it the possibility that the delicate balance achieved in American society through the Constitution of the United States will be upset. Each person, young or old, is to be respected for who he or she is, for his or her human nature, and not just for the contribution that person has made to society from a work-ethic point of view. The person should be supported by society and be free of the fear of being manipulated and controlled by the government in life-and-death matters. The right to life applies to older people as well as to younger people. In this regard, the rights of the older population are to be protected and preserved from violation by society, governmental agencies, or other citizens.

Personhood. Personhood (the totality of physical, psychosocial, and spiritual components constituting the personality of a human being) may be understood as the basic ethical construct to be considered in the question of whether age makes a difference in making decisions in ethical situations. Davis (1979); Benjamin and Curtis (1981); Bahr (1991) address the value of human nature in itself. A person has intrinsic value because of the humanity possessed by that person. Personhood is described by Buscaglia (1970, 4)* as a common bond of humanness in which persons possess the traits of a "deep need to survive, to realize their experience, to love and be loved, to overcome loneliness and isolation, to use their creative endeavors to make things more comfortable and beautiful for themselves and their loved ones, to attempt to understand their world and their part in it." He noted further that personhood "is not a gift, it is an inalienable right" (147). Davis (1979) reported that ethicists such as Fletcher are describing some of

the concrete indicators of personhood and noted that personhood could be identified with the following characteristics: intelligence, self-awareness, self-control, use of time, future time frame, capacity to relate, concern for others, control of existence, curiosity, capacity for change and changeability, and a balance of responsibility and feelings. These elements of personhood are associated with a fully functioning mature person who is continually growing and becoming the person potentially present from the moment of conception. Each phase of life, from infancy to old age, is important and has its unique tasks of development and growth. As the person develops, insight is gained about the unique self and purpose in life. The developmental tasks of the older adult are as important to that phase of life as those of the earlier years of development. Consequently age in terms of chronological years is an unimportant factor when viewed from the perspective of the beauty of the human being and his or her contribution to life merely through being.

Age and Equal Distribution of Resources. Age, however, has become an ethical issue in relation to justice. Justice is concerned with the common good: all people should be treated with respect and dignity and should be given an equal share in the distribution of resources so that a meaningful and a high quality of life is sustained. This point is important in the light of the limited resources available to older adults in American society. Once again it should be remembered that the fixed income of the majority of older adults is the crucial factor in the major difficulties experienced by them—insufficient food; inadequate housing; inappropriate temperature regulation (too hot or too cool); inaccessible transportation leading to isolation—that affect the life of the older person and have ethical implications. An example of this problem, reported by a client in a clinical setting, involved a 91-year-old Mexican man living with his 59-year-old daughter. He had worked for a large meatpacking corporation for more than forty years. He had retired when he was 65, according to company policy, although he was in good health and could have worked longer. The retirement pension

---

*Buscaglia LF. *Personhood, The Art of Being Fully Human*, Thorofare, NJ: Slack, Inc., 1979. Used with permission.

from that long employment record is $42.50 monthly. Obviously subsistence on this amount is impossible in the current period of inflation. Fortunately the man also receives approximately $200 in Social Security benefits. But the total amount is insufficient for the medical expenses he incurs, for the repair of his home, and for transportation needs, since he does not have a car at his disposal (Branson 1979). What rights or respect have his golden years given him? The resources available to him are extremely limited. Age has a negative ethical effect in this case.

Callahan (1987), of the Hastings Center of Bioethics, in *Setting Limits: Medical Goals in Aging Society* suggests that age is a legitimate factor for rationing of care and reduction of health care resources. His premise is that a person who has reached the age of 72 years should be considered as an individual who has been afforded a lifetime of productivity. He purports that allowing the natural life span of chronicity and illness to consume the remainder of the earthly life of these older adults without major consumption of health care resources is in the best interest of American society, given the present condition of limited resources available for all. His argument is that basic health care is being denied to millions of American citizens while the increasing older population is consuming more and more resources (Bahr 1991). Callahan suggests that the solution to the ethical dilemma of limited resources is the rationing of care with age as a criterion for that rationing.

Age-Related Decisions in the Hospital. Turning now to the other end of the spectrum, in terms of ethical situations, what effect does the age of the individual who is hospitalized and in need of special treatments have on the decision-making process? A number of factors must be considered here. The wishes of the patient or the right to independence (e.g., the Patient Self-Determination Act, 1991) in making decisions about one's self (Davis 1979) must take precedence over all other desires expressed by family members, physician, nurse, or other supportive personnel. The patient, if able and in communication with others, takes the responsibility for making an informed decision regarding his or her own well-being. Knowing the risks, the person accepts the consequences that may result from his or her decision. In this case, age may or may not be a factor in the final analysis. Suc-

cessful elective or emergency surgical procedures demonstrate that age is no longer considered a major deterrent to health care needs of older adults.

Other factors to be considered are the availability of the medical treatment and the benefits to be accrued from the procedure. The risk factors for the older person may be prohibitive in light of the drastic effects of the treatment or the limited good that can be expected from the prescribed therapy. In determining the decision regarding treatment, the value systems of the client, family, nurse, and physician play an important role. Basically the decision is made by the client and the family with the assistance of the nurse and the physician who can provide information about the advantages and disadvantages of the decision to be made. Once again informed consent is essential so that the best ethical decision is made regarding an older person.

Still another factor is that of the monetary expenditure, if money is a problem for the older person and family. Many medical procedures are costly. These forbidding costs may draw heavily on the savings of the older person and family and/or those of the adult children, producing a deleterious effect (Grau and Kovner 1986). Consequently the element of age must enter into the ethical decision-making process. The value of prolonging for a short time a life that has been lived to its fullest extent must be weighed against the suffering and hardship that will be felt by both the patient and the family, especially if all their savings are expended in the process. This principle of justice to all must be considered as well.

The consideration of age has relevance in the discussion of age and its effect on decisions in ethical situations (Office of Technology Assessment 1987). The older human being should be given respect and dignity during all the days of his or her life. That is the first ethical principle and should be the right of every human being. However, other factors must be considered in light of justice for the person, the family, and the rest of the community in terms of the use of resources and the benefits accrued to the older person. Age in and of itself is not the issue. The matter of proper distribution of resources so that all may benefit is the crux of the problem.

Because of the complexity of ethical dilemmas facing families and health professionals in terms of safety and autonomy issues of community-based older adults (e.g., falls, restraints, frailness of older persons, memory deficits, middle-aged child/older parent conflicts), ethical dilemmas are important to resolve to the best advantage of all parties involved (Hogstel and Gaul 1991). Each situation must be individually analyzed according to the ethical principles of justice, beneficence, autonomy, and nonmaleficence to bring resolution to the conflict that is present in each case. When fairness is used as the overriding approach, all parties can agree to the solution that seems preferable and beneficial, making the best informed ethical decision possible at the given time (Hogstel and Gaul 1991).

Older People as Research Subjects: The Issue of Informed Consent. Research is a vehicle for bringing about change and improvement in the health care system and for correcting injustices committed against older adults (that is, abusive practices and inadequate nursing care). These injustices may be corrected by obtaining valid data through research. These data can be used to present documentation for improvement of client care. Without research, new knowledge about clinical problems and how to cope with them would be unavailable to the practitioner. Research is essential for the furtherance of any discipline.

In the field of gerontology, research in which older people are used as subjects poses some interesting dilemmas (Reich 1978; Perry and Miller 1986; Harper 1990). Although the ethical principles that apply to the older person are no different from those for other research subjects, older adults who are chosen are usually poor, impaired, institutionalized, and often have no family. Consequently these older people are more vulnerable to research abuse. Who speaks on their behalf?

Two major ethical principles should be exercised in conducting research with older subjects: *(1)* the principle of autonomy and *(2)* the principle of familial justice (Davis 1979). The principle of autonomy implies that the older person has a right to self-determination and describes the act of potentiating the totality of personality to become fully human. The older person may be dependent on the health care system for care, but that does not give anyone in the system the right to violate his or her personhood. The freedom to participate or not to participate in a study belongs to each person. The principle of familial justice identifies the right of a family member to speak on behalf of an older person on the issue of

participation in a research study. The family member must weigh the benefits to be accrued from the study against the burden placed on the older member by such participation. Patients should be neither coerced nor treated paternalistically by the institution, the family, or the researcher regarding the patients' proposed roles as subjects in a research study.

The question then is: How does one obtain informed consent from the older person who may be vulnerable and frail? Makarushka and McDonald (1979) noted that in 1966 the United States Public Health Service identified the need for establishing an Institutional Review Committee (IRC) in every university to monitor the ethical components of any research proposal submitted for funding. This structure has been imposed on all institutions seeking federal funding from the Department of Health and Human Services. Through this structure it was hoped that the individual and the rights of personhood would be protected. The main issue, of course, is informed consent, which indicates the willingness of the subject to participate in the study and protects the rights of the older people who are participants. The main tenets of informed consent are that the subject

1. Participates on a voluntary basis;

2. May withdraw from the study at any time even after he or she has signed the consent form;

3. Is informed of the purposes, procedures, benefits, and risks of the research;

4. Agrees that the benefits will outweigh any investment to be made, e.g., time;

5. Understands that the research will be conducted by a qualified person;

6. Will receive answers to any questions regarding procedures.

Each research proposal therefore has a written consent form for the older person or a family member to read and sign. Each proposal is carefully reviewed by the IRC before its approval for data collection and analysis. This type of institutional protection assures that the older person's rights are preserved and that no undue risk will be forced upon that person.

The signature on the informed consent form may be either that of the older person, if in a position to assume that kind of responsibility, or of a family member or legal guardian when that arrangement is appropriate. In no case should research be conducted without first obtaining the appropriate consent. Davis (1979) noted that each person has a right to aid in the discovery of truth if it will benefit society. No one group in society should be denied the opportunity to aid humankind.

Availability of Health Care to Older Adults

The problem of the availability of health care raises such basic questions as: What is health? By what standards does a person judge if she or he is healthy? What type of health care system is presently in vogue in the United States? Is it capable of caring adequately for all people—young, middle-aged, and old? Is health a right, the responsibility of each person, or an obligation that society must fulfill for its citizens? Who determines when enough health care has been made available to any one group of citizens?

The concept of health has many connotations. It ranges from not only the absence of disease, but also physical, mental, and social well-being (World Health Organization 1947) to a state of high-level wellness (Dunn 1973). Health is, from a holistic point of view, more than just a physical state. Mental, social, and spiritual health must also be considered to form a four-dimensional view. Discussions have been held in relation to what could justifiably be considered *health*, given our present resources of health professionals and economics. Should the emphasis be on the physical aspect only? Who decides what component should be emphasized in our present health delivery model? Or should a holistic approach to total needs of a person be implemented?

Presently in the United States, older adults are the misfits in terms of health care and its delivery. For the most part, health care is conducted within the walls of large medical centers removed from the neighborhoods where older clients live. The burden of seeking health care is on the older person, who may be in frail condition and without adequate transportation. The long trip to the medical facilities and the long wait to see personnel are detrimental to the efficient use of health care resources. The physician and staff generally consider the physical problems of the older patient their primary concern. Little if any attention is given to the other components of the person, namely, the psychosocial and spiritual dimensions. Often only

a short period of time is spent with the older person because the chronic nature of the illness is perhaps less "exciting" than other critical conditions would be to the physician. This attitude may stem from the personnel's ignorance of the subtleties of the geriatric person's condition, which may require astute, highly sophisticated investigation and diagnostic abilities to uncover. Concern for these problems is voiced by such activist groups as the Grey Panthers, the American Association of Retired Persons, and the National Retired Teachers Association. As numbers of older people increase in the population, so too will the need for additional health services and nursing care. Nurses must also become more qualified to care for clients with the complex conditions that accompany the aging process, whether the care is given in institutions or in homes (Bahr 1987). The federal government is investigating ways to initiate more home health care, especially for the older population. It is now recognized through research findings that the cost is lower for home health care than for hospitalization and that it is more beneficial to the older patient to remain at home. As the availability of home health care increases, the demand for more qualified nursing personnel with preparation in gerontological nursing and community health will become critical (Nursing's Agenda for Health Care Reform 1990).

The health care delivery system is geared primarily for the middle-class, white, young-adult population. The emphasis is on acute conditions that are short, episodic, and catastrophic in nature and that require short-term hospitalization and insurance coverage for entry into the system. Difficulty is experienced by the older client who is on Medicare or Medicaid or who lacks insurance coverage of any kind. The health care system has little to offer a person with limited financial resources. The right to health care, basic to the value of personhood, is often denied to people who happen to be in a class other than those just described. The right to life is intrinsic in each human being (Bernardin 1986). Health in the four-dimensional sense is essential to life. Without health, life is not sustained. Ethically therefore the question of health care becomes of great importance for the vast majority of older adults who are denied their basic right to health merely because they are old and unable to pay the inflated bills of affluent medical professionals who do not perceive their responsibility to offer their medical expertise to all citizens.

Ironically in earlier years these same older citizens may have supported, through their tax dollars, the education of the medical personnel from whom they now seek health care. The system as it now operates cannot continue without beginning to exhibit the cruelty and inhumanity of an uncivilized society. A society is judged on the basis of how it treats its older citizens. This thought should arouse concern about the lack of progress that has been made in this regard, as the numbers of older people continue to increase while the available resources appear to be decreasing.

It is recognized through personal and professional observation that the mental and spiritual dimensions of older people become more prominent as their age increases. The activity of the mind and spirit is the substance of the inner resources that give older adults the strength of character and the will to live a meaningful and purposeful life (Gress and Bahr 1984). In recent years some attention has been given in nursing homes to activity programs for older adults. These activities cover a broad range, but for the most part they include handiwork such as crafts, crocheting, and knitting. These activities may serve a purpose, but they offer little mental stimulation to keep the patient's thought processes active and current and keep the patient in touch with reality. In some institutions current events are read aloud from the newspaper each day; but only the high points of the news are read, and there is no opportunity for in-depth discussion. Also, only those items that interest the reader may be chosen. Older adults are thus deprived of selecting their own reading material. The same is true for the selection of television or radio programs. Little if any consideration is given to programs of interest to older people. They are usually selected by the nursing personnel. Evidence of disinterest in the television programs is readily apparent in the television room of a nursing home; the older clients are usually sleeping in their chairs. Indeed the lack of mental stimulation is all too evident.

Many nurses are uncomfortable in dealing with patients' spiritual needs unless they have had preparation in this area. Nurses who ignore an older patient's desire for spiritual sustenance can be considered negligent. The older person's religious feelings may be a key to that person's survival. Readings from Scripture may have been a source of sustenance throughout such a person's lifetime and therefore may be an important source of comfort and solace to these older adults at this time in their lives. The spiritual dimension of the older person's life can give that life meaning and a sense of purpose. The nurse is in a key position to support this important aspect. How can support be given?

The nurse should consult with critically and chronically ill older people who are hospitalized for medical treatment to determine if they want the presence of a person who will pray with them, offer counsel and advice, and aid in making ethical decisions regarding proposed medical treatments. In addition the nurse might pray with older patients if requested to do so (and if the act does not conflict with or impose on the nurse's beliefs) and listen attentively to their faith experiences. Older people will sense a nurse's discomfort immediately and will not continue to request such services from the nurse. Such preparation in the basic educational program of the nurse becomes more and more imperative if the nurse is to be effective in ministrations with older adults. Nurse educators should be attuned to this need in curricular offerings. Supervision of nursing students as they interact with older people is important so that they can become familiar with effective approaches in helping older people with their spiritual needs (Gress and Bahr 1984; Bahr 1991).

Another difficulty encountered in the present health care delivery system is the inattention of nursing personnel to the cultural beliefs and health practices that are significant in the lives of the older members of minority groups who seek access to the health care delivery system (Harper 1991; Hines-Martin 1992). These people have incorporated the heritage of their ancestors into the fabric of their lives. Without these cultural practices, life becomes meaningless to them. Nursing personnel who are of a different ethnic origin than their clients should study the clients' cultural practices and language when ministering to their needs. Many of these older people do not speak English and have difficulty complying with their medical regimens, not because they do not appreciate the efforts made on their behalf but because they do not understand the reasons for the procedures (Hays, Guttman, Ooms, and Mahon-Stetson 1986). They are fearful of the unknown. The priorities established for them by the medical and nursing staff may not be the priority of values they embrace. Consequently conflict may arise and the older person may feel rejected and mistreated and may be labeled unjustly. Sometimes such patients become the victims of retaliation by the health professionals through such actions as withholding care, handling the client roughly in such a way that causes fear in the older person, or by ignoring legitimate requests for care. Nurses, in adopting the Code for Nurses, have voluntarily embraced the concept that they will give care to all people regardless of race, creed, or color. The acceptance of this code implies that nurses assume the responsibility of understanding those whose cultures differ from their own and attempt to understand the patients' cultural health beliefs, practices, and concepts according to their value system, not the nurses'. Prejudice may be found in anyone. People whose background is different than one's own may be seen as inferior. Consequently they are treated in a manner unbecoming to human beings. Minority older adults, because they are vulnerable and usually poor, become victims of the system that has been established to deliver health care to all human beings in the attempt to secure a meaningful, quality lifestyle for all. Ethically the health care delivery system in the United States has a long way to go before its services are truly adequate for them. An appreciation of each culture's contributions and traits is needed so that members of different cultures may be respected as citizens with rights. They must not be treated as victims who are to be punished (Gress and Bahr 1984; Hays, Guttman, Ooms, and Mahon-Stetson 1986; Harper 1991; Nursing's Agenda for Health Care Reform 1990).

Health Care Decisions for the Disoriented Older Adult: Whose Responsibility?

Human life is valuable whatever a person's mental, physical, or spiritual condition may be. This moral principle is basic to American society and should be preserved. Without such moral fiber, society can become chaotic, dehumanized, and brutal in its decisions regarding the lives of its citizens.

A number of problems must be resolved regarding the welfare of older people who, through the ravages of time and the aging process, suffer from the deterioration of their mental faculties. Questions that must be considered include: What can be done to maintain the dignity and respect of such people? What responsibility do older people have to provide for their basic needs? If they are unable to provide for their own basic needs, should the family, friends, neighbors, health care personnel, or the state assume this responsibility? Does the health care system offer adequate care to the older person who becomes disoriented and out of touch with reality? What responsibilities should the nation assume for citizens who, throughout their productive years, contributed so much to the country and preserved it for today's generation?

As noted previously, the older person should enjoy all the rights and privileges of a member of the human species. This should be an inherent right that cannot be destroyed or denied.

One of the key and basic rights of a person is the right to health. With it goals may be accomplished and a high quality of life enjoyed. What a person does throughout life by way of health practices will have an effect on that person's health status during the later years. Even if the person's health habits have not always been adequate, he or she is entitled to the best and most suitable health care available (Bahr 1991).

As people age, they may exhibit symptoms that present serious ethical problems for the health professional in relation to accurate assessment, diagnosis, and treatment. In the case of apparent impaired mental functioning or confusion, for example, a diagnosis of organic mental disorder should be withheld until valid evidence for the existence of this condition is obtained and verified. To fulfill the older person's right to health in this instance, a thorough examination is needed to determine if the person is truly disoriented or merely suffering from such reversible conditions as malnutrition, overdosage of medication, lack of sleep, confusion due to removal from the familiar surroundings of home, a prolonged grieving process due to the loss of spouse and friends, or concern regarding money for subsistence (Ebersole and Hess 1990). Any of these factors may contribute to what seems at first glance to be disorientation or confusion (Wolanin and Phillips 1981). Alleviating these problems may clear the confusion to the point where the person may resume living independently and responsibly without further difficulty.

If, however, the older person is suffering from irreversible organic brain damage, further investigation is needed to fulfill the health professional's moral responsibility for the older person's health care decisions. The investigation should elicit certain data.

- Is there a living will in existence to direct the family or health care team in decisions regarding health care ministrations?

- Is there a family member who can be reached for direction in decisions to be made, e.g., a legal guardian or trustee?

- If no family members are available, does the client have a friend or neighbor who could assist in the decision-making process so that the older patient will be taken care of properly?

- Is it necessary for the nurse and the physician to make decisions together, taking into consideration the policies of the hospital and/or nursing home, their respective ethical codes, and the legal directives of the state in which the institution is located and in which the citizen now resides?

- Is it necessary to seek guidance from the appropriate state agency so that the patient who has no support system of family or friends can be declared incompetent to manage his or her affairs and life and can be admitted to an institution where adequate care would be available?

The last action is, of course, the last resort in caring for an older person who may be disoriented (Harper 1990).

The Family's Decision-Making Responsibilities. Family members, nuclear and extended, are the legitimate people to make decisions about health care for the disoriented older adult (Harper 1990). They must assume responsibility of the familial ties that bind them to this older person. Ideally they are charged with the care and concern for this human being through the bonding of love. In loving concern they should attempt to make a decision based on information provided them by the health care team and, if they desire, a member of the clergy, realizing that at the same time their financial and human resources must be weighed against the benefits to be accrued from the suggested health measures. The age of the family member who needs care may or may not play a major part in the determination of the health care needed and requested. The family has an obligation to the older member to see that all reasonable care

will be given, but the family is not obligated to such a degree of indebtedness that its well-being is jeopardized as well. The principle of justifiable means and ends is used to guide the final determination of what care is feasible in a particular situation with the particular patient. At best, such a determination often calls for uncomfortable and difficult decisions. The family may weigh the options for a long time before they make the final decision. Health care professionals should not attempt to hurry the process unless an emergency exists.

Mr. Zeros, age 92, was admitted to the ICU of Morning Star Hospital by ambulance. He was cyanotic and experiencing respiratory distress. He also was hemorrhaging from the rectum. Miss Ray, the newly assigned R.N. in charge of the unit, was called to the area. The man was in a semicomatose condition and appeared unable to communicate clearly regarding orientation to time, date, and place. Dr. Rojas was called and an assessment of the situation was made. The ethical decision facing this health team was: How should this situation be handled? Only one daughter accompanied her father to the hospital. In requesting information from her regarding her father's treatment, she became very frightened because there were seven children in the family but all were not immediately available for an emergency decision. She began to cry and said she could not assume responsibility for a decision regarding whether to treat or not to treat the condition of her father.

What should the role of the nurse be in such a dilemma? Miss Ray, first of all, needs to collect as much data as possible from the daughter about her father and attempt to ascertain who in the family is the decision maker. If this information can be obtained, an immediate call to that individual must be made as quickly as possible to obtain a decision regarding surgical intervention *or* a decision to utilize ordinary means of comfort measures as palliation for the discomfort experienced by Mr. Zeros. The nurse must respect whatever decision is made by the family and support their decision in every way. If spiritual assistance is needed, the nurse should coordinate those efforts. This case is typical of the types seen with older individuals whose family has not made an attempt to obtain a clear decision about personal wishes. The principle of autonomy had to be compromised in this situation because a family member had to make the decision regarding treatment. What was the decision? Only to offer ordinary means of nourishment by tube feeding and comfort measures as needed. Mr. Zeros died within ten days of admission.

Decision-Making Responsibilities of Friends and Neighbors. In the event that the older person has no family members who can serve as consultants in decision making when the older person is not capable of such activity, the professional nurse should check to see if any friends or former neighbors have been informed about the Durable Power of Attorney as designated by the Patient Self-Determination Act of 1991 or are interested in assisting the person at this time. Often a friend who is not in the vicinity can be traced and his or her assistance can be requested. The nurse must become a detective, working through an informal community network to uncover any link between such a friend and the older person. The nurse should also evaluate whether or not the friend's actions are in the best interest of the patient.

Decision-Making Responsibilities of Professional Nurse and Physician. In rare instances when no family, friend, or neighbor is available or no advance directives exist for making decisions for the health care of the disoriented older adult, the task falls to the health care professionals. They are obligated by their respective codes of ethics to analyze the situation to determine the benefits to be gained and the resources available. Each older person should be reviewed individually. Avoid the paternalistic view that it is the institution that knows best (Cicarelli 1992). Decide according to the idea that each life is to be respected and treated with appropriate resources, loving care, and concern for this "family member" of the institution.

Ethically each patient must be treated as a person, not just as a number in a room with a diagnosis of dementia. This attitude will keep the problem of paternalism from creeping into the decision-making process. Paternalism is the easiest approach when little effort is made to provide more than minimal care for disoriented older patients. Instead such patients should be considered as part of the "family" of the institution and the health care team should choose the care they think is best.

Ashley and O'Rourke (1978) noted that in cases where ethical decisions regarding the care of the client are needed, the professional nurse should take the lead in the decision-making process. This should be done within the context of an Ethics Committee, if one exists in the facility (Enderlin and Wilhite 1991). It is the nurse who takes responsibility for the care of the older person twenty-four hours a day and knows best the intricate details of that person's life and care requirements. The nurse must assume an important role in the discussion of the effects of the proposed treatment plan and its psychologic, physical, and spiritual consequences for the older client. The nurse should be viewed as an advocate, particularly when the client is incapable of making decisions (Bahr 1991).

Resuscitation Decisions

When an older person encounters serious illness, such as cancer, heart disease, or stroke, or meets with an accident in which severe injury is sustained, a serious question arises: What ministrations are ethical to maintain life? This question raises the issue of ordinary and extraordinary measures and their application to the seriously or terminally ill person.

From a medical point of view, *ordinary means* are defined as the usual measures that help an ill person to overcome his or her physical problems (Ashley and O'Rourke 1978). These measures might include injections of penicillin and the administration of oxygen. Such measures offer a reasonable assurance of benefit and may be implemented without unreasonable expense, pain, or other untoward effects. *Extraordinary means*, on the other hand, are those measures that are considered heroic or cannot be obtained without great expense, pain, or other inconvenience and do not offer much hope for reversal of the terminal condition of the client (Ashley and O'Rourke). Ethical decision making is essential when applying these two measures to any client, young or old.

Who really determines whether a measure is ordinary or extraordinary? The medical personnel, in gathering data regarding the person's health status, determine whether the condition is reversible by the use of various measures, ordinary or extraordinary. This information should be shared with the client and the family members in the context of an Ethics Committee. If the client is capable of making decisions, he or she, in conjunction with the family and health care team, should decide what is best regarding the use of ordinary and extraordinary means. Certain factors must be considered: the price to be paid for the measure, the benefit accrued, and the availability of the resources to the physician. The family members play an important role in the final determination. However, the patient has the right to make the final decision (Ashley and O'Rourke 1978).

When the patient is comatose and incapable of participating in the decision, it is the responsibility of the family, in consultation with the health care team and a member of the clergy if the family desires, to determine what course of action is best for their relative. In this case the main focus for the decision is the benefit to the patient, not the benefit to the family (Ashley and O'Rourke 1978).

Therefore the initiation of measures for resuscitation when a cardiac or respiratory arrest occurs in an older client is not an automatic decision by the health care team. If an arrest occurs and is the first such emergency, and if no directives have been mandated by the patient, family, or physician, the nurse should immediately implement measures and policies that have become for the most part ordinary means in hospital wards. If, however, the physician, in consultation with the family and client, has come to the decision that, *not because the older person is advanced in age* but because of the hopelessness, trauma, and expense resulting from such drastic measures, no resuscitation should be carried out and the patient should be allowed to die with dignity and respect, the professional nursing team must, from an ethical point of view, respect those wishes and orders. For this reason, it is important for the professional nurse to be included in the final decision-making process, because it is the nurse who provides the continuity of care for patients twenty-four hours a day during their hospitalization or institutionalization.

Enderlin and Wilhite (1991) suggested that an institutional policy on DNR (Do Not Resuscitate) orders should contain statements about the following:

- Resuscitation as a standing order that is initiated unless there is a no resuscitation order

- The resident's wishes (The courts have held that a competent resident has the right to refuse treatment. The resident has the primary responsibility for such decisions.)

- The medical conditions that shall be present to justify an order not to resuscitate (DNR orders are appropriately recommended when the resident suffers from a terminal and irreversible illness.)

- The role of the family or close significant others (The family does not have the right to make a DNR decision for a competent patient.)

- The protocols describing the process for a DNR order (These include how the DNR order is entered in the resident's chart, reasons for the DNR order, and comments about the decision made with residents, family, or legal guardian.)

- The scope of the DNR order (An order not to resuscitate refers only to cardiopulmonary resuscitation and does not imply the omission of any other type of medical order.)

- The frequency with which the order is reviewed, and how and under what circumstances the order is rescinded.

The right to life, health, and death with dignity belongs to every person. Each person should decide what is best in any circumstance. Nursing personnel must continually strive to be advocates for their clients, particularly those advanced in age, so that their personhood is respected and preserved throughout the process of living and dying. Each human being needs the support of another person, particularly when faced with the crucial decisions about measures that may or may not prolong life. No one in the health care field has the right to jeopardize another's life in any way.

Because of recent concern by the Congress of the United States regarding ethical decision making facing the health professions and older adults, a charge was given to the Office of Technology Assessment to study implications for the use of medical technologies that can sustain life in older people who are critically or terminally ill. An advisory committee comprised of physicians, nurses, lawyers, economists, and ethicists was formulated and a study conducted. A report entitled *Life-Sustaining Technologies and the Elderly* was completed and submitted to Congress in August 1987. An important component of the study is the listing of ethical principles composed by the advisory committee and offered to the Congress and the public for consideration. These ethical principles for decision making regarding the use of life-sustaining technologies for older persons include the following:

- An adult patient who is capable of making decisions has the right to decline any form of medical treatment or intervention. However, an individual does not necessarily have a right to unlimited medical treatment or intervention.

- Decisions regarding the use of life-sustaining treatments must be made on an individual basis and should never be based on chronologic age alone. Chronologic age *per se* is a poor criterion on which to base individual medical decisions. However, age may be a legitimate modifier regarding appropriate utilization of life-sustaining medical technologies.

- Diagnosis alone is a poor criterion for decisions about the use of life-sustaining technologies. Because of the great variability among patients with the same diagnosis, patient assessment must also include measures of functional impairment and severity of illness.

- Cognitive function is an important marker of the quality of life.

- The courts are not and should not be the usual route or determinant for making decisions about the use of life-sustaining technologies or for resolving the dilemmas these technologies may create.

- There is little need or room for federal legislation concerning the initiation, withholding, or withdrawal of specific life-sustaining technologies.

- There is a major need for a clear, workable definition of the appropriate role of surrogates in health care decision making, including the nature of their responsibilities and their suitability to make decisions.

- There is a need to recognize that a process exists, or should exist, for making decisions about the use of life-sustaining technologies. The process described by the President's Commission for the Study of Ethical Problems in Medicine and Biomedical and Behavioral Research could serve as a model.

- A physician or other health professional who does not want to follow the wishes of a patient who is capable of making decisions regarding his or her treatment should withdraw from that case.

- Socioeconomic status should not be a barrier to access to health care, including life-sustaining technologies.

- There is an important need for education of the public and health care providers regarding the nature and appropriate use of life-sustaining technologies.

- There is a specific need for improved clinical information that would predict the probability of a critically or seriously ill patient's survival, functional status, and subsequent quality of life.

- There is a wide range of medical and legal disagreement and varying levels of emotional strain and moral conflict about the appropriate use of life-sustaining technologies. The great heterogeneity of the American population makes consensus difficult and increases the likelihood of formal institutional decision-making procedures (Office of Technology Assessment 1987).

Euthanasia

Euthanasia is a highly controversial ethical issue in America today. Although euthanasia is presently illegal and many groups feel that because it is unethical and immoral it should remain so, other groups are convinced that it should be legalized. (From this latter opinion it can be inferred that these groups consider euthanasia ethical and moral.)

Good death or *happy death* is a translation of the Greek word *euthanasia* (Ashley and O'Rourke 1978). It is a word that for centuries was used to describe the putting to death, in as painless a manner as possible, of people who were suffering from a disease believed to be incurable or who were in a comatose condition that was thought to be irreversible (*Euthanasia: An Annotated Bibliography* 1979). It is often referred to as mercy killing or death with dignity (Ashley and O'Rourke 1978). In these words the thought is conveyed that a life is intentionally ended—either by oneself or by another person who becomes an accomplice to the action. In reality, euthanasia may take three forms: suicide, in which the person ends life because he or she feels that it is not worth living; active euthanasia, in which another person willfully commits an action to end another's life, e.g., assisted suicide; and passive euthanasia, in which the decision is made to leave the patient or person to die without further medical assistance and without implementing extraordinary measures. Thus euthanasia, in the Judeo-Christian tradition, "without the patient giving consent, would be murder and with the consent would be considered both murder and suicide" (Ashley and O'Rourke 1978, 380).

Active Euthanasia

In active euthanasia a person requests that life be terminated by some other person through some means that fully assures the termination of that life. Ashley and O'Rourke (1978) state that to believe that one is terminating another's life out of compassion for that person is false compassion. According to these authors, nothing is gained by such an action by either the person whose life is to be terminated or by the accomplice to the act, which is described as murder, or the taking of the life of another (Ashley and O'Rourke 1978). In contrast, although active euthanasia is presently illegal and seen as homicide by the courts, other viewpoints prevail in society that advocate the ending of life if the individual or others directly involved encourage it. Such viewpoints promote the idea that life may be ended by the individual if he or she no longer views life as purposeful or meaningful. A variety of value systems and ethical viewpoints are in operation in society today that view life as an entity to be manipulated at will.

Health professionals must rank their ethical principles and values regarding life and health in proper order. The Code for Nurses (American Nurses' Association 1985) embraced by professional nurses clearly makes the point that nothing will be done to harm another person through the nurse's ministrations. Consequently when working with persons of all ages, but especially the older population, nurses must be on guard that other health team members do nothing to cooperate in what might be considered active euthanasia. Medical technology today is continuing to advance and bring innovations to the relief of pain and distress so that a degree of comfort can be achieved, even for the most seriously ill person (Office of Technology Assessment 1987). Nurses must be on guard so that older adults are not subjected to treatments for the pure sake of experimentation or to provide nursing and medical students with practice to achieve their clinical goals. The nurse who knows a patient well should always be the coordinator of services and should attend to the planning for the continuity of care of the patient in an institution (Gunter et al. 1979).

Situations that are intolerable to nurses because of their ethical principles must be reported to a supervisor. The nurse in such a situation will need to document clearly the activities that give cause for concern and should present the data to the appropriate authorities. In addition the nurse should be free to request a transfer to another unit in the institution, if possible, to preserve personal integrity. These options are within the nurse's rights as a professional and as a person.

Active euthanasia is a serious ethical dilemma. Older people, because they are frail, vulnerable, and usually financially disadvantaged, often say, "I want to die." But health professionals are not ethically permitted to take another's life. Older adults have entrusted their state of well-being to the health professionals as they move into the health care system.

Passive Euthanasia

Passive euthanasia connotes the fact that no active and immediate intervention is undertaken to terminate a life, merely that no extraordinary means are used to prolong a life that is in the process of terminating through grave illness or old age. Comfort and supportive measures can be used to sustain life until such time as the forces of life are overcome by the forces contributing to death. In terms of passive euthanasia the health care team may become entangled in the ethical decision about when to remove life-support systems and allow the person to die, as in the highly publicized Quinlan case in New Jersey and the Curzan case in Missouri in 1989.

The decision should be made by the patient and/or family, in consultation with the health care team members, primarily the physician, professional nurse, and a member of the clergy if desired. The family has the right to determine whether prolongation of life through the initiation of ordinary or extraordinary means is valuable and valid from an ethical point of view. These wishes must be respected, because neither the physician nor the nurse owns the patient. Family members ultimately have the responsibility for the welfare of their relative.

Euthanasia, then, whether active or passive, deals with questions about the lives of others. These lives, although dependent to a great extent on the health care team, are not under the control of the team, and therefore cannot be mutilated or destroyed at will.

The health care team functions under the aegis of ethical codes that dictate the team's conduct regarding preservation of life and health, which it is bound to do to the best of its ability. It is the opinion of some that without this respect for life, genocide might soon be the fate of certain groups—the mentally retarded and the older adults, who are likely to be the first to be considered unessential to society.

SUMMARY

Older adults, the family, and society face many ethical dilemmas in the care of older people. In discussing the meaning of ethics and its relationship to the health care professional and health care system, it becomes clear that the value system of the individual takes precedence over that of the institution and society. The right to life of the individual is an all-important and pervasive right to be enjoyed by each person. People have a right to demand respect and dignity from others because of their humanness and the bonding of humanity.

Ethical decision making is a process that must be engaged in by the person, the family, and the health care team, with the goal of preservation of life. Some authors believe that several types of ethical thinking mechanisms are erroneous: *(1)* that morality and practicality are synonymous; *(2)* that morality and opinion are the same; and *(3)* that morality and subjectivity can cloud the essence of the ethical decision to be made. Still other viewpoints promote these lines of thinking as feasible and compatible in resolving ethical issues facing individuals in our society. Professional nurses must be aware of these modes of thinking and attempt to avoid the pitfalls of such thought processes. The value system of the professional nurse is embodied in the ANA Code for Nurses, which guides the nurse in deliberations each day when caring for people, sick or well. With the

Code for Nurses as a guide, professional nurses can enter into the ethical decision-making process with a greater understanding of the ethics involved in the profession of nursing.

Six major areas cover the dilemmas faced by older people in today's society.

1. Quality of life versus quantity of life

2. Age: its effect on decisions in ethical situations

3. Availability of health care to older adults

4. Health care decisions for the disoriented older adult: whose responsibility?

5. Resuscitation decisions

6. Euthanasia: active and passive

Each of these is a gray area that creates conflict in terms of the values of the individual, the family, and society. The whole person—mind, body, and spirit—is the concern of nursing. To continue to kindle the spark of life in these three areas is to remind the person continually of the tremendous dimension of personhood. The older people of this country are a precious resource. If some of the ethical dilemmas they face can be resolved, everyone will experience much joy and a sense of reward from helping other human beings continue to live life fully.

STUDY QUESTIONS

1. How is the term *ethics* defined from a philosophical perspective?

2. Identify three common errors in ethical thinking that influence ethical decision making.

3. Discuss the ANA Code for Nurses.

4. Describe the major points in the process of ethical decision making as outlined by Wheelock.

5. Name the rights and responsibilities of older Americans as identified in the Bicentennial Charter Statement.

6. What is meant by "quality of life?" Why is this component so important when considering any type of ethical decision?

7. Whose responsibility is it to make decisions for disoriented older people and in what rank order

is authority assumed for such decisions? What is the role of the nurse in these circumstances?

8. Define *ordinary means* and *extraordinary means* of health care for the older person. Give examples of each type of measure. Discuss the ethical principles regarding life-sustaining technologies.

9. Explain the meaning of euthanasia. Where does this word originate? Give the rationale for its prominence in the thinking of health professionals and legislators in contemporary society.

10. Compare and contrast active and passive euthanasia. Describe situations that could be examples of each type.

REFERENCES

American Nurses' Association. 1985. *Code For Nurses with Interpretive Statements*. Kansas City, MO: American Nurses' Association.

Aroskar, M. 1987. The interface of ethics and politics in nursing. *Nursing Outlook* 35(6):268–72.

Ashley, O.P. and K.D. O'Rourke. 1978. *Health Care Ethics: A Theological Analysis*. St. Louis: The Catholic Hospital Association.

Bahr, R.T. 1987. Ethiolegal issues in the gerontological nursing curriculum. *Journal of Gerontological Nursing* 13(3):3–6.

Bahr, R.T. 1991. Selected ethical and legal issues in aging. In *Perspectives on Gerontological Nursing*, edited by E.M. Baines. Newbury Park, CA: Sage Publications, Inc.

Benjamin, M. and J. Curtis. 1981. Moral dilemmas and ethical inquiry. *Ethics in Nursing*. New York: Oxford University Press.

Bernardin, J. 1986. The consistent ethic: What sort of framework? *Origins* 16(20):346–50.

Branson, M. 1979. Clinical log in graduate course. *Nursing Process and Care of the Aging I*. Kansas City, KS: The University of Kansas School of Nursing.

Buscaglia, L.F. 1979. *Personhood, the Art of Being Fully Human*. Thorofare, NJ: Slack, Inc.

Callahan, D. 1987. *Setting Limits: Medical Goals in an Aging Society*. New York: Simon and Schuster.

Cicarelli, V.C. 1992. *Family Caregiving: Autonomous and Paternalistic Decision-Making*. Newbury Park, CA: Sage Library of Social Research, 186, Sage Publications, Inc.

Davis, A.J. 1979. Theoretically realistic. *Clinical and Scientific Sessions*. Kansas City, MO: ANA, Division of Practice.

Dunn, H.L. 1979. *High Level Wellness*. Arlington, VA: Beatty.

Ebersole, P. and P. Hess. 1985. Environmental considerations as they affect safety and security. *Toward Healthy Aging: Human Needs and Nursing Response*. 3d ed. St. Louis: C.V. Mosby.

Ebersole, P. and P. Hess. 1990. *Toward Healthy Aging*. St. Louis: C.V. Mosby.

Enderlin, A. and M. Wilhite. 1991. Establishing incidence and administrative protocols for do not resuscitate orders. *Journal of Gerontological Nursing* 17(3):12–16.

Euthanasia—An Annotated Bibliography, May 1979. New York: Euthanasia Fund, 1979.

Federal Council on Aging. 1976. *Bicentennial Charter for Older Americans: Statement of Rights and Responsibilities of Citizens*. Washington, DC: United States Government Printing Office.

Grau, L. and C. Kovner. 1986. Comorbidity and length of stay: A case study. *Nursing and Health Care* 7(8):427–30.

Gress, L. and R.T. Bahr. 1984. *The Aging Person: A Holistic Perspective*. St. Louis: C.V. Mosby.

Gunter, L., L. Heckman, D. Moser, and M. Fasano. 1979. Issues and ethics in gerontic nursing. *Journal of Gerontological Nursing* 5(6):15–20.

Harper, M.S. 1991. *Managing Care of the Elderly: Psychosocial Perspectives*. Newbury Park, CA: Sage Publications, Inc.

Harper, M.S. 1990. Mental health and older adults. In *Geropsychiatric Nursing*, edited by M.O. Hogstel. St. Louis: C.V. Mosby.

Hays, C.L., D. Guttman, T. Ooms, and P. Mahon-Stetson. 1986. *The Euro-American Elderly in the United States: A Manual for Service Providers and Ethnic Leaders*. Washington, DC: The Catholic University of America, The Center for the Study of Pre-Retirement and Aging.

Hines-Martin, V. 1992. A research review: Family caregivers of chronically ill African-American elderly. *Journal of Gerontological Nursing* 18(2):25–29.

Hogstel, M. and A. Gaul. 1991. Safety or autonomy:

An ethical issue for clinical gerontological nurses. *Journal of Gerontological Nursing* 17(3):6–11.

House Subcommittee on Health and the Environment, Committee on Energy and Commerce. *Health Care for the Homeless: A Congressional Hearing*. (Serial No. 99-139). March 26, 1986.

House Subcommittee on Health and the Environment, Committee on Energy and Commerce. *Health Care for the Homeless: A Congressional Hearing*. December 15, 1986.

Hunter, S. 1992. Adult day care: Promoting quality of life for the elderly. *Journal of Gerontological Nursing* 18(2):13-16.

Husted, G.L. and J.H. Husted. 1991. *Ethical Decision-Making in Nursing*. St. Louis: C.V. Mosby.

Ketefian, S. 1987. A case study of theory development: Moral behavior in nursing. *Advances in Nursing Science* 4(1):10–19.

Killeen, M.L. 1986. Nursing fundamental texts: Where's the ethics? *Journal of Nursing Education* 25(8):334–46.

Kosnik, A.R. 1976. Ordinary and extraordinary means of prolonging life. *Ethical Issues in Nursing: A Proceedings*. St. Louis: The Catholic Hospital Association.

Makarushka, J.L. and R.D. McDonald. 1979. Informed consent, research and geriatric patients: The responsibility of institutional review committees. *The Gerontologist* 19(1):61–66.

Maslow, A. 1970. *Motivation and Personality*. 2d ed. New York: Harper and Row.

Mosely, R. 1989. DNR: The continuing ethical problem. *Florida Nursing Review* 3(4):8–14.

National Conference of Catholic Bishops. 1979. *To Live in Christ Jesus: A Pastoral Reflection on the Moral Life*. 11(3); Washington, DC: United States Catholic Conference.

National Conference of Catholic Bishops. *Putting Children and Families First: A Challenge for Our Church, Nation and World*. A statement approved at the general meeting, Washington, DC, November 13, 1991.

Nursing's Agenda for Health Care Reform. 1990. Washington, DC: ANA-NLN-AACN.

Office of Technology Assessment. 1987. *Life-Sustaining Technologies and the Elderly: A Summary Report*. Washington, DC: United States Government Printing Office.

Payton, R. 1979. Pluralistic ethical decision-making. *Clinical and Scientific Sessions*. Kansas City, MO: ANA Division on Practice.

Perry, C.B. and S.T. Miller. 1986. Ethical considerations of clinical research. *J Am Geriatr Soc* 34(1):49–51.

Reich, W.T. 1978. Ethical issues related to research involving elderly subjects. *The Gerontologist* 18(4):326–37.

Rigali, N.J. 1979. Morality and historical consciousness. *Chicago Studies* 18:161–68.

Selby, P. and M. Schechter. 1982. Ensuring suitable housing. *Aging 2000: A Challenge for Society*. Boston: MTP Press Limited.

Synod of Bishops. 1974. *Statement on Rights of Individuals*. Washington, DC: United States Catholic Conference.

Tobin, S.S., J.W. Ellor, and S.M. Anderson-Ray. 1986. *Enabling the Elderly*. Albany, NY: State University of New York Press.

U.S. Congress. *Patient Self-Determination Act*, Omnibus Reconciliation Budget Act of 1990. Effective date of implementation: December 1, 1991.

Weber, L.J. 1976. What is ethics? *Ethical Issues in Nursing: A Proceedings*. St. Louis: The Catholic Hospital Association.

Wheelock, R.D. 1976. Nursing and pastoral care. *Ethical Issues in Nursing: A Proceedings*. St. Louis: The Catholic Hospital Association.

Wolanin, M.O. and L.R. Phillips. 1981. *Confusion: Prevention and Cure*. St. Louis: C.V. Mosby.

World Health Organization. 1947. Constitution of the world health organization. *Chronicle of the World Health Organization* 1:29–43.

Yeaworth, R. 1985. The ANA code: A comparative perspective. *Image* 17(3):94–98.

Appendix A

Sociocultural Assessment, Intervention, and Teaching Guide

I. Asian and Pacific Islanders

A. Demographics

1. Comprise 11 million persons in the United States population.

2. Ethnic subgroups are very diverse and speak over thirty different languages.

3. Three-fourths are immigrants or refugees.

4. Broad cultural group composed of the following ethnic subgroups: Laotians, Cambodians, Pacific Islanders, Vietnamese, Hawaiians, Asian Indians, Thais, Samoans, Koreans, Filipinos, Chinese, Japanese, Guamanians, and other Asian groups (unspecified)

B. General characteristics

1. Great economic contrast exists among ethnic subgroups. Those who are acculturated are economically stable and may have incomes above the United States median. Recent immigrants may be among the poorest of the United States poor.

2. Family relationships are highly valued, as is filial piety. Behavior of individuals reflects on the family as a group and the needs of individuals are subordinated to the needs of the family lineage.

3. Individuals, within the family and in society at large, are assigned roles according to the superordinate/subordinate model (e.g., husband/wife; parent/child). Women are subordinate to men.

4. Older family members have more authority than younger family members and are respected (in some groups, revered).

5. Deference is shown to older persons and their authority is not subject to question.

6. Deference is also shown to those perceived to be in a superior position (e.g., employers and physicians).

7. High cultural value is placed on respect and deference.

8. In some groups, eye contact with superiors is avoided as a sign of respect (e.g., among the Vietnamese). In other groups, eye contact is a prerequisite for establishing functional relationships (e.g., among the Filipinos).

9. High premium is placed on harmony in relationships. There is a great desire not to disappoint, upset, embarrass, or cause another to lose face.

10. Open disagreement destroys harmony and is to be avoided.

11. Great value is placed on self-control and emotional restraint. Public displays of emotion are avoided and are considered a personal weakness.

12 Cultural values dictate against openly expressing thoughts and feelings, particularly to outsiders.

13. Smiles may be used as an apology for a social offense, to cover emotional pain, and/or to indicate that another has been heard. Smiles do not necessarily imply agreement with others.

14. A response of "yes" to a question or communication indicates that it has been heard but cannot be construed to mean assent.

15. Asians are a quiet people. They feel that those who talk a lot do not think much and may be seeking attention. They would rather say nothing at all than to say something not well thought-out (Freebaim and Gwinup 1979).

16. At best, responses to questions may be brief and succinct. Therefore health care providers desiring to collect data will want to avoid questions that can be answered yes or no.

17. Decisions are carefully weighed and based on many variables. They may depend on signs, symbols, and correlations with life or cosmic events.

18. Depending on the ethnic subgroup, individuals may follow the religious practices of Taoism, Buddhism, Islam, Confucianism, or Christianity.

19. Shrines may be maintained in the home for ancestor worship.

20. Value is placed on material sharing.

21. Modesty, confidentiality, and privacy are valued.

22. Outcome of life situations may be viewed as destined or inevitable.

23. Diseases can have both natural and supernatural causes.

24. Illness may result from an imbalance in "Yin" (the negative, inactive female force, the cold force) and "Yang" (the positive, active male force, hot force). These opposites are considered complementary. Imbalance is treated by applying agents or actions to counter the one considered out of balance. (For example, if a disorder is caused by too much "Yin," it will be treated with "Yang" interventions to restore balance.)

25. Illness may also relate to "Ch'i." "Ch'i" as an energy force that flows through the body in meridians. "Ch'i" and blood may be considered vital life forces. When the flow of "Ch'i" is blocked, it can be returned to normal by acupuncture or acupressure.

26. Asians may fear having blood drawn or removed from the body for fear that the body cannot compensate for the alteration in life force.

27. Illness may not be viewed as a result of germs but as a result of imbalance due to faulty diet or strong emotional feelings. Body harmony is restored through self-restraint, use of a corrective diet, and herbal treatments.

28. Illness can also occur as a result of offending God or a spirit or violating a moral or religious code.

29. Due to the value placed on emotional control, mental illness may be unacceptable in many Asian subgroups. Therefore anxiety and mental stress may find their only acceptable expression in somatic complaints.

30. Western and Asian medicine may be used simultaneously.

31. Filipinos may subscribe to the theory of the four humors: phlegm or mucus, air or vapors, bile, and blood. Illness is caused by air or wind (mal aire). Three concepts underlie health beliefs and

practices: flushing (to keep the body from debris), heating (to maintain a balanced internal temperature), and protection (to guard the body from outside influences). Vinegar is often used in the preparation of home remedies (Giger and Davidhizer 1991).

32. Herbs and folk medicines purchased in Asian communities and used in the practice of folk medicine may

    a) potentiate the effect of Western medications (e.g., ginseng and antihypertensives)
    b) contain heavy metals (lead, mercury, and arsenic) and become toxic with heavy use
    c) be labelled inadequately and contain harmful chemicals (e.g., phenylbutazone, aminopyrine)

33. Asians may use large amounts of monosodium glutamate in cooking as well as soy, miso, fish, and oyster sauce. The large amounts of sodium in these products may need to be taken into consideration if the individual client has hypertension.

34. Pain may be present but not visibly expressed due to rigid emotional control.

35. Metals such as jade, copper, and brass may be worn for their symbolic power to prevent disease, promote long life and good health, or to control pain.

36. Special practices may surround death. Some ethnic subgroups will prefer that an individual die at home because those who die away from home are believed to become wandering souls who can find no place to rest. Other subgroups, who believe in reincarnation, may believe it to be important for the individual's state of mind to be calm, hopeful, and clear at the time of death. This state of mind will facilitate reincarnation into a better being.

37. In contrast to customary restraint, great emotional display may be allowed by some subgroups as a part of bereavement.

38. Asians may experience vasomotor symptoms and facial flushing after alcohol consumption.

C. Folk medicine healers

   1. Shamans

   2. Curers

D. Folk medicine practices

   1. Acupuncture

   2. Acupressure

   3. Giac cupping

   4. Moxibustion

   5. Skin scraping or coin rubbing (cao gio)

   6. Massage

E. Causes of morbidity and mortality

   1. Hepatitis B

   2. Tuberculosis

   3. Liver cancer

   4. Smoking

   5. Diabetes

6. G-6-P-D deficiency

7. Alpha-thalassemia (Hemoglobin H disease)

8. In addition recent immigrants may suffer from: intestinal parasites, malaria, malnutrition, and anemia.

II. African-Americans

A. Demographics

1. Comprise 12.4 percent of the United States population.

2. One-third of African-Americans live in poverty.

3. Fifty percent live in inner cities.

4. African-Americans have a life expectancy of 69.4 years, compared to 75 years for the overall population.

5. Black Americans are represented in the following ethnic subgroups: native born or of Haitian, Jamaican, or Bahamian descent.

B. General characteristics

1. The ancestors of native born African-Americans originally immigrated to America under the system of slavery. They were the only American immigrant group brought to the United States involuntarily.

2. There is a dichotomy in the African-American population. There is a growing middle class with representation in the highest occupational ranks, contrasted with a disproportionate number of the nation's poor and illiterate (Yee 1990).

3. Families are organized around kinship networks rooted in blood ties.

4. "Fictive" kin or "play" parents, children, siblings, aunts, or uncles may be included in the family system on an equal basis with blood relatives.

5. The family is often matrifocal, oriented around women. Over half of families are headed by females.

6. The African-American marital dyad has been described as egalitarian because the African-American female has not been dependent on the African-American male from the time of slavery on through the present (Yee 1990).

7. The role of the African-American grandmother is pivotal. She is often the primary caregiver for her grandchildren and other relatives.

8. The family matriarch plays an important role in decision making, caregiving, and dissemination of health information.

9. Older African-Americans display a high degree of involvement in religious activities. They attend church frequently, hold offices in the church, and define themselves as religious (Burnside 1988).

10. Older African-American women may define work as the central organizing feature of their existence. Work may have commenced in early childhood and continued throughout life to promote the survival of their families. Much resourcefulness may have been required to sustain survival because wages and opportunities were limited. Therefore in old age these women may prove to be very self-reliant (Allen and Chin-Sang 1990).

11. Older African-American women may see self-reliance and the freedom to spend time as they

please in old age as significant accomplishments to be valued and protected (Allen and Chin-Sang 1990). A lifetime of work and care for others may transfer to caring for peers in their own community well into late life.

12. African-American males may be overprotected within the family unit due to high mortality from all causes (especially homicide).

13. Individuals may use African-American dialect (African-American English or Ebonics), which is a combination of pidgin-creole-English in all African-American settings or when they do not wish to be understood by non African-Americans. African-American dialect services as a cultural unifier. It arose out of and endures because of conditions related to servitude, segregation, and discrimination.

14. Great importance is placed on nonverbal elements of communication.

15. Time may be handled polychronically, i.e., individuals may engage in multiple activity involvement simultaneously (Giger and Davidhizer 1991).

16. Distinctions may not be made between physical, mental, and spiritual illness.

17. Illness may be viewed as a disharmony or conflict in some aspect of an individual's life.

18. The causes of disease may be linked to an alteration in blood volume and may be described as "high blood" or "low blood." These disorders are not associated with hypertension or hypotension.

19. A belief in opposites may be present (e.g., for every birth there will be a corresponding death).

20. Individuals may respond to pain stoically out of a desire to be a perfect patient or because they believe that pain and trouble are a part of God's will for them.

21. In some sections of the country, voodoo and witchcraft may be a compliant of folk medicine.

C. Folk healers

1. "Granny" or "old lady"—treats with home remedies; refers to others when disorders are beyond her skill

2. "Spiritualist"—uses combination of rituals, spiritual beliefs, herbal medicines

3. "Hougan"—Voodoo priest or priestess who treats the most difficult cases

4. "Root doctor"

5. "Herb doctor"

D. Causes of morbidity and mortality

1. Heart disease

2. Stroke

3. End-stage renal disease

4. Cancer

5. Homicide

6. Hypertension

7. Substance abuse

8. AIDS

9. Poor nutrition

III. Hispanic Americans

  A. Demographics

    1. Comprise 8 percent of the total United States population.

    2. Seventy percent of Hispanic-Americans were born in the United States.

    3. Eighty-seven percent live in urban areas.

    4. The largest group of migrant farm workers are Hispanic. For migrants the average life expectancy is forty-nine years.

    5. Hispanics are divided into five ethnic subgroups: Mexican-Americans, Puerto Ricans, Cuban-Americans, Central and South American immigrants, and other (unspecified).

    6. Mexican-Americans are concentrated in California and Texas; Puerto Ricans in the east coast states; and Cuban-Americans in Florida.

  B. General characteristics

    1. The Hispanic population has a strong extended-family orientation.

    2. Family needs supersede individual needs.

    3. Actions of individuals reflect on the family as a unit and individuals are expected to contribute positively to the collective achievement of the family as a group.

    4. Definitions of family may include close friends and the children's godparents (Patrinos or Compadrazgos), who share the social support network and have the responsibilities of family members.

    5. Family structure is age-graded, with the young subordinate to older persons.

    6. Older persons are shown respect and viewed as wise.

    7. Aging and the realities of aging are accepted and culturally sanctioned.

    8. As Hispanics age, role shifts are allowed. Those no longer able to perform hard physical labor assure family continuity by being transmitters of accumulated wisdom, nurturers of small children, religious teachers, or family historians (Yee 1990).

    9. Strong gender roles are upheld. Women may play a significant role in the home, but men exercise the major authority, particularly in matters outside the home.

    10. Machismo, the male role, requires that males act as head of the household, breadwinner, primary decision maker, protector, and provider for dependent family members.

    11. Machismo may prevent men from admitting illness or seeking treatment until severe functional impairment occurs.

    12. Wellness is based on a belief in equilibrium—a balance between man and nature.

    13. Illness may be viewed as having natural or supernatural causes.

    14. The presence of family members is very important during illness.

    15. Disease is caused by "hot" and "cold" imbalance. To treat illness, agents having the opposite quality of the causative agent must be applied.

    16. Religion is very important. The major religion of most Hispanic-Americans is Catholic.

    17. "Last rites" are seen as essential preparation for dying but may be delayed as long as possible to prevent the client from believing that the family has given up hope.

18. Hispanic individuals may believe that the outcome of circumstances is controlled by external forces.

19. A high value is placed on modesty; caregiving by persons of the opposite sex may be resisted.

20. Sex is a sensitive topic. Care of male genitals by females is generally not acceptable.

21. Multiple senses are used in communication. Problems that have emotional components may be described using dramatic body language.

22. Small talk or informal social interaction needs to precede the collection of health care data or the delivery of health care services to establish trust and interest. Self-disclosure is reserved only for the trusted and the client must be given time to size up health care providers.

23. Kidding will be viewed as rude and offensive.

24. Clients will respond better to nondirective, open-ended questions. If translators are used, they should be the same sex as the client.

25. Herbs and herbal teas are used in the practice of folk medicine. Careful history should be taken to determine what is being used. These folk remedies may counteract or potentiate prescription medications.

C. Folk healers

    1. Family folk healer

    2. Jerbero

    3. Yerbero

    4. Santero

    5. Curandero or curandera (practices white magic)

    6. Brujos or Brujas (witches who practice black, red, or green magic)

    7. Sobodoras (masseuses)

D. Folk illnesses

    1. Diseases can be a result of: mal puesto ("evil put on")—witchcraft; mal ojo ("evil eye")—magical disorder caused when a strong person exerts influence over a weak one; susto (fright)—an unsettling experience that causes one's soul to detach from the body; empacho—dysfunction of the digestive tract; sea por Dios (the will of God)—disorder as a punishment for wrongdoing.

E. Causes of morbidity and mortality

    1. Diabetes

    2. Obesity

    3. Smoking

    4. Cerebrovascular disease

IV. Native Americans and Alaska Natives

A. Demographics

    1. Comprise 1.6 million persons in the United States population.

    2. Broad cultural group is divided into four hundred federally recognized nations.

3. One-third live on reservations or historic trust lands.

4. Fifty percent of this population group live in urban centers.

5. Twenty-five percent live on incomes below the poverty threshold.

B. General characteristics of American Indians (Native Americans)

1. Extended family network with strong kinship ties is important.

2. Older Native Americans are family leaders.

3. Older members play a central role in family life by providing guidance to the young, exercising spiritual leadership, and maintaining cultural heritage.

4. Among reservation Indians, the older adult's pension or Social Security check may relieve the poverty of younger family members (Yee 1990).

5. Family gender roles may be rigid, with women responsible for "kin keeping" and men for employment activities.

6. High mortality rates exist before age 45; the median age of American Indians is 23. Therefore there are proportionately fewer older people in comparison to the White population.

7. Human beings and nature are viewed as interrelated. Harmony is vital to both.

8. Medicine and religion are considered inseparable.

9. Death is considered a natural part of life. After death the soul returns to one's ancestors.

10. Native Americans may not subscribe to the germ theory of disease.

11. Health is defined as the interrelationship of social, physical, psychologic, and spiritual forces.

12. Entire family will be involved in selected folk healing rites.

13. Indians value responsibility to the tribe.

14. They have great respect for individual rights and believe that no person has the right to interfere in another's life unless specifically asked.

15. Native Americans believe that no one can speak for another or reveal personal things about another. Therefore health care providers may have difficulty obtaining information from family members regarding clients.

16. Individuals will not share confidences or personal information until trust is well established.

17. Sharing and generosity are more important than owning material things. Individuals are more valued than possessions.

18. Great significance is placed on keeping one's word or promise. Native American groups note with disappointment that the White man has broken all major treaties made with Indians and that promises of Whites are not readily or consistently kept.

19. Groups may believe that many events cannot be changed by human action.

20. Listening is highly valued.

21. Indian clients may avoid eye contact as a courtesy to the health care provider. Direct eye contact is considered an invasion of privacy and is therefore considered impolite.

22. Modesty is valued.

23. Handshakes are brief or may be marked by a passing or brushing of hands. Vigorous or prolonged handshaking may be viewed as an aggressive act.

24. Time focus tends to be present oriented. Time is seen as having no beginning and no end.

25. The concept of "just being" may be important. One's value is not measured by constant activity.

26. Native Americans resent things being forced on them. Each family member is given the opportunity to participate in family decision making and problem solving.

27. Directions may be considered a power source in daily life: the east represents positive thinking; the west represents life; the south represents planning; and the north represents hope (Marchione and Stearns 1990).

C. American Indian folk healers

1. Medicine man or woman

2. Shaman

D. Causes of morbidity and mortality among American Indians

1. Alcoholism (As many as 95 percent of Native American families are affected directly or indirectly by alcohol abuse.)

2. Unintentional injury

3. Diabetes or complications of diabetes

4. Cirrhosis

5. Homicide

6. Suicide

7. Pneumonia

8. Tuberculosis

9. Obesity

E. General characteristics of Alaska Natives

1. Place a high value on modesty.

2. The extended family is the primary social unit.

3. Family rights take precedence over individual rights.

4. Individual choice in behavior is valued so long as the integrity of the group is not jeopardized.

5. Older Eskimos may view illness as a disease of the spirit or as the result of a violation of a taboo.

6. Value periods of silence and thinking in conversation.

7. Place a high value on interpreting body language; evaluate others based on their body language.

8. Modesty is highly valued, particularly among older persons.

9. The handshake is an expression of mandatory politeness.

10. Eskimo language contains no terminology that recognizes the future—their language describes all actions in the present.

11. The Eskimo language has no vehicle for the transmission of abstract ideas.

12. Eskimos refer to themselves as well as to others in the third person.

F. Causes of morbidity and mortality among Alaska Natives

1. Lactose intolerance

2. Sucrose intolerance

3. Susceptibility to narrow angle glaucoma

4. Endemic haemophilus, type b

Appendix A was compiled from the following: Allen and Chin-Sang 1990; Dr. Clement Au M.D., Chinatown, Philadelphia, PA; Burnside 1988; Clavon 1986; Downes 1986; Freebairn and Gwinup 1979; Giger and Davidhizer 1991; Marchione and Stearns 1990; Reinhart 1983; Ross and Cobb 1990; Tien-Hyatt 1987; United States Department of Health and Human Services 1990; and Yee 1990.

Appendix B

Psychosocial Assessment Guide

Name _____ Sex _____ Birth date _____

I. Questions in this section are designed to obtain basic identification data and to establish the purpose of contact with the health care facility or worker.

Current address _____

Permanent address _____

Phone numbers at which you can be reached: Home _____

Business _____ Other (friend, relative) _____

Marital status: S   M   D   W   Other (live with friend, common-law spouse) _____

If married, name of spouse _____

Address _____ Phone number _____

Social Security number _____

Other hospital/medical insurance policy _____

Medicare number _____

Religious preference _____

Name of person to be contacted in case of an emergency_____

Relationship to client _____ Phone number _____

Address _____

Name of family physician _____

Names of other physicians currently involved in your care _____

Brief description of initial impression of the client (include dress, speech patterns, gait, manner, and attitude toward the interviewer): _____

_____

_____

_____

_____

_____

II. Data collected in this section will be directed toward examination of the chief complaint. An attempt will be made to determine whether the chief complaint represents "signal behavior" or is an accurate representation of the older adult's needs. Questions asked will also allow the nurse to identify the health belief system of the client which may impact nursing care.

_____

Chief complaint _____

When did it start? _____

What do you think caused your problem? _____

Why do you think it started when it did? _____

What do you think your illness has done to you? _____

How does it work? _____

How bad do you think your illness is? _____

Do you think it will last a long time or improve soon? _____

What kind of treatment have you tried? _____

What kind of treatment do you think you need now? _____

What results do you expect from treatment? _____

What problems has your illness caused for you? _____

What frightens you most about your illness? _____

Who is helping you manage with your illness?_____

How did you hope I could help you today?_____

III. Questions in this segment of the assessment guide are designed to obtain information concerning the past medical history of the client. See chapter 6, Health Assessment, for a detailed review.

IV. This section of the assessment guide focuses on obtaining data through a review of systems (ROS) history. See chapter 6, Health Assessment, for a detailed review.

V. Questions in this sequence are designed to obtain a picture of the current health status and preventive health practices of the client. These questions include some that ask for the respondent's evaluation of his or her own health status. This technique has proven accurate when used with older clients (Idler and Kasl 1991).

A. At the present time, how would you rate your health—excellent, good, fair, poor, or bad? Explain.

B. Are you presently being treated by a physician or other health practitioner for any condition or chronic illness? Please describe.

C. If chronic illness exists, how has your illness affected your lifestyle? Your family?

D. Have you noted any change in or impairment of

| _____ sight | _____ taste | _____ hearing |
| _____ smell | _____ touch | _____ balance |

E. Do you have any difficulty getting around? Sitting? Standing? Turning self in bed? Getting in and out of tub or shower?

F. Are you able to perform the following activities of daily living alone or do you need assistance? (Mark *S* for self-performed, *A* for assistance needed)

Self-care activities:

_____ Feeding self	_____ Bathing _____ tub _____ shower
_____ Dressing	_____ sponge bath
_____ Toileting	_____ Combing/arranging hair _____ Driving car
_____ Dialing phone	_____ Applying makeup _____ Reading
_____ Shaving	_____ Climbing stairs
_____ Washing hair	_____ Opening doors

Home maintenance activities:

_____ Vacuuming	_____ Food preparation _____ Shopping
_____ Dusting	_____ Washing dishes
_____ Scrubbing	_____ Laundry
_____ Garbage disposal	_____ Ironing
_____ Mowing/maintaining yard	_____ Minor household repairs

G. Do you have, wear, or use any of the following appliances or supportive devices?

_____ Artificial limb	_____ Insulin pump
_____ Braces	_____ IPPB machine
_____ Cane	_____ Large-print/talking books
_____ Contact lenses	_____ Mechanical lift
_____ Crutches	_____ Nebulizers
_____ Dentures	_____ Oxygen concentrator, portable tanks, units
_____ Glasses (reading, bifocals, trifocals)	_____ Pacemaker
_____ Hospital bed	_____ Parenteral nutrition support
_____ Hearing aid	_____ Phone amplifier

If any of the preceding are used by the client, the nurse should determine when their use commenced, whether the devices were prescribed by a physician or were self-prescribed, the date they were last evaluated by a physician or nurse, problems or difficulties encountered in their use, and existence of insurance coverage.

H. Which of the following health care providers do you use?

_____ Chiropractor	_____ Pharmacist
_____ Companion/sitter	_____ Podiatrist/chiropodist
_____ Dentist	_____ Psychologist
_____ Home health aide	_____ Psychiatrist
_____ Homemaker	_____ Physical therapist
_____ LVN/LPN	_____ Physician/M.D., D.O.
_____ Native/ethnic practitioner	_____ Registered nurse
_____ Neighbor/friend	_____ Social worker
_____ Nutritionist/dietitian	_____ Speech-language pathologist
_____ Occupational therapist	_____ Spiritual healer

The nurse should secure data concerning the frequency and reason for contacts with any of these personnel, the benefits sustained from their treatment or care, and duration of the treatment plan authorizing their use.

I. Are you disturbed by pain or discomfort? (Include the location, intensity, duration, activities with which pain is associated, and methods commonly used to relieve pain.)

J. Patterns of medication usage. Ask client to take you to the place where he or she stores medications and look at all of them. Medications are a major problem in management of care and the nurse will learn more by observation than by report.

1. What medications are you presently taking regularly? (Include date of onset of therapy, dosage ordered, dosage taken, reason for use, results obtained, side effects, allergic responses, and the date last evaluated by M.D.)

   Prescription medications (Example: Digoxin, Lasix):

   Over-the-counter drugs (Example: aspirin, laxatives, vitamins):

   Mood-altering drugs (Example: marijuana, cocaine, amphetamines, alcohol):

   Other:

2. What medications do you keep on hand for periodic use? Reason for use? Expiration date on these drugs?

3. Are you presently receiving prescription medications from more than one physician? Are these physicians aware of each other's participation in your care?

4. Do you have difficulty remembering when to take medications or if you have already taken them? Have you ever accidentally taken an overdose? ever omitted a dose? ever increased a dose?

5. Do you understand the reason you are taking current medications? the importance of taking them as prescribed? the side effects or allergic responses for which you must notify the physician? Do you need additional information concerning these medications?

6. Do you have difficulty opening medication containers? reading print on the labels? obtaining prescriptions or refills?

7. Do you store medications in an area where they cannot be confused with household chemicals or another person's medications?

8. How much do your medications cost each month? Are you having any difficulty paying for the medications you need?

K. Current immunization history

Type of immunization, date, unusual response or reaction:

_____ Diphtheria toxoid	_____ Polio
_____ Tetanus toxoid	Salk
_____ DT toxoid	Sabin
_____ Tetanus antitoxin	_____ Tuberculin skin test
_____ Mumps	_____ Typhoid
_____ Measles	_____ Influenza
Rubeola	_____ Homemaker
Rubella	_____ Other:
_____ Pneumonia	

L. Do you have any routines or practices that you follow to maintain your health? (Example: breast self-examination, colorectal cancer screening, diet, exercise, annual physical examination, semiannual dental examination, fasting, purging)

M. For what reasons do you usually seek health care?

N. How would you describe the health of your spouse? Has there been any recent change in his/her health? Do you provide physical care for your spouse?

VI. Questions in this section are designed to obtain data regarding personal habits and patterns of living. These patterns may be used as a basis for planning nursing care that will produce the least disruption in the client's life or that may indicate present or potential problems that will require alteration in long-standing habit patterns.

A. Dietary patterns

1. Do you follow a special diet? If so, was it presecribed by a physician or was it self-prescribed?

2. Please describe a typical daily plan for meals (twenty-four hour recall). In addition to regular meals, include any snacks.

3. What foods do you especially enjoy (include snacks)?

4. What foods are avoided? For what reason?

5. Have you noticed any difference in the taste of foods? smell of foods? If so, do you find yourself trying to correct these deficits by adding seasonings, salt, or making other changes?

6. Do you have any difficulty chewing? swallowing? Do you have episodes of choking?

7. How would you describe your appetite? The volume or amount of food consumed?

8. Are meals usually eaten alone or with others?

9. Are meals eaten at home? in restaurants? senior citizen centers? at home with the aid of home-delivered meals programs? with relatives?

10. Are you able to shop for and prepare your own food? How many hot meals do you eat per week?

11. Approximately what percentage of your income is used for food? Are you receiving food stamps? Do you have difficulty purchasing the foods you need and want?

12. What beverages are consumed? number of glasses or cups per day? Do you find it difficult to remember to drink enough fluids? Which fluids are preferred? which avoided? Do you prefer beverages cold, temperate, or hot?

13. Do you use alcoholic beverages?

    a. Type of beverages enjoyed (mixed drinks, beer, wine, whiskey)

    b. Pattern of use: occasional cocktail? daily drinks? with meals? throughout the day?

    c. Number of glasses, cans, jiggers, or shots consumed per day? per week?

    d. Have any physical changes occurred as a result of your use of alcohol? (Example: forgetfulness, confusion, amnesia during periods of use, malnutrition, injury)

    e. Have any social changes occurred as a result of your use of alcohol? (Example: divorce, alienation from children, arrest)

14. What is your usual weight? Has there been any recent gain or loss? Do you consider yourself overweight? underweight?

B. Patterns of elimination

1. How frequently do you have bowel movements (elimination)?

2. Color, shape, and consistency of stool? Experience any difficulty passing stool? Usual time of day for evacuation?

3. Are there any special routines used to maintain bowel regularity? (Example: laxatives, enemas, digital removal of feces, prune juice)

4. Are you bothered with flatus (gas)? If so, what do you do for this problem?

5. What is the frequency of urinary elimination? amount eliminated per time? color? odor? quality of stream?

6. Do you have any difficulty initiating and maintaining urinary stream? Do you experience pain when voiding?

7. Do you have any difficulty with dribbling or seepage of urine especially when laughing, coughing, or physically straining? Do you ever experience urinary incontinence or loss of bladder control?

C. Patterns of rest and sleep

1. How many hours of sleep and rest do you require per day? Do you feel rested after sleep? What do you do to rest when not planning sleep? What time do you go to bed? Get up?

2. Have you noticed any changes in patterns of sleep and wakefulness as compared with your younger years?

3. Do you take "cat naps" during the day?

4. Do you experience any difficulty in falling asleep? Maintaining sleep?

5. Do you have wakeful periods during the night? What initiates these?

6. Have you noticed or have you been told about any changes in your behavior at night? Do you ever become confused or disoriented? Have difficulty remembering where you are?

7. Do you use items that provide a protective environment at night? (Example: nightlights, bedrails, bedside commode)

8. Are any special bedtime rituals used to facilitate sleep? (Example: warm milk, warm bath, reading, sleeping medications)

9. What equipment is used on the bed to provide comfort? (Example: bedboard, number of blankets, number of pillows)

10. Do you sleep alone or share a bed (or bedroom)? Does having another person in bed or bedroom interfere with your ability to sleep?

D. Patterns of exercise and activity

1. Tell me about the type and amount of exercise you have in a typical day; in a week.

2. Are you involved in any special exercise program? Has this program been prescribed by your physician or is it self-prescribed?

3. Do you tire easily or become winded upon exertion?

4. Do you have any difficulty pacing yourself to complete necessary daily tasks? How does your physical stamina compare with that of your younger years?

5. Do you find that you have more leisure time than you did before retirement (if retired)? Have you had any difficulty adjusting to the use of this time?

6. What activities do you engage in during the day (or evening)? Which of these activities do you find most meaningful? (Example: visiting with others, travel, television, volunteer work, participating in social groups, learning new skills, caring for grandchildren, gardening)

7. Can you think of any activities you have lost interest in or have given up as a result of changes due to aging?

8. Have you changed any of your activities due to changes in senses? (Example: decreased vision, decreased hearing)

9. Do you have transportation available to take you to activities? (Example: church, senior centers)

10. Are activities limited by your environment? (Example: high-crime neighborhood, no recreational resources)

E. Patterns of sexual activity

1. At what age did you experience the onset of sexual activity?

2. Are you presently sexually active? with one partner? more than one?

3. Are your sexual partners about the same age as yourself? older? younger? Is birth control or family planning information desired?

4. How do your present sexual interest and activity compare with the patterns followed during your younger years?

5. Have any of the physical changes of aging created difficulty in having sexual intercourse? (Example: slower erection, slower ejaculation, decrease in sensual experience, pain, difficulty achieving orgasm)

6. Has there been any recent change in your patterns of sexual activity? Do you have any special concerns about your present level of sexual functioning?

7. Do you find pleasure in nongenital forms of sexual expression, such as cuddling, touching, kissing?

8. Female client:

   a. How old were you at onset of menses (menarche)? At onset of menopause? At cessation of menses? Were you troubled by any physical or emotional changes that accompanied menopause?

   b. Date of last Pap smear?

   c. Do you perform monthly breast self-examination?

   d. How many pregnancies have you experienced? Number of live births? Miscarriages? Types of birth? Complications of pregnancies or deliveries? Any residual effects of childbearing?

   e. Have you experienced any difficulty with your female organs? Had a hysterectomy?

9. Male client:

   a. Have you noted changes in the size or anatomic position of genitalia?

   b. Have you had a vasectomy? Date?

   c. Do you perform self-examination for testicular cancer?

10. If currently sexually active, what methods are you using to protect yourself from sexually transmitted diseases?

11. Are you taking any medications that have affected sexual performance?

F. Patterns of tobacco utilization

   1. Have you ever used tobacco? Do you presently use tobacco? On a periodic basis? Daily basis?

   2. What form or forms of tobacco do you use? (Example: cigarettes, cigars, pipe, snuff)

   3. If tobacco is smoked, number of cigarettes, cigars, pipes smoked per day?

   4. Have you experienced any physical changes as a result of your smoking? Have any conditions been aggravated by your tobacco habit?

VII. Questions in this section will explore the relationship of the client to others—family, friends, and support groups. Satisfaction in later adulthood seems to depend closely upon the existence and quality of relationships with significant others. The nurse will wish to involve these individuals in planning care for and with clients.

A. Tell me about the family from which you came: Parents, grandparents, siblings? Cultural background? Level of education? Health status? History of disease and causes of death of family members?

B. Present family

   1. Tell me about the family you formed:

      a. How long have you been married to your present spouse? Is your marital partner younger or older? Have there been previous marriages? Length of these marriages and reason for termination?

      b. Tell me about children and grandchildren: Names, ages, sex, occupation, state of health?

      c. What are the roles and responsibilities of present family members? Who makes the major decisions in the family?

      d. Have there been any major problems in the family? How has the family responded to these stressful situations?

2. What present responsibilities do you have for your parents? Spouse? Children? Siblings? Do you share these responsibilities with other family members?

3. Are you responsible for caring for a parent or child who is a senior adult?

4. If you are responsible for dependent relatives, have you made alternate plans for them should you become incapacitated?

5. Have your responsibilities within the family changed in recent years? In what way?

6. Does your family support you in your decisions? (Example: to live alone, to marry or remarry, to travel) Do members of your family provide support for one another in crisis situations?

7. Do you live near the members of your family? How are family contacts maintained? (Example: visits, phone calls, letters) How often do you have contact with other family members?

8. If you are a grandparent, what is the nature of your relationship to your grandchildren? Amount and type of involvement?

9. If you are living with children or another relative, has this had any effect on your lifestyle? (Example: limitation of customary activities, lack of privacy, feelings of dependency) Do you expect this arrangement to be permanent?

10. What activities are enjoyed by and include the whole family?

11. How do you think the members of your family would describe you (spouse's, children's, siblings' and parents' views)?

12. Tell me about friends. Are there friends who are especially significant? Are these friendships of long standing? Are they new friendships? Do you hear from friends on a daily basis?

13. Do you belong to any groups or organizations? (Example: church, civic, professional) Are you presently active in these groups? What has been your role in the past? What is your weekly schedule of activities?

14. Are there people upon whom you feel you can rely? Are there special people you would want summoned in case of an emergency?

15. Are pets present in your home? What type? Are they a source of pleasure or annoyance to you?

16. Do you find your physician and local medical facility to be supportive in meeting your needs?

17. What type of help are you able to give to others? family? friends? organizations?

18. If living alone, are you frightened? lonely? bored? victim of a crime?

VIII. Questions in Section VIII center around cultural identity and socioeconomic status. These are often the chief qualities used by people to evaluate life performance and to determine success or failure. Roles are often defined in terms of jobs held and positions achieved. Loss or change in a defined role and a lowering of the standard of living due to retirement often form the major crises for the older client.

A. Economic data

1. In what range, approximately, does your annual income fall?

   _____ Below $5,000   _____ $20,000–$29,999
   _____ $5,000–$9,999   _____ $30,000–$39,999
   _____ $10,000–$14,999   _____ $40,000–49,999
   _____ $15,000–$19,000   _____ $50,000 or above

2. What are current sources of income?

   _____ Social Security   _____ Supplemental Security
   _____ Pension plan   Income (SSI)
   _____ Return on investments   _____ Disability
   _____ Life insurance   _____ Public assistance
   _____ Full-time employment   _____ Spousal support
   _____ Part-time employment   _____ Family contributions
   _____ Veterans' benefits   _____ Other: _____

3. What methods are used to pay for your health care? (Example: Medicare, Medicaid, private insurance, direct payment) What percentage of your income must be used to meet medical expenses?

4. Is your income adequate to meet financial needs for items such as

   _____ rent or house payments, taxes   _____ clothing
   _____ food   _____ operation and upkeep on car
   _____ insurance (life, health, home, car) _____ utility bills
   _____ pet care   _____ recreation
   _____ medical care, dental care   _____ gifts

5. Are there any major expenses or debts that concern you?

6. Does your family have a special system for allotting money to members, such as allowances?

7. If you are retired, how would you describe the change in your income from that received during the years of full employment? What effect has this change had on your standard of living?

8. Are you presently managing your own financial affairs? Are you having any difficulty in this area?

9. Have you designated someone to manage your affairs should you become seriously ill or disabled?

10. Has there been any conflict in your family regarding the use of your current assets or their perceived patterns of inheritance?

11. If you should become incapacitated, do you have assets that could be used to provide care for you?

B. Educational background

1. Tell me about your education. Schools attended? Age span during educational involvement? Degrees or certificates awarded? Attitude toward education?

2. Are you presently involved in educational or creative endeavors? If so, are you pursuing education as a goal to facilitate a career change, for self-enrichment, or for social interaction?

C. Work or employment history

1. Tell me about the jobs you have had since you first began working until your retirement. Job titles? Duties performed? Positions achieved? (*Note to nurse*: Job history will often indicate exposure to occupational or industrial hazards that may have initiated the process of a long-term chronic disease.)

2. Was retirement voluntary or mandatory? When did you retire? When did spouse retire? Did you plan ahead for the transition from work to retirement?

3. Are relationships continuing with friends and colleagues at former place(s) of work?

4. Has retirement had any effect on your marriage?

5. Have friends been helpful as you make the transition into the years of retirement?

D. Cultural history

1. In what country, state, town were you born?

2. To which ethnic or cultural group do you belong? Has identification with this group changed or evolved in your lifetime? Has this been a source of conflict for you?

3. Are special ethnic or cultural practices maintained in the family unit and conveyed to subsequent generations?

4. What is your native language? What other languages do you speak? What language is primarily used in the home? When you are under stress?

5. What place do you consider home? (Example: house, neighborhood, country, state)

IX. The questions in this section seek to explore the older adult's self-image, spiritual strength and resources, perception of the effect aging is having on his or her present life, and plans and goals for the future. Aging is accompanied not only by role losses but also by losses of family members, friends, and support systems essential to identity. In addition the older person is often concerned with participation in and control over planning for his or her own death. Nursing support is indicated as the client seeks to evaluate the meaning of his or her own life and a satisfactory style for concluding it.

A. Self-concept

1. How would you describe yourself?

2. Have you identified any changes in your personality or sense of values since your younger years?

3. What things in life are now especially important to you?

4. What do you consider the most significant events in your life? (Example: marriage, first job, birth of children, winning Pulitzer prize)

5. As a young adult did you set any specific goals for your life? At this point how do you view your progress in relation to these goals?

6. What do you enjoy most about this stage of your life? Compared with that of your younger years, how would you rate your present level of happiness and satisfaction?

7. How would you describe your physical appearance? Are there changes in your appearance that please or displease you? Are they what you expected?

8. Do physical changes make it difficult for clothes to fit like they once did? Do you have trouble with waistlines? Hems? Are you able to make alterations yourself or do you need assistance?

9. How do you compare yourself physically and mentally to other adults your age?

10. As you think about the aging process and its effects on you, do you have any special concerns or fears?

11. Do you find that you now enjoy thinking about or reviewing events from your past? Are you able to share those reflections with others?

12. Has "life review" created any special problems for you? Has it led to any personal action? (Example: reestablishing broken relationships)

13. What have been the pleasant "surprises" in your life? The unexpected events that had a major impact on who you are?

14. What are your future goals or plans?

B. Attitude toward loss and death

(*Note to nurse*: Very often the client's attitude toward the aging process and death are developed from perceptions of these aspects of life as applied to his or her own parents or significant others. It is not unusual for the older adult to experience "anniversary reactions" on the date of death of a loved one or to unconsciously program his or her own demise on the basis of these perceptions [Burgess 1976].)

1. Tell me about aging as it applied to your parents.

2. Did you or your siblings provide care for a parent before death?

3. How old were your parents at the time of death? Did their deaths come after long illness or suddenly? Did they die at home or in a hospital?

4. Do you experience any grief or other reaction on the anniversary date of a loved one's death?

5. Have you thought about your own death? Did you have any thoughts about what it will be like? Have you any special concerns regarding your own death?

6. Have you made any special arrangements regarding your own death? (Example: burial plot, will, prepaid funeral arrangements)

7. Do you have an attorney? Will you need assistance with legal matters, such as wills, living wills, power of attorney?

8. Have you discussed your wishes regarding extraordinary life-support measures, organ donorship, and burial with members of your family? With your physician?

C. Response to loss of spouse, friends

1. Have you lost a spouse? How long ago? What changes did this loss make in your life? How did you react to this loss? How are you presently reacting?

2. Was spouse ill before death? Who provided the necessary care for him or her?

3. Has your health changed since being widowed? Have you had any major episodes of illness since bereavement?

4. Has the death of any other relative or friend had a great impact on you?

5. Can you identify any new relationships that have emerged or old ones that have become stronger since bereavement?

6. Do you ever have feelings of loneliness and depression? If so, how do they affect you? What steps do you take to alleviate these feelings?

7. Do you have any special religious preference? Are you a member of a church? Do you participate in religious activities?

8. Are you interested in spiritual matters even though you are not a member of an established church?

9. Is there clergy or a spiritual counselor you would like to have involved in your care or called in case of an emergency?

X. Questions in this section are used to ascertain mental status and orientation to reality. If the client appears confused, the nurse may wish to conduct this portion of the assessment at the outset. If all has gone well in earlier sections of the interview, the nurse may wish to omit this segment.

A. Reality orientation (state of consciousness and sensory awareness)

1. What is your name?

2. How old are you?

3. Can you tell me the day? Month? Year?

4. Where are you? city? State? Nation?

5. Who is president of the United States?

6. Name the parts of your body as I point to them. (Example: head, foot, knee)

7. Please identify the odors as I present them. (Example: onion, lemon)

8. What time of day is it?

9. What color is this? (Example: identify red, green, yellow, blue)

10. What are the names of these objects? (Present: pencil, key, glass)

11. Tell me how this feels. (Example: ice, warm water, sandpaper, plastic)

B. Speech: What language is spoken? Are speech patterns congruent with the educational status of the client? Are words distinct and is speech-flow fluid? Is the client's use of language appropriate for the situation? Is there any impairment in speech? Evidence of aphasia? Do ideas flow in a logical sequence?

C. Is client interested in and aware of his or her surroundings?

D. Does client demonstrate culturally correct responses in social situations? (Example: shake hands)

E. Is affect appropriate for content discussed?

F. Is the ability to abstract present? (Example: Client can explain meaning of "a bird in the hand is worth two in the bush.")

G. Is computational ability intact? (Example: Can client subtract multiple 7s from 100 to reach 0 or solve a problem such as "If you bought a brush that cost 75¢ and you gave the clerk $1.00, how much change would you receive?")

H. Does client demonstrate the ability to hear and process information by responding to instructions?

I. Is recent memory intact? (Examiner may test by presenting a series of five digits and asking the client to repeat them)

J. Is remote memory intact? (Ask about date of marriage, birth of children)

K. Do family members or caregivers describe troublesome or abnormal behavior patterns?

L. Level of anxiety during interview?

M. Score on Depression Scale or Mini Mental Status Exam.

XI. Items in Section XI may be used by the nurse in assessment of the institutionalized client. Some of the items are presented in the form of questions to be asked of the client. Other items are observations to be made by the nurse. If evidence of behavioral change due to isolation and dehumanization exists, immediate nursing action is indicated.

A. Process of institutional admission

1. Who made the decision that extended care/skilled nursing home or hospital was needed? To what extent was the client involved in this decision?

2. How was this institution selected? By client? By family? By physician? By social worker?

3. Was visit made before selection and admission to facility? By client? By family?

4. What present feelings does client express concerning presence in the institution? Does he or she view tenure as long-term or of short duration?

B. Adjustment to the institution

1. Has the client's behavior regressed since admission? Can the nurse identify factors contributing to this regression?

2. What losses (role, possession, self-esteem) have occurred as a result of admission to the facility?

3. What are the client's patterns of interaction with other residents?

4. Does the client evidence increased depersonalization through such behaviors as hoarding of food, "pack ratting"?

5. Who comes to visit? How long do they stay? How often do they come? What is the client's reaction to the visit? What do they do with or for the client during the visit?

6. Does client receive mail? How often? From whom?

7. If lonely, does the client attempt to deny that there is no one who is concerned about him or her?

8. Are the client's social contacts limited, contributing to the phenomenon of body monitoring and hypochondriasis?

9. Does the client express feelings of shame at present state and express the opinion that he or she is "useless" or a "burden" to others?

10. Is there visible evidence of depression? (Example: apathy, withdrawal, loss of appetite, constipation, chronic fatigue, frequent somatic complaints)

11. Is there evidence of the client attempting to commit benign suicide through *(a)* refusal of medications or food, *(b)* inability to retain food, *(c)* stating he or she is tired of living, *(d)* repeatedly placing self in dangerous situation, *(e)* apathy?

12. Is the client predicting his or her own death?

13. Is there behavioral evidence of anxiety or fear? (Example: manipulative behavior, rigid behavior patterns, rage, chronic irritability, delusions, paranoia, denial, garrulousness, hostility, anger)

14. Does the client engage in destructive behavior toward self or others?

15. Does the client participate in activities of the institution?

16. Is the client able to verbalize his or her feelings about institutionalization?

17. Has the client formed positive relationships with selected staff members?

XII. The single question in Section XII is designed to give the client a chance to clarify information, express serious concerns of his or her own, or to simply ask questions.

---

1. Is there anything you would like to ask me?

GUIDE FOR FAMILY ASSESSMENT

The guide that follows may be used in obtaining information from members of the family and significant others (friends) of the client.

1. Family composition: names, relationship to client.

2. How would you describe relationships within the family?

3. How does the family as a whole cope with stress?

4. Have there been recent changes in family composition that have created stress, such as marriage of older adult?

5. What role does the older adult play in decisions regarding his or her care?

6. How do you view the ability of the client to make important decisions concerning
   a) independent living arrangements?
   b) health care?
   c) self-care?
   d) financial affairs?
   e) property management?

7. How would the family feel about and who would make important decisions regarding the older adult should he or she become incompetent to do so? (Such decisions might include admission to nursing home, sale of house, disposal of personal possessions.)

8. How would you describe the client's personality?

9. Have there been any changes in the client's personality in recent years?

10. How would you describe the client's present state of health?

11. What do you see as the greatest assets of character or physical development possessed by client?

12. How would you describe physical or psychologic limitations of your older relative?

13. How would you describe the client's typical response to stress?

14. Has the client developed or exhibited any behaviors that are disturbing to the family?

15. Has there been any change in the parent/child, sibling/sibling, spouse/spouse relationship in recent years?

16. What is the present family role of the older adult?

17. How would you describe your relative's ability to adapt to a new environment? new people? new situations?

18. Are you receiving income from the older adult? How does that affect your lifestyle? How does it affect the client's lifestyle?

19. What services does the older adult provide for you? (Example: babysitting with grandchildren)

20. What services are you presently providing for the older adult? How are these viewed by the rest of the family?

21. Who bears primary responsibility for the financial support of the older adult?

22. Who bears primary responsibility for the physical care of the older adult? housing?

23. Are you providing financial support to your older relative?

24. If yes, has this provision of financial assistance been difficult? What effect has it had on meeting the needs of your own family? How do other family members view this?

25. Is financial support of the older adult shared by sibling children or the adult's own siblings? If so, how were these arrangements determined? How do family members who are involved feel about them?

26. Does the older adult live with your family? What effect has this had on the lifestyle of your family? On each individual in the family, especially children?

27. Has the older adult experienced difficulty adjusting in one relative's home and subsequently been moved to another?

28. Are there other relatives or friends who can be relied on in a crisis or emergency or who would be actively interested in or involved with the client?

29. Are family members able to give physical care to the client if needed? If a medical condition exists, does the family understand its present status? How it may change in the future? What treatments and medications are prescribed?

30. Does the family desire information and assistance in learning to provide care for acute or chronic conditions of the client?

31. Will outside assistance be needed in caring for the client? Maid? Skilled nursing care? Home health aide? Homemaker?

32. Does the family need information concerning available community resources to help maintain client at home? (Example: Visiting Nurse Association, equipment supply agencies, senior center programs, home-delivered meals, Alcoholics Anonymous, welfare department, cancer society, financial assistance programs, budget counseling, physical therapy, occupational therapy, speech therapy)

33. What recreational pursuits are followed by the family that is caring for an older adult? Do caregivers have a chance to get away for awhile? Who cares for the older adult while the family is gone? Are services such as adult day care, respite care, or personal care boarding homes used?

34. What preparation does the older relative receive before the family leaves for vacations or extended trips?

35. What activities does the family engage in with client?

36. Recreation for client (trips, movies)?

37. Has there been any difficulty within the family over proposed dispersal of assets and property after the death of the older adult?

38. Does a family member have the client's power of attorney? How do other members view this situation?

39. If the older adult is ill, was the onset of illness gradual? Sudden?

40. What type of treatment was given by health care personnel? Did the family feel treatment was effective? ineffective?

41. What is the degree of involvement of the physician in the care plan? Does the physician see the client in hospital or as outpatient?

42. If the family has admitted the older adult to an institution
    a. What feelings have been experienced by the family since the decision was made to place the older adult in the hospital? Nursing home? Extended care facility?
    b. Do you find the staff in the institution supportive? Hostile?

    c. Do you feel you are getting sufficient information concerning the client's care?

    d. Does the staff listen to your ideas and suggestions concerning care?

    e. Do you want to assist with the care of your relative? Does the institution allow this?

    f. What does the family expect of the client? Of the institution? Of the physician? Of the nurses?

43. If the family cares for the older adult at home or has placed family member in an institution, are they or do they wish to be involved in family support groups?

Appendix C

Home Environment Assessment Guide

CRITERIA FOR EVALUATION

General Information

1. Does the client live alone? With others?

2. In what type of home does client live? (Example: single-family dwelling, apartment, condominium, hotel, rooming house)

3. Brief description of home. (Size? One- or two story? Number of bedrooms? State of repair?)

4. Does client own or rent home?

5. How long has client lived in present home?

6. Brief description of environment in which the home is located. (Rundown neighborhood? High-crime area? Parks? Age-segregated?)

7. How far from home must client travel to

visit friends	visit physician
visit family	visit beauty/barber shop
shop	attend house of worship
bank	reach hospital

8. What type of water supply is available? (City? Well? Spring?)

9. What type of sewage disposal is present? (City? Septic tank?)

10. Are screens present on windows?

11. What type of heating is available? (Furnace—coal, oil, electric, gas? Wood stove? Fireplace? Oven? Space heater? electric blankets?)

12. How is home cooled? (Fans? Central air? Evaporative coolers?)

13. Is home supplied with electricity?

14. Does client own his or her own car? Age of car and state of repair? Does client presently drive car? Is license current? Are limitations noted on license? Does client use seat belts, shoulder harnesses? Has client had any recent accidents? Does client report any difficulty driving?

15. Is public transportation available? What type? (Bus? Taxi?) Does client use public transportation? Are special rates in effect for senior citizens?

Attributes Present in Environment:

Characteristics Facilitating Maintenance of Older Adult at Home

Check (✔) if Present

_____ 1. Doorways and passageways wide enough to accommodate wheelchair and other assistive equipment.

_____ 2. If assistive equipment is used, ramp is available to at least one entrance of home.

_____ 3. Telephone is present or an emergency signaling system has been developed to alert neighbors in case of an emergency.

_____ 4. Phone amplifiers are used if the client is hard of hearing.

_____ 5. Emergency phone numbers are clearly written in large numbers and letters and posted near the phone. Numbers listed include physician, ambulance, fire, police, relative, friend.

_____ 6. Neighbor, friend, or relative checks on client daily, in person if possible. If not, phone contact is made.

_____ 7. Client has clearly developed plan of action in case of an emergency such as fire, medical crisis, or criminal attack.

_____ 8. Adequate lighting is available both inside and outside of dwelling; lighting is of sufficient brightness to offset decreased visual acuity of older adult.

_____ 9. Sidewalks are in good repair and well illuminated.

_____ 10. Street lights and exterior house lights are present and placed in appropriate positions to deter breaking and entering.

_____ 11. Porch lights clearly illuminate steps and doors.

_____ 12. All stairs are well illuminated and top and bottom stairs are indicated by color coding (red, yellow, or orange) or illuminated stripes.

_____ 13. Stair risers are covered with or made of nonskid substance; all carpet runners on stairs are tacked firmly into place.

_____ 14. Handrails are present on at least one side of stairway, if not both.

_____ 15. Night lights are present in rooms and passageways to reduce confusion and disorientation at night.

_____ 16. Doors at stairwells are closed to decrease likelihood of accidental fall.

_____ 17. Locks are present on doors and windows to protect against burglary but can be opened easily from inside in case of fire; keys are stored for easy access and a spare set is kept. (Assessment of such locks is important because many older people cannot open doors and windows for ventilation. In summer heat waves they may die from heat exhaustion as a result of orifices sealed to prevent crime.)

_____ 18. Spare house keys are left with a neighbor or friend so that senior citizen may re-enter dwelling if accidentally locked out.

_____ 19. Windows and doors are properly caulked and sealed to reduce drafts that might contribute to hypothermia.

_____ 20. Furnace provides adequate warmth at an affordable price and is cleaned, oiled, and maintained yearly. Other devices used for heating are checked for safety hazards.

_____ 21. Senior citizen is cautioned about the danger of fire with wood stoves and space heaters. Flues, chimneys, and grates are checked frequently.

_____ 22. Older adult is warned about danger of burns if electric blanket or heating pad is used for heat and is cautioned to set heating devices in low position.

_____ 23. Ventilation is available in all rooms.

_____ 24. Exits are easily accessible and marked so they can be seen clearly at night in an emergency.

_____ 25. Smoke alarms are properly installed and working.

_____ 26. Stickers are affixed to windows, indicating to firefighters the rooms in which senior citizens sleep; this precaution aids emergency rescue in case of fire.

_____ 27. Fire extinguisher available in kitchen, or resident has been instructed in alternate methods of extinguishing kitchen fires.

_____ 28. Bathroom easily accessible and near sleeping quarter.

_____ 29. Toilet lids and seat tops affixed tightly.

_____ 30. Side rails and grip bars available near commode and tub to aid in mobility and transfer.

_____ 31. Bathtub and shower equipped with nonskid strips.

_____ 32. Equipment such as bath seats affixed firmly and free of rough or jagged edges.

_____ 33. Shower curtains and stalls are adequate to prevent water splashes on floors, which could precipitate a fall.

_____ 34. Water heater set to provide adequate heat for washing dishes but not hot enough to produce instant third-degree burns. (Faucets have adapters to control water temperature.)

_____ 35. Resident owns and knows how to use a bath thermometer and verifies temperature before bathing.

_____ 36. Floors level, smooth, and free of defects such as warped boards or torn linoleum.

_____ 37. Furniture sturdy and provides adequate support; no wobbly chairs or tables.

_____ 38. Furniture arranged to provide for clear, unimpeded lanes for moving from one room to another.

_____ 39. Throw rugs and area carpeting have been removed or are secured to flooring by suction cups or nonskid backing.

_____ 40. No electrical cords meander across floor to cause tripping.

_____ 41. Appliances in good repair and resident knows how to use them; absolutely no frayed cords.

_____ 42. Food storage and preparation facilities are present and in proper working order.

_____ 43. Beds at proper height to facilitate entry and exit; mattress provides firm, even support for spine. Side rails, if used, are in good repair.

_____ 44. Equipment or assistive devices (crutches, walkers, mechanical lifts, hospital beds, wheelchairs) are in good repair and the client or significant other has been instructed in their proper use and maintenance. Client has demonstrated safe use of any assistive devices in carrying out ADLs.

_____ 45. Sensory stimulation is available (books, radio, television). Telephone conveniently placed.

_____ 46. Medications stored away from cleansers and household chemicals.

_____ 47. Expired medications discarded and all current medications bear large-print labels; client can remove caps or gain access to medication containers without difficulty.

_____ 48. Laundry facilities are positioned to decrease the necessity for the older adult to carry heavy loads up and down stairs, or alternate plans are made to reduce size of loads or request assistance.

_____ 49. Lawn equipment (mowers, edgers, clippers) is lightweight, easy to use, and kept in good repair.

_____ 50. Preparations have been made to secure assistance for removal of ice and snow from walks and steps.

_____ 51. Garage door posts painted contrasting color or with luminous paint to decrease accidental collision.

_____ 52. Support systems are available in the community for the client who remains at home (visiting nurses, homemaker, home health aide, occupational therapist [OT], physical therapist [PT], speech-language pathologist, home-delivered meals, senior centers).

_____ 53. Client has been taught safe techniques for standing on stools and chairs to reach for objects.

_____ 54. Client has been taught to "fall safely" to reduce injury once a slip occurs.

_____ 55. Adaptations have been made in cleaning equipment and techniques to reduce fatigue in performing household chores. (Example: stool provided so that client can sit to iron).

_____ 56. Crime-stopper techniques have been taught. (Example: hooking shoulder bag over arm and then putting on jacket to prevent purse snatching.)

_____ 57. Alternate systems have been explored for the safekeeping of valuable papers and possessions; resident is discouraged from storing them in old handbags and mattresses.

_____ 58. System for taking medications that safeguards against overdose has been developed.

_____ 59. Client has been taught procedure for performing Heimlich maneuver on self or other older adult in an emergency.

_____ 60. Client has been taught to identify symptoms of heart attack and ventilatory insufficiency and understands importance of securing emergency aid. If physically able, older adult has been taught CPR if living with a spouse subject to these disorders.

_____ 61. Client has periodic assistance from caregivers or significant others in removing accumulated clutter and trash from home.

_____ 62. Pets and pet-care equipment do not pose a hazard to the psychological and physical safety of the client.

Appendix D

CRITERIA FOR EVALUATION

Check (✔) if Present

_____ 1. Environment leaves a pleasant first impression.

_____ 2. Orientation to the institution is available for the resident and family. Orientation includes tour, briefing on services available, privileges, restrictions, fees for services rendered, and method of payment expected.

_____ 3. Owner and administration are actively involved in and committed to quality care for the residents. Personal interest in residents and staff is displayed by these people and they demonstrate an awareness of the day-to-day operation of the institution.

_____ 4. The institutional philosophy is quality care at a reasonable cost.

_____ 5. Evidence of active community involvement in and commitment to quality of care in the institution. This reduces likelihood of residents being cast aside and isolated. Such involvement may be through volunteer service, patient advocacy, sponsorship of foster grandparents, or support and encouragement for staff, which serves to boost morale of residents and staff alike.

_____ 6. Stable staff/resident contact is maintained as opposed to a rapid changing of staff faces.

_____ 7. Staff members call patient by surname and correct title to foster patient's validation of identity.

_____ 8. If individual accommodations are unavailable, care is taken in the selection and assignment of roommates to foster the formation of warm, supportive, interpersonal relationships.

_____ 9. Personal territory is provided and delineated (bed, closets, tables, chests, bathroom). Territory is not invaded by staff or other residents without consent of client.

_____ 10. Resident can have personal possessions in the institution. Adequate space is provided for storage or display of these items, such as photographs of family.

_____ 11. Possessions are secure from theft or abuse by others. If not, provision is made for such security and at the same time resident is allowed access to cherished items upon request.

_____ 12. Clothing and other personal possessions are where resident can see and have easy access to them.

_____ 13. Staff members are aware of individual ownership of possessions and do not indiscriminately use private possessions for other clients. (Example: taking a gown out of the closet and putting it on the wrong resident.)

_____ 14. Privacy is provided for entertaining family members and guests (includes bedroom or overnight accommodations for resident and spouse).

_____ 15. Individual dignity is recognized through provision of privacy for toileting, bathing, treatments, and confidentiality of personal information.

_____ 16. Conversation areas are provided in the client's room, in public areas, and out-of-doors to encourage social interaction.

_____ 17. Residents are encouraged to feel needed by relating to others or performing services that are within their area of interest, desire, and competence.

_____ 18. Families are encouraged to interact with resident, visit frequently, assist with development of plan of care, and participate in the delivery and implementation of nursing care.

_____ 19. A wide range of services is available to resident and is used to meet individualized needs (PT, OT, speech therapy, personal grooming, social services).

_____ 20. Resident care routines are flexible and allow for individual decision making regarding time for bathing, snacking, going to sleep. Thus the resident is able to exercise some control over the environment and continue using decision-making skills that are the prerogative of adults.

_____ 21. Activities, provided on site or within the community, cater to a variety of interests. (Example: educational classes, crafts, or creative endeavors, volunteer service, musical performance and practice, library service, religious services, games, dance)

_____ 22. Contact with the "outside" world is maintained through newspapers, magazines, television, newscasts, and discussion of these by residents and staff; excursions are provided to shopping centers, plays, historic sites, educational facilities.

_____ 23. Religious activities are available, ranging from consultation with a member of the clergy chosen by the resident to attendance at religious services on site and within community.

_____ 24. Resident provided with opportunity to conduct business. (Example: visits with attorney, banker, financial advisor)

_____ 25. Residents (except those not legally competent) have access to money for meeting personal needs and have access to banking services for larger monetary transactions.

_____ 26. Presence of a "resident council," composed of residents, that can articulate the needs of residents to staff and administration.

_____ 27. Written schedules of institutional routines and times for activities and special events are provided.

_____ 28. Large-faced clocks and large-numbered calendars are readily evident to facilitate residents' orientation to time, day, week, and season.

_____ 29. Holidays are celebrated and marked by decorations and special meals to reinforce residents' orientation to time and investment in life as a part of the larger community.

_____ 30. Birthdays of residents (anniversaries of couples) are recognized and celebrated in some fashion (example: a birthday party) to recognize and support individual value and worth.

_____ 31. Staff members consistently encourage appropriate social behavior and demonstrate same in dealing with residents to reinforce participation in the "real" world of socially determined and censored behavior.

_____ 32. Facility provides variety in colors to relive monotony and to facilitate resident orientation to place.

_____ 33. Room doors and floors are color coded for easy identification and to facilitate orientation to place. Floors may be specifically color coded along important routes to reduce disorientation.

_____ 34. Mirrors are readily available for assessment of personal grooming status and evaluation and re-validation of body image.

_____ 35. Nonskid floors, side bars, and railings are present in bath, halls, and stairwells and are kept clean and free of debris to reduce possibility of falls and enhance security.

_____ 36. Doors and passageways are adequate for the accommodation of wheelchairs and other assistive equipment.

_____ 37. Lighting is sufficient and planned to reduce glare.

_____ 38. Stair surfaces are covered with a nonskid covering and the top and bottom stairs are clearly delineated by differentiating colors.

_____ 39. Instructions are given to resident by staff member before any nursing procedures or treatments are performed in recognition of every intelligent human being's right to know and consent to invasion of his or her body and personal space.

_____ 40. Residents are encouraged to complete activities of daily living as far as possible within the limits of their abilities and are given sufficient time to complete tasks. Supplemental assistance is given as needed.

_____ 41. Care is planned to minimize stress and energy of immobile bed resident. (Example: bedmaking efficient and done with minimum number of movements)

_____ 42. Residents' nails are trimmed and cleaned and perineal area is cleaned after toileting. Bed linens are changed after incontinence (voiding or defecating).

_____ 43. Residents' hair is clean, cut, and arranged in a fashion appropriate to age and sex. (Example: Pony tails and bows do not increase the dignity and self-image of an older woman and indicate a lack of respect for her individuality on the part of the staff, who are meeting their own needs with such actions)

_____ 44. Variety of fluids are offered frequently throughout the day and water is kept in a place accessible to the resident.

_____ 45. Range-of-motion exercises and therapeutic body positioning are provided routinely to reduce the hazards of immobility.

_____ 46. Immobile bed residents are turned at least every two hours, more often if indicated by condition.

_____ 47. Odors and noise level controlled to provide an environment conducive to social interaction and pride in one's environment.

_____ 48. Food patterns of residents are constantly evaluated and staff knows when food is not eaten and attempts to evaluate why.

_____ 49. Companionship is provided at meals either in communal dining hall or in resident's room to provide a time of socialization and a pleasant environment to stimulate appetite.

_____ 50. Food served in dining room and on trays is varied, appetizing, visually appealing, and tasty.

_____ 51. Snacks and "afternoon tea" are provided in recognition of individual variations in the need for nourishment and satiety.

_____ 52. Staff decreases sensory loss through therapeutic and thoughtful use of touch, such as light touches on the hand, spontaneous hugs, and loving administration of backrubs and massage to pressure areas.

_____ 53. Programs in sensory stimulation, reality orientation, and remotivation are available for those residents who need them.

_____ 54. Safety and security of residents is fostered by provision of equipment in good repair and proper preparation of staff in use of equipment available.

_____ 55. Protection of the resident's health and safety is evidenced by protocols for action in an emergency situation such as fire or cardiac arrest.

_____ 56. Medical care of the resident is monitored by a personal physician who visits frequently. If physician visits lag, nursing personnel takes steps to encourage such visits by physician or meet with family and resident to discuss revision of care. The resident has worth and value and does not warrant such neglect.

_____ 57. The value of life is promoted through provisions of emergency equipment (fire extinguishers, fire doors, sprinklers, CPR cart, tornado shelters) and drills for residents; staff check behavior expected in an emergency situation.

_____ 58. Sufficient personnel (including the administrator) are present to meet resident needs and are appropriately prepared to meet the complex physical and psychosocial needs of residents. Emphasis is given to continuing education. Insufficiently prepared staff members are not given responsibilities beyond their limited preparation and are closely supervised by appropriately prepared staff in the delivery of these limited aspects of nursing care. Properly prepared staff provides twenty-four-hour coverage.

_____ 59. Staff members exhibit a positive self-image in dress and manner. Feeling good about themselves facilitates feeling good about the residents and establishes an environment of positive image promotion.

_____ 60. Personnel use positive reinforcement and express appreciation to older adults for common courtesies in recognition of individual's need to be considered a being of value. "Please" and "thank you" are used frequently.

_____ 61. Staff maintains eye contact when communicating with the resident and displays an awareness of his or her individuality.

_____ 62. Staff frequently checks on and "visits" with resident, as opposed to clustering at nursing station as needs go unmet.

_____ 63. Staff sits, talks, eats, and plays games with residents to provide stimulus to social interaction.

_____ 64. Staff responds quickly and appropriately to call lights and resident requests for assistance.

Appendix E

Helpful Resources for Maltreatment of Older Adults

The following agencies, organizations, and facilities provide aid and assistance with prevention, identification, assessment, investigation, treatment, recovery and rehabilitation, and prosecution of maltreatment of older adults.

Abuse Hotline*: *1-(800)-252-5400

- Twenty-four hour hotline for reporting suspected abuse or neglect of older persons.

- Investigates complaints, assists with treatment referrals and case management, assists with treatment and prosecution of perpetrators.

American Public Welfare Association
810 First Street, N.E.
Suite 500
Washington, DC 20002

- Offers financial assistance and resources for qualifying individuals.

- Investigates complaints.

Attorneys (available in your local area)

- Perform litigation for abuse and neglect of older adults.

Better Business Bureau
[local agencies available; for out-of-state offices, call 1-(703)-276-0100]

- Receives complaints on poor and fraudulent business practices, but has no power to prosecute.

Bureau of Long-Term Care, State Department of Health

- Performs routine inspections on nursing homes.

- Performs unannounced nursing home inspections on complaints.

Consumer Affairs (local and city branches available in most areas)

- Assists with investigations of consumer complaints and consumer fraud.

Crime Prevention Association (many available locally and statewide)
Washington State Crime Prevention Association
111 N.E. Olympia Avenue
Olympia, WA 98501

- Provides education and referral for crime protective resources.

Department of Health (local city or county health departments)

- Provides health inspections for nursing homes.

- Provides low-cost health care and immunizations. Services vary with each area.

Federal Trade Commission
Correspondence Branch
Washington, DC 20580

- Investigates complaints; prosecutes advertisement fraud and investment fraud.

Hospitals (available locally)

- Provide acute care for health care problems.

- Can assist in referrals to physicians, health care support services, and protective services.

Legal Aid (local offices available in most areas; check with local Area Agency on Aging)

- Assists in mediation and litigation with consumer issues, health and care concerns, family law; does not assist with criminal cases.

National Futures Association
200 W. Madison Street
Ste. 1600
Chicago, IL 60606
1-(800)-621-3570 (in Illinois, 1-(800)-572-9400)

- Self-regulatory organization for brokers and brokerage firms selling commodities.

- Investigates complaints of fraud.

Nursing Home Association (state sponsored organization)

- Investigates complaints on nursing homes.

Police/Sheriff Departments (local branches available in each area)

- Assist with prevention, protection, and prosecution of crimes.

Protective Agencies (Titles vary per locality and/or state. May be found in local directories under listings such as Department of Human Services, Department of Human Resources, Department of Health and Social Services, Department of Public Welfare, or Department of Health and Human Services.)

- Receive complaints on all forms of maltreatment of older adults.

- Investigate complaints. (Complaints often are investigated on priority of danger, due to staffing limitations.)

- Provide case management with treatment, referrals to resources, and follow-up.

- Maintain files on complaints.

- Assist with prosecution and treatment recommendations for perpetrators.

Senior Citizen Centers (available locally)

- Provide support groups, activities, classes, information, and resource referrals for older persons.

Social Security Administration (local offices available)

- Reviews Medicare cases.

- Investigates complaints for Medicare.

United People for Better Nursing Home Care—Katherine Bates, Chief Executive Officer.

- Supplies information and support for investigations of complaints on nursing home care.

United States Postal Service (contact Postal Inspector or local postmaster; available locally; listing under "U.S. Government, Postal Service" in telephone directory).

- Investigates complaints on mail-order fraud and fraudulent businesses that use mail advertisement or sell through the mail.

Appendix F

Sample Advance Directive to Physicians

"Directive made this _____ day of _____ (month, year).

"I _____, being of sound mind, willfully and voluntarily make known my desire that my life shall not be artificially prolonged under the circumstances set forth in this directive.

"1. If at any time I should have an incurable or irreversible condition caused by injury, disease, or illness certified to be a terminal condition by two physicians, and if the application of life-sustaining procedures would serve only to artificially postpone the moment of my death, and if my attending physician determines that my death is imminent or will result within a relatively short time without application of life-sustaining procedures, I direct that those procedures be withheld or withdrawn, and that I be permitted to die naturally.

"2. In the absence of my ability to give directions regarding the use of those life-sustaining procedures, it is my intention that this directive be honored by my family and physicians as the final expression of my legal right to refuse medical or surgical treatment and accept the consequences from that refusal.

"3. If I have been diagnosed as pregnant and that diagnosis is known to my physician, this directive shall have no effect during my pregnancy.

"4. This directive is in effect until it is revoked.

"5. I understand the full import of this directive and I am emotionally and mentally competent to make this directive.

"6. I understand that I may revoke this directive at any time.

"Signed _____"
(City, County, and State of Residence)

"I am not related to the declarant by blood or marriage. I would not be entitled to any portion of the declarant's estate on the declarant's death. I am not the attending physician of the declarant nor an employee of the attending physician. I am not a patient in the health care facility in which the declarant is a patient. I have no claim against any portion of the declarant's estate on the declarant's death. Furthermore, if I am an employee of a health facility in which the declarant is a patient, I am not involved in providing direct patient care to the declarant and am not directly involved in the financial affairs of the health facility.

"Witness _____"

"Witness _____"

Sample Durable Power of Attorney for Health Care

Appendix G

DESIGNATION OF HEALTH CARE AGENT

I, _____ appoint
(insert your name)

Name: _____

Address: _____

_____ Phone: _____

as my agent to make any and all health care decisions for me, except to the extent I state otherwise in this document. This durable power of attorney for health care takes effect if I become unable to make my own health care decisions and this fact is certified in writing by my physician.

LIMITATIONS ON THE DECISION-MAKING AUTHORITY OF MY AGENT ARE AS FOLLOWS:

_____

_____

DESIGNATION OF ALTERNATE AGENT

(You are not required to designate an alternate agent but you may do so. An alternate agent may make the same health care decisions as the designated agent if the designated agent is unable or unwilling to act as your agent. If the agent designated is your spouse, the designation is automatically revoked by law if your marriage is dissolved.)

If the person designated as my agent is unable or unwilling to make health care decisions for me, I designate the following persons to serve as my agent to make health care decisions for me as authorized by this document, who serve in the following order:

A. First Alternate Agent

Name: _____

Address: _____

_____ Phone: _____

B. Second Alternate Agent

Name: _____

Address: _____

_____ Phone: _____

The original of this document is kept at _____

_____

_____

The following individuals or institutions have signed copies:

Name: _____

Address: _____

_____

Name: _____

Address: _____

_____

DURATION

I understand that this power of attorney exists indefinitely from the date I execute this document, unless I establish a shorter time or revoke the power of attorney. If I am unable to make health care decisions for myself when this power of attorney expires, the authority I have granted my agent continues to exist until the time I become able to make health care decisions for myself.

(If Applicable) This power of attorney ends on the following date: _____

PRIOR DESIGNATIONS REVOKED

I revoke any prior durable power of attorney for health care.

ACKNOWLEDGMENT OF DISCLOSURE STATEMENT

I have been provided with a disclosure statement explaining the effect of this document. I have read and understand that information contained in the disclosure statement.

(You must date and sign this Power of Attorney.)

I sign my name to this Durable Power of Attorney for Health Care on this ____ day of

_____, 19 ____ , at _____

(City and State)

_____

(Signature)

_____

(Print Name)

STATEMENT OF WITNESSES

I declare under penalty of perjury that the principal has identified himself or herself to me, that the principal signed or acknowledged this Durable Power of Attorney in my presence, that I believe the principal to be of sound mind, that the principal has affirmed that the principal is aware of the nature of the document and is signing it voluntarily and free from duress, that the principal requested that I serve as witness to the principal's execution of this document, that I am not the person appointed as agent by this document, and that I am not a provider of health or residential care, an employee of a provider of health or residential care, the operator of a community care facility, or an employee of an operator of a health care facility.

I declare that I am not related to the principal by blood, marriage, or adoption and that to the best of my knowledge I am not entitled to any part of the estate of the principal on the death of the principal under a will or by operation of law.

Witness Signature: _____

Print Name: _____ Date: _____

Address: _____

Witness Signature: _____

Print Name: _____ Date: _____

Address: _____

NOTE:

Appendix F, "Sample Advance Directive to Physicians," and Appendix G, "Sample Durable Power of Attorney for Health Care," are only examples of typical forms. The specific format for such forms will vary from state to state and among health care settings. Similar forms may be obtained from physicians and/or most health care facilities or purchased in many local-office supply stores. See chapter 23, "Legal Concerns," for specific instructions regarding the use of such forms. These sample forms have been provided through the courtesy of the Texas Hospital Association.

Appendix H

Journals and Other Publications Relating to Older Adults

(Write to the addresses listed for subscription prices and frequency of publication.)

AARP News Bulletin
   AARP Fulfillment
   AARP Publications
   3200 East Carson Street
   Lakewood, CA 90712

Age Page
   National Institute on Aging
   US Department of Health and Human Services
   US Government Printing Office
   Washington, DC 20402

Aging
   Office of Human Development Services
   Department of Health and Human Services
   200 Independence Avenue, SW
   Washington, DC 20201

Generations
   American Society on Aging
   833 Market Street
   Room 512
   San Francisco, CA 94103

Geriatric Nursing
   Mosby Year-Book, Inc.
   Journal Circulation Fulfillment
   11830 Westline Industrial Drive
   St. Louis, MO 63146

Geriatrics
   For the Primary Care Physician
   Harcourt Brace Jovanovich Publications
   1 East First Street
   Duluth, MN 55802

The Gerontologist
   1275 K Street, NW
   Suite 350
   Washington, DC 20005-4006

Gerontology Newsletter
   Institute of Human Development
      and Family Studies
   Main Building 2300
   University of Texas at Austin
   Austin, TX 78712

Home Healthcare Nurse
   680 Route 206 North
   Bridgewater, NJ 08807

The International Journal of Aging and Human Development
   Baywood Publishing Co., Inc.
   26 Austin Avenue, P.O. Box 337
   Amityville, NY 11701

Journal of Gerontologic Social Work
Haworth Press, Inc.
10 Alice Street
Binghampton, NY 13904

Journal of Gerontological Nursing
Charles B. Slack, Inc.
6900 Grove Road
Thorofare, NJ 08086

Journal of Gerontology
1275 K Street NW
Suite 350
Washington, DC 20005-4006

Journal of Nutrition for the Elderly
The Haworth Press
12 West 32nd St.
New York, NY 10001

Journal of Religion and Aging
28 E. 22nd St.
New York, NY 10010

Long-Term Care Currents
Ross Laboratories
625 Cleveland Avenue
Columbus, OH 43216

Long-Term Care Quarterly
American Nurses' Association
600 Maryland Ave., S.W.
Suite 100 West
Washington, D.C. 20024-2571

Modern Maturity
(Publication of the American Association
of Retired Persons)
3200 E. Carson Street
Lakewood, CA 90712

Research on Aging
(A Quarterly of Social Gerontology
and Adult Development)
Sage Publications, Inc.
2111 West Hillcrest Drive
Newbury Park, CA 91320

Organizations Providing Resources and Information for and about Older Adults

Appendix I

Administration on Aging
330 Independence Avenue, SW
Washington, DC 20201

Alzheimer's Disease and Related Disorders
  Association, Inc.
70 East Lake Street
Chicago, IL 60601

American Association for Geriatric Psychiatry
P.O. Box 376-A
Greenbelt, MD 20770

American Association of Homes for the Aging
1129 20th Street, NW, Suite 400
Washington, DC 20036-3489

American Association of Retired Persons
601 East Street NW
Washington, DC 20049

American Association of Retired Persons
Andrus Foundation
601 East Street, NW
Washington, DC 20049

American College of Nursing Home Administrators
4650 East-West Freeway
Washington, DC 20014

American Geriatrics Society
770 Lexington Avenue, Suite 400
New York, NY 10021

American Health Care Association
1200 L Street, NW
Washington, DC 20005

American Nurses' Association
Division on Gerontological Nursing Practice
600 Maryland Ave., S.W.
Suite 100 West
Washington, DC 20024-2571

American Society on Aging
833 Market Street, Room 516
San Francisco, CA 94103

Association for Gerontology in Higher Education
1001 Connecticut Ave. NW
Suite 410
Washington, DC 20036-5504

Children of Aging Parents
1609 Woodbourne Road 302-A
Box KC-791
Levittown, PA 19057

The Gerontological Society of America
1275 K Street, NW Suite 350
Washington, DC 20005-4006

Grey Panthers
311 South Juniper Street, Suite 601
Philadelphia, PA 19107

National Association of Home Care
519 C Street, NE
Stanton Park
Washington, DC 20002

National Association of Area Agencies on Aging
600 Maryland Avenue, SW, Suite 208
Washington, DC 20024

National Association of Directors of Nursing
 Administration in Long Term Care
 (NADONA/LTC)
10999 Reed Hartman Highway, Suite 229
Cincinnati, OH 45242

National Caucus and Center on the Black Aged, Inc.
1424 K Street, NW, Suite 500
Washington, DC 20005

National Council of Senior Citizens, Inc.
925 15th Street, NW
Washington, DC 20005

The National Council on the Aging, Inc.
600 Maryland Avenue, SW
West Wing 100
Washington, DC 20024

National Gerontological Nursing Association
7250 Parkway Drive, Suite 510
Hanover, MD 21076

National Institute on Aging
Information Center
Federal Building, Room 6C12
9000 Rockville Pike
Bethesda, MD 20892

National League for Nursing
350 Hudson Street
New York, NY 10014

Older Women's League
730 Eleventh Street, NW, Suite 300
Washington, DC 20001

Social Security Administration
6401 Security Boulevard
Baltimore, MD 21235
1-800-772-1213

The Society for the Right to Die
250 W. 57th Street, Room 323
New York, NY 10107

Veterans Administration
810 Vermont Avenue NW
Washington, DC 20420

Index

Note: Page numbers in **bold** type reference non-text material. Titles in **bold** type reference publication titles.